Step-Up to USMLE Step 1

A High-Yield, Systems-Based-Review for the USMLE Step 1, Fourth Edition

Sonia Mehta, MD
Resident Physician
Department of Ophthalmology
Scheie Eye Institute
University of Pennsylvania
Philadelphia, Pennsylvania

Sonul Mehta, MD
Resident Physician
Department of Ophthalmology
Georgetown University/Washington Hospital Center
Washington, District of Columbia

Samir Mehta, MD
Assistant Professor
Department of Orthopaedic Surgery
Chief, Orthopaedic Trauma Service
The Hospital of the University of Pennsylvania
Philadelphia, Pennsylvania

LCDR Edmund A. Milder, MC USNR
Department of Pediatrics
Naval Medical Center
San Diego, California

Adam J. Mirarchi, MD
Assistant Professor
Department of Orthopaedic Surgery
Oregon Health & Science University
Portland, Oregon

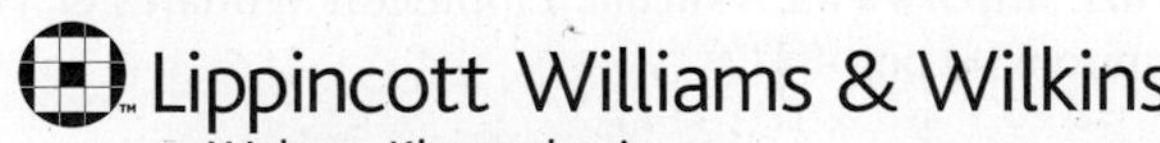
Lippincott Williams & Wilkins
a Wolters Kluwer business
Philadelphia • Baltimore • New York • London
Buenos Aires • Hong Kong • Sydney • Tokyo

Acquisitions Editor: Charles W. Mitchell
Managing Editor: Jennifer Verbiar
Marketing Manager: Jennifer Kuklinski
Designer: Holly McLaughlin
Compositor: SPi

351 West Camden Street
Baltimore, MD 21201
530 Walnut Street
Philadelphia, PA 19106

Printed in China

First Edition, 1999
Second Edition, 2003
Third Edition, 2007

Library of Congress Cataloging-in-Publication Data

Step-up to USMLE step 1 : a high-yield, systems-based-review for the USMLE step 1 / Sonia Mehta ... [et al.]. — 4th ed.
p. ; cm.
Rev. ed. of: Step-up to USMLE step 1 / Sonia Mehta, Sonul Mehta, Samir Mehta. 3rd ed. c2007.
Includes bibliographical references and index.
ISBN 978-1-60547-470-0
1. Medicine—Examinations, questions, etc. 2. Physicians—Licenses—United States—Examinations—Study guides. I. Mehta, Sonia. II. Mehta, Sonia. Step-up to USMLE step 1.
[DNLM: 1. Clinical Medicine—United States—Outlines. WB 18.2 U8275 2010]

R834.5.M45 2010
616.0076—dc22 2009022072

To purchase additional copies of this book, call our customer service department at **(800) 638-3030** or fax orders to **(301) 223-2320**. International customers should call **(301) 223-2300**.

Visit Lippincott Williams & Wilkins on the Internet: http://www.LWW.com. Lippincott Williams & Wilkins customer service representatives are available from 8:30 am to 6:00 pm, EST.

06 07 08 09 10
1 2 3 4 5 6 7 8 9 10

CCS0909

Dedication

To our parents, Sudesh, and Shobha

—Samir, Sonia, and Sonul Mehta

To my parents, James and Phyllis, and my siblings Eugene, Shannon, and Robert

—Edmund A. Milder

To my parents, Anthony and Andrea, my brother Alan, and my wife Sharon

—Adam J. Mirarchi

To our teachers
To our friends
And to the physicians of the future

Preface to the Fourth Edition

The fourth edition of Step-Up: *A High-Yield, Systems-Based Review for the USMLE Step 1*, while retaining the essential features of the first three editions, has been changed in some important ways. First, an introduction to the USMLE Step 1 exam and an effective guide to preparation have been added to provide the student with strategies for success. To reinforce and ease student preparation, the authors have created an online question bank available with purchase of the book consisting of greater than 350 questions in USMLE Step 1 format. The popularity of the case studies text "Step-Up to the Bedside" led to our development of clinical vignettes within the body of each chapter. These vignettes, following the format of the rest of the book, are integrated within each chapter, discussing topics and concepts as they arise. We have further expanded coverage of the therapeutics portion of each system by integrating more pharmacology directly into each system at the appropriate areas within the text. However, we retained the "Drug Index" at the end of the text for reference. In fact, we have added a "Crunch Time Review" to the end of the book to facilitate last-minute studying and keep the reader organized. Each chapter also has mnemonics integrated into the body of the text to help the reader remember vital facts that are presented. Finally, figures, tables, and text have been revised to reflect the most current thinking in medicine. Many of these changes were implemented as a result of feedback from readers like you, and we hope to continue this relationship with our readers who use this text and future texts in the Step-Up series. Good luck!

Samir Mehta
Sonia Mehta
Sonul Mehta
Edmund A. Milder
Adam J. Mirarchi

Acknowledgments

We extend our thanks to all the reviewers and contributors to this and previous editions, including our editor for the second edition, Eugene Milder. Special thanks go to our editors and marketers at Lippincott Williams and Wilkins—Sharon Zinner, Emilie Moyer, Jennifer Verbiar, Charley Mitchell, and especially to Elizabeth Nieginski and Julie Scardiglia without whom the Step-Up series would not be possible. It is through the co-operation and vision of LWW that this series was able to move from concept to a practical, useful tool.

Student Contributors

We extend our special thanks to the student contributors to this edition, who are in the trenches helping us constantly evolve and innovate.

Salvatore Docimo
Medical Student IV
New York College of Osteopathic Medicine
New York City, New York

Zi Yang Jian
Medical Student IV
University of Illinois College of Medicine
Chicago, Illinois

Andrea W. Schwartz
Medical Student III
Mount Sinai School of Medicine
New York City, New York

Santina Wheat
Medical Student III
University of Illinois College of Medicine
Chicago, Illinois

Faculty Contributors

We extend our warm thanks to the faculty contributors to this edition, who continue to push students to do their best.

David R. Burt, Ph. D
(retired) Professor of Pharmacology
University of Maryland School of Medicine
Baltimore, Maryland

Susan Cline, Ph. D
Assistant Professor of Biochemistry
Division of Basic Medical Sciences
Mercer University School of Medicine
Macon, Georgia

Bruce A. Fenderson, Ph. D
Professor of Pathology
Department of Pathology, Anatomy, and Cell Biology
Jefferson Medical College
Thomas Jefferson University
Philadelphia, Pennsylvania

Barbara Goodman, Ph. D
Professor of Physiology
Director of SD Biomedical Research and Infrastructure Network
Sanford School of Medicine of the University of South Dakota
Vermillion, South Dakota

Arthur Johnson, Ph. D
Professor Emeritus
Department of Anatomy, Pathology, and Microbiology
University of Minnesota School of Medicine
Duluth, Minnesota

How to Contribute

Interested in medical publishing? Contribute to Step-Up!

Student suggestions and feedback are always welcomed and appreciated by the Step-Up team. Please send feedback and suggestions for new study material and test taking strategies by writing the authors on the website below. Students can also directly submit new mnemonics, quick hits, tables, and figures. For each original entry incorporated into the text, students' names will be listed and personally acknowledged in the next edition. If duplicate entries are received, the first to submit will be acknowledged.

To make an entry or provide feedback and suggestions, simply visit the Step-Up website below. Learn more about becoming a student contributor to the next edition of Step-Up. Applications are available online on the Step-Up website.

http://www.lww.com/step-up

To apply to become an LWW student representative and to learn more about this position, visit the LWW website below.

http://www.lww.com/student-incentive-program

Disclaimer:
Please note: submissions become the property of LWW.

Contents

Preface iv
Acknowledgments v

Strategies for Success: A Guide to Effective Preparation for the USMLE Step 1 1
The Exam: The USMLE Step 1 1
Preparing for the Exam: Study Strategies 5
Online Resources 9
Personalized Study Schedule 10

System 1. Basic Concepts 11
DNA, RNA, and Protein 11
Bacterial Morphology and Genetics 15
Viral Genetics 20
Concepts in Pharmacology 22
Anti-infective Agents 26
Enzyme Kinetics 37
Biostatistics and Epidemiology 39

System 2. The Nervous System 44
Development 44
Congenital Malformations of the Nervous System 45
Major Receptors of the Nervous System 45
Meninges, Flow of Cerebrospinal Fluid, and Pathologic Trauma 46
Blood Supply to the Brain 46
Lesions of the Cerebral Cortex 52
Important Pathways of the Spinal Cord 52
Important Pathways of the Brain Stem and Cerebrum 54
Common Ocular Pathology 59
Classic Lesions of the Spinal Cord 60
Hypothalamus 60
Thalamus 61
Cranial Nerves 61
Contents of the Cavernous Sinus 63
Sleep 63
Seizure Types 64
Degenerative Diseases 65
Demyelinating Diseases 68
Diseases that Cause Dementia 69
Acute Meningitis 69
Nervous System Tumors 70
Headache 71
Psychiatry and Behavioral Science 71
Ethics and the Role of the Physician 78

System 3. The Cardiovascular System 80
Development 80
Physiology and Pathology of Heart Function 81
Arrhythmias 87
Antiarrhythmics 87
Atherosclerosis 91
Familial Dyslipidemias 92
Lipid-lowering Agents 93
Hypertension 93
Antihypertensive Agents 94
Aneurysms 98
Ischemic Heart Disease 99
Congestive Heart Failure 101
Intrinsic Diseases of the Heart 105
Cardiac Neoplasms 109
Diseases of the Pericardium 109
Shock 110
Cardiovascular Manifestations of Systemic Diseases 110
Drugs that Cause Adverse Effects to the Cardiovascular System 111

System 4. The Respiratory System 112
Development 112
Physics and Function of the Lung 113
Control of Breathing 118
Lung Defenses 120
Adult Respiratory Distress Syndrome and Neonatal Respiratory Distress Syndrome 120
Pneumothorax 121
Pulmonary Vascular Diseases 121
Chronic Obstructive Pulmonary Disease 122

Interstitial Lung Disease ... 125
Environmental Lung Diseases (Pneumoconiosis) ... 126
Respiratory Infections ... 126
Cystic Fibrosis ... 132
Lung Neoplasms ... 133
Drugs that Cause Adverse Effects to the Respiratory System ... 134

System 5. The Gastrointestinal System ... 135
Innervation and Blood Supply of the Gastrointestinal Tract ... 135
Hormones of the Gastrointestinal System ... 136
Important Congenital Malformations of the Gastrointestinal System ... 136
The Oropharynx, Esophagus, and Stomach ... 137
The Small Intestine, Large Intestine, and Rectum ... 140
Location of Absorption of Vitamins, Minerals, and Nutrients ... 143
Common Clinical Disorders of the Small Intestine, Large Intestine, and Rectum ... 143
Malabsorption Syndromes of the Small Intestine ... 148
Neoplastic Polyps ... 149
The Hepatobiliary System ... 150
The Pancreas ... 158
Bugs of the Gastrointestinal Tract ... 159
Therapeutic Agents for the Gastrointestinal System ... 159

System 6. The Renal System ... 164
Development ... 164
Gross Description of the Kidney ... 164
Normal Kidney Function ... 165
Glomerular Diseases ... 172
Urinary Tract Infections ... 177
Major Causes of Acute Renal Failure ... 177
Chronic Renal Failure and Uremia ... 180
Kidney Stone Formation ... 182
Adult Polycystic Kidney Disease Versus Normal Kidney ... 182
Renal Cancers ... 183
Therapeutic Agents ... 184

System 7. The Endocrine System ... 187
Development ... 187
Congenital Malformations ... 188
Hormones ... 188
Calcium Homeostasis ... 191
Insulin and Glucagon ... 191
Blood Glucose Levels ... 194
Diabetes Mellitus ... 197
Obesity ... 202
Pituitary Disorders ... 202
Diabetes Insipidus ... 202
The Adrenal Glands ... 204
Therapeutic Agents for the Hypothalamus, Pituitary, and Adrenal Glands ... 207
Thyroid ... 207
Parathyroid Pathology ... 212
Multiple Endocrine Neoplasia (MEN) Syndromes ... 213

System 8. The Reproductive System ... 214
Determination of Sex ... 214
Female Reproductive System Development ... 214
Male Reproductive System Development ... 214
Congenital Malformations ... 215
Genetic Abnormalities ... 216
Menarche, Menstruation, and Menopause ... 216
Pregnancy and Its Associated Complications ... 227
Gynecologic Diagnostic Tests ... 229
Sexually Transmitted Diseases ... 230
Female Gynecologic Neoplasms ... 230
Breast Pathology ... 230
The Prostate ... 233
Testicular Pathology ... 233
Human Immunodeficiency Virus ... 235
Psychosocial Development ... 240
Timeline of the Developmental Stages of Life ... 240
The Family Unit and Related Concepts ... 240
Sexuality ... 241
Rape ... 243
Suicide ... 243
Therapeutic Agents for the Reproductive System ... 244

System 9. The Musculoskeletal System ... 247
Development ... 247
Bone Function and Metabolism ... 249
Bone, Cartilage, and Joint Disease ... 251
Metabolic and Infectious Skeletal Disease ... 252
Systemic Lupus Erythematosus (SLE) ... 256
Other Connective Tissue Disorders ... 256
Brachial Plexus ... 258
Lumbosacral Plexus ... 259
Pain Management ... 259
Muscle Function and Dysfunction ... 266
The Inguinal Canal ... 269
Skin Disorders ... 272

System 10. The Hematopoietic and Lymphoreticular System 274

Development 274
The Cells.................................... 274
The Organs of the Lymphoreticular System.................................... 274
Red Blood Cell Physiology................ 277
Lymphocyte Differentiation............... 278
Immunoglobulins 279
Complement System 280
Hypersensitivity Reactions................ 282
Immunodeficiencies........................ 284
Immunosuppressants 286
Thrombosis and the Clotting Cascade 287
Antithrombotic Therapeutic Agents...... 289
Coagulation Disorders 292
Lymphoma................................ 295
Leukemia 295
Anemia.................................... 295
Myeloproliferative Disorders 302
Chemotherapeutics 303

Crunch Time Review.................... 307

Appendix I: Drug Index 321
Appendix II: Bug Index..................... 381
Glossary.................................... 399
Index 405

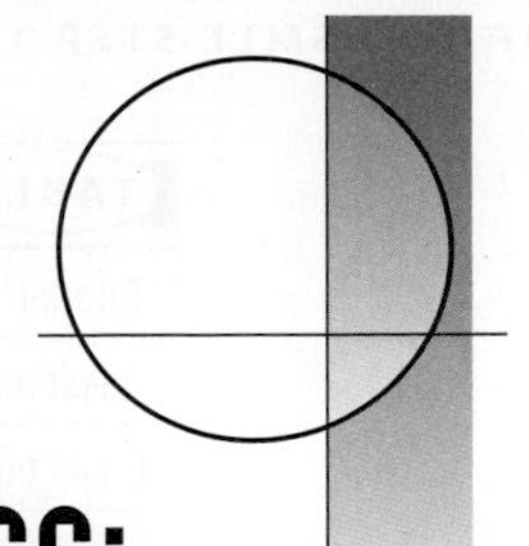

Strategies for Success: A Guide to Effective Preparation for the USMLE Step 1

As the first national licensure exam encountered during a medical career, the USMLE Step 1 is often a source of anxiety for the medical student.

As with most things in life, having a systematic plan can be helpful in approaching what at first seems like an enormous task—preparing for the boards. The authors of *Step-Up to the USMLE Step 1* have created this guide below to direct you in effectively preparing for and excelling on the boards.

The first section of the guide will introduce you to the exam and the test makers. It will also familiarize you with the exam structure, content, testing environment, and interface. Finally, it will review how the test is scored and how to register for the exam.

The second section of the guide details successful preparation strategies. In this section, you will learn tips for creating study schedules and gathering study materials, as well as strategies for effective studying. At the end of this section, you will find a blank study schedule you can use as a basis for creating your personalized study schedule.

THE EXAM: THE USMLE STEP 1

The National Board of Medical Examiners

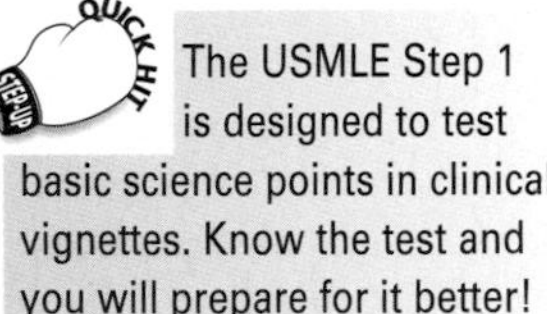

The USMLE Step 1 is designed to test basic science points in clinical vignettes. Know the test and you will prepare for it better!

The USMLE is a joint endeavor by the National Board of Medical Examiners (NBME) and Federation of State Medical Boards (FSMB). Step 1 is the first of three exams medical students and graduates need to pass in order to become licensed physicians in the United States. The NBME was founded in 1915 in Philadelphia, PA, and administered its first exam in 1916. The first exams were largely essay-based and organized around testing the basic science subjects of anatomy, physiology, biochemistry, pathology, pharmacology, microbiology, and behavioral science. The exam has evolved over the years. In the early 1990s, after years of culminated efforts, the USMLE was introduced. This test embraced the systems-based practice of medicine and adopted a clinically oriented question format. In 1992, Step 1 replaced the FLEX exam and now serves as the single exam for international medical graduates seeking US medical licensure. In 1999, the test became computer based and in 2005 the FRED software was adopted.

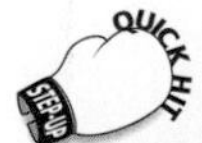

After the seventh block, a screen appears to move on to the eighth block. The eighth block is not a question block. It is a survey of your testing experience consisting of 11 questions. Don't be fooled!

Test Structure

The exam consists of 350 questions administered in seven blocks of 50 questions each with 60 minutes per block (Table 1). The eighth block is a survey consisting of 11 questions. Students are allotted a minimum of 45 minutes of authorized break time that can be taken anytime between blocks. At the beginning of the exam, you will be presented with

TABLE 1 Time Breakdown of the USMLE Step 1 Exam

Tutorial	15 minutes (added to break time if skipped)
Question blocks	7 hours (60 minutes per block)
Break time	45 minutes (includes time for lunch)

QUICK HIT: Prior to test day, take the exam tutorial offered on the NBME website. On exam day, skip the tutorial and gain an extra 15 minutes of break time.

a 15-minutes tutorial. This tutorial is also available on the NBME website: http://www.usmle.org/Orientation/2009/menu.html. If the tutorial is taken prior to the exam date, it can be skipped on exam day—allowing you an **extra 15 minutes for break time. You can also gain extra break time by finishing blocks earlier.**

Breaks can be taken between blocks when you wish. Figure 1 shows two suggested test day schedules. The first schedule is the traditional one break schedule made for the student who likes one large mid day break (Figure 1). The second schedule is for those students who prefer a break following each block as a reward for finishing the block and as a time to refresh and recuperate before the beginning of the next block. Both schedules may be modified to individual preferences.

FIGURE 1 Structure of the USMLE Step 1 Exam

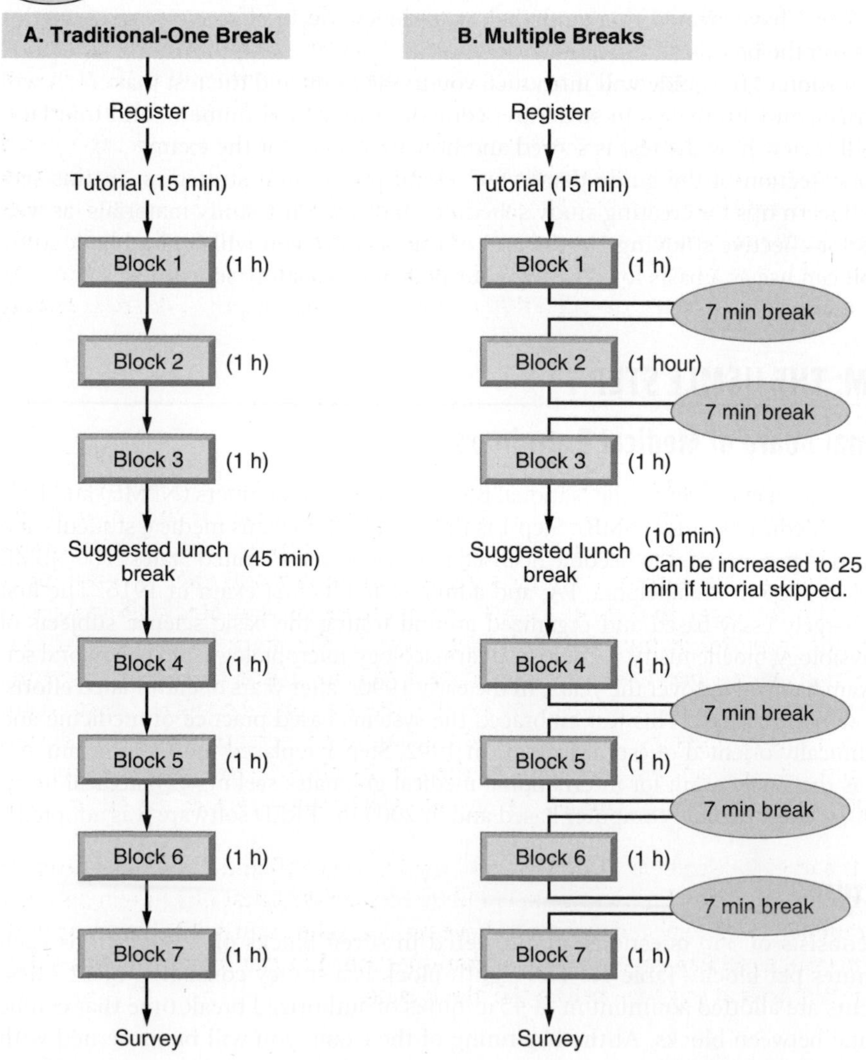

Test Content

The exam consists of multiple-choice questions; each question contains a question stem followed by five or more answer choices. Nearly 75% of questions begin with a clinical vignette or patient scenario. Students may also be asked direct questions. What kinds of questions are **not** seen on the test? Question stems including "all of the following except," "not," and matching-style questions are **never** included in Step 1 exams.

Often, examinees will be presented with answer choices that are partially correct. In these instances, it is important to pick the option that **best** answers the statement in the question stem and move on.

Questions may range in difficulty from medium to hard. While the questions vary from test to test and year to year, the proportion of question difficulty does not.

Something important for you to remember: Anywhere from 10% to 20% of questions seen on exam day are experimental questions that are not scored. Therefore, when presented with a difficult question with options that seem partially correct, it is important to select an answer that best fits and move on.

Test Environment

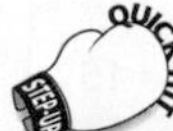

Not everyone will be taking the Step 1. All types of testing take place at the Prometric center and tests are started at different times of the day. Don't be surprised when other test-takers come and go at different times than you do.

In general, Prometric centers share a generic design. There is the reception area where you will register on the morning of the exam, place your belongings in a locker, and return to take breaks. Beyond this is the examination area where only certain items are allowed: a government issued identification card (typically a driver's license or passport) and a locker key. Everything else, including cell phones, pagers, digital watches, PDAs, books, notes, wallets, food, and beverages, goes into the locker. The examination area consists of a series of cubicles with computers. Test-takers are given noise reducer muffs, a dry erase board, markers, and a dry eraser to use as needed during the exam. Proctors walk through the rooms periodically to make sure test rules are obeyed. When taking an authorized break after a block is completed, you will need to leave the examination area, present an identification card, and sign a book. The process is repeated when you return to the testing area after the break. When you return to the cubicle, the computer will ask for your candidate identification number, which is written at the top of the dry erase board. As soon as you enter the candidate identification number into the computer, the next testing block begins.

Test Interface

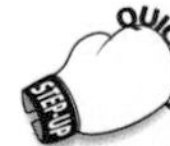

The testing interface allows you to annotate text in the question stem. These can be helpful tools, but be wary of the clock; they can also cause you to waste valuable testing time.

The NBME offers an online tutorial that reviews exam procedures and the testing interface. Briefly, the testing interface for each block consists mainly of a single question and answer choices below it (Figure 2). Above this is a panel with several icons. Clicking on the appropriate icons allows you to perform that specific function. Clicking on the **mark button** will mark the question for that block allowing you to return to the question at the end of the set. Next to the mark button are navigation buttons including a **previous button** and **next button**. These move you back one question or forward one question. Clicking on the **labs button** displays the normal lab values screen. Four options are offered: blood, hematologic, cerebrospinal, and sweat/urine/BMI. You can also write a note next to the text by clicking on the **notes button**. Finally, clicking the **calculator button** brings up a calculator to use for basic math functions.

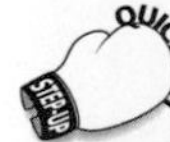

There is no penalty for guessing or benefit in leaving a question blank on the USMLE Step 1. Select answer choices as you move through and complete the block. If you are unsure of your answer, mark the question. If you have time at the end of the block, you can easily return to it and reconsider your initial response.

On the left part of the screen is a panel with a running list of 50 questions. The question that is currently being viewed is highlighted in blue. Incomplete questions have a dot next to the item number and completed questions have no dot. When you mark questions with the mark function, a red flag appears next to that question. You can directly click on that question to return to it at any time before the block ends.

FIGURE 2 **Testing interface**
(Adapted from http://www.usmle.org/Orientation/2009/menu.html.)

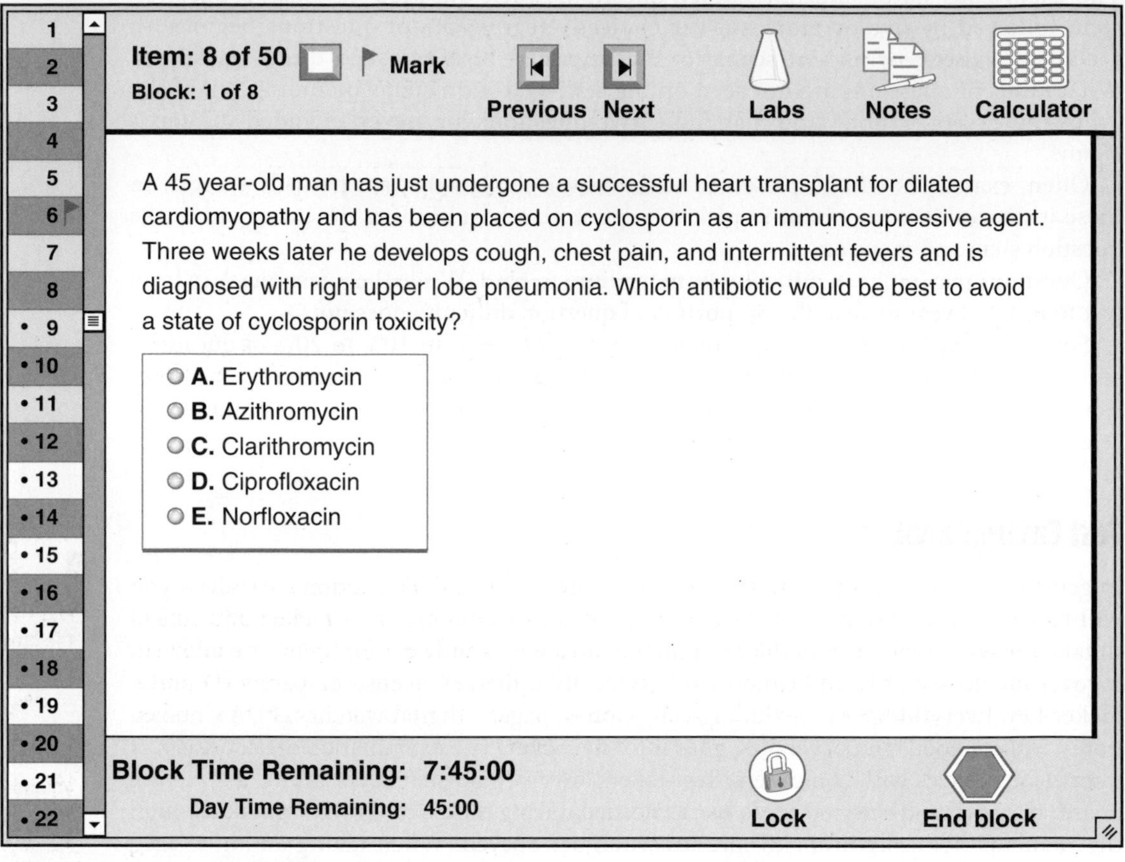
Item: 8 of 50
Mark
Block: 1 of 8
Previous
Next
Labs
Notes
Calculator
A 45 year-old man has just undergone a successful heart transplant for dilated cardiomyopathy and has been placed on cyclosporin as an immunosupressive agent. Three weeks later he develops cough, chest pain, and intermittent fevers and is diagnosed with right upper lobe pneumonia. Which antibiotic would be best to avoid a state of cyclosporin toxicity?
A. Erythromycin
B. Azithromycin
C. Clarithromycin
D. Ciprofloxacin
E. Norfloxacin
Block Time Remaining: 7:45:00
Day Time Remaining: 45:00
Lock
End block
1
2
3
4
5
6
7
8
• 9
• 10
• 11
• 12
• 13
• 14
• 15
• 16
• 17
• 18
• 19
• 20
• 21
• 22

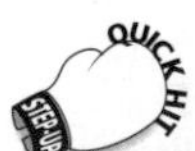

If you have concerns about or fear of taking computer-based tests, consider visiting a Prometric center ahead of time to take a practice exam with the testing interface.

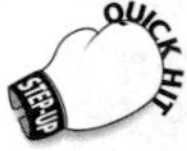

The minimum passing score on the USMLE Step 1 is 185. This number generally corresponds to getting 60% to 70% of exam questions right.

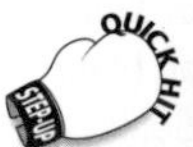

94% to 95% of the United States and Canadian medical students pass the exam on their first attempt. Compare this to the US bar exam, which has a passing rate of 67%.

Test Scoring

Examinees receive their score via an electronic score report 3 to 6 weeks after taking the exam. The score report consists of three key pieces of information. First, it states whether the examinee has passed or failed. Second, it displays a score in a three-digit scale and two-digit scale that reflects how well the examinee performed on the content of the exam. The mean score on the exam is 217 with a standard deviation of 20. **Passing on the three-digit scale is 185, which corresponds to 75 on the two-digit scale.** The minimum passing score is subject to change by the NBME, although it is not expected to change for a few years. Finally, there is a table depicting the examinee's performance profile by basic science subject and organ system. The examinee's medical school also receives a report containing pass/fail status, digit score, and group performance profile. During the residency application process, residency programs receive a transcript containing pass/fail status and the digit score without the performance profile (Figure 3).

When preparing for the exam, the goal is two-tiered. Your first objective should be to **pass the exam** so that you can be on your way to becoming a licensed physician in the United States. Also, passing the exam is often linked to proceeding to the third year of medical school and getting your medical degree. The second objective is doing the best you can so that you can make yourself a **competitive applicant for the residency of your choice**. Certain highly competitive residency programs such as orthopaedic surgery and ophthalmology use Step 1 scores in the selection process.

It is important to note that the Step 1 score is only one of many factors that weigh in on the residency selection process. Programs make use of other applicant characteristics such as clinical rotation grades, research, publications, and reference letters. Having insight into your academic portfolio and defining your personal goals may be helpful in guiding your studies for Step 1.

FIGURE 3 **Median scores for matched US seniors by specialty. The numbers displayed are median values for USMLE Step 1 Score for matched US Seniors by specialty. The vertical lines reflect interquartile ranges, the range of scores for applicants excluding the top and bottom quarters of the distribution**

(Adapted from http://www.nrmp.org/data/chartingoutcomes2007.pdf.)

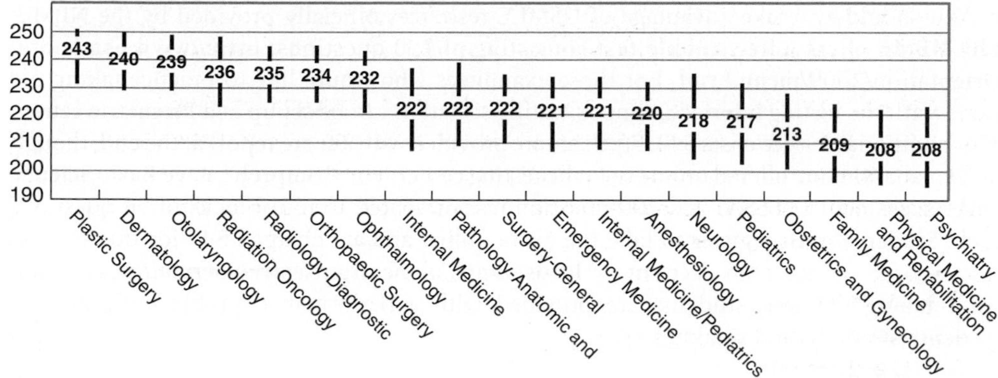

Registering to Take the Exam

Six to eight months prior to the anticipated exam date, you will likely be prompted by your school to begin the registration process for taking the exam. The Step 1 application packet can be downloaded from the USMLE web site: http://www.usmle.org. Applicants must select a 3-month time period to take the exam (e.g., April–May–June, June–July–August). The application includes a form requiring a passport-sized photo that must be certified by the school registrar. The NBME processes the submitted application and sends out a scheduling permit.

> You should register for the exam six to eight months prior to your anticipated exam date.

The scheduling permit contains a unique candidate identification number, which is necessary in order to schedule the exam and take the exam. After receiving the scheduling permit, you should attempt to schedule your exam as soon as possible in order to receive the location and time of your choice. Scheduling occurs on a first-come, first-served basis, and testing centers fill up quickly during popular testing times of the year. Specific instructions on scheduling the test are delineated on the scheduling permit and require calling Prometric 1-800-633-3926 or logging into the Prometric site at www.prometric.com. A list of Prometric testing centers nearest you can be found on the Prometric web site. Of note, testing centers are closed the first 2 weeks of January, during major holidays, and generally on Sundays. Also, the exam can be started at different times of the day for those preferring the early or late hours of the day. Generally, Step 1 is taken by second year medical students finishing their second year of medical school. Some relevant information to consider when scheduling your exam is your second year end date and third year start date. Because most curricula end in May, and students allow themselves a study time of 1 month, most students take the exam in June.

> Schedule your test as soon as possible after receiving the scheduling permit in order to receive the location and time of your choice.

> The scheduling permit needs to be presented on the day of the exam. Put it in a safe place. Copies will not be accepted.

If for some reason you need to reschedule your exam, you will need to call or visit the Prometric web site. The rescheduled date must fall within the 3-month eligibility period selected earlier during the registration process (also found on your scheduling permit). Also, to avoid a rescheduling fee, Prometric should be contacted before noon EST 5 business days prior to the testing date.

> To avoid a rescheduling fee, contact Prometric before noon EST 5 business days before the scheduled testing date.

PREPARING FOR THE EXAM: STUDY STRATEGIES

Study Materials

The first step to preparing for the exam is collecting and familiarizing yourself with study materials. You can start this step years before you actually take the exam. When starting medical school, consider purchasing a comprehensive review text such as *Step-Up to the USMLE Step 1*. The purpose of this is to begin reading, annotating, and familiarizing yourself with the test and content of the book. You might also consider investing early in subject-based reviews as you study those subjects in medical school. Finally, consider purchasing one or a series of question banks. Question banks allow you the opportunity to practice and apply learned concepts, solidifying the exam preparation process.

You should also take advantage of USMLE resources officially provided by the NBME. **The NBME offers a free sample test consisting of 150 questions: http://www.usmle.org/Orientation/2009/menu.html**. For those examinees who would like to practice taking the exam with the testing interface, a mock testing situation can be set up at a Prometric center. This additional service costs $42. Students are provided with a score report at the end, though no explanations are offered online or at the testing center. The **Comprehensive Basic Science Self Assessment** (CBSSA) is a 200-question test presented in four blocks of 50 questions each. Students must register to take the exam online and are charged $45 for this service. The website to create an account is: **https://apps.nbme.org/nsasweb/servlet/mesa_main.** After taking the test, students are provided with a performance profile outlining the student's strengths and weaknesses.

Study Schedule

After collecting study materials, the next step is creating a study schedule. Preparation for the USMLE Step 1 can start years before actually taking the exam. As mentioned earlier, as you prepare for your medical school classes, read and annotate review texts along with studying syllabi and textbooks for classes. The purpose of this is to familiarize yourself with the text.

In the months prior to the exam, you should register for the exam, schedule the exam, and collect study materials including a question bank. Familiarize yourself with your study materials and attend campus review sessions.

The month before the exam, create and follow a **study schedule**. The purpose of the study schedule is to cover each of the disciplines tested on the exam. Typically, most medical students are provided 1 month to study for the exam. When students are creating a study schedule, oftentimes the most challenging feat is determining how many days to allocate toward one discipline. Suggested study schedules that have been successful for students in the past are included in this guide (Figures 4 and 5, at the end of this section). The first study schedule is organized by organ system and the second by basic science discipline. These schedules are only suggested schedules. Individual schedules should be tailored to your needs, keeping in mind your individual strengths and weaknesses, high yield topics for the exam, and available time to study.

FIGURE 4 **Suggested study schedule: Organ systems based**

Sunday	Monday	Tuesday	Wednesday	Thursday	Friday	Saturday
1 NER	2 VOUS	3	4	5 CAR	6 DIO	7
8 RES	9 PIR	10 GAS	11 TRO	12 REN	13 AL	14
15 ENDO	16	17 REP	18 RO	19 MUSC	20 ULO	21 HEME
22 LYMPH	23 BASIC	24 CONCEPTS	25 WRAP	26 UP	27 DAYS	28
29	30					

FIGURE 5 Suggested study schedule: Basic science based

Sunday	Monday	Tuesday	Wednesday	Thursday	Friday	Saturday
1 PAT	2 HOLO	3 GY	4	5 PHYS	6 IOL	7 OGY
8	9 PHA	10 RMA	11 COL	12 OGY	13 MIC	14 RO/
15 IMM	16 UNO	17 BIO	18 CHEM	19	20 BEHAV	21 SCI
22 ANATOMY (including embryology, histology)	23 NEURO	24	25 WRAP	26 UP	27 DAYS	28
29	30					

The suggested study schedules in Figures 4 and 5 assume 28 days available for study, including the day before the USMLE. If you have more or fewer days, adjust the schedule accordingly. For example, if you have 31 days, add ½ day to Behavioral Science, ½ day to Gross Anatomy/Embryology, 1 day off, and 1 day to wrap-up. In these suggested schedules, 2 to 3 days are allocated for wrap-up before the exam, 1 to 2 days are scheduled as days off as rewards for doing your work, and 24 days are full study days. In general, when determining the order of subjects to study, the general strategy should be longer-term memory subjects early and shorter-term memory subjects late (Table 2). Also, when determining how many days to allocate certain subjects or organ systems, provide more days for heavily tested subjects like pathology and physiology (Table 3).

TABLE 2 Order for Organ System and Basic Science Schedule

Order for Organ System Schedule	Order for Basic Science Schedule
Basic concepts/general	Physiology
Endocrine	Pathology
Nervous	Behavioral science
Cardiovascular	Microbiology/Immunology
Respiratory	Pharmacology
Renal	Biochemistry
Gastrointestinal	Neuroanatomy
Musculoskeletal	Gross Anatomy/Embryology/ Histology
Reproductive	
Heme/Lymph	

TABLE 3 **Allocation of Days**

Allocation of Days by Organ System		Allocation of Days by Basic Science	
Organ System	**Days**	**Basic Science**	**Days**
Nervous	3.5	Pathology	4
Cardiovascular	3	Physiology	4
Respiratory	2.5	Pharmacology	4
Gastrointestinal	2	Microbiology/Immunology	4
Renal	2.5	Biochemistry	3
Endocrine	2.5	Behavioral Science	1.5
Reproductive	2	Gross Anatomy/Embryology/Histology	1.5
Musculoskeletal	2	Neuroanatomy	2
Heme/Lymph	2		
Basic Concepts/General	2		

In the month prior to the exam, you should also create and follow a **daily schedule**. Table 4 contains a sample daily study schedule. The daily schedule should allot time for **studying review texts**, **reading cases/clinical vignettes**, and **doing questions**. While studying texts, you should not only read, but also spend time **understanding concepts** and **memorizing key facts**. Tools that help with understanding and memorizing information include organizing information into **tables**, **charts**, and **figures**, using **mnemonics**, and **applying information in daily practice**, such as in clinics and caring for patients. Books with clinical cases and vignettes are based on this premise and provide an opportunity to integrate studied information. Doing questions is another excellent method of reinforcing and remembering learned information. An online question bank of more than 450 USMLE format questions based on commonly tested facts has been included with this text and can be accessed via this website: www.thePoint.lww.com/StepUp4e. Moreover, clinical vignettes and questions simulate the test day experience. Make sure you also include in your schedule **time to relax** and do other things that are important to you (work out, spend time with friends and family, etc.).

The **night before the exam**, relax and gather your **required materials (orange permit slip, government issued photo ID)**. Make sure you know how to get to the testing center and have confirmed with the testing center your test time and date. Get a good night's rest!

TABLE 4 **Suggested Daily Study Schedule**

Time	Activity
8:00 am–Noon	Study
Noon–1:00 pm	Lunch
1:00 pm–5:00 pm	Study
5:00 pm–8:00 pm	Exercise, dinner, errands, phone calls
8:00 pm–10:00 pm (or 11:00 pm)	Questions

Study Strategies

Studying is a two-stage process. First, learn the basic definitions and concepts. The best method of accomplishing this is reading. Second, recognize and remember key facts. This is the hardest stage and one that most students neglect. Helpful strategies include:

1. **Memorization**—Use study aids like mnemonics, tables, and figures.
2. **Active learning**—Engage in active learning by applying the concepts to scenarios, clinical settings, and mini-case presentations.
3. **Questions**—Apply learned concepts by doing questions.
4. **Study groups**—Discuss studied material and quiz each other; these activities are helpful in retaining information.

ONLINE RESOURCES

Table 5 summarizes important NBME websites and online resources available to you as you prepare for the USMLE.

TABLE 5 Important Websites for Preparing for the USMLE Step 1

	Website	Description	Cost
NBME	http://www.nbme.org	Find general information and updates on the USMLE Step 1	N/A
Application materials	http://www.usmle.org	Apply to take the USMLE Step 1	$
Scheduling the exam	http://www.prometric.com	Schedule your exam	N/A
FRED software tutorial and practice questions	http://www.usmle.org/Orientation/2009/menu.html	Select option "Multiple-Choice Tutorial and Practice Test Items-Version: Fred V2."[a] This contains a tutorial on the FRED software, familiarizes you with the testing interface, and contains over 100 sample questions. After taking this tutorial, you may skip the tutorial on test day, providing yourself with an extra 15 minutes in break time	Free
CBSSA	https://apps.nbme.org/nsasweb/servlet/mesa_main	The CBSSA contains USMLE Step 1 format questions designed by the NBME. There are 200 questions in four blocks of 50 questions each. Register to create an account and then follow instructions for CBSSA	$
Step Up to the USMLE Step 1 Question Bank	www.thePoint.lww.com/StepUp4e	Includes more than 350 questions in USMLE format with explanations preparing you for the most commonly tested facts on the USMLE	Free
Step Up to the USMLE Step 1 Website	http://www.lww.com/Step-Up	Ask the authors questions, become a student contributor for the next edition, provide feedback on this text	N/A

[a]In 2009, the USMLE Step 1 migrated from FRED version V1 to version V2. This may have changed further after publication of this text. Please refer to the NBME website for the latest changes in test delivery software.

PERSONALIZED STUDY SCHEDULE

Use the blank study schedule on this page to build your own based on the tips included in this chapter and your own areas of strength and weakness (Figure 6).

FIGURE 6 **Blank study schedule**

PERSONALIZED STEP 1 STUDY SCHEDULE

Use this blank calendar to create your own personalized Step 1 study schedule. Determine your preference for systems-based review or subject-based review, identify your strong areas and weak areas, and create your study schedule.

______ SYSTEMS-BASED ______ SUBJECT-BASED

Strong Areas: ____________________

Weak Areas: ____________________

Sunday	Monday	Tuesday	Wednesday	Thursday	Friday	Saturday
1	2	3	4	5	6	7
8	9	10	11	12	13	14
15	16	17	18	19	20	21
22	23	24	25	26	27	28
29	30					

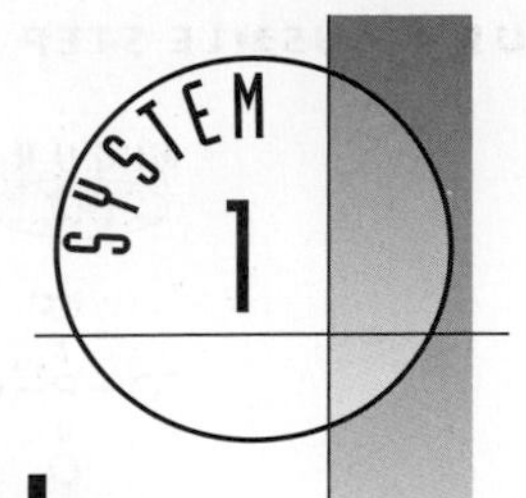

Basic Concepts

DNA, RNA, AND PROTEIN

I. Chemical components of DNA and RNA

A. Deoxyribonucleic acid (DNA) and ribonucleic acid (RNA) are made up of nucleotides, which contain

1. A **nitrogenous base**—either a purine or pyrimidine (Figure 1-1)
   a. **Purines** are formed from
      - Aspartate
      - Carbon dioxide (CO_2)
      - Glutamate
      - Glycine
      - N10-formyl-tetrahydrofolate

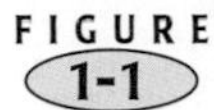

Bases
C, carbon; H, hydrogen; N, nitrogen; O, oxygen

Purines

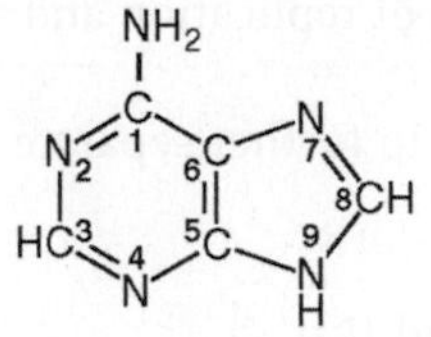

Adenine (A)

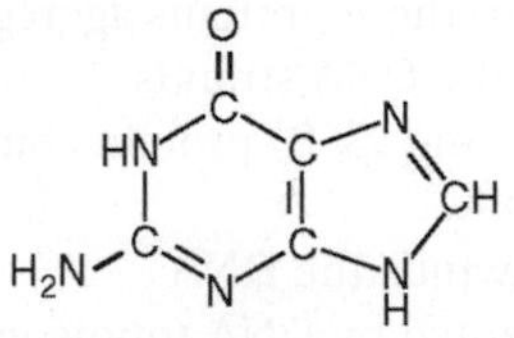

Guanine (G)

Pyrimidines

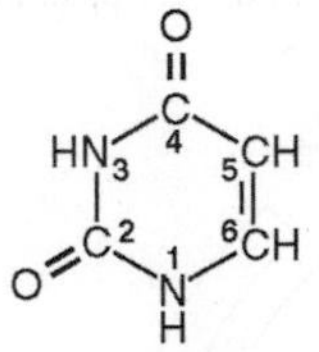

Uracil (U)

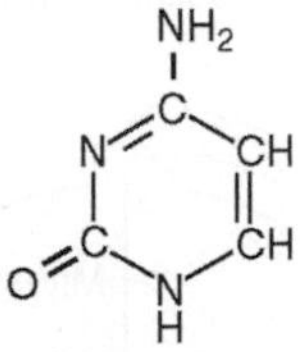

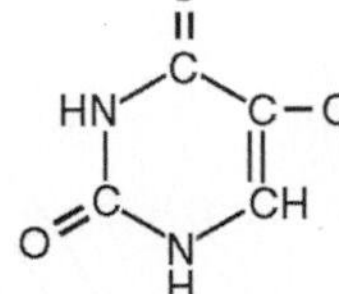

Cytosine (C)

Thymine (T)

   b. **Pyrimidines** are formed from
      - Aspartate
      - CO_2
      - Glutamate
2. A **pentose sugar**—either a **ribose** for RNA or a **2-deoxyribose** for DNA
3. One, two, or three phosphate groups forming a -monophosphate, -diphosphate, or -triphosphate, respectively (Figure 1-2)

FIGURE 1-2 **Nucleotide structure**

C, carbon; H, hydrogen; O, oxygen; P, phosphate.

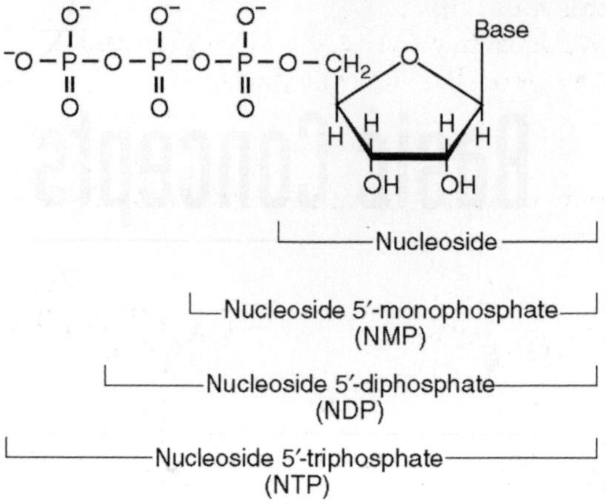

$^{-}O-P(=O)(O^{-})-O-P(=O)(O^{-})-O-P(=O)(O^{-})-O-CH_2$ — ribose (O, H, H, H, H, OH, OH) — Base

Nucleoside

Nucleoside 5′-monophosphate (NMP)

Nucleoside 5′-diphosphate (NDP)

Nucleoside 5′-triphosphate (NTP)

B. Nucleoside triphosphates (NTP) are linked together by a 3′–5′ phosphodiester bond to form single-stranded RNA or DNA.

C. **Adenine** (A) binds to **thymine** (T), while **guanine** (G) binds to **cytosine** (C) in DNA. **Uracil** (U) replaces thymine (T) in RNA.

> QUICK HIT: DNA synthesis can be prevented by nucleoside analogs such as cytosine arabinoside, zidovudine, and acyclovir. These types of drugs are useful in antiviral and anticancer therapy.

II. DNA replication

A. It is **semiconservative**—When two DNA molecules are created from the original helix, one strand of parental DNA is incorporated with each new daughter strand.

B. It takes place in the S **phase** of the cell cycle (Figure 1-3).

C. DNA strand separation requires several proteins.

1. **DnaA**—20 to 50 of these proteins aggregate at the origin of replication and begin to separate the DNA strands.
2. **Single-strand binding** (SSB) proteins bind cooperatively to further separate the two strands of DNA.
3. **DNA helicase** unwinds the DNA.

D. Supercoiling is prevented by DNA **topoisomerase** types I and II.

FIGURE 1-3 **The cell cycle**

(Adapted from Bhushan V, Le T, Amin C. First Aid for the USLME Step 1. Stamford, CT: Appleton & Lange, 1999:165.)

M: Mitosis: Prophase–metaphase–anaphase–telophase

G_1: Growth

S: Synthesis of DNA

G_2: Growth

G_0: Quiescent G_1 phase

G_1 and G_0 are of variable duration. Mitosis is usually the shortest phase. Most cells are in G_0. Rapidly dividing cells have a shorter G_1.

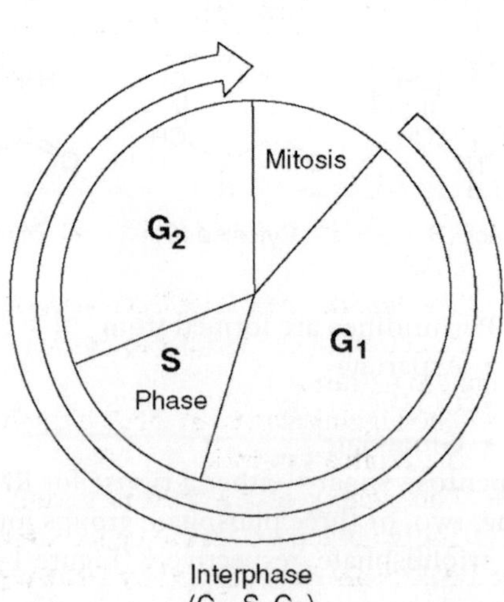

E. Replication process in prokaryotic cells (Figure 1-4)
1. An RNA primer is placed on the separated DNA strands by RNA polymerase (also called **primase**) before replication can begin.
2. Only one RNA primer is needed on the leading strand; on the lagging strand, however, a new primer is required as the replication fork opens.

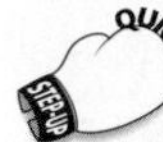

In eukaryotic cells, replication is accomplished by POL enzymes similar to those in prokaryotic cells. POL α performs primase activity like prokaryotic primase; POL δ synthesizes the leading DNA strand; POL ε synthesizes the lagging strand; and POL β repairs and excises primers, similar to DNA polymerase I.

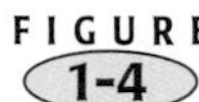

FIGURE 1-4 DNA synthesis
(Adapted from Marks DB. BRS Biochemistry. 3rd Ed. Baltimore, MD: Williams & Wilkins, 1999. Used by permission of Lippincott, Williams & Wilkins.)

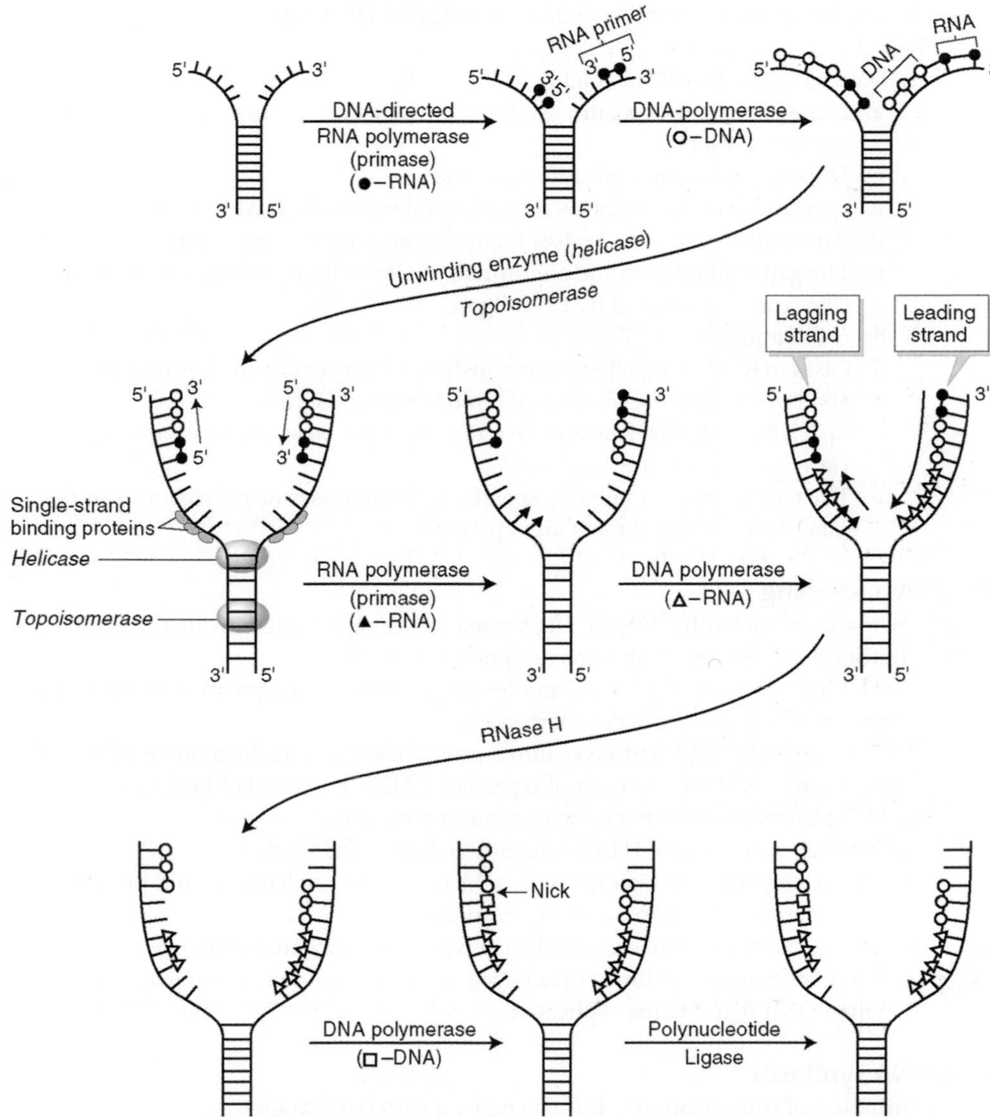

a. Leading strand
- The leading strand produces a continuously elongating strand of new DNA.
- The leading strand of DNA is copied continuously from 5′ to 3′ in the direction of the replication fork.

b. Lagging strand
- The lagging strand of DNA is copied piecewise in the direction opposite of the replication fork.
- The lagging strand produces small pieces of new DNA with RNA interspersed, which are called Okazaki fragments.

3. The DNA chain is elongated by DNA polymerase III, which adds nucleotides with energy provided by breaking of the triphosphate bond.

4. When DNA strand synthesis is complete, it is proofread.
    a. The proofreading function of DNA polymerase III (3′–5′ exonuclease) allows it to correct mismatched base pairs.
    b. The improperly placed base is hydrolytically removed and replaced with the appropriate one.
5. RNA primers are removed from the Okazaki fragments and leading strand.
    a. DNA polymerase I or III has **3′–5′ exonuclease** activity that allows it to remove the RNA primer.
    b. Once the primer is removed, the space is filled with DNA.
6. The break in the strand backbone is sealed by **DNA ligase**.

F. Repair

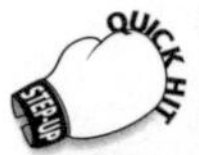

Xeroderma pigmentosum is a genetic disease in which cells cannot repair damaged DNA. People suffering from this disease cannot repair skin damage caused by sunlight and are predisposed to skin cancer.

1. Damage caused by ultraviolet light.
    a. Ultraviolet light exposure results in pyrimidine dimers (especially thymine–thymine dimers).
    b. Dimers inhibit the replication process.
    c. Specialized **endonucleases** recognize a dimer and cleave it at its 5′ end.
    d. An **exonuclease** then excises the dimer and leaves a gap in the DNA strand.
    e. The gap is filled with the appropriate nucleotides by DNA polymerase I.
    f. The strand is resealed by DNA ligase.
2. Base alterations.
    a. Bases may be changed spontaneously or slowly over time because of **alkylating agents** (cyclophosphamide and nitrosoureas).
    b. Specialized **glycosylases** remove the improper base and leave an empty (apyrimidinic or apurinic) space.
    c. The empty space is filled by specific endonucleases or polymerases in the same manner that dimers are repaired.

III. DNA packaging

A. Owing to its incredible length, DNA must be properly coiled inside the cell.

B. **Histones** are a group of proteins designed to coil DNA.
1. The high content of arginine and lysine gives histones a positive charge, which attracts them to negatively charged DNA.
2. Histones organize themselves into a group of eight to make a **nucleosome** core; each core contains two each of types H2A, H2B, H3, and H4 histones.
3. DNA twists approximately twice around each core.
4. Between cores, a type H1 histone is attached to the DNA.
5. The arrangement of histones and DNA is called a nucleosome and produces a characteristic "beads-on-a-string" appearance.
6. The nucleosomes coil around themselves to produce nucleofilaments.
7. **Nucleofilaments** are further packaged and coiled into more compact structures when DNA is not being replicated.

IV. mRNA synthesis

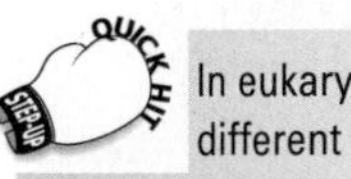

In eukaryotes, different RNAs are synthesized by different RNA polymerases. RNA polymerase I synthesizes ribosomal RNA; RNA polymerase II synthesizes messenger RNA; and RNA polymerase III synthesizes transfer RNA.

A. Initiation of transcription is influenced by a variety of factors.
1. **RNA polymerase** binds to the promoter region of the DNA.
2. The TATAAT nucleotide sequence is a section of the promoter located upstream from the start of transcription; it is contained in the Hogness box of eukaryotes and the Pribnow box of prokaryotes.
3. The CAAT box, found in eukaryotes, and the ~35 sequence, found in prokaryotes, are located further upstream from the TATAAT sequence and have promoter function.

B. After recognition of the promoter region by RNA polymerase, elongation begins.
1. Elongation of RNA occurs in a manner similar to DNA replication, but does not require a primer for initiation.
2. RNA polymerase does not have a proofreading function, so it cannot correct mismatched base pairs that may occur.

C. In eukaryotic cells, RNA undergoes **post-translational** modification; in prokaryotic cells, transcription and translation occur simultaneously.
   1. RNA synthesized by eukaryotic **RNA polymerase II** is called **heterogeneous nuclear RNA (hnRNA)** and is found in the nucleus of the cell.
   2. This hnRNA is **capped at the 5′ end** by a 7-methylguanine molecule provided by *S*-adenosylmethionine (SAM).
   3. **A poly-A nucleotide tail is added to the 3′ end.**
   4. Introns are cleaved out.
   5. The molecule is now mature messenger RNA (mRNA) and is transported to the cytoplasm.

V. Protein synthesis (Figure 1-5)

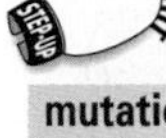

Point mutations include **silent mutations** (the same amino acid), **missense** mutations (a new amino acid), and **nonsense mutations** (stop codon). Insertions are the addition of extra amino acids, and deletions are the loss of amino acids.

A. Initiation is started with the binding of the ribosomal subunits to the mRNA.
B. The start codon **AUG** is the first codon to be recognized and translated; initiation factor 2 (**IF-2** in prokaryotes, **eIF-2** in eukaryotes) and guanosine 5′-triphosphate (GTP) are required.
C. A methionine is added as the first amino acid.
D. Elongation requires a transfer RNA (tRNA) with the appropriate **anticodon** to the codon on the mRNA, elongation factors, and GTP.
E. Termination requires a **UAA**, **UAG**, or **UGA** codon.
F. Regulation of RNA synthesis.
   1. Eukaryotes
      a. Control is accomplished by gene **methylation**, **amplification**, and **rearrangement**.
      b. Histones play a role in gene suppression.
      c. Inducers activate gene expression.
      d. Some eukaryotic genes are regulated at transcription.
   2. Prokaryotes
      a. Protein synthesis is controlled at the level of transcription using operons.
      b. An **operon** is a set of adjacent genes that are activated or deactivated.
      c. Each operon has a **promoter** region upstream from the genes, an operator that activates or deactivates the genes, and a **repressor** protein that can bind to the operator and deactivate transcription (Figure 1-6).

VI. Post-translational folding of proteins

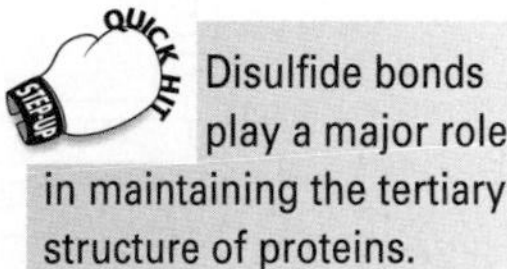

Disulfide bonds play a major role in maintaining the tertiary structure of proteins.

A. Newly synthesized proteins have a linear structure (**primary structure**).
B. On the basis of interactions between amino acids, these linear structures can assume **secondary structures**, such as an **α-helix** or a **β-pleated sheet**.
C. The **tertiary structure** incorporates the secondary structures into a complete three-dimensional configuration. This is the final conformation of many proteins.
D. A **quaternary structure** is formed when several tertiary structures are arranged together. This occurs in hemoglobin, for example, in which two α and two β globular proteins form the complete hemoglobin molecule.

BACTERIAL MORPHOLOGY AND GENETICS

I. Cell Wall—The Outermost Component of all Bacteria

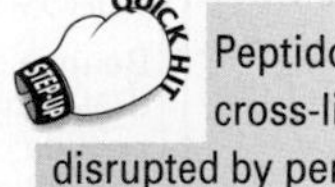

Peptidoglycan cross-linking is disrupted by penicillin and cephalosporins.

A. Cell wall components
   1. Peptidoglycan, which provides rigid support and protects against osmotic pressure changes, is thick and multilayered in Gram-positive organisms, and thin and single layer in Gram-negative organisms.
   2. Gram-positive outer membrane is made up of teichoic acid.

(text continues on page 19)

FIGURE 1-5 **Protein synthesis**

A, adenine; Arg, arginine; C, cytosine; EF, elongation factor; fMET, formyl methionine; G, guanine; GDP, guanine diphosphate; GTP, guanine triphosphate; IF, initiation factor; Phe, phenylalanine; P_i, inorganic phosphate; RF, release factor; T, thymine; tRNA, transfer ribonucleic acid; U, uracil. (Adapted from Champe PC, Harvey RA. Lippincott's Illustrated Reviews: Biochemistry. 2nd Ed. Philadelphia, PA: Lippincott-Raven Publishers, 1994:396–397. Used by permission of Lippincott, Williams & Wilkins.)

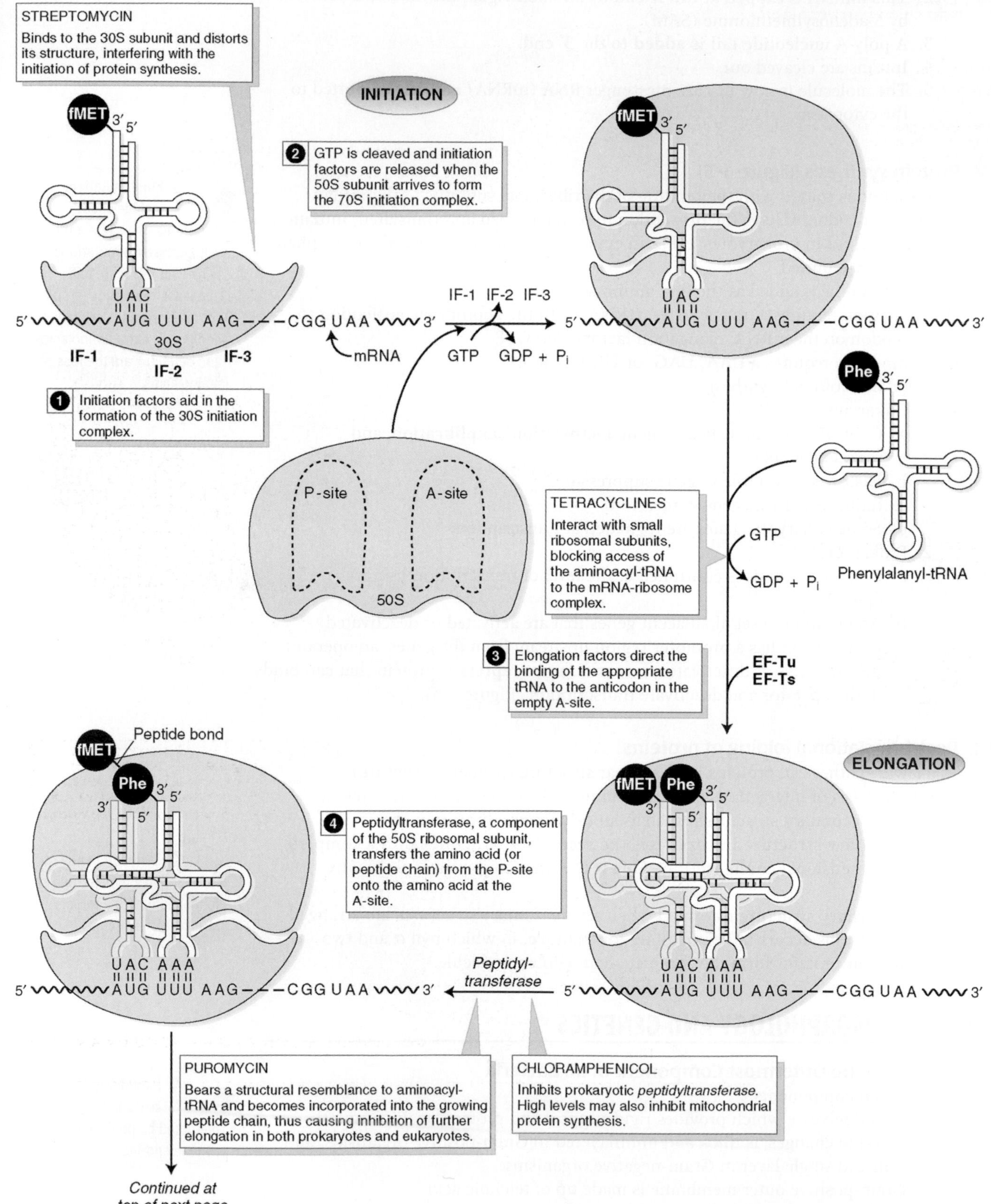

Continued at top of next page

FIGURE 1-5 *(Continued)*

5 The ribosome moves a distance of three nucleotides along the mRNA in the 5′→ 3′ direction.
fMET
Phe
3′ 5′
CLINDAMYCIN and ERYTHROMYCIN
Bind irreversibly to a site on the 50S subunit of the bacterial ribosome, thus inhibiting translocation.
GTP GDP + P$_i$
Translocation
EF-G
A A A
5′ AUG UUU AAG – – – CGG UAA 3′
3′ 5′
UAC
DIPHTHERIA TOXIN
Inactivates the eukaryotic elongation factor, eEF-2, thus preventing translocation.
6 Steps 3, 4, and 5 are repeated until the growing peptide is complete.
fMet
Phe
Lys
Arg
3′ 5′
TERMINATION
UAC
5′ AUG UUU AAG – – – CGG UAA 3′
Termination codon
RF-1
RF-2
RF-3
fMet
Lys
Phe
Arg
Completed peptide
7 A termination codon is recognized by a release factor (RF), which activates the release of the newly synthesized peptide and dissolution of the synthesized complex.
AUG UUU AAG – – – CGG UAA 3′
Recycled

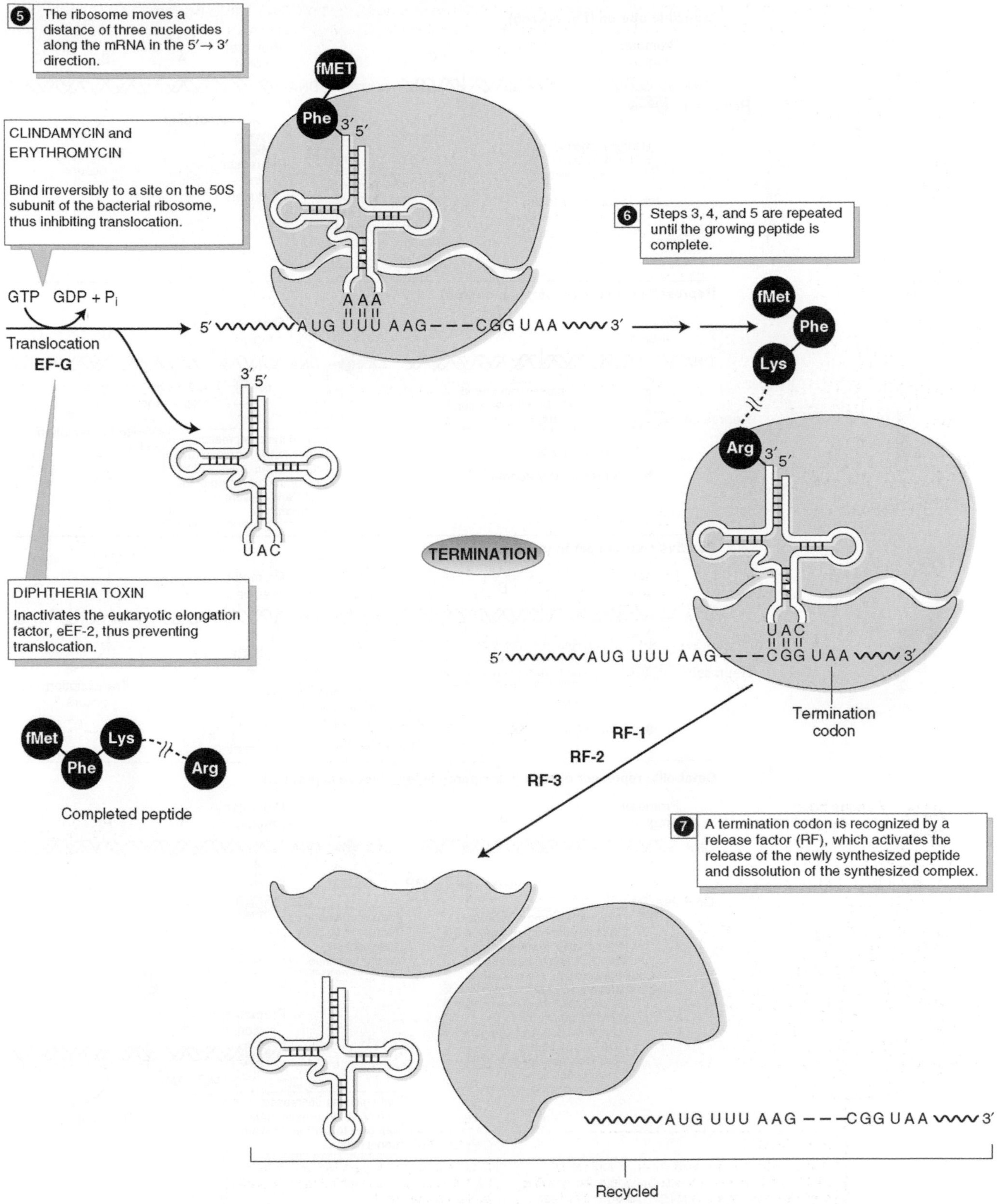

FIGURE 1-6 **Operons**
cAMP, cyclic adenosine monophosphate.

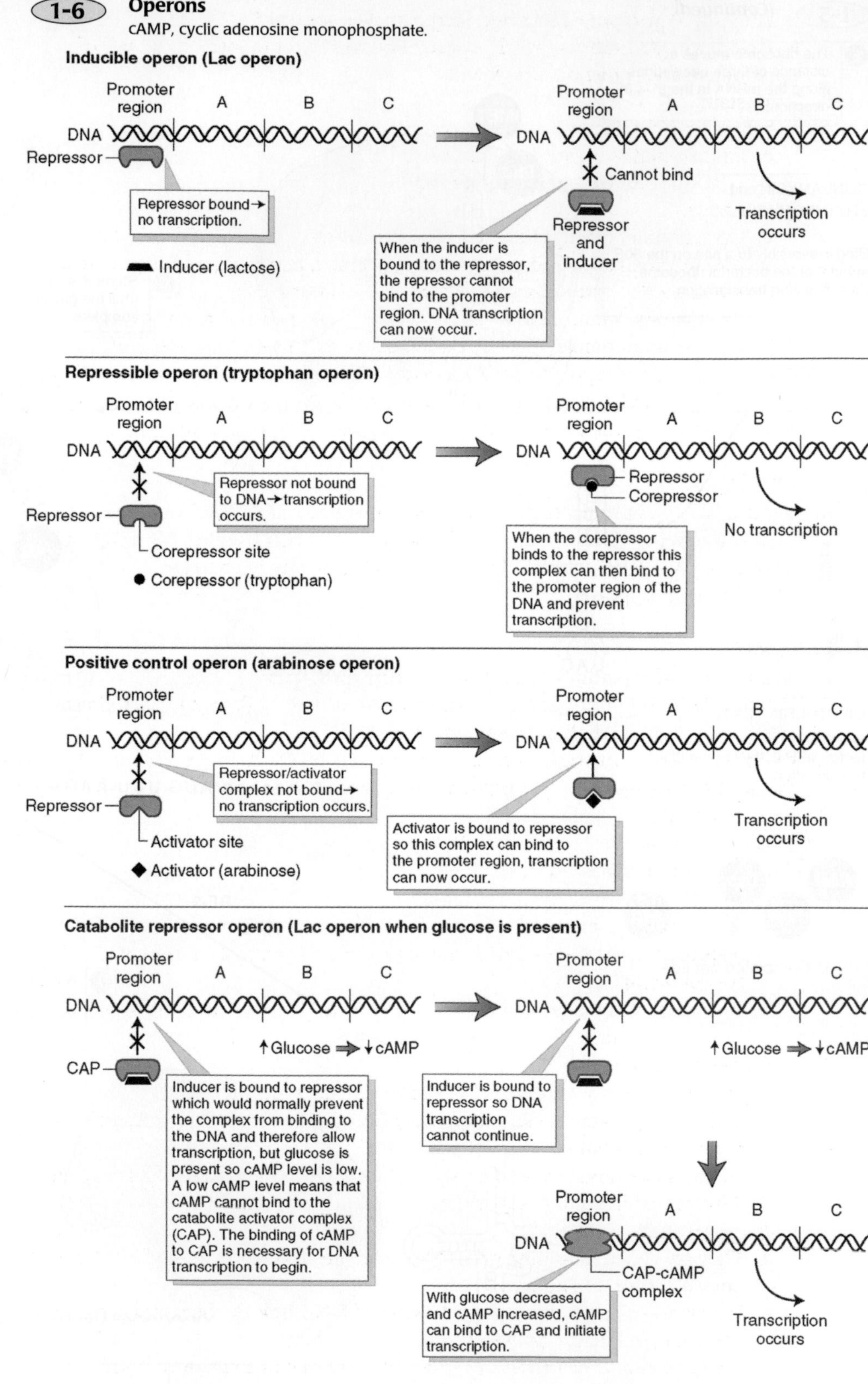

3. Gram-negative outer membrane is made up of lipid-A (toxic component of endotoxin) and polysaccharide (major surface antigen).
4. Cytoplasmic membrane is a lipoprotein bilayer without sterols, the site of oxidative and transport enzymes.

B. Gram stain
1. Separates most bacteria into two groups
   a. Gram-positive organisms stain blue.
   b. Gram-negative organisms stain red.
2. Procedure
   a. Crystal violet dye applied to the specimen stains all bacterial cells blue.
   b. Iodine, when added to the specimen, acts as a mordant and forms crystal violet–iodine complexes. Cells continue to appear blue.
   c. An organic solvent, such as ethanol, added to the specimen extracts the crystal violet–iodine complexes from Gram-negative organisms. Gram-negative organisms now appear colorless, whereas Gram-positive organisms remain blue.
   d. Safranin (red dye) is applied, staining the Gram-negative organisms red, while the Gram-positive organisms maintain their blue color.

II. Bacterial genome

A. Bacteria have a **haploid** genome, whereas humans have a **diploid** genome.

B. A typical bacterial cell has a **circular** DNA molecule with a molecular weight of approximately 2×10^9 with about 5×10^6 base pairs, which code for ~ 2,000 proteins.

III. Mutation

A. Several types of mutations occur that can alter the bacterial genome.

B. Mutation is an important factor in bacterial survival as it allows the bacteria to change and adapt to their environment.

C. Mutations may be caused by a mistake committed by DNA polymerase, a chemical mutagen, ultraviolet light, a virus, or other cause.

D. Types of mutations
1. **Base substitution**
   a. One base replaces another.
   b. Occurs at DNA replication.
   c. Can generate a missense mutation, which causes the wrong amino acid to be placed in the protein, or it can generate a nonsense mutation, which is read as a stop codon.
   d. Also occurs in eukaryotic cells, but can be repaired by the processes described earlier.
2. **Frameshift mutation**
   a. One or more bases are added or removed (not a multiple of 3).
   b. The reading frame is shifted on the mRNA molecule, causing massive errors in translation.
   c. Often causes protein to end prematurely as a result of creation of a stop codon
   d. Also occurs in eukaryotic cells.
3. **Transposons** (Figure 1-7)
   a. They are called "jumping genes" because they transfer pieces of DNA from one bacterium to another.
   b. Transposons can integrate small pieces of DNA into the bacterial genome, plasmids, or bacteriophages.
   c. Integration of transposon DNA into the host genome can occur within a preexisting gene and render the host gene useless.
   d. Each transposon has four domains:
      - **Inverted repeats**—appear at the ends and mediate integration of the transposon into a DNA molecule
      - **Transposase**—the enzyme that controls integration and removal of the transposon

FIGURE 1-7 **Transposons**
IR, inverted repeats.

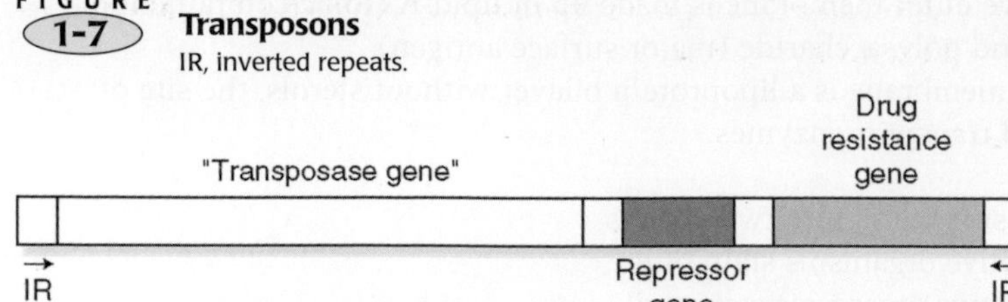

- **Repressor gene**—controls synthesis of transposase and whichever gene is in the fourth domain
- **Drug-resistance gene**—often appears in the fourth gene domain

e. Transposons replicate with the host DNA and are not capable of independent replication.
f. When transposons integrate and remove themselves from a DNA molecule, they can cause profound mutations.

IV. Genetic transfer

A. Transfer within a cell
1. Transposons can transfer information between different areas of the same DNA molecule.
2. **Programmed rearrangements**
   a. These are performed by certain organisms, including *Neisseria*, *Borrelia*, and trypanosomes.
   b. Programmed rearrangements cause a silent gene to be expressed. Programmed rearrangements also allow the organism to evade the immune system.

B. Transfer between cells (Table 1-1)

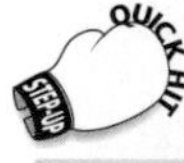

QUICK HIT: Conjugation is performed by fertility plasmid (F plasmid). A bacterium containing the F plasmid (the male) has a sex pilus, which can attach to an F plasmid-deficient bacterium (the female). Once attached, the female is reeled in and DNA is transferred.

TABLE 1-1 Genetic Transfer Between Prokaryotic Cells

Mode	Mechanism	Notes
Transduction	Transfer of DNA from one cell to another using a viral vector	Generalized transduction can transfer any gene and contains no viral DNA; specialized transduction can transfer only certain genes and contains viral DNA
Conjugation	Transfer of DNA from one bacterium to another via contact and exchange	Can transfer chromosomes or plasmids; uses a sex pilus

VIRAL GENETICS

- Comparison of Cells and Viruses (Table 1-2)

QUICK HIT: **Prions** lack most of the features associated with cells or viruses. Prions are thought to be abnormally folded proteins that are capable of catalyzing similar folding in the host's proteins. Accumulation of these abnormally folded proteins can cause spongiform diseases characterized by vacuolization of brain tissues, such as kuru or Creutzfeldt-Jakob disease.

TABLE 1-2 Comparison of Cells and Viruses

	Eukaryotes	Prokaryotes	Viruses
Size (in μm)	7	2–6	0.01–0.2
Membrane-bound organelles	Present	Absent	Absent
Ribosomes	80S	70S	Absent
DNA	46 chromosomes	1 circular chromosome	DNA or RNA; circular, single-strand, or multiple segments
Replication	Mitosis or meiosis	Binary fission	Production and assembly

In contrast to infectious bacteria and fungi, viruses are not cells. They do not have a nucleus or organelles and are not capable of reproducing independently. Current antiviral agents, such as acyclovir and foscarnet, can only suppress viral replication. Viral elimination requires a functioning host immune response.

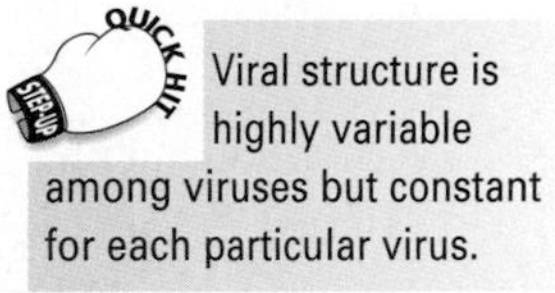

QUICK HIT
Viral structure is highly variable among viruses but constant for each particular virus.

I. Viral structure (Figure 1-8)

A. Nucleic acid
   1. May be DNA or RNA, but never both
   2. May be single- or double-stranded
   3. May be linear, segmented, or circular
   4. Most are haploid, but retroviruses are diploid

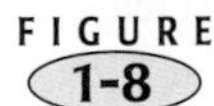

Structure of viruses. (A) Icosahedral capsid; (B) helical capsid

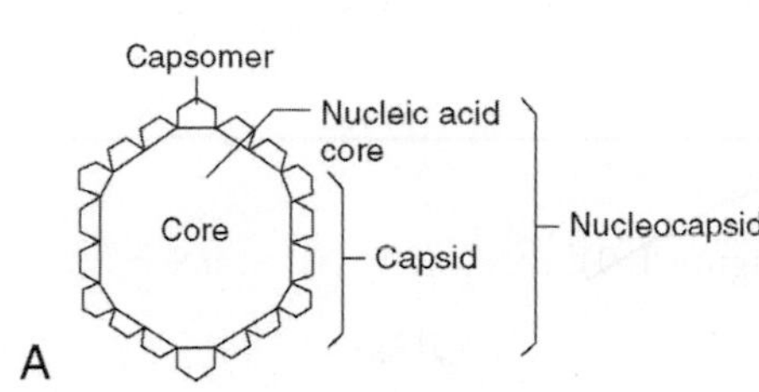

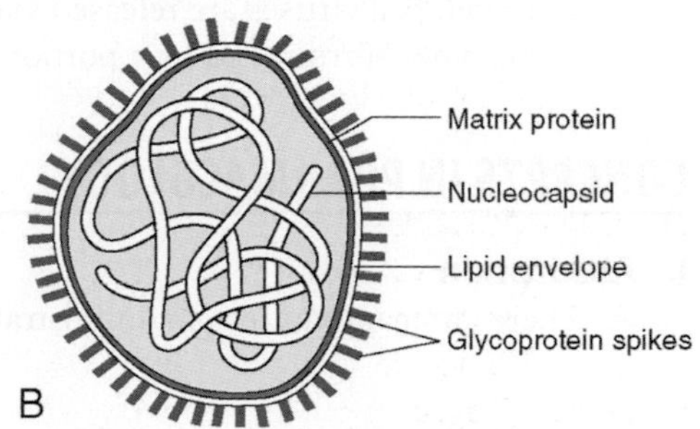

B. Capsid
   1. The protein coat around the nucleic acid core is composed of repeating units called **capsomeres**.
   2. The capsid assumes one of two shapes:
      a. **Helical**—hollow rod shape
      b. **Icosahedral**—multiple triangles arranged into a small sphere
   3. The capsid functions to protect the viral nucleic acid.

C. Envelope
   1. Surrounds the capsid of some viruses.
   2. Causes the virus to be more susceptible to drying and lipid solvents.
   3. Composed of virus-specific proteins and cell-derived lipids.
   4. Most **DNA viruses** derive their envelope from the host cell's **nuclear membrane**, whereas most **RNA viruses** derive their envelope from the host's **plasma membrane**.

II. Replication

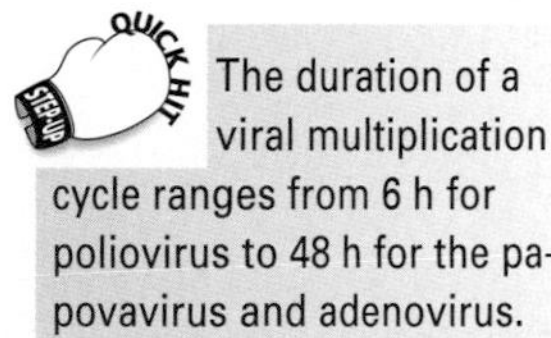

QUICK HIT
The duration of a viral multiplication cycle ranges from 6 h for poliovirus to 48 h for the papovavirus and adenovirus.

A. Attachment
   1. Viral surface proteins specifically attach to receptor proteins on the cell surface.
   2. The noncovalent interaction of proteins determines host range.

B. Penetration
   1. The virus may be engulfed by the host via a pinocytotic vesicle (**viropexis**).
   2. Nonenveloped viruses may slip through the host membrane by direct **translocation**.
   3. The viral **envelope may fuse with the host cell membrane**.

C. Uncoating
   1. DNA viruses partially uncoat in the cytoplasm and undergo final uncoating in the nucleus (to protect the DNA from endonucleases in the cytoplasm).
   2. RNA viruses uncoat in the cytoplasm.

D. **Expression and replication**

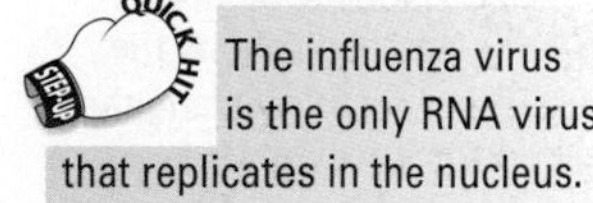

QUICK HIT
The influenza virus is the only RNA virus that replicates in the nucleus.

   1. DNA viruses replicate in the nucleus (except poxvirus) using the host cell's RNA polymerase and other proteins.
   2. **Positive single-stranded RNA viruses** contain an mRNA genome, which interacts **directly with host ribosomes** for translation of a viral RNA polymerase, which completes replication.

3. **Negative single- and double-stranded RNA viruses** are packaged with a **viral RNA polymerase, which produces positive RNA** for transcription.
4. Thousands of copies of viral proteins are produced.
5. For the retrovirus life cycle, see discussion of human immunodeficiency virus (HIV) (System 8).

E. **Assembly**
1. DNA viruses are assembled in the nucleus (except for the pox viruses).
2. RNA viruses are assembled in the cytoplasm (except for the influenza virus, which is assembled in the nucleus).

F. **Release**
1. Nonenveloped viruses usually **rupture the host cell membrane**, which releases mature particles.
2. Enveloped viruses are released via budding, in which each mature particle becomes surrounded by a portion of the host cell's membrane.

CONCEPTS IN PHARMACOLOGY

QUICK HIT: When infusing a drug, it takes 4.3 half-lives to achieve 95% of the steady-state concentration.

I. Absorption

A. There are many routes of administration (Figure 1-9).

FIGURE 1-9 **Routes of drug administration**
IM, intramuscular; IV, intravenous; SC, subcutaneous. (Adapted from Mycek M, Harvey RA, Champe PC. Lippincott's Illustrated Reviews: Pharmacology. 2nd Ed. Philadelphia, PA: Lippincott-Raven Publishers, 1996:2. Used by permission of Lippincott Williams & Wilkins.)

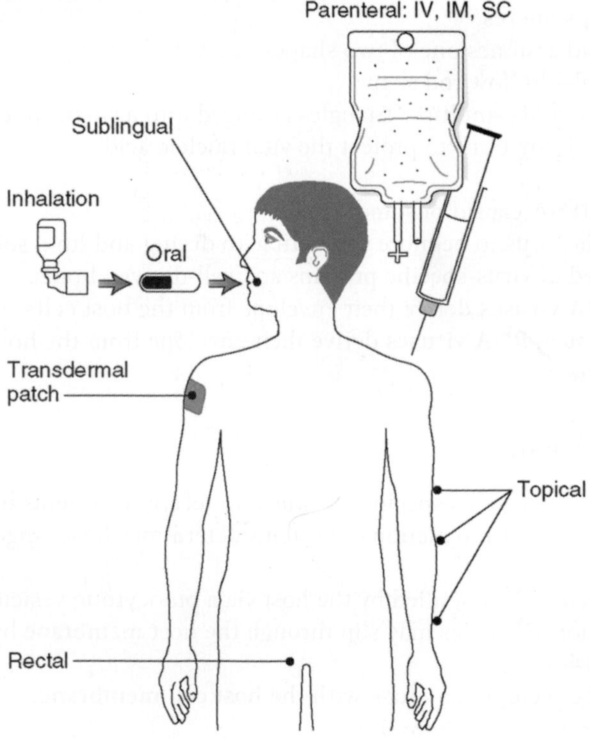

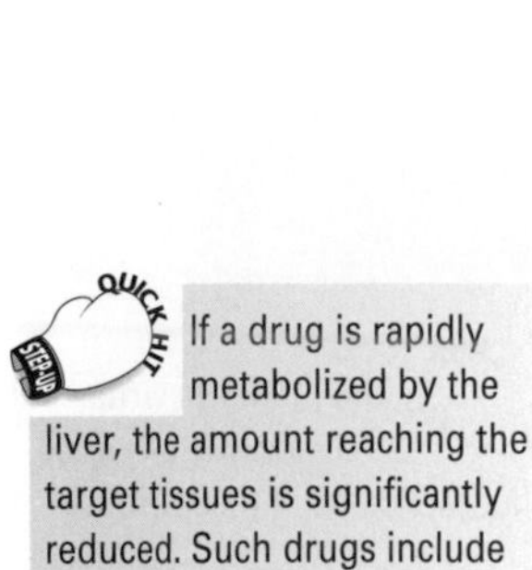
QUICK HIT: If a drug is rapidly metabolized by the liver, the amount reaching the target tissues is significantly reduced. Such drugs include propranolol, lidocaine, verapamil, and meperidine.

B. Oral administration is the most common route.

C. Most drugs are absorbed in the **duodenum**.
1. Drugs enter the portal circulation.
2. They are subject to **first-pass metabolism** by the liver.

D. Other factors that affect absorption are
1. Intestinal pH.
2. Whether taken with food (slows transit allowing for further acid digestion).

3. Whether the drug is a sustained-release preparation.
4. Whether gastrointestinal diseases or malabsorption syndromes are present.

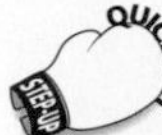

Charged species do not cross the gastrointestinal membrane as readily as uncharged species. Therefore, the percent of drug in the uncharged state determines the rate of absorption

$$pH = pK_a + \log \frac{\text{protonated}}{\text{unprotonated species}}$$

II. Distribution

$V_d = TD/C$

A. V_d, volume of distribution; TD, total drug in body; C, plasma concentration.
B. Distribution occurs more rapidly with high blood flow, high vessel permeability, and a **hydrophobic drug**.
C. Binding to **plasma proteins** (albumin and globulins) accelerates absorption into plasma but slows diffusion into tissues.
D. Many disease states alter distribution:
   1. Edematous states (e.g., cirrhosis, heart failure, nephrotic syndrome) prolong distribution and delay clearance.
   2. Obesity allows for greater accumulation of lipophilic agents within fat cells, increasing distribution and prolonging half-life.
   3. Pregnancy increases intravascular volume, thus increasing V_d.
   4. Hypoalbuminemia allows drugs that are protein-bound to have increased availability because of lack of albumin for binding.

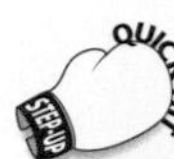

Acidophilic drugs bind to albumin, whereas basophilic drugs bind to globulins. The administration of a drug that binds to sites already occupied by a drug can displace the first drug. This leads to a surge in free drug, which, in turn, leads to increased activity and elimination.

III. Pharmacokinetics

A. The effect an agonist has on its receptors depends on concentration.
B. **Efficacy** is a measure of the maximum effect a drug can produce.
C. **Potency** is a measure of the amount of drug needed to produce a given effect (Figure 1-10).

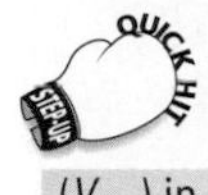

Efficacy is equivalent to maximum velocity (V_{max}) in enzyme kinetics.

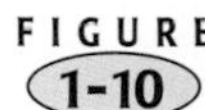

FIGURE 1-10 Dose–response curve
ED_{50}, dose effective in 50% of population

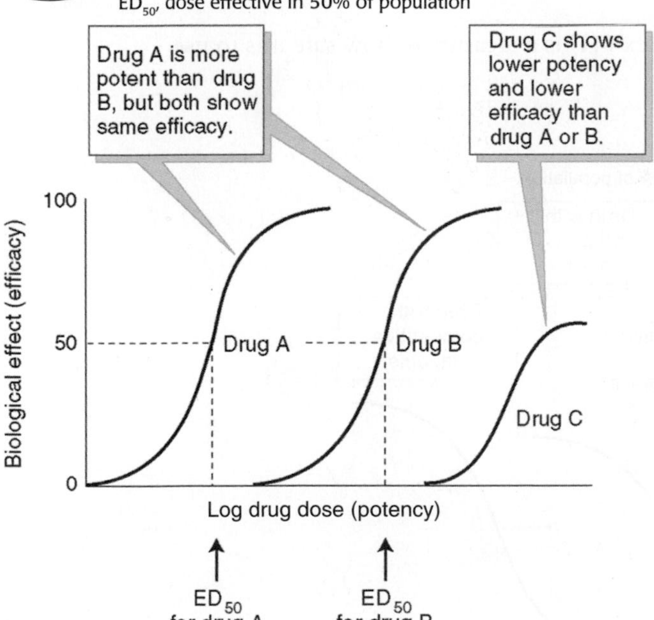

D. Effective dose (ED) and lethal dose (LD)
   1. ED is the dose of the drug that produces the desired effect.
   2. ED_{50} is the dose of the drug that produces the desired effect in 50% of the population.
   3. LD is the dose of the drug that produces death.
   4. LD_{50} is the dose of the drug that produces death in 50% of the population.
   5. Separation of ED and LD determines therapeutic range (Figure 1-11).

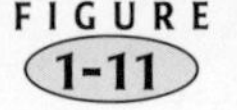

FIGURE 1-11 **Therapeutic range**

ED_{50}, dose effective in 50% of population; LD_{50}, dose that is lethal in 50% of population.

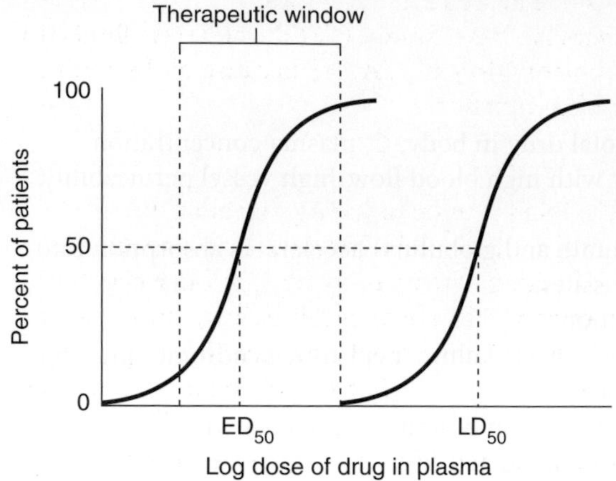

E. Antagonists (Figure 1-12)
   1. **Competitive antagonist**: competes for the same binding site as the agonist or drug
   2. **Noncompetitive antagonist**
      a. Prevents binding of the agonist or drug to the receptor or prevents activation of the receptor by the agonist
      b. Decreases the efficacy of the agonist
   3. **Complete antagonist**: prevents all pharmacologic action(s) of the agonist or drug
   4. **Partial agonist**: binds to the same receptor site as the agonist or drug, but has a lower efficacy

F. A drug's **therapeutic index (TI)** is a measure of how safe it is to use.

FIGURE 1-12 **Drug antagonism**

ED_{50}, dose effective in 50% of population.

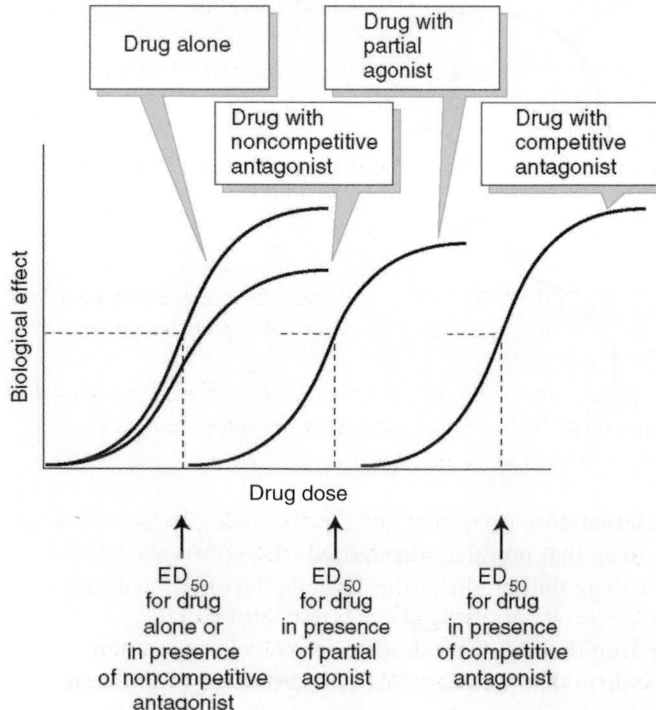

G. Pharmacokinetics is affected by disease states:
   1. Hyperthyroidism increases the heart's sensitivity to catecholamines.
   2. Cirrhosis patients are more sensitive to sedative-hypnotics.
   3. Patients with cirrhosis and congestive heart failure (CHF) will retain fluids if taking nonsteroidal anti-inflammatory drugs (NSAIDs) because of the role of prostaglandins in maintaining renal function.

IV. Metabolism

A. Drugs may be chemically altered, varying activity or aiding excretion.
B. The enzymatic transformation of drugs usually follows one of two kinetics:
   1. **First-order kinetics**: a constant **fraction** of drug is metabolized in a certain unit of time, by far the most common. This arises because drugs have higher affinities for their receptors (K_d) than their metabolizing enzymes (K_m).
   2. **Zero-order kinetics**: a constant **amount** of drug is metabolized in a certain unit of time (e.g., ethanol), rare.
C. The liver is the primary site of metabolism and uses two sets of reactions:
   1. **Phase 1**: drugs are modified or portions are removed (cytochrome P450 oxidation, enzymatic reduction, hydrolysis)
   2. **Phase 2**: conjugation reactions add chemical groupings to the drug (e.g., glucuronidation, sulfate or glutathione conjugation, acetylation, methylation)
D. **Prodrugs** are drugs that are administered in an inactive form and are metabolically activated by the body.
E. Some drugs are metabolized to toxic products (e.g., acetaminophen).

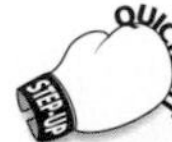

Ethanol, barbiturates, and phenytoin induce cytochrome P450 enzymes, whereas cimetidine and ketoconazole inhibit cytochrome P450 enzymes, increasing and decreasing the metabolism of other drugs, respectively (e.g., warfarin). The macrolide antibiotics (e.g., erythromycin) inhibit cytochrome P450 enzymes and increase the cardiac toxicity of cisapride.

V. Elimination

A. Most drugs are eliminated in the urine or bile.
B. Volatile drugs (e.g., ethanol) can be eliminated through the lungs.
C. **Renal excretion**
   1. Substances with a molecular weight (MW) <5,000 that are free in the plasma are filtered in the glomerulus.
   2. Higher concentrations of a substance within the tubules may favor some reabsorption.
   3. The proximal convoluted tubule (PCT) may actively secrete a drug.
   4. Urine pH, the molecular size, lipid solubility, and negative logarithm of the acid ionization constant (pK_a) of the drug affect renal excretion.
D. Biliary excretion
   1. Hepatocytes actively take up the drug from plasma, store it or metabolize it, and release it into the bile duct.
   2. Some drugs are excreted in feces.
   3. Some drugs are reabsorbed in the terminal ileum (enterohepatic cycling).

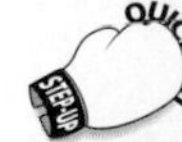

Filtration is dependent on the amount of free drug in the blood, whereas active secretion is dependent on the total plasma concentration (free and bound drug).

VI. Special circumstances

A. **Older patients**
   1. These patients often use multiple prescriptions and over-the-counter medications.
   2. Decreased body size, body water, and serum albumin, along with increased body fat, alter drug distribution.
   3. **Decreased phase 1 reactions**, liver mass, and liver blood flow all slow metabolism.
   4. Decreased kidney mass, renal blood flow, glomerular filtration rate, and tubular function hamper drug excretion.
B. **Pediatric patients**
   1. **Most drugs cross the placenta** to some extent, and their possible effects on the fetus are ranked as category A, B, C, D, and X (A = no risk, X = risk outweighs benefit).
   2. Absorption
      a. High gastric pH and delayed emptying affect enteral absorption.
      b. High surface area-to-volume ratio affects transdermal administration.
      c. Low muscle mass limits intramuscular (IM) administration to the **vastus lateralis** in infancy.

3. Albumin does not reach adult levels until 1 year of age.
4. Both phases of metabolism are deficient to varying degrees until 12 years of age.
5. Specific antibiotics avoided in childhood include **quinolones** (articular cartilage erosion and tendon damage) and **tetracycline** (depression of bone and teeth formation).

C. **Pharmacogenetics**
1. Acetylation of isoniazid
   a. **In patients who are slow acetylators**, there is increased incidence of neuropathy, bladder cancer, and familial Parkinson disease.
   b. **Patients who are rapid acetylators** are the majority of the population.
   c. It also affects metabolism of hydralazine, dapsone, and phenytoin.
2. Succinylcholine sensitivity
   a. Atypical **pseudocholinesterase** does not hydrolyze succinylcholine effectively.
   b. It leads to prolonged paralysis (succinylcholine apnea).
   c. It is **autosomal recessive.**
3. Ethanol metabolism
   a. Aldehyde dehydrogenase shows diminished activity in certain patients (50% of Chinese and Japanese).
   b. Acetaldehyde accumulation leads to facial flushing, headache, nausea, and vomiting.

D. **Toxicology** (Table 1-3)

TABLE 1-3 Toxicology

Poison	Therapy
Acetaminophen	*N*-Acetylcysteine
Aspirin	Alkalinization of urine
Benzodiazepine	Flumazenil
Carbon monoxide	100% oxygen
Cyanide	Sodium nitrite
Digitalis	Digitalis antibody or potassium (if serum potassium level is low)
Ethylene glycol, methanol, isopropyl alcohol	Ethanol
Heavy metals	Calcium EDTA (for lead); dimercaprol (for arsenic, mercury); penicillamine (for copper); deferoxamine (for iron)
Heparin	Protamine sulfate
Opioids	Naloxone
Propranolol	Glucagon
Tricyclic antidepressants	Gastric lavage, alkalinization of serum
Warfarin	Vitamin K

EDTA, ethylenediaminetetraacetic acid.

ANTI-INFECTIVE AGENTS

I. Antibiotics (Table 1-4)

A. **β-Lactam agents**
1. Specific agents
   a. Penicillins (e.g., penicillin G, ampicillin, piperacillin)
   b. Cephalosporins (e.g., cefazolin, ceftriaxone)
   c. Monobactams (e.g., aztreonam)
   d. Carbapenems (e.g., meropenem)

(text continues on page 31)

TABLE 1-4 Antibiotics

Therapeutic Agent (common name, if relevant) [trade name, where appropriate]	Class–Pharmacology and Pharmacokinetics	Indications	Side Effects or Adverse Effects	Contraindications or Precautions to Consider; Notes
Cell wall inhibitors				
Penicillin	**β-Lactam—binds PBP → inhibits transpeptidase** cross-linking of cell wall **→ inhibits bacterial cell wall synthesis → activates autolytic enzymes**; bactericidal	**Gram-positive cocci, Gram-positive rods, Gram-negative cocci, some anaerobes, enterococci**, and **spirochetes**	**Hypersensitivity reactions; platelet aggregation problems; hemolytic anemia; CNS effects, superinfection** (pseudomembrane colitis)	Not penicillinase resistant
Methicillin, nafcillin, dicloxacillin	**β-Lactam, penicillin derivative**—same mechanism as penicillin; distinguished by activity against **penicillinase producing Staphylococcus**; bactericidal	**Staphylococcus infections** (except MRSA)	**Hypersensitivity reactions**; interstitial nephritis (methicillin)	Penicillinase resistant; MRSA is resistant to methicillin because of altered PBP target site
Ampicillin, amoxicillin	**β-Lactam penicillin derivative**—same mechanism as penicillin; distinguished by activity against **Gram-negative rods**; bactericidal	Gram positive cocci, Gram-positive rods, Gram negative cocci, and **Gram negatives rods–extended spectrum**: *E. coli*, Proteus, Salmonella, Shigella, *Haemophilus influenzae*	**Hypersensitivity reaction, pseudomembrane colitis, rash when given to mononucleosis patients**	Not effective against penicillinase resistant Staphylococcus, **combined with clavulanic acid** (pencillinase inhibitor) to enhance spectrum. Amoxicillin is used as oral agent and ampicillin as IV agent
Ticarcillin, carbenicillin, piperacillin	**β-Lactam penicillin derivative**—same mechanism as penicillin; distinguished by activity against **Pseudomonas**; bactericidal	**Extended spectrum**—Pseudomonas, Proteus, Enterobacter species	**Hypersensitivity reactions**, decreased platelet function	Not effective against penicillinase resistant Staphylococcus, **combined with clavulanic acid** (pencillinase inhibitor) to enhance spectrum; **resistant to β-lactamase**; administered IV.
Cephalosporin	**β-Lactam**—same mechanism as penicillin, **from first generation to third generation**: a. **Gram-positive** coverage **decreases** b. **Gram-negative** coverage **increases** c. **CNS penetration increases** d. β-lactamase **resistance increases**; bactericidal	**First generation: Gram-positive cocci and PEcK** (*Proteus mirabilis, E. coli*, and Klebsiella) **Second generation:** same as first generation + **HENPEcK** (*H. flu*, Enterobacter, Neisseria), **Third generation: cephalosporins are used for meningitis, *Klebsiella*, Lyme disease, and Gram-negative bacteria**	**Hypersensitivity reaction; pain at injection site; nephrotoxicity; intolerance to alcohol** (cefamandole, cefotetan, moxalactam, cefoperazone), **hypothrombinemia** (cefamandole, cefoperazone, moxalactam due to vitamin K inhibition); **thrombophlebitis; positive Coombs test**	**First generation**: cefazolin, cephalexin; **second generation**: cefaclor, cefoxitin, cefuroxime; **third generation**: ceftriaxone, cefoperazone, ceftazidime; **fourth generation**: cefepime **Pseudomonas coverage**: ceftazidime, cefoperazone, cefepime; **cross-hypersensitivity with penicillins occurs in 5% to 10% of patients**

(continued)

TABLE 1-4 Antibiotics *(Continued)*

Therapeutic Agent (common name, if relevant) [trade name, where appropriate]	Class–Pharmacology and Pharmacokinetics	Indications	Side Effects or Adverse Effects	Contraindications or Precautions to Consider; Notes
Aztreonam [Azactam]	**Monocyclic β-lactam** —same mechanism as penicillin (binds to PBP3); bactericidal	**Gram-negative bacteria esp. Pseudomonas, Klebsiella, Serratia, and Enterobacteriaceae. No activity against Gram-positives or anaerobes.**	Skin rash, GI distress (nausea, vomiting)	**Does not cross-react with penicillin; synergistic with aminoglycosides;** can be used in patients with **penicillin allergies** and **renal insufficiency who cannot take aminoglycosides**
Imipenem/ cilastin	**Carbapenem**—same mechanism as penicillin; bactericidal	**Broad spectrum—Gram-positive cocci** (MSSA and Streptococcus), **Gram-negative rods** (Pseudomonas and Enterobacter species), **anaerobes**, dormant bacteria	Hypersensitivity reaction, **seizure**, confusion state, superinfection (pseudomembrane colitis)	Significant side effects limit use to when other drugs have failed or life-threatening infections; always administered with cilastin (inhibits renal dihydropeptidase) to reduce inactivation in renal tubules
Meropenem	**Carbapenem**—same mechanism as penicillin; bactericidal	**Broad spectrum—Gram-positive cocci** (MSSA and Streptococcus), **Gram-negative rods** (Pseudomonas and Enterobacter species), **anaerobes**, dormant bacteria	Reduced risk of seizure compared to imipenem.	Stable to dihydropeptidase I, unlike imipenem
Vancomycin	**Cell wall inhibitor**—binds to D-alanyl-D-alanine portion of cell wall → inhibits cell wall glycopeptide polymerization → stops bacterial cell wall synthesis; bactericidal	**Serious infections by Gram-positive bacteria: Streptococcus, Staphylococcus, Pneumococcus, and some anaerobes (especially *C. difficile*)**	**Ototoxicity, nephrotoxicity, thrombophlebitis, diffuse flushing—"red man syndrome"; caused by histamine release**	Can prevent red man syndrome by pretreatment with antihistamines and slow infusion; resistance occurs when bacteria change amino acid in cell wall to *D*-ala *D*-lac
Protein synthesis inhibitors				
Streptomycin, gentamicin, tobramycin, amikacin, spectinomycin	**Aminoglycosides—irreversibly bind 30S ribosome** subunits; **bacteriostatic** at low concentration; **bactericidal** at high concentration	**Broad-spectrum**: Gram-negative rods; good for **bone** and **eye** infections; Proteus, Pseudomonas, Enterobacter, Klebsiella, *E. coli*	**Ototoxicity; renal toxicity; neuromuscular blockade**; nausea; vomiting; vertigo; allergic skin rash; superinfections	
Tetracycline, doxycycline, demeclocycline, minocycline	**Tetracyclines—bind 30S ribosome subunits** → prevent attachment of tRNA; bacteriostatic	**Broad-spectrum including atypical pathogens: Chlamydia, Rickettsia, and *Mycoplasma pneumoniae, Vibrio cholerae, Ureaplasma urealyticum,* Tularemia, *H. pylori, Borrelia burgdorferi* (Lyme disease), Rickettsia**	**Liver toxicity; GI distress; depression of bone/teeth development** (less with doxycyline); **photosensitivity** (less with doxycyline); **superinfections owing to broad-spectrum; Fanconi syndrome**	**Contraindicated in pregnancy and children; divalent cations inhibit gut absorption, therefore cannot be taken with milk, antacids, or iron-containing preparations. Tetracycline is renally eliminated; Doxycyline is fecally eliminated and must not be taken by patients with renal insufficiency**

Erythromycin [E-Mycin], clarithromycin, azithromycin	**Macrolide**—binds to the 23S RNA of the 50S ribosome subunits → block translocation → prevents protein synthesis; bacterostatic	**First choice for cell wall-deficient bugs: Mycoplasma, Rickettsia, Chlamydia, Legionella; *Corynebacterium diphtheria;*** Gram-positive cocci (Streptococcus)	GI discomfort, **acute cholestatic hepatitis**, **eosinophilia**, **skin rashes**. Increases concentration of **oral anticoagulants** and theophyllines	Can be used in patients with **streptococcal infections** and **penicillin allergies**
Chloramphenicol [Chloromycetin]	**Protein synthesis inhibitor—inhibits 50S peptidyltransferase activity; bacteriostatic**, but bactericidal versus *H. influenzae* and *Neisseria meningitidis*	Menigitis (*H. influenza, N. meningitidis, S. pneumoniae*); typhoid fever; Salmonella; rickettsia (Rocky Mountain spotted fever in children); bacteroides	**Fatal aplastic anemia; bone marrow suppression; gray baby syndrome** (cyanosis, vomiting, green stools, vasomotor collapse due to insufficient glucuronidase in neonatal liver)	Interacts with phenytoin, warfarin, or coumadin; inhibits cytochrome P450; used to treat serious infections after other antibiotics have failed given side effects
Clindamycin [Cleocin]	**Protein synthesis inhibitor—binds to 50S subunits** → blocks peptide bond formation; bacteriostatic or bactericidal depending on concentration, site, and organism	**Gram-positive bacteria (Streptococcus, Pneumococcus, Staphylococcus); Treat anaerobic** infections (*Bacteroides fragilis, Clostridium perfringens*)	Severe diarrhea; **potentially fatal pseudomembranous colitis caused by *C. difficile***	
DNA synthesis inhibitors				
Sulfamethoxazole, sulfisoxazole, sulfadiazine	**Sulfonamide—competitive inhibitor of dihydropteroate synthetase (blocks folic acid synthesis)**; bacteriostatic	**Broad-spectrum; Gram-positive UTI; Chlamydia infection of genital tract and eye; treatment of nocardiosis**	**Form crystals in kidney and bladder causing damage; hypersensitivity reaction; photosensitivity; kernicterus (in infants); hemolysis (in G6PD deficiency)**	Displaces other drugs such as warfarin from albumin
Trimethoprim [Proloprim, Trimpex]	**Antibiotic—competitive inhibition of dihydrofolate reductase** (blocks folic acid synthesis); bacteriostatic	**Gram-negative UTI; combined with sulfonamides to treat UTI, otitis media, chronic bronchitis, shigellosis, Salmonella, and PCP**	Megaloblastic anemia, leukopenia, granulocytopenia	Supplementation with folic acid may help pancytopenia
Ciprofloxacin [Cipro], norfloxacin, ofloxacin, Levofloxacin [Levaquin], Moxifloxacin	**Quinolone antibiotic—Inhibits DNA gyrase** (topoisomerase II) and **topoisomerase IV** → blocks DNA synthesis; bactericidal	**Gram-negative infections (esp. UTI and bone): Pseudomonas, Enterobacteriaceae, Neisseria; Gram-positive infections** (Staphylococcus, Streptococcus); **intracellular: Legionella**	**GI disturbances; headache; dizziness; phototoxicity; cartilage damage (children, fetus); tendonitis** and **tendon rupture (adults); myalgias (children)**	**May elevate theophylline to toxic levels causing seizure**; **contraindicated in pregnant women**

(continued)

TABLE 1-4 Antibiotics *(Continued)*

Therapeutic Agent (common name, if relevant) [trade name, where appropriate]	Class–Pharmacology and Pharmacokinetics	Indications	Side Effects or Adverse Effects	Contraindications or Precautions to Consider; Notes
Metronidazole [Flagyl]	**Antibiotic, Antiprotozoal**—penetrates cell membrane and gives off nitro moiety → forms toxic metabolites → react and damage DNA; bactericidal	***Bacteroides fragilis*** (esp. for endocarditis and CNS); **Pseudomembrane colitis** (*C. difficile*); **amebiasis; giardiasis; trichomoniasis, bacterial vaginosis** (*Gardnerella vaginalis*), **peptic ulcer disease** (part of *H. pylori* triple therapy)	Nausea; vomiting; **disulfiram-like reaction to alcohol**; metallic taste; paresthesia; stomatitis; carcinogenic and mutagenic	**Contraindicated in pregnancy**
Cell membrane inhibitor				
Polymyxins [Aerosporin]	**Antibiotic—bind to cell membranes** → disrupt osmotic properties; bactericidal	**Gram-negative bacteria: Pseudomonas and coliforms; topical only; intrathecal for Pseudomonas meningitis**	**Neurotoxic; nephrotoxic** (acute renal tubular necrosis)	

MSSA, methicillin sensitive *Staphylococcus aureus*; MRSA, methicillin resistant *Staphylococcus aureus*, PBP, penicillin-binding protein.

2. Mechanism of action: bactericidal
   a. **Inhibit cell wall synthesis**
   b. Act on penicillin-binding proteins (PBPs) in bacterial cell walls
   c. Require active cell division for bactericidal effect
3. Spectrum of action varies for each particular drug
   a. Gram-positive and Gram-negative bacteria
   b. Anaerobes and spirochetes
4. Side effects/adverse reactions
   a. **Allergic reactions** (especially a rash with penicillins)
   b. Platelet aggregation dysfunction
   c. Thrombophlebitis (cephalosporins)
   d. Direct central nervous system (CNS) toxicity
   e. Superinfections including *Clostridium difficile* and yeasts such as *Candida* spp.
5. Mechanisms of resistance
   a. Inactivation by **β-lactamase enzymes**
   b. Failure to reach PBP targets
   c. Poor binding to PBPs

B. **Aminoglycosides** (e.g., gentamicin, tobramycin, neomycin)
1. Mechanism of action: bactericidal
   a. Bind to the **30S ribosomal subunits of bacteria**
   b. Subsequently interfere with protein synthesis
2. Spectrum of action
   a. Broad-spectrum activity against Gram-negative bacilli
   b. Some activity against Gram-positive bacteria
   c. No anaerobic activity
3. Side effects/adverse reactions
   a. Ototoxicity
   b. Nephrotoxicity
4. Mechanisms of resistance
   a. Enzymatic modification of the aminoglycoside
   b. Altered ribosome binding sites
   c. Altered antibiotic uptake

C. **Tetracyclines** (e.g., tetracycline, demeclocycline, doxycycline)
1. Mechanism of action: **bacteriostatic**
   a. Reversibly bind to the 30S ribosomal subunit
   b. Prevent the addition of new amino acids onto growing peptide chain
2. Spectrum of action: broad-spectrum activity
   a. Gram-positive and Gram-negative bacteria, anaerobes, spirochetes, mycoplasma, rickettsia, and chlamydia
   b. Some protozoa
3. Side effects/adverse reactions
   a. Teeth discoloration
   b. **Depression of skeletal growth**
   c. Gastrointestinal distress
   d. **Hepatotoxicity**
   e. Photosensitivity
4. Mechanisms of resistance
   a. Reduction of tetracycline influx
   b. Active tetracycline export from within the bacterial cell

D. **Chloramphenicol**
1. Mechanism of action: usually bacteriostatic but bactericidal in some organisms
   a. Binds to the 50S ribosomal subunit
   b. Prevents the addition of new amino acids onto growing peptide chain
2. Spectrum of action
   a. Gram-positive and Gram-negative bacteria
   b. Spirochetes, rickettsia, chlamydia, and mycoplasma

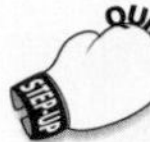

"-floxacin" suffix = quinolone derivative. Ciproflaxacin, norfloxacin, ofloxacin = 2nd generation; Levofloxacin = 3rd generation; Moxifloxacin = 4th generation.

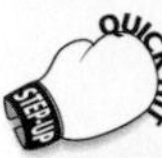

β-Lactam inhibitors, which have weak bactericidal activity but greatly inhibit β-lactamase, are used in combination with some penicillins to enhance their effectiveness (e.g., amoxicillin–clavulanate, ampicillin–sulbactam, piperacillin–tazobactam).

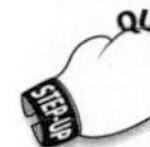

Tetracyclines are contraindicated in pregnancy and in children because of their effect on the teeth and bones.

Remember the following drugs as **bacteriostatic**: tetracyclines, erythromycin, clindamycin, chloramphenicol, sulfonamides, trimethoprim. Remember these drugs as **bactericidal**: penicillin, cephalosporin, vancomycin, aminoglycosides, fluroquinolones, metronidazole, polymyxin.

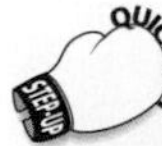

Avoid the following drugs in pregnancy: **Aminoglycosides** (ototoxicity), **Tetracyclines** (tooth discoloration and decreased bone growth), **Erythromycin** (acute cholestatic hepatitis in mother), **Clarithromycin** (embryotoxic), **Chloramphenicol** (gray baby syndrome), **Sulfonamides** (kernicterus), **Fluroquinolones** (cartilage damage), **Metronidazoles** (mutations), **Ribavirin** (teratogenic), **Griseofulvin** (teratogenic).

3. Side effects/adverse reactions: chloramphenicol is rarely a first choice because of its adverse reactions
   a. **Aplastic anemia**
   b. Reversible bone marrow depression
   c. **Gray baby syndrome**: abdominal distention, vomiting, flaccidity, cyanosis, circulatory collapse, and death
4. Mechanisms of resistance
   a. Impermeability of bacteria to drug
   b. Production of enzymes that inactivate the antibiotic

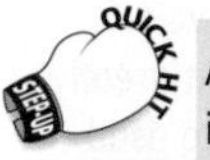

Although clindamycin is typically associated with pseudomembranous colitis (*C. difficile* infection), cephalosporins cause more cases of pseudomembranous colitis because of their greater use.

E. **Macrolides** (e.g., erythromycin, azithromycin, clarithromycin) and lincosamides (e.g., clindamycin)
1. Mechanism of action: bactericidal activity is relative to dose, and these agents are generally considered bacteriostatic.
   a. Bind to the bacterial 50S ribosomal subunit
   b. Consequently inhibit RNA-dependent protein synthesis
2. Spectrum of action: broad-spectrum activity
   a. Gram-positive and Gram-negative bacteria. **Clindamycin is especially effective against anaerobes (chiefly *Bacteroides fragilis*).**
   b. Treponemes, mycoplasma, chlamydia, and rickettsia. Erythromycin is a good choice for cell wall–deficient organisms such as *Mycoplasma, Rickettsia, Chlamydia*, and *Legionella.*
3. Side effects/adverse reactions
   a. Gastrointestinal distress
   b. Allergic reactions
   c. Superinfections
      - Candida with erythromycin
      - *C. difficile* (pseudomembranous colitis) with clindamycin
4. Mechanisms of resistance
   a. Decreased permeability into bacterial cells
   b. Active efflux out of cells
   c. Alteration in a 50S ribosomal protein
   d. Enzymatic inactivation of antibiotic

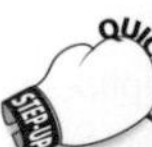

The **sulfa-containing drugs** are sulfonamides, sulfasalazine, sulfonylureas, thiazide diuretics, and furosemide. These drugs should not be given in patients with sulfa drug allergies.

F. **Sulfonamides** (e.g., sulfamethoxazole) and trimethoprim
1. Mechanism of action: The **bacteriostatic** action is potentiated when sulfonamides and trimethoprim are used together.
   a. Competitively inhibits dihydrofolate reductase (trimethoprim)
   b. Competitively inhibits dihydropteroate synthetase (sulfonamides)
   c. **Blocks folic acid synthesis** in this way
2. Spectrum of action: broad-spectrum activity
   a. Gram-positive and Gram-negative bacteria, *Chlamydia*
   b. *Actinomyces, Plasmodium, Toxoplasma*

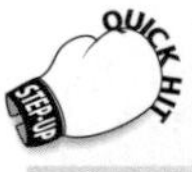

Sulfonamide–trimethoprim is used primarily for urinary tract infections.

3. Side effects/adverse reactions
   a. Gastrointestinal distress
   b. Acute hemolytic anemia, aplastic anemia, agranulocytosis, and thrombocytopenia in individuals with glucose-6-phosphate dehydrogenase (G-6-PD) deficiency
   c. Hypersensitivity reactions, including erythema multiforme (Stevens–Johnson syndrome)
4. Mechanisms of resistance
   a. Bacterial mutation resulting in microbial overproduction of folic acid precursors
   b. Structural change in bacterial enzymes, with lowered affinity for sulfonamides and trimethoprim
   c. Decreased bacterial cell permeability

Quinolones are a good choice for urinary tract infections; the sexually transmitted diseases, gonorrhea and chlamydia; and respiratory and gastrointestinal infections.

G. **Quinolones** (e.g., ciprofloxacin)
1. Mechanism of action: bactericidal
   a. **Inhibit DNA gyrase** and DNA topoisomerase
   b. Block DNA synthesis in this way

2. Spectrum of action: aerobic Gram-negative bacilli and Gram-negative cocci
3. Side effects/adverse reactions
   a. Gastrointestinal distress
   b. Headache, dizziness
   c. Phototoxicity
   d. **Damages developing cartilage and tendons (contraindicated in children and pregnancy)**
   e. Some prolong QT_c interval
4. Mechanisms of resistance
   a. Mutation of bacterial enzymes
   b. Decreased permeability of bacterial wall to antibiotic

H. **Other agents**: vancomycin, teicoplanin, and the streptogramins quinupristin/dalfopristin
1. Mechanism of action
   a. Vancomycin and teicoplanin—**inhibit cell wall assembly**
   b. Quinupristin/dalfopristin—can be bactericidal or bacteriostatic depending on the organism; bind to the 50S bacterial ribosomal subunit
2. Spectrum of action
   a. Vancomycin and teicoplanin: serious Gram-positive infections and some anaerobic infections
   b. Quinupristin/dalfopristin: serious infections caused by Staphylococcus or Enterococcus
3. Side effects/adverse reactions
   a. Vancomycin and teicoplanin
      (1) **Red man syndrome** (flushing of the face, neck, and torso)
      (2) Fever, chills, and phlebitis at injection site
   b. Quinupristin/dalfopristin
      (1) Gastrointestinal distress
      (2) Pain at injection site
      (3) Arthralgia, muscle weakness
4. Mechanisms of resistance
   a. Vancomycin and teicoplanin: gene-mediated alteration in cell wall peptidoglycans
   b. Quinupristin/dalfopristin
      (1) Drug-modifying enzymes
      (2) Efflux of antibiotic out of bacterial cell

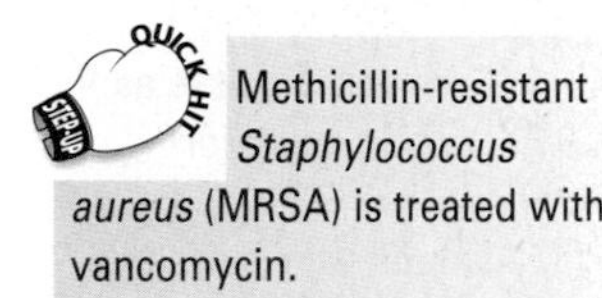

QUICK HIT: Methicillin-resistant *Staphylococcus aureus* (MRSA) is treated with vancomycin.

II. Antimycobacterial and antifungal agents

A. **Antimycobacterial agents**: drugs active against *Mycobacterium tuberculosis* (Table 1-5)
1. **First-line agents**: isoniazid, rifampin, pyrazinamide, ethambutol, and streptomycin
2. Bactericidal, except for ethambutol
3. Initial therapy: three first-line agents for **6 to 9 months**

B. **Antifungal agents** (Table 1-6)
1. **Amphotericin B**
   a. Disrupts fungal membrane, leading to increased permeability
   b. Used for serious systemic fungal infections
   c. **Nephrotoxic**
2. **Triazoles** (e.g., fluconazole)
   a. **Disrupt synthesis of ergosterol**, which is necessary for fungal membranes
   b. Fluconazole is used for candida infections and cryptococcal meningitis

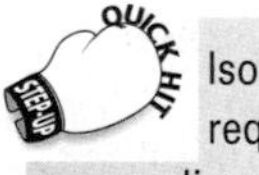

QUICK HIT: Isoniazid therapy requires vitamin B_6 as an adjunct.

MNEMONIC

To remember the **mechanism of action of griseofulvin** think **"greasy tubes."**

MNEMONIC

To remember the **side effects of amphotericin B** think **"shake and bake"**: convulsions and fever.

III. Antiviral agents (Table 1-7)

A. **Antiretrovirals** (see System 8)
1. Reverse transcriptase inhibitors (e.g., zidovudine [azidothymidine; AZT], didanosine [ddI], nevirapine)
   a. Act as either nucleoside/nucleotide analogs or inhibit the reverse transcriptase enzyme itself
   b. **Prevent creation of DNA copy of viral RNA**

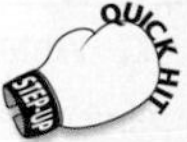

QUICK HIT: Both acyclovir and ganciclovir are effective against herpes virus, but ganciclovir is also effective against cytomegalovirus.

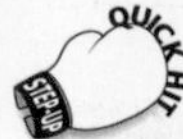

Isoniazid, rifampin, ethambutol, and **pyrazinamide** are used in the treatment of **tuberculosis. Azithromycin, rifampin, ethambutol,** and **streptomycin** are used in the treatment of **MAC. Dapsone, rifampin,** and **clofazimine** are used in the treatment of **leprosy.**

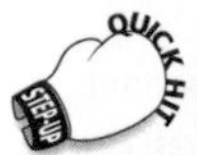

Isoniazid is used as a solo agent for *M. tuberculosis* (TB) prophylaxis. **Azithromycin** is used as a solo agent for *M. avium intracellulare* (MAC) prophylaxis.

2. Protease inhibitors (e.g., saquinavir, indinavir)
   a. **Block the cleavage of viral polyproteins**
   b. Result in the production of immature, defective viral particles

B. **Acyclovir and ganciclovir**
   1. Inhibit viral DNA polymerase, which blocks viral DNA synthesis
   2. **Suppress symptoms of herpes simplex virus infections** but **are not a cure**

C. **Amantadine and rimantadine**
   1. Inhibit the replication of **influenza A**
   2. Can be used prophylactically and therapeutically

D. **Ribavirin**
   1. Alters viral messenger RNA formation
   2. Used to treat **respiratory syncytial virus and pneumonia in children**

E. **Interferons (IFNs)**
   1. Most cells produce IFN-α and IFN-β in response to viral infection.
   2. IFN-γ mediates the inflammatory response and has less antiviral action.
   3. IFNs are not directly antiviral but stimulate cellular mechanisms of viral resistance.
   4. IFNs also may cause some of the symptoms and tissue damage associated with viral infections.
   5. Used for hepatitis B, hepatitis C, and some types of cancer.

TABLE 1-5 Antimycobacterial

Therapeutic Agent (common name, if relevant) [trade name, where appropriate]	Class–Pharmacology and Pharmacokinetics	Indications	Side or Adverse Effects	Contraindications or Precautions to Consider; Notes
Isoniazid [INH, Nydrazid]	**Antibiotic**—inhibits synthesis of mycolic acids	**Mycobacterium treatment (*M. tuberculosis* and *M. kansasii*); *M. tuberculosis* prophylaxis**	**Peripheral and CNS effects as a result of pyridoxine deficiency; liver damage; hemolytic anemia in G-6-PD deficiency; SLE-like syndrome**	Pyridoxine (vitamin B_6) can prevent neurotoxicity
Rifampin [Rifadin]	**Antibiotic—inhibits DNA-dependent RNA polymerase**	**Mycobacterium; reduces resistance to dapsone when used in treatment of leprosy; meningococcal prophylaxis in contacts of children with *H. influenza* type b**	**Turns body fluid orange in color; liver damage**	**Interferes with birth control pills by increasing estrogen metabolism; induces cytochrome P450**
Ethambutol [Myambutol]	Antibiotic—unknown mechanism	Mycobacterium	**Optic neuropathy (red-green color blindness)**; tolerance develops	
Streptomycin	**Antibiotic—aminoglycoside; binds 30S ribosome subunits; bacteriostatic at low concentration; bactericidal at high**	**Tuberculosis and other mycobacteria**		
Pyrazinamide	Antibiotic-postulated mechanism involves inhibition of enzyme pyrazinamidase → inhibition of fatty acid synthesis	Mycobacterium	Impairs liver function	

MAC, *Mycobacterium avium intracellulare.*

TABLE 1-6 Antifungals

Therapeutic Agent (common name, if relevant) [trade name, where appropriate]	Class–Pharmacology and Pharmacokinetics	Indications	Side or Adverse Effects	Contraindications or Precautions to Consider; Notes
Amphotericin B [Fungizone]	**Antifungal—binds to cell membrane sterols** (esp. ergosterol); forms pores in membrane; fungicidal	**Wide spectrum fungal coverage: Candida, Histoplasma, Cryptococcus, Blastomyces, Aspergillus, Coccidioides, *Sporothrix, Mucor***	**Impairment of renal function; hypersensitivity; flushing; fever; chills;** hypotension; **convulsions**; thrombophlebitis; anemia; arrythmias	**Does not enter CNS;** poor GI absorption so given IV; administered intrathecal for meningitis
Nystatin [Mycostatin]	Antifungal—binds to cell membrane sterols (esp. ergosterol) → disrupting fungal membranes; fungicidal	**Mucosal candida** infections (skin, vaginal, GI)	Few	Used topically or as mouth rinse; too toxic for systemic use
Ketoconazole [Nizoral]	**Antifungal—inhibits ergosterol synthesis, preventing cell membrane formation; inhibits adrenal and gonadal steroid synthesis**	**Chronic mucocutaneous candidiasis; blastomycosis; histoplasmosis; coccidioidomycosis; hypercortisolism; prostate carcinoma**	**GI irritation; gynecomastia; thrombocytopenia; hepatotoxic; rash; fever, chills**	**Inhibits cytochrome P450**
Fluconazole [Diflucan]	**Antifungal—inhibits ergosterol synthesis, preventing cell membrane formation**	**Cryptococcal meningitis; oral candidiasis in AIDS**	**Abdominal pain; nausea**	
Itraconazole [Sporanox]	**Antifungal—inhibits ergosterol synthesis,** preventing cell membrane formation	**Oral for fungal infections (esp. dermatophytoses and onychomycosis)**	**GI disturbances; hepatotoxicity**	
Miconazole [Monistat IV], clotrimazole [Lotrimin, Mycelex]	Antifungal—inhibits ergosterol synthesis, preventing cell membrane formation	**Topical use against yeasts, dermatophytes, ringworm, fungi, mold, and oral candidiasis in AIDS**	Burning, itching, and redness when used topically; thrombophlebitis; nausea; vomiting; anaphylaxis when used IV	
Flucytosine [Ancobon]	Antifungal—competitive inhibitor of thymidylate synthetase; impairs DNA synthesis	Candida; Cryptococcus; Aspergillus	Nausea; vomiting; diarrhea; rash; bone marrow and liver toxicity; enterocolitis	Imported in the fungus via permease
Caspofungin	Inhibits cell wall synthesis	Invasive aspergillosis or Candida	GI irritation, flushing	Administered IV
Terbinafine [Lamisil]	Antifungal—inhibits squalene-2,3-epoxidase	Orally for onychomycosis; topically for dermatophytes	Hepatotoxicity	
Griseofulvin [Fulvicin, Grifulvin, Grisactin]	**Antifungal—inhibits cell mitosis by disrupting mitotic spindles; binds to tubulin**	**Dermatophytes (esp. *Trichophyton rubrum*)**	**Headache; mental confusion; rash; GI irritation; hepatotoxic; photosensitivity; carcinogenic; teratogenic**	Increases **cytochrome P450** and warfarin metabolism

TABLE 1-7 Antivirals

Therapeutic Agent (common name, if relevant) [trade name, where appropriate]	Class–Pharmacology and Pharmacokinetics	Indications	Side or Adverse Effects	Contraindications or Precautions to Consider; Notes
Amantadine [Symmetrel]	**Antiviral—antiparkinsonian;** inhibits fusion of lysosomes; inhibits viral penetration and uncoating; increases release of endogenous dopamine	**Influenza A** (prophylaxis and treatment); **Parkinson disease**	**CNS effects** (ataxia, dizziness, slurred speech, nervousness, seizure); **anticholinergic;** orthostatic hypotension; **livedo reticularis** (skin rash)	Mechanism of viral resistance is mutated M2 protein
Zanamivir, oseltamivir [Tamiflu]	**Antiviral—Inhibits neuraminidase →** decreases release of progeny viruses	**Influenza A and B treatment and prophylaxis**		Begin within 2 days of onset of flu symptoms to decrease duration and intensity of symptoms
Ribavirin	**Antiviral—guanosine analog;** inhibits IMP dehydrogenase → decreases synthesis of guanine nucleotides	**RSV in children; hepatitis C when given with interferon**	**Hemolytic anemia, teratogen**	
Acyclovir [Zovirax]	**Antiviral—guanosine analog;** monophosphorylated by **viral thymidine kinase**; triphosphorylated form **inhibits viral DNA polymerase**	**HSV, VZV, EBV, CMV** (at high doses); **HSV-induced mucocutaneous, genital lesions**, and **encephalitis**	**Side effects depend on route of administration: IV—neurotoxicity, renal problems,** tremor **Oral—diarrhea,** headache **Topical—local skin irritation**	**Resistant forms lack thymidine kinase**
Valacyclovir [Valtrex]	**Antiviral—guanosine analog;** inhibits DNA polymerase	**HSV, VZV, EBV, and CMV at high doses**	**GI disturbances; CNS and renal problems; headache; tremor; rash**	**Longer lasting than acyclovir**
Ganciclovir [Cytovene]	**Antiviral—guanosine analog;** inhibits viral DNA polymerase	**CMV (esp. CMV retinitis in AIDS)**	**Bone marrow suppression** (leukopenia, neutropenia, thrombocytopenia), **renal impairment, seizures**	**Resistance from lack of thymidine kinase or mutation of viral DNA polymerase. More toxic than acyclovir**
Foscarnet [Foscavir]	**Antiviral**—nonnucleoside inhibitor of DNA polymerase	**CMV retinitis (resistant to ganciclovir), HSV (resistant to acyclovir)**	Hypocalcemia; CNS, cardiac, and **renal toxicity**; anemia	**Does not require activation by viral kinase**
Interferon α-2a (Roferon A), α-2b (Intron A), and α-n3 (Alferon-N)	**Antiviral—glycoproteins → block viral RNA, DNA, and protein synthesis**	**Genital warts; chronic hepatitis B and C; AIDS-related Kaposi sarcoma; laryngeal papillomatosis; hairy cell leukemia**	**Flulike symptoms; neutropenia**	
Interferon β	**Antiviral—glycoproteins → block viral RNA, DNA, and protein synthesis**	**Multiple sclerosis**	**Flulike symptoms; neutropenia**	
Interferon γ	**Antiviral—glycoproteins → block viral RNA, DNA, and protein synthesis**	**NADPH oxidase deficiency**	**Flulike symptoms; neutropenia**	

IMP, Inosine-5'-monophosphate.

ENZYME KINETICS

I. Enzymes

A. An enzyme is a protein or nucleic acid molecule that decreases the **energy of activation for a reaction** (Figure 1-13).
B. Enzymes interact specifically with substrates at an enzyme active site.
C. By lowering the energy of activation, enzymes increase the rate of reaction.
D. Enzymes **do not alter the equilibrium** of substrates and products, which is concentration dependent or the free energy released from the reaction.
E. Enzymatic reactions generally require cofactors, such as metals, derivatives of vitamins, or small organic molecules. The vitamins and small organic molecules are often referred to as coenzymes.

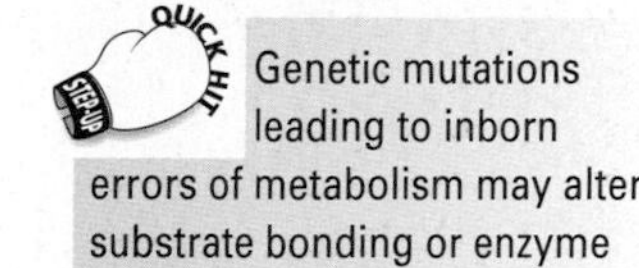

Genetic mutations leading to inborn errors of metabolism may alter substrate bonding or enzyme activity on a substrate.

FIGURE 1-13 Enzyme effect on a chemical reaction

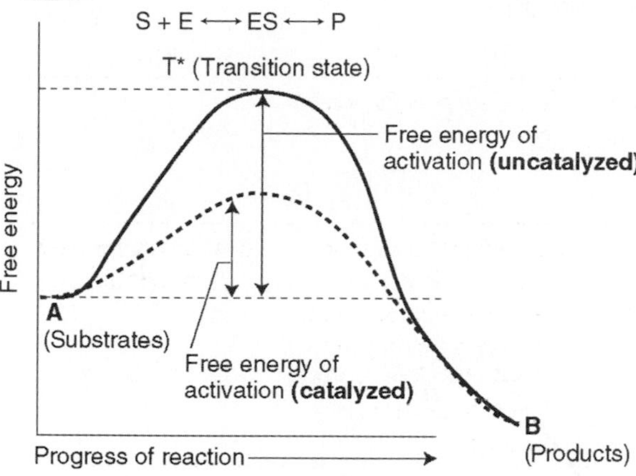

II. Kinetics

A. **Velocity** (V) is the rate of reaction and is dependent on enzyme concentration, substrate concentration, temperature, and pH.
   1. Enzyme concentration: increased enzyme concentration leads to faster rate of reaction.
   2. Substrate concentration: increased concentration leads to increased rate of reaction, until a maximum is reached when all enzyme receptor sites are saturated.
   3. Temperature: increased temperature leads to increased rate of reaction up to a maximum, after which enzymes denature.
   4. pH: velocity of a reaction is maximum at its optimal pH. A pH that is either too high or too low leads to a slower reaction or may denature the enzyme.

B. Michaelis–Menten equation
   1. Enzymatically catalyzed reactions can be characterized by the Michaelis–Menten equation:

      $V = V_m \times [S]/(K_m + [S])$

      where V is the velocity of the reaction.

      V_m is the maximum velocity of the reaction.
      $[S]$ is the substrate concentration.
      K_m is the Michaelis constant (the substrate concentration at which velocity is one-half of the maximum velocity of a given reaction; $V = V_m/2$)
   2. Effect of substrate concentration on reaction velocity (Figure 1-14)

C. Lineweaver–Burk plots (Figure 1-15)
   1. A Lineweaver–Burk plot is a linear representation of the Michaelis–Menten equation, which allows for easier interpretation of the maximum velocity of an equation.

FIGURE 1-14 **Effect of substrate concentration on reaction velocity**

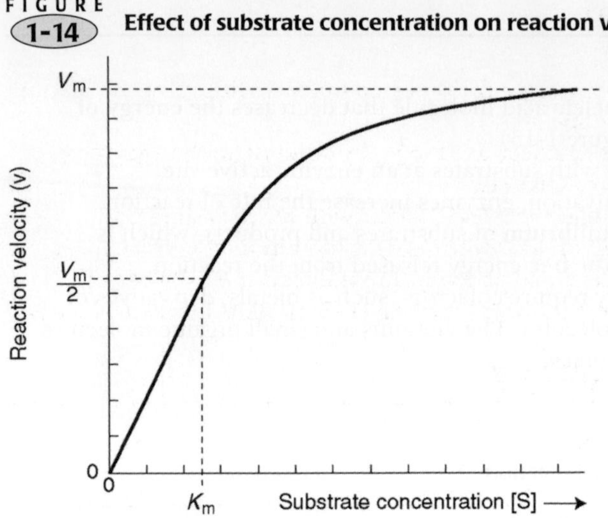

V_m = Maximum velocity
V = Velocity
K_m = Michaelis constant, where $V = 1/2\ V_m$

FIGURE 1-15 **Lineweaver–Burk plot**

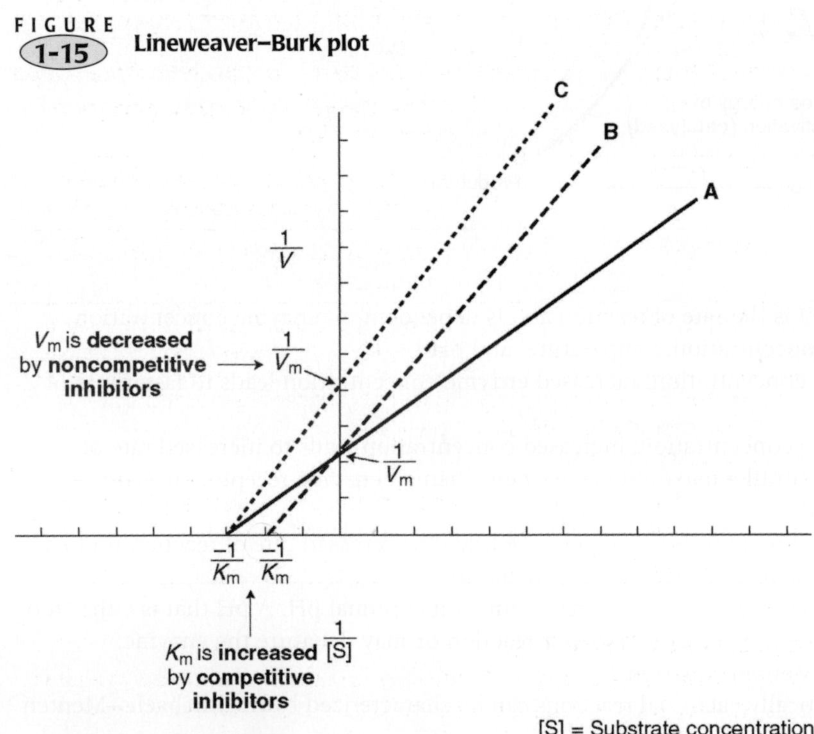

A = No inhibitor
B = Competitive inhibitor
C = Noncompetitive inhibitor

[S] = Substrate concentration
V = Reaction velocity
V_m = Maximum velocity
K_m – Michaelis constant

$\frac{1}{V_m}$ is where the plot crosses the y-axis

$\frac{-1}{K_m}$ is where the plot crosses the x-axis

2. Lineweaver–Burk equation:
   $1/V = K_m/(V_m \times [S]) + 1/V_m$
   a. Competitive inhibitors increase the K_m by competing with substrate binding to enzyme at the active site.
   b. Noncompetitive inhibitors decrease the V_m by bonding to the enzyme (E or ES) outside of the active site.
   c. Irreversible inhibitors inactivate the enzyme with kinetics similar to noncompetitive inhibition. Example: Aspirin inhibition of cyclooxygenases.
3. Regulatory enzymes in metabolic pathways are influenced by allosteric interactions and will have nonlinear Lineweaver–Burk plots for their kinetics.

BIOSTATISTICS AND EPIDEMIOLOGY

I. Sensitivity and specificity (Table 1-8)

TABLE 1-8 Sensitivity and Specificity

Disease States			
		Have disease	Do not have disease
Test Results	+	True Positive (TP)	False Positive (FP)
	–	False Negative (FN)	True Negative (TN)

Terminology	Equation	Definition
Sensitivity (positive in disease)	TP/(TP. FN)	Probability that a person having a disease will be correctly identified
Specificity (negative in healthy)	TN/(TN. FP)	Probability that a person who does not have a disease will be correctly identified
Positive-predictive value	TP/(TP. FP)	Probability that an individual who tests positive has the disease
Negative-predictive value	TN/(TN. FN)	Probability that an individual who tests negative does not have the disease
Prevalence	TP FN/(TP. FP. TN. FN) Generally calculated by: incidence × duration of disease	Total number of cases in a population at a given time
Incidence	Generally calculated by: number of new cases/susceptible population	Number of new cases of disease in the population over a given time

QUICK HIT: For chronic conditions (e.g., diabetes or cirrhosis), the prevalence is higher than the incidence because the long length of the disease process increases prevalence. For conditions that resolve quickly (e.g., strep throat) or are rapidly fatal (e.g., pancreatic cancer), the incidence and prevalence are approximately equal.

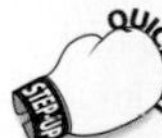

QUICK HIT: A screening test is more useful in a population where the disease is highly prevalent. As prevalence increases, PPV increases, and clinical usefulness is reflected in PPV.

II. Incidence and prevalence (Table 1-8)

A. Incidence rate is the number of new individuals who develop an illness in a given time period divided by the total number of individuals at risk for the illness.
B. Prevalence is the number of individuals in the population who have an illness divided by the total population.
C. Example: **Incidence** is the number of drug abusers newly diagnosed with HIV in 2007 divided by the number of drug abusers in the population in 2007. **Prevalence** is the number of people in the United States who are currently HIV-positive divided by the total population.

III. Key relationships among statistical variables

A. **Sensitivity (Sn), false-negative ratio (FNR), negative predictive value**
   1. Sn and FNR are inversely related: Sn = 1 – FNR.
   2. Therefore, increasing the sensitivity of a test decreases the FNR (the number of false negatives) and increases the negative predictive value.

MNEMONIC

To remember which statistical variables affect each other, think of the rule of Ns and Ps: **Sn** and **FNR** are inversely related. **Sp** and **FPR** are inversely related.

3. Example: A FBS <125 mg/dL is used to diagnose diabetes. If we lower the threshold to 110 mg/dL, then we will catch more individuals with diabetes. Statistically, this means decreasing the number of false negatives (those individuals who test negative but actually have the disease) and increasing sensitivity.

B. **Specificity (Sp), false-positive ratio (FPR), positive predictive value (PPV)**
   1. Sp and FPR are inversely related: Sp = 1 − FPR
   2. Therefore, increasing the specificity of a test decreases the FPR (the number of false positives) and increases the positive predictive value.
   3. Example: Western blot testing is used as a confirmatory test for HIV. Improving the technique such that the number of false positives (those individuals who tested positive but did not have the disease) were reduced would increase the specificity of the test.

C. **Specificity and sensitivity**
   1. Specificity and sensitivity are inversely related: as specificity increases, sensitivity decreases and vice versa.

QUICK HIT

High-sensitivity tests are better suited for screening purposes, whereas high-specificity tests are used as confirmatory tests.

D. **Treatment**
   1. Treatment decreases prevalence by shortening duration (remember that prevalence = incidence × duration of disease) (Table 1-8).
   2. Treatment has no effect on incidence.
   3. Adherence, therapy, physician access, early detection → decreases duration → decreases prevalence.

IV. Research study designs (Table 1-9)

A. **Cohort studies**
   1. Observational and can be prospective or retrospective
   2. After assessment of exposure to a risk factor, subjects are compared with each other for a period of time
   3. Clinical treatment trial
      a. Highest-quality cohort study
      b. Compares the therapeutic benefits of two or more treatments
   4. **Relative risk**
      a. Calculated only for cohort studies
      b. Compares incidence rate in exposed group with incidence rate in unexposed individuals

QUICK HIT

The most rigorous form of a clinical trial is the **double-blind study** in which neither the subject nor the examiner knows which drug the subject is receiving. Single-blind, double-blind, randomization crossover, and placebo studies are done to reduce bias.

B. **Case-control studies 1**
   1. Retrospective and observational
   2. Subjects with and without disorder are identified, and information on exposure to risk factors is assessed
   3. **Odds ratio** (Table 1-8)
      a. Used to determine relative risk in case–control studies
      b. Based on disease occurring with or without exposure
      c. Odds ratio = TP × TN/FP × FN

where

TP, true positives;
TN, true negatives;
FP, false positives;
FN, false negatives.

V. Biases—A systematic tendency to produce an outcome that differs from the underlying truth

A. **Sampling bias**—Volunteer subjects in a study may not be representative of the population being studied; as a consequence, the results of the study may not be generalizable to the entire population.

B. **Selection bias**—Occurs when the subject chooses to enter a drug group or a placebo group rather than being randomly assigned (or the investigator purposely chooses to put a subject in a drug or placebo group). One method of decreasing this bias is randomization.

TABLE 1-9 **Research Study Designs**

Study	Purpose	Notes
Case series	A study reporting on a consecutive collection of patients treated in a similar manner; no control group	
Case–control	Retrospective study designed to determine the association between an exposure and outcome: patients are sampled by outcome (e.g., patients with the disease are compared to patients without the disease); the investigator then examines the proportion of patients with the exposure in the two groups	Information reported as odds ratio. Example: Individuals with and without lung cancer are identified (outcome = lung cancer). The number of individuals who smoke within each group are counted (exposure = smoking)
Cohort	Prospective study of the factors that might cause a disorder; begins with identification of a specific population (cohort) free of outcome; one cohort is exposed to the putative cause and compared with a concurrent cohort not exposed to the putative cause; both cohorts are then followed to compare the incidence of the outcome of interest	Information reported as relative risk. Example: Two groups are made: one is exposed to UV radiation, the other is not (exposure = UV radiation). The number of individuals developing skin cancer is then counted within each group (outcome = skin cancer)
Crossover	A study design in which all patients receive both experimental and control treatments in sequence	Subjects act as own control
Cross-sectional	Provide information on possible risk factors and health status of a group of individuals at one specific point in time	Assess prevalence
Meta-analysis	Pooling data from several studies to achieve greater statistical power: often done via literature searches	
Controlled trial	Type of cohort study in which a cohort receiving one treatment/intervention is compared with a cohort receiving a different treatment or placebo	Example: Two groups are made: one is applied sunscreen the other is applied a placebo cream (intervention = sunscreen). The number of individuals developing skin cancer is then counted within each group (outcome = skin cancer)

C. **Expectancy bias**—Occurs when a physician knows which patients are in treatment versus placebo group, causing the physician to interact with the patients differently. *Note*: This type of bias can only occur in an intervention and can never occur in an observation study. One method of decreasing this bias is a double-blind design.

D. **Late-look bias**—Occurs in gathering data about a severe disease; the more severe cases may be dead or inaccessible.

E. **Measurement bias**—Describes how information gathered affects information collected. For example, the Hawthorne effect describes how people act differently when being watched.

F. **Proficiency bias**—This is an issue when comparing the effects of different treatments administered at multiple sites. Physicians at one site may have more skill, thereby providing better treatment, causing the results to reflect more skill than the pill.

G. **Recall bias**—Patients who experience an adverse outcome have a different likelihood of recalling an exposure than do patients who do not have an adverse outcome, independent of the true extent of the exposure.

VI. Disease prevention

A. **Primary prevention** stops disease occurrence; for example, encouraging use of sun protection to prevent skin cancer.

B. **Secondary prevention** detects disease early; for example, physician checking for suspicious growths.

C. **Tertiary prevention** decreases devastating complications of the disease; for example, administering insulin to a diabetic.

VII. Testing and statistical methods

A. Reliability versus validity

1. **Reliability** refers to the reproducibility of test results either among examiners or among test takers.
2. **Validity** refers to the appropriateness of a test's measurements (i.e., the test measures what it is supposed to).
3. **Sensitivity** and **specificity** constitute validity.

B. **Bell curve** (Figure 1-16)

1. In a **normal distribution**, the mean, median, and mode are equal.
   a. Mean: average
   b. Median: middle value in a sequentially ordered group of numbers
   c. Mode: number that appears most often in a group

FIGURE 1-16 **Bell curve**

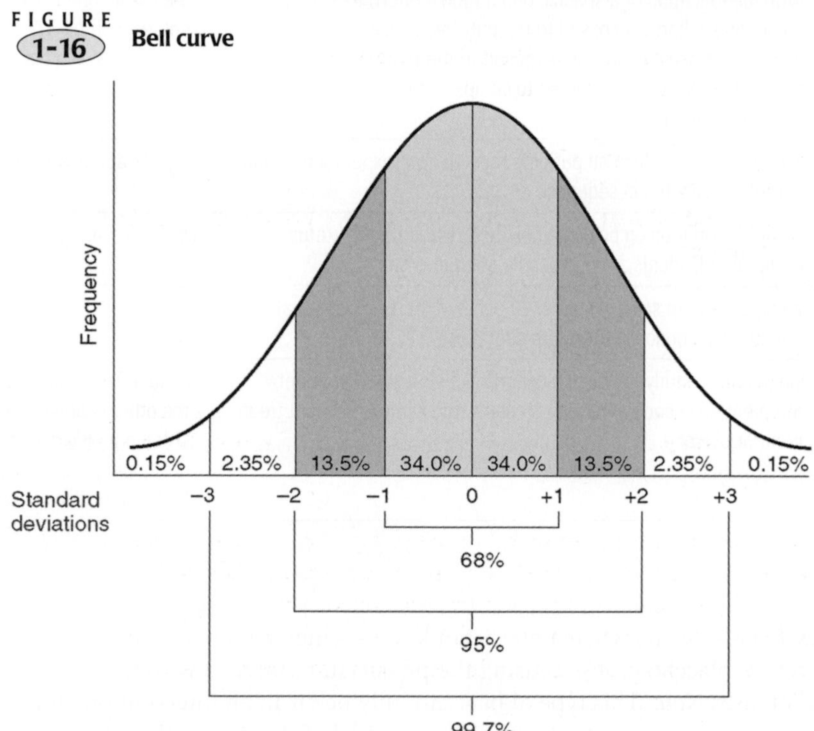

2. A bimodal distribution has two peaks.
3. Skew refers to the way a peak may be offset.
   a. **Positive skew**: peak is to the left (most scores at low end; mean > median > mode)
   b. **Negative skew**: peak is to the right (most scores at high end; mean < median < mode)

C. The **null hypothesis** (H_0)

1. Postulates that there is no significant difference between groups.
2. A **type I error** occurs when the null hypothesis is rejected when it is true. Probability (*p*) value is the chance of making a type I error.
3. A **type II error** occurs when the null hypothesis is accepted when it is not true. β is the chance of making a type II error.
4. **Power** is the probability of rejecting the null hypothesis when the null hypothesis is false. Power = 1 – β. Increasing the sample size increases power. If $p < 0.05$, then the null hypothesis can be rejected
5. Example
   a. A study is conducted on the influence of medical school on dating frequency.
   b. The null hypothesis would be that medical school students, when compared with 22- to 26-year-olds in the working population, have no difference in dating frequency.

c. If the *P* value of the study is less than 0.05 (meaning that there is a statistical difference), then the null hypothesis can be rejected.
d. Furthermore, it can be stated that medical school decreases dating frequency.

VIII. General statistics

A. Leading causes of **mortality**
1. Ages 1 to 14 years: injuries
2. Ages 15 to 24 years: accidents (majority are motor vehicle)
3. Ages 25 to 64 years: cancer (lung > breast/prostate > colon)
4. Ages 65 years: heart disease
5. **Acquired immunodeficiency syndrome (AIDS) is the leading cause of death in males between 25 and 44 years of age**

B. **Aging**
1. The elderly constitute 12% of the US population.
   a. They incur 30% of healthcare costs.
   b. 5% are in nursing homes.
   c. They commit **25% of suicides.**
   d. 15% suffer from dementia.
2. 75% of men and 50% of women 60 to 65 years of age continue to be interested in sex.
3. Life expectancy is 8 years longer for women.

C. **Family**
1. 95% of people in the US marry.
2. Approximately 50% of marriages end in divorce.
3. 50% of children live in an environment with two working parents.
4. 20% of all families are single-parent households, but 50% of Black families are single-parent households.
5. Abuse
   a. 32% of children younger than 5 years of age are physically abused.
   b. 25% of children younger than 8 years of age are sexually abused.
6. First sexual intercourse usually occurs around 16 years of age.

D. **Disorders**
1. At least 25% of the people in the United States are obese.
2. Insomnia occurs in 30% of people.
3. Alcohol
   a. Highest use is by people 21 to 34 years of age.
   b. 13% of adults abuse alcohol.
4. There is a 1.5% chance of becoming schizophrenic (equal occurrence rate in men and women, and Whites and Blacks).
5. 10% of men and 15% to 20% of women have unipolar disorder (depression).
6. 1% of all individuals have bipolar disorder.

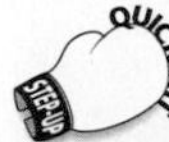

Hard and fast statistical numbers are rarely sought after as answers on the USMLE Step 1 Examination. However, having a general idea of some select statistics may assist one in answering the vignette-style questions.

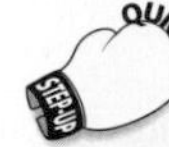

Suicide is the second leading cause of death for people 15 to 24 years of age.

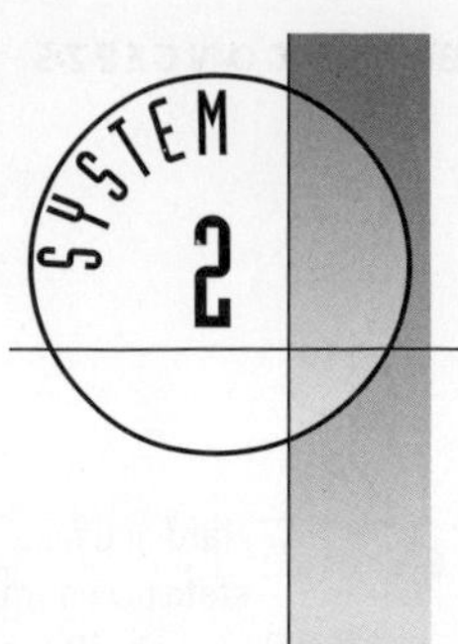

The Nervous System

DEVELOPMENT

> **QUICK HIT** Symptoms of a disk herniation are referred to the myotome and dermatome **below** the lesion. For example, a herniation of the C4–C5 disk would cause impingement of the C5 nerve root.

I. Central nervous system (CNS)

A. The CNS includes the **brain** and **spinal cord**.

B. The CNS forms **from the neural tube**

1. The **basal plate** of the neural tube forms **motor neurons**.
2. The **alar plate** of the neural tube forms **sensory neurons**.
3. The basal and alar plates are **separated** by the **sulcus limitans**.

C. **Oligodendrocytes** are responsible for **myelination**, which begins 4 months after conception and is completed by the second year of life.

D. The distal end of the spinal cord, the conus medullaris, is at the level of the third lumbar vertebra (L3) at **birth**. As the body grows, the cord "ascends" to its final resting position at the first lumbar vertebra (L1) (Figure 2-1).

FIGURE 2-1 Adult derivatives of embryonic structures in the nervous system

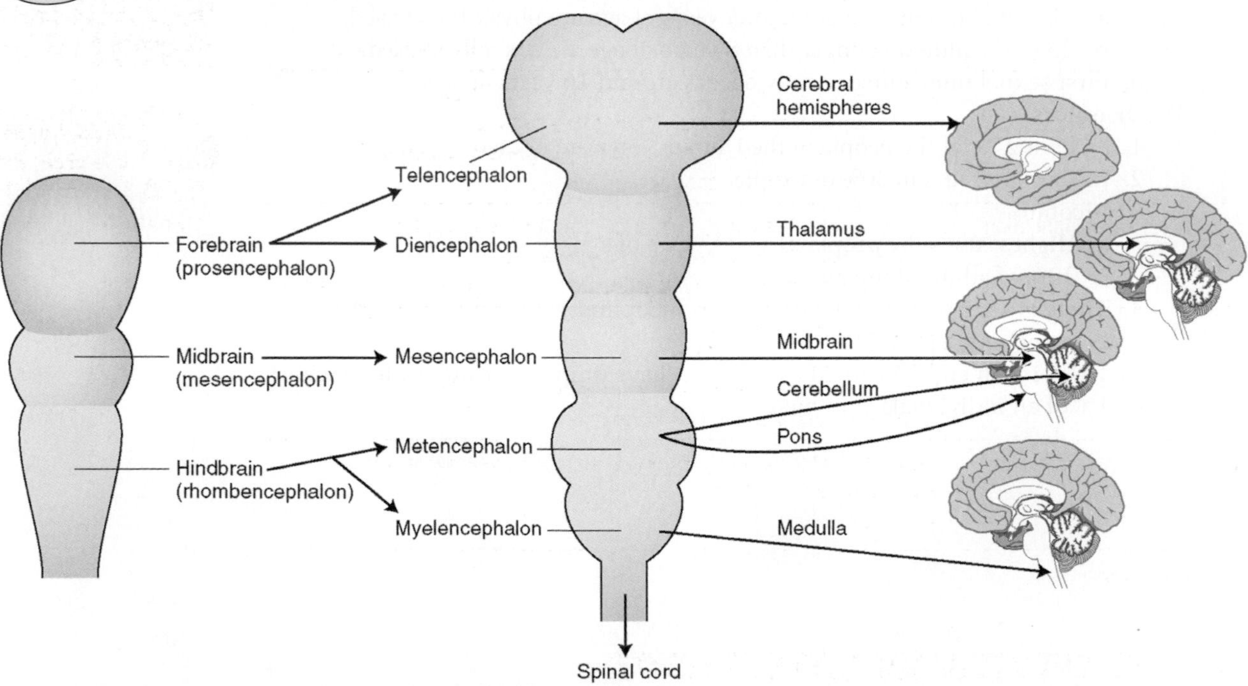

> **QUICK HIT** Each oligodendrocyte can myelinate several axons, whereas each Schwann cell can only myelinate one axon.

II. Peripheral nervous system (PNS)

A. The PNS includes the **peripheral nerves** and the **autonomic** and **sensory ganglia**.

B. It is **derived from neural crest cells**, which give rise to

1. Schwann cells
2. Pseudounipolar cells of the spinal and cranial nerve ganglia

3. Multipolar cells of the autonomic ganglia
4. Pia and arachnoid mater (not part of PNS)
5. Melanocytes (not part of PNS)
6. Epinephrine-producing chromaffin cells of the adrenal gland (not part of PNS)

C. **Schwann cells** are responsible for **myelination**, which begins 4 months after conception and is completed by the second year of life.

CONGENITAL MALFORMATIONS OF THE NERVOUS SYSTEM

Abnormal development of the embryonal components of the nervous system can result in some of the malformations described in Table 2-1.

TABLE 2-1 Congenital Malformations of the Nervous System

Condition	Clinical Features
Fetal alcohol syndrome	• **Most common cause of mental retardation** • **Cardiac septal defects** • Facial malformations including widely spaced eyes and long philtrum • Growth retardation

Spina bifida	• Improper closure of posterior neuropore
	• Several forms
	  • **Spina bifida occulta** (mildest form)—failure of vertebrae to close around spinal cord (tufts of hair often evident)
	  • Spinal meningocele (spina bifida cystica)—meninges extend out of defective spinal canal
	  • Meningomyelocele—meninges and spinal cord extend out of spinal canal
	  • Rachischisis (most severe form)—neural tissue is visible externally

Hydrocephaly	• Accumulation of CSF in ventricles and subarachnoid space • Caused by congenital blockage of cerebral aqueducts • May be caused by **cytomegalovirus or toxoplasma infection** • Increased head circumference in neonates
Dandy–Walker malformation	• Dilation of fourth ventricle, leading to hypoplasia of cerebellum • Failure of foramina of Luschka and Magendie to open • May result from riboflavin inhibition, posterior fossa trauma, or viral infection
Anencephaly	• Failure of brain to develop • Caused by lack of closure of anterior neuropore • Associated with increased maternal α-fetoprotein (AFP) • Decreased head circumference in neonates
Arnold–Chiari malformation	• Herniation of the **cerebellar vermis** through the foramen magnum • Hydrocephaly • Myelomeningocele

CSF, cerebrospinal fluid.

QUICK HIT: The risk of spina bifida can be decreased by taking folate supplements prior to conception and during pregnancy.

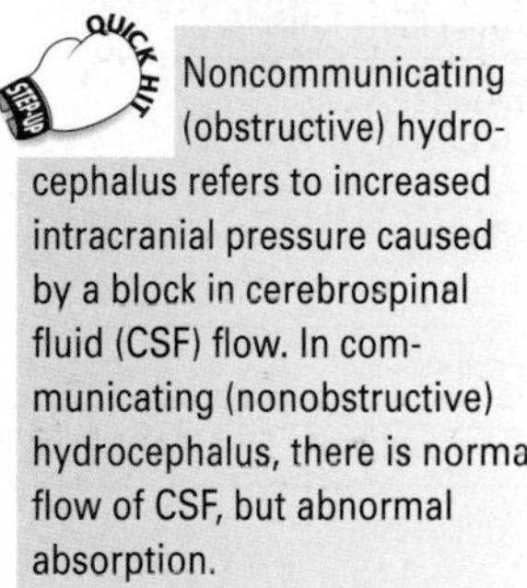
Noncommunicating (obstructive) hydrocephalus refers to increased intracranial pressure caused by a block in cerebrospinal fluid (CSF) flow. In communicating (nonobstructive) hydrocephalus, there is normal flow of CSF, but abnormal absorption.

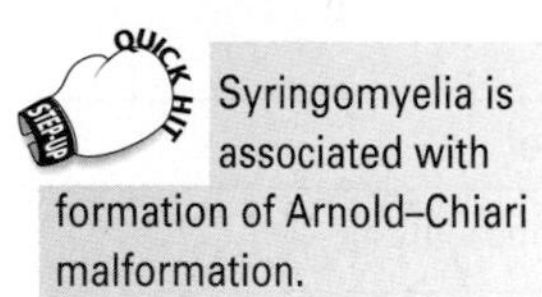
Syringomyelia is associated with formation of Arnold–Chiari malformation.

MAJOR RECEPTORS OF THE NERVOUS SYSTEM

I. Receptors of the sympathetic and parasympathetic nervous systems

A. The sympathetic and parasympathetic nervous systems exert their effects via various receptors scattered throughout the body (Table 2-2).

B. These effects are mediated by the substances shown in Figure 2-2.

TABLE 2-2 Receptors of the Sympathetic and Parasympathetic Nervous Systems

	Sympathetic Nervous System		Parasympathetic Nervous System	
Site of Action	**Receptor**	**Effect on Site**	**Receptor**	**Effect on Site**
Smooth muscle; skin and viscera	α_1	Contract	Muscarinic	Relax
Smooth and skeletal muscle	α_1 β_2	Contract Relax	Muscarinic	Relax
Smooth muscle of the lung	β_2	Relax	Muscarinic	Contract
Smooth muscle of the gastrointestinal tract	β_2 α_1	Relax intestinal wall Contract sphincters	Muscarinic	Contract intestinal wall; relax sphincter
Heart; SA node	β_1	Increase heart rate	Muscarinic	Decrease heart rate
Heart; ventricles	β_1	Increase contractility and conduction velocity	Muscarinic	Small decrease in contractility
Eye; radial muscle	α_1	**Mydriasis** (dilation of pupil)	N/A	N/A
Eye; sphincter muscle	N/A	N/A	Muscarinic	**Miosis** (constriction of pupil)
Eye; ciliary muscle	β_2	**Relax**	Muscarinic	**Contract** (near vision)
Bladder	β_2 α_1	Relax wall Contract sphincter	Muscarinic	Contract wall; relax sphincter
Uterus	α_1 β_2	Contract Relax	Muscarinic	Contract
Penis	α_2	Ejaculate	Muscarinic	Erection
Sweat glands	Muscarinic	Secrete	N/A	N/A
Pancreas	α_2 β_2	**Decrease insulin secretion** **Increase insulin secretion**	N/A N/A	N/A N/A
Liver	α_1, β_2	Glycolysis, gluconeogenesis	N/A	N/A
Adipose tissue	β_1, β_3	Lipolysis	N/A	N/A

N/A, not applicable; SA, sinoatrial.

II. Neurotoxins and their effects (Figure 2-3)

MENINGES, FLOW OF CEREBROSPINAL FLUID, AND PATHOLOGIC TRAUMA (Figure 2-4)

BLOOD SUPPLY TO THE BRAIN (Figure 2-5)

Cerebrovascular disease is the most common cause of CNS pathology and the third major cause of death in the United States (Table 2-3).

(text continues on page 52)

FIGURE 2-2 **Major receptors of the nervous system**

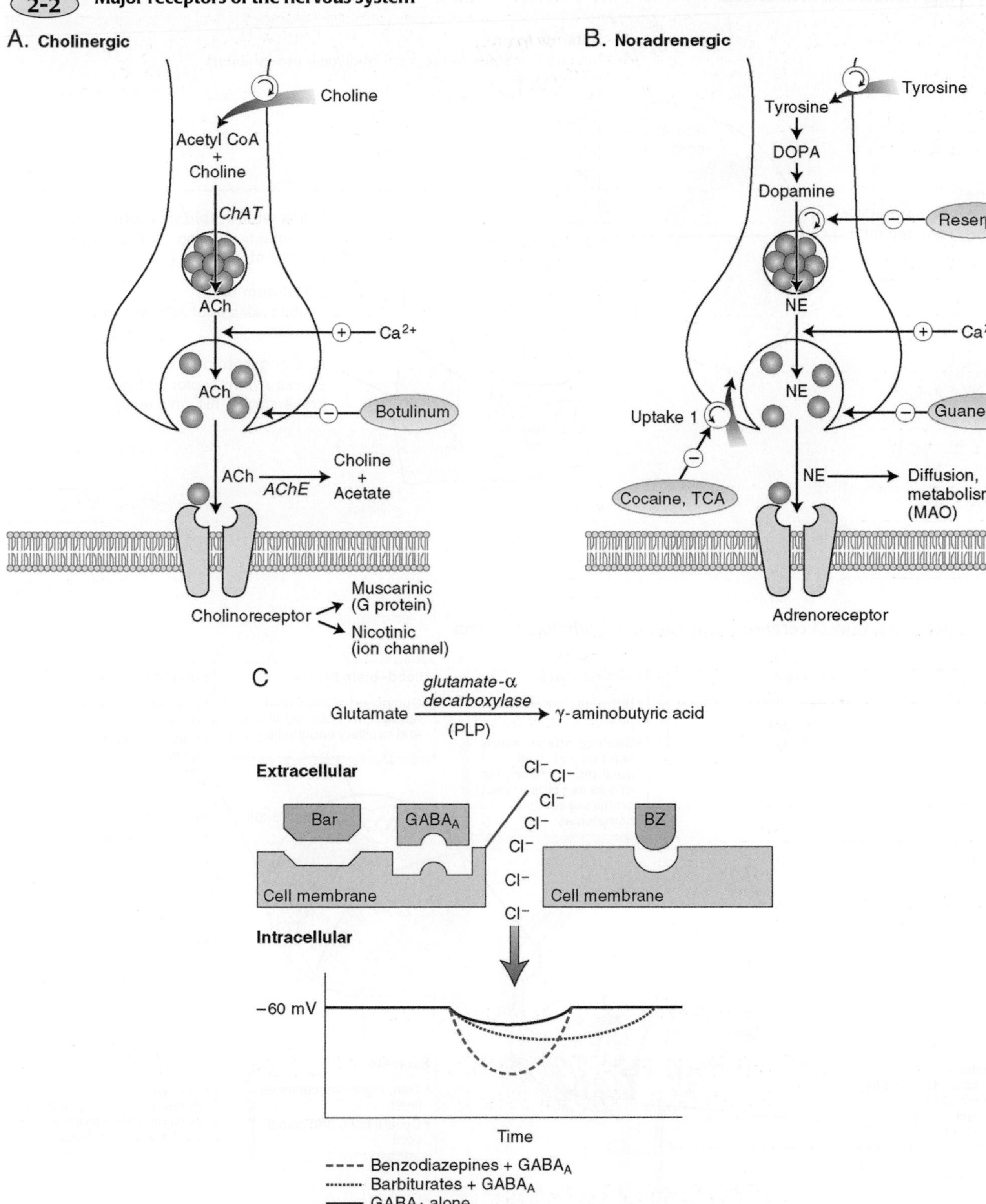

Binding of barbiturates or benzodiazepines to the GABA ionophore increases chloride ion conductance. Barbiturates increase the duration of chloride channel opening while benzodiazepines increase the amplitude of depolarization.

FIGURE 2-3 Neurotoxins and their effects

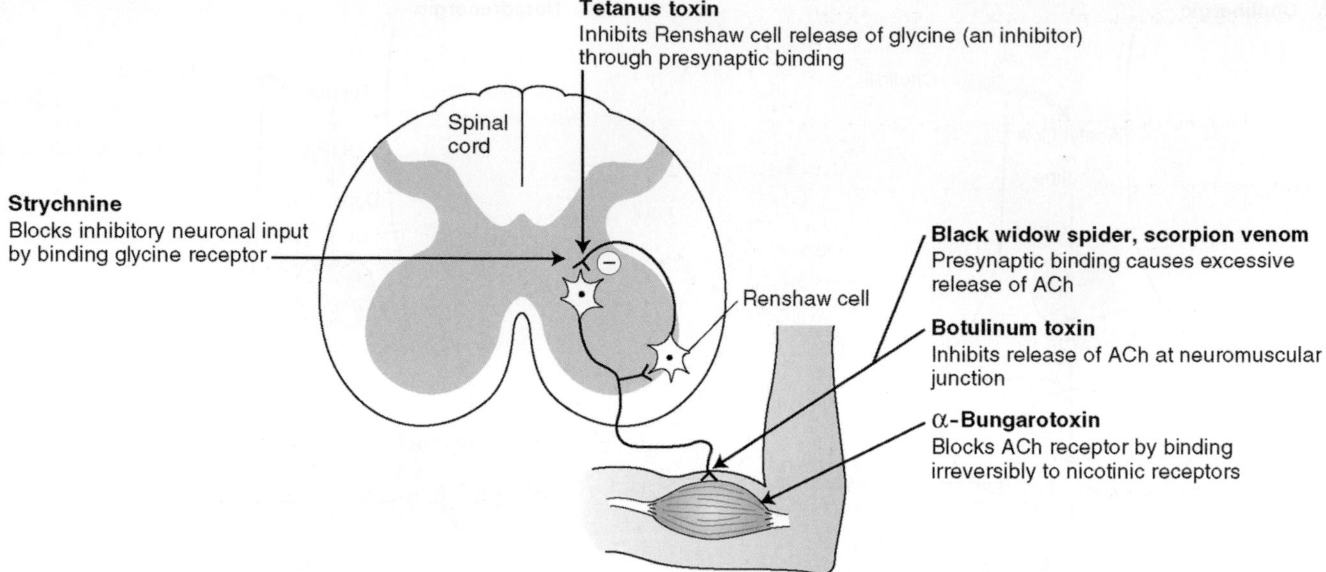

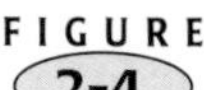

Inhibits Renshaw cell release of glycine (an inhibitor) through presynaptic binding

Blocks inhibitory neuronal input by binding glycine receptor

Black widow spider, scorpion venom
Presynaptic binding causes excessive release of ACh

Blocks ACh receptor by binding irreversibly to nicotinic receptors

FIGURE 2-4 Meninges, flow of cerebrospinal fluid, and pathologic trauma

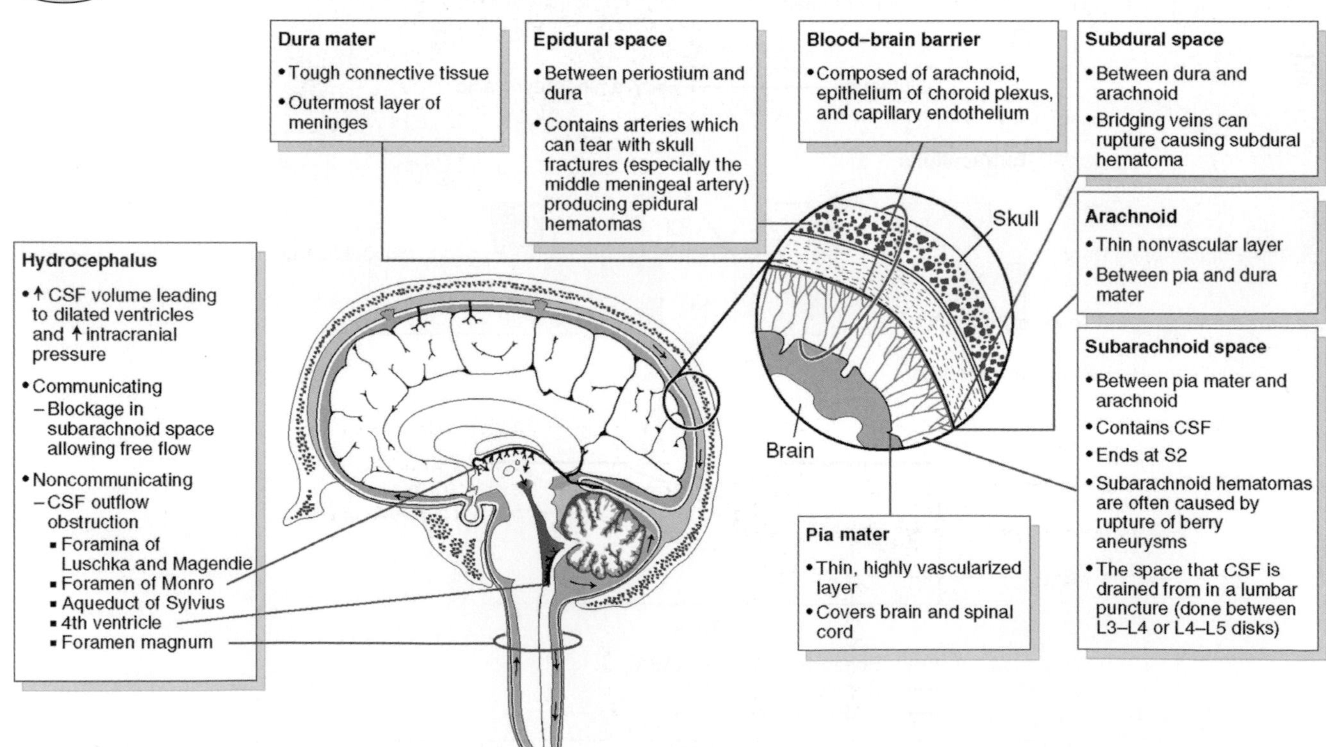

Dura mater
• Tough connective tissue
• Outermost layer of meninges
Epidural space
• Between periostium and dura
• Contains arteries which can tear with skull fractures (especially the middle meningeal artery) producing epidural hematomas
Blood–brain barrier
• Composed of arachnoid, epithelium of choroid plexus, and capillary endothelium
Subdural space
• Between dura and arachnoid
• Bridging veins can rupture causing subdural hematoma
Skull
Arachnoid
• Thin nonvascular layer
• Between pia and dura mater
Subarachnoid space
• Between pia mater and arachnoid
• Contains CSF
• Ends at S2
• Subarachnoid hematomas are often caused by rupture of berry aneurysms
• The space that CSF is drained from in a lumbar puncture (done between L3–L4 or L4–L5 disks)
Brain
Pia mater
• Thin, highly vascularized layer
• Covers brain and spinal cord
Hydrocephalus
• ↑ CSF volume leading to dilated ventricles and ↑ intracranial pressure
• Communicating
– Blockage in subarachnoid space allowing free flow
• Noncommunicating
– CSF outflow obstruction
▪ Foramina of Luschka and Magendie
▪ Foramen of Monro
▪ Aqueduct of Sylvius
▪ 4th ventricle
▪ Foramen magnum

FIGURE 2-5 **Blood supply to the brain**

A. **Arteries of the base of the brain and brain stem**

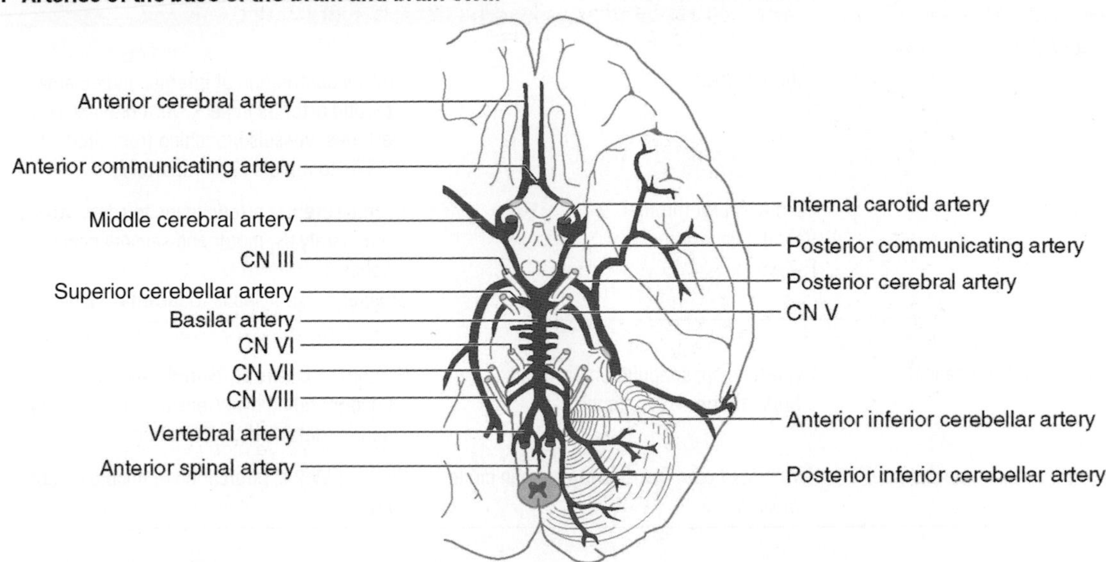

B. **Arterial blood supply to the cortex**

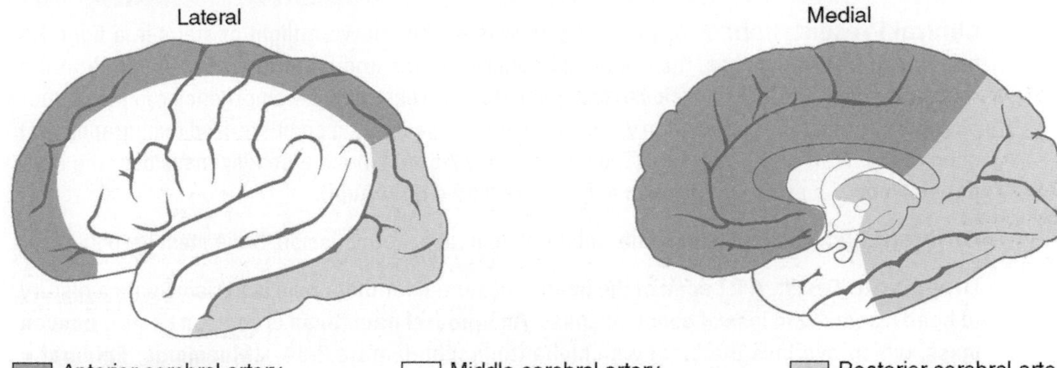

C. **Venous drainage of the brain**

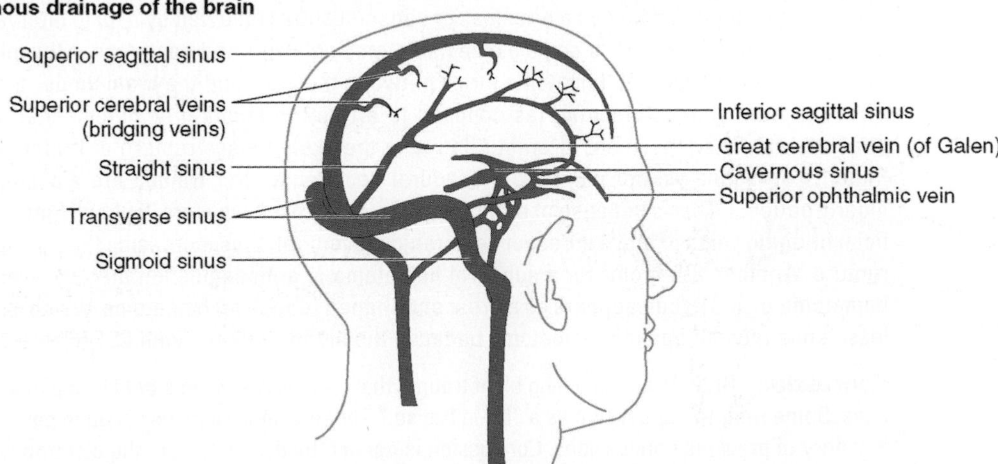

TABLE 2-3 Cerebrovascular Disease

Disease	Predisposing Factor	Common Sites
Infarction *(more frequent than hemorrhage)*		
Thrombosis	Atherosclerosis	Arterial obstruction of internal and external carotid arteries in neck, vertebral and basilar arteries, vessels branching from circle of Willis to middle cerebral artery
Embolus	Cardiac mural thrombi Valvular vegetation Fat emboli	Middle cerebral artery: leads to contralateral paralysis, motor and sensory deficits, aphasias Smaller vessels: leads to **lacunar strokes**
Hemorrhage		
Intracerebral (bleeding into brain substance)	Hypertension, coagulation disorders, hemorrhage within tumor	Rupture of **Charcot–Bouchard** aneurysms (long-standing hypertension), basal ganglia, pons, frontal lobe, cerebellum
Subarachnoid (bleeding into subarachnoid space)	Associated with **berry aneurysm** in circle of Willis	Circle of Willis, bifurcation of middle cerebral artery

Clinical Vignette 2-1

Clinical Presentation: A 26-year-old man was pushed down a flight of stairs in a fight. He **briefly lost consciousness,** then regained consciousness and went to dinner. **After 1 h** at the restaurant, the man lost consciousness again. He was rushed to the emergency room and after airway, breathing, and circulation were assessed and secured, a computerized tomography (CT) scan of the head was performed. The scan (Figure 2-6A) showed a convex mass over the right parietal lobe. An eye exam showed a fixed and dilated **right pupil**.

Differentials: Epidural hematoma, subdural hematoma, concussion, brain stem herniation.

Diagnostic Tests: A **CT scan of the head** is essential for diagnosis in patients with a history of head trauma with loss of consciousness. **An epidural hematoma** is seen on CT as a **convex mass,** which overlays the brain with high attenuation (Figure 2-6A). (**Mnemonic: Epidural = convEx**). An epidural hematoma is a blood clot between the skull and the dura, caused by laceration of the **middle meningeal artery** when the temporal bone is fractured. The "classic" presentation is a patient who has a brief loss of consciousness followed by a lucid interval, after which the patient goes into a coma as the hematoma enlarges and compresses the midbrain.

In contrast, a **subdural** hematoma forms between the dura and the brain (under the dura). It results from **venous bleeding** (as opposed to arterial in epidural hematomas) after blunt head trauma. The movement of brain relative to the skull causes rupture of **bridging veins**. Patients at higher risk for incurring a subdural hematoma after trauma are alcoholics and elderly patients. This is because of brain atrophy, which results in more "space" for the superficial bridging veins to move in response to rapid movement, thus increasing the risk of vessel rupture. Another risk factor for a subdural hematoma is anticoagulation therapy. A subdural hematoma on a CT scan appears as a crescent-shaped (**concave**) hematoma, which is usually less dense than an epidural hematoma because the blood is diluted with CSF (Figure 2-6B).

Concussion: Brain injury following blunt trauma that usually results in a brief loss of consciousness. Some refer to concussion as a "brain bruise." Those at increased risk include patients with a history of previous concussions. Concussion is caused by dysfunction of the electrophysiology of the midbrain secondary to impact. Patients experience confusion, dizziness, problems with concentration, and inability to answer questions (or a delay in answering) after awakening.

Management: Treatment for an epidural hematoma includes rapid surgical decompression. Conversely, an acute subdural hematoma can be managed by observation or craniotomy with evacuation, depending on size and severity of symptoms. There is no treatment for a concussion.

FIGURE 2-6 **A. Epidural hematoma**

(Reproduced from Daffner RH, ed. Clinical Radiology: The Essentials. 2nd Ed. Philadelphia, PA: Lippincott Williams & Wilkins, 1999:513, with permission.)

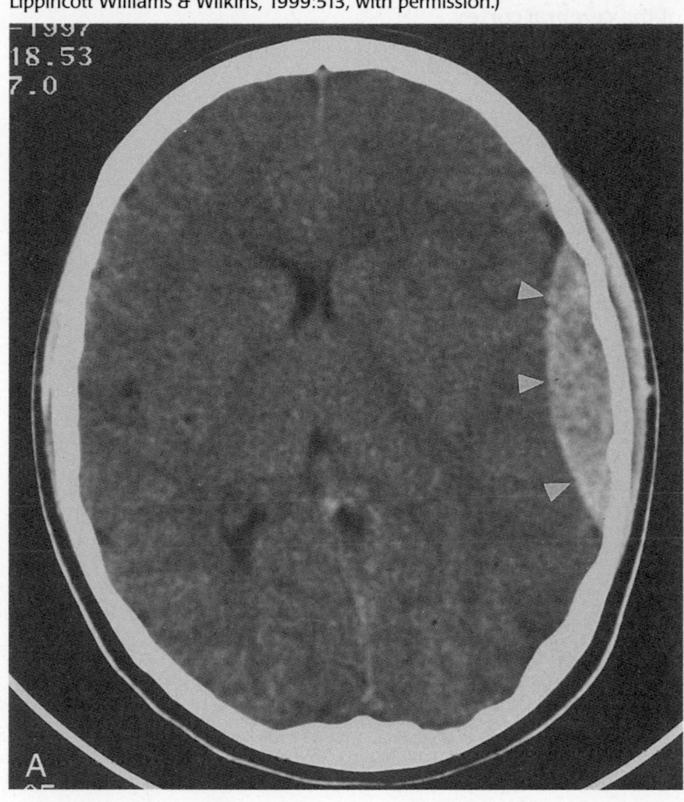

FIGURE 2-6 **B. Subdural hematoma**

(Reproduced from Daffner RH, ed. Clinical Radiology: The Essentials. 2nd Ed. Philadelphia, PA: Lippincott Williams & Wilkins, 1999:513.9, with permission.)

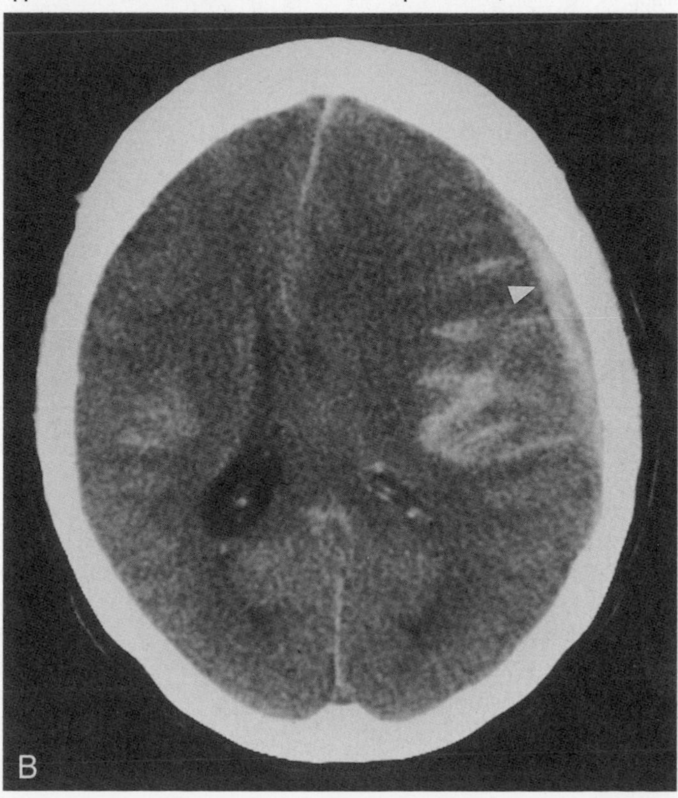

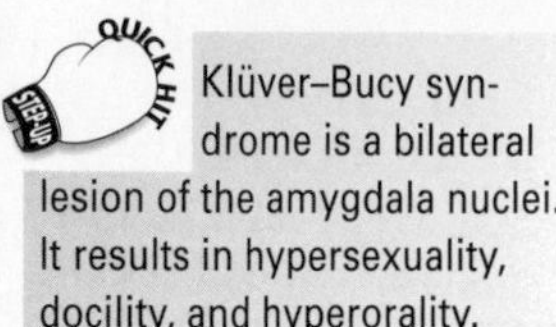
QUICK HIT

Klüver–Bucy syndrome is a bilateral lesion of the amygdala nuclei. It results in hypersexuality, docility, and hyperorality.

LESIONS OF THE CEREBRAL CORTEX (Figure 2-7)

FIGURE 2-7 **Lesions of the cerebral cortex**

(Adapted from Fix JD. High-Yield Neuroanatomy. Baltimore, MD: Williams & Wilkins, 1995:102, with permission.)

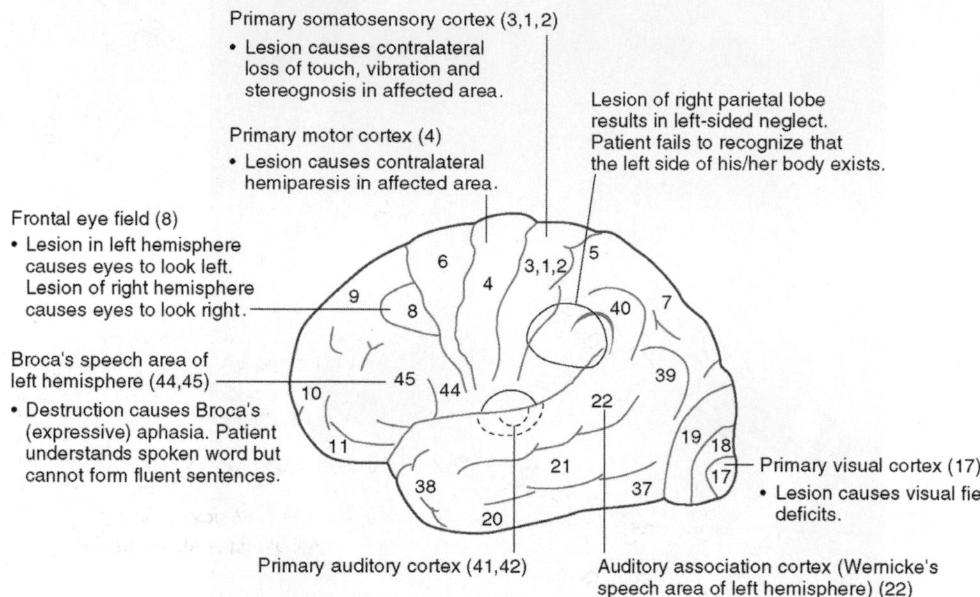
A. Lateral view
Primary somatosensory cortex (3,1,2)
• Lesion causes contralateral loss of touch, vibration and stereognosis in affected area.
Lesion of right parietal lobe results in left-sided neglect. Patient fails to recognize that the left side of his/her body exists.
Primary motor cortex (4)
• Lesion causes contralateral hemiparesis in affected area.
Frontal eye field (8)
• Lesion in left hemisphere causes eyes to look left. Lesion of right hemisphere causes eyes to look right.
Broca's speech area of left hemisphere (44,45)
• Destruction causes Broca's (expressive) aphasia. Patient understands spoken word but cannot form fluent sentences.
6
4
3,1,2
5
9
8
40
7
45
44
10
39
22
11
19
18
17
21
38
37
20
Primary visual cortex (17)
• Lesion causes visual field deficits.
Primary auditory cortex (41,42)
Auditory association cortex (Wernicke's speech area of left hemisphere) (22)
• Destruction causes Wernicke's aphasia. Patient cannot understand spoken word and speech is fluid but does not make sense.

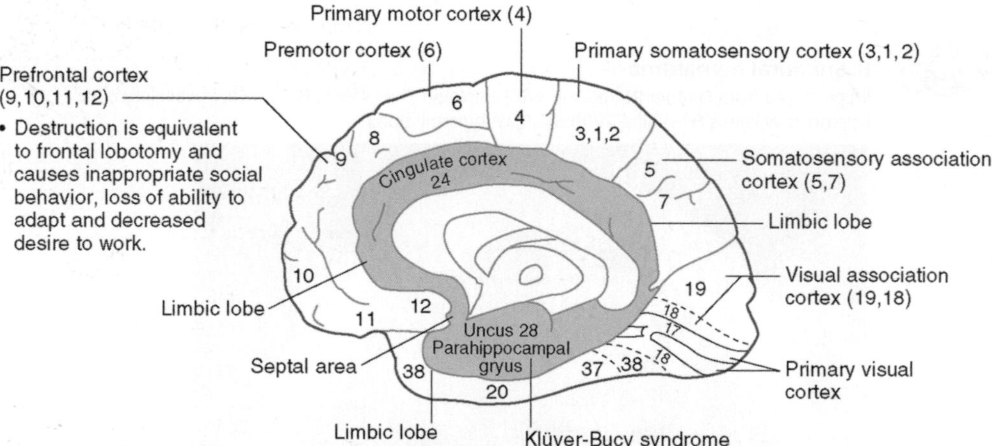
B. Medial view
Primary motor cortex (4)
Premotor cortex (6)
Primary somatosensory cortex (3,1,2)
Prefrontal cortex (9,10,11,12)
• Destruction is equivalent to frontal lobotomy and causes inappropriate social behavior, loss of ability to adapt and decreased desire to work.
6
4
8
3,1,2
9
Cingulate cortex 24
5
7
Somatosensory association cortex (5,7)
Limbic lobe
10
19
Visual association cortex (19,18)
Limbic lobe
12
11
18
17
18
Uncus 28
Parahippocampal gryus
Septal area
38
37
38
20
Primary visual cortex
Limbic lobe
Klüver-Bucy syndrome

IMPORTANT PATHWAYS OF THE SPINAL CORD (Figure 2-8)

I. Posterior white column (dorsal column medial lemniscus pathway)

A. The posterior white column is the ascending pathway that conveys **discriminatory touch (two-point touch)**, **vibration**, **proprioception**, and **stereognosis.**

B. The posterior white column receives information at all spinal cord levels from pseudounipolar cells of dorsal root ganglia. This information is conveyed from a variety of receptors:

1. Meissner corpuscles (rate of applied stimulus)
2. **Pacinian corpuscles (vibration stimulus)**
3. Joint receptors (joint position; proprioception)
4. Muscle spindles (length of a muscle)
5. **Golgi tendon organs** (**tension** on a muscle)

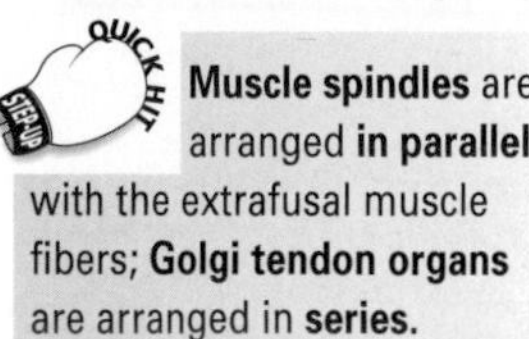
QUICK HIT

Muscle spindles function as the afferent limb of the myotactic (stretch) reflex (e.g., tapping knee with reflex hammer). Ventral horn motor neurons function as the efferent limb.

QUICK HIT

Muscle spindles are arranged **in parallel** with the extrafusal muscle fibers; **Golgi tendon organs** are arranged in **series.**

FIGURE 2-8 **Important pathways of the spinal cord**

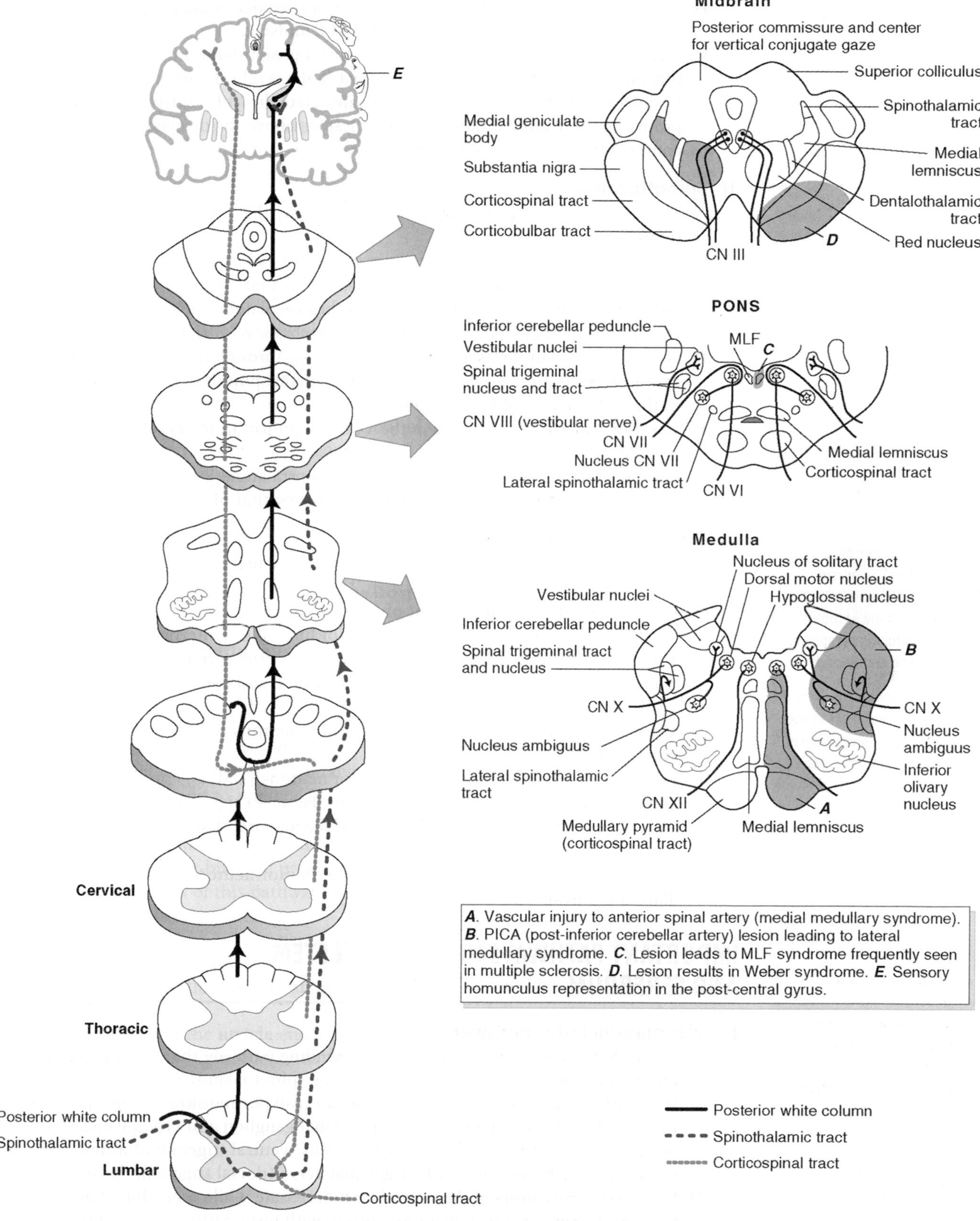

A. Vascular injury to anterior spinal artery (medial medullary syndrome). ***B***. PICA (post-inferior cerebellar artery) lesion leading to lateral medullary syndrome. ***C***. Lesion leads to MLF syndrome frequently seen in multiple sclerosis. ***D***. Lesion results in Weber syndrome. ***E***. Sensory homunculus representation in the post-central gyrus.

MNEMONIC

Remember **COWS**: cold opposite, warm same side for the direction of movement during fast phase of caloric nystagmus.

TABLE 2-4 Direction of Movement in Types of Nystagmus

Form of Nystagmus	Direction of Movement During Fast Phase	Direction of Movement During Slow Phase
Rotary nystagmus (i.e., while spinning in a circle)	Same as direction of rotation	Opposite direction of rotation
Postrotary nystagmus (i.e., after spinning in a circle)	Opposite direction of rotation	Same as direction of rotation
Caloric nystagmus		
• Warm water placed in one ear	Toward the ear with warm water placed in it	Away from the ear with warm water placed in it
• Cold water placed in one ear	Away from the ear with cold water placed in it	Toward the ear with cold water placed in it

V. Visual pathways (Figure 2-9)

A. Muscles of the eye (Figure 2-10)

B. **Horner syndrome**

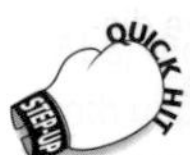

Horner syndrome is often caused by **Pancoast tumor,** a lung neoplasm that invades the cervical sympathetic chain.

1. It is caused by a lesion of the sympathetic trunk in the neck.
2. Clinical features of the syndrome include ipsilateral **ptosis**, **anhydrosis**, **flushing of skin**, and **miosis**.

C. **Argyll Robertson pupil**

1. A pupil that **accommodates** to near objects but **does not react to light**
2. Seen in syphilis, systemic lupus erythematosus (SLE), and diabetes mellitus

D. **Marcus Gunn pupil**

The Marcus Gunn pupil can be diagnosed using the **swinging flashlight test.** Shining a flashlight in the normal pupil causes constriction of both pupils. Swinging the flashlight quickly to the affected eye causes paradoxical dilation of the pupils.

1. It is caused by a relative deficit in the afferent portion of the light reflex pathway.
2. Shining a light in the affected pupil causes minimal bilateral constriction, but shining light in the unaffected pupil causes normal constriction of both pupils.

E. **MLF syndrome**

1. Caused by a lesion of the medial longitudinal fasciculus and can be unilateral or bilateral.
2. **Clinical features**
   a. The ipsilateral eye (the eye on the side of the MLF lesion) is unable to adduct and the contralateral eye (the opposite eye) has nystagmus. For example, in the cases of right MLF lesions, the right eye is unable to adduct and the left eye has nystagmus when looking left.
   b. Convergence is unaffected.
3. Often seen in **multiple sclerosis (MS).**

F. **Uncal herniation**

1. The uncus of the temporal lobe is forced through the opening of the tentorium.
2. Clinical features include (Figure 2-9)
   a. Compression of CN III occurs, leading to fixed and dilated ("blown") pupil on ipsilateral side
   b. Ophthalmoplegia (paralysis of one or more of the ocular muscles)
   c. Compression of the corticospinal tract leading to ipsilateral hemiparesis
   d. Compression of the posterior cerebral artery leading to contralateral homonymous hemianopsia

FIGURE 2-9 **Visual pathways. A. Legend for lesions: (1) total blindness; (2) bitemporal hemianopsia—common lesion caused by superiorly growing pituitary tumor; (3) right hemianopsia; (4) right upper quadrantanopia; (5) right lower quadrantanopia; (6) right hemianopsia with macular sparing. B. Light shined in one eye causes constriction of both pupils. C. Abduction of one eye results in adduction of the other eye in individuals with an intact medial longitudinal fasciculus, and normal lateral conjugate gaze**

(Adapted from Chung, Kyung Won. BRS Gross Anatomy. 2nd Ed. Baltimore, MD: Williams & Wilkins, 1991:302, with permission.)

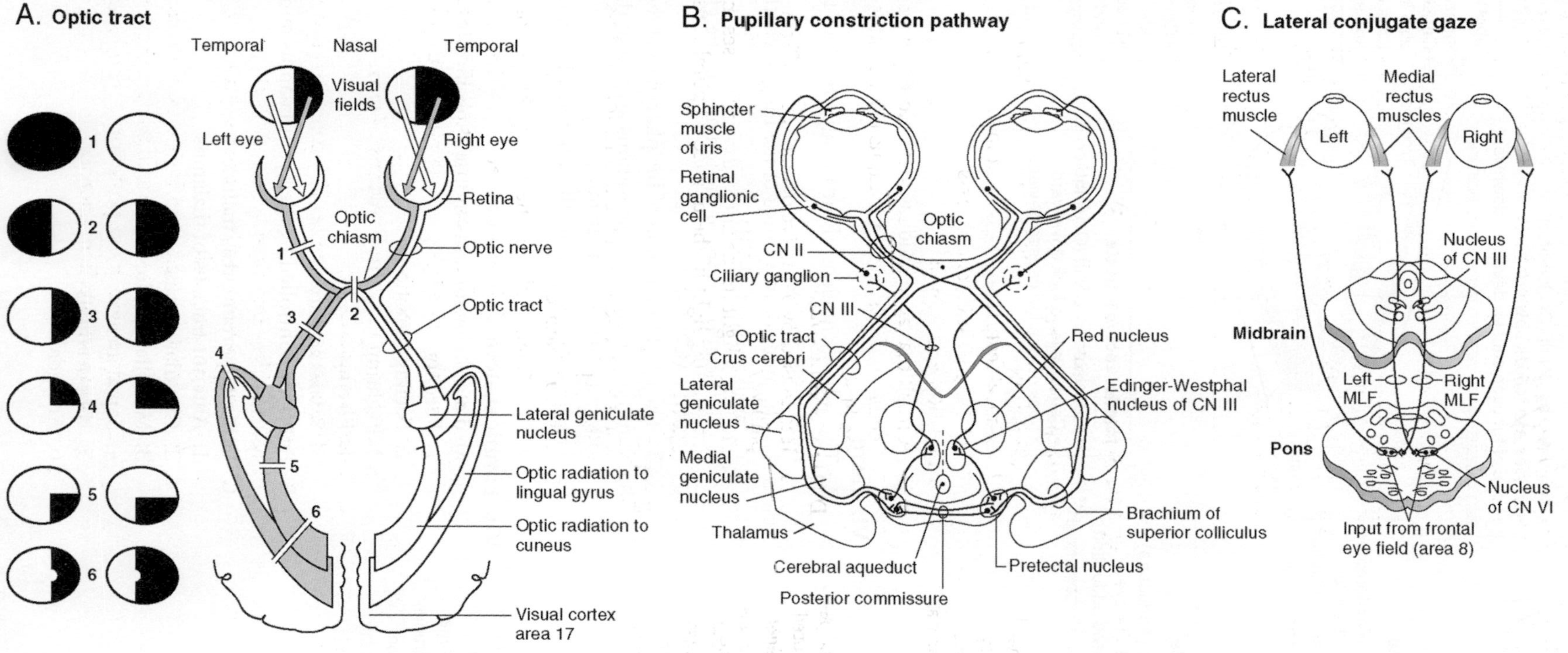

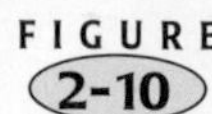

FIGURE 2-10 **Muscles of the eye**
(Adapted from Chung, Kyung Won. BRS Gross Anatomy. 2nd Ed. Baltimore, MD: Williams & Wilkins, 1991:302, with permission.)

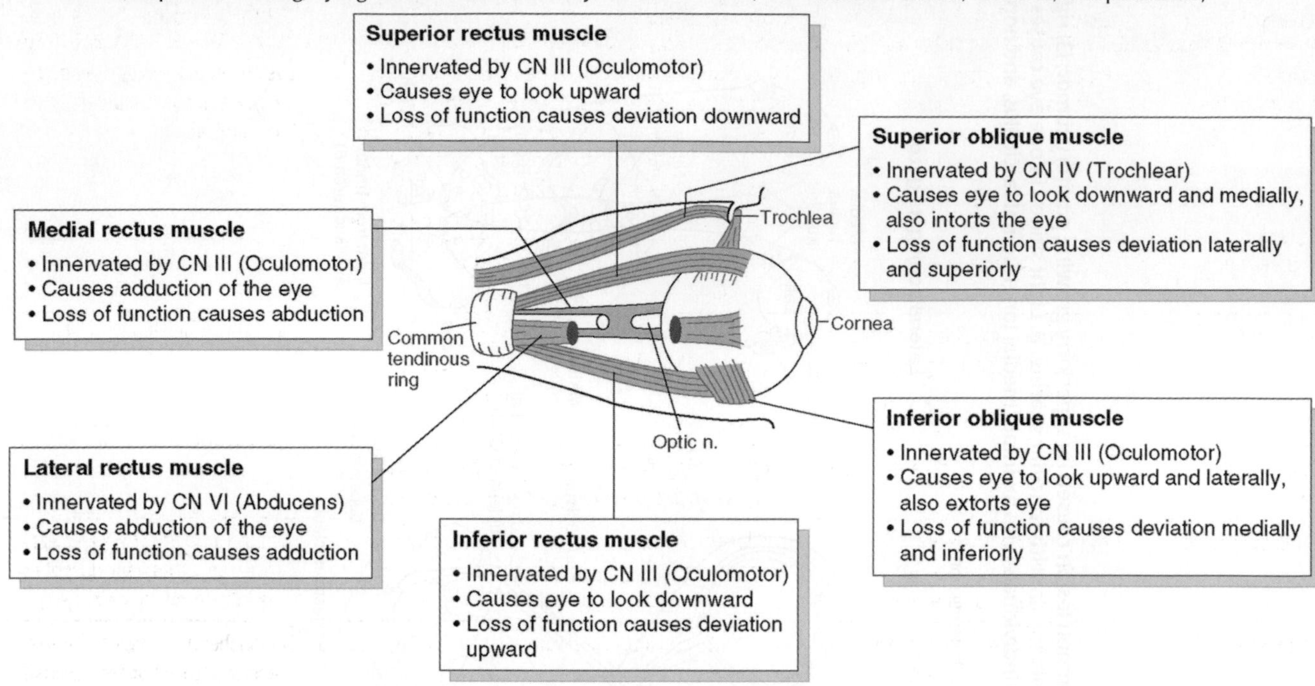

Superior rectus muscle
• Innervated by CN III (Oculomotor)
• Causes eye to look upward
• Loss of function causes deviation downward
Superior oblique muscle
• Innervated by CN IV (Trochlear)
• Causes eye to look downward and medially, also intorts the eye
• Loss of function causes deviation laterally and superiorly
Trochlea
Medial rectus muscle
• Innervated by CN III (Oculomotor)
• Causes adduction of the eye
• Loss of function causes abduction
Cornea
Common tendinous ring
Inferior oblique muscle
• Innervated by CN III (Oculomotor)
• Causes eye to look upward and laterally, also extorts eye
• Loss of function causes deviation medially and inferiorly
Optic n.
Lateral rectus muscle
• Innervated by CN VI (Abducens)
• Causes abduction of the eye
• Loss of function causes adduction
Inferior rectus muscle
• Innervated by CN III (Oculomotor)
• Causes eye to look downward
• Loss of function causes deviation upward

VI. Taste

A. The **solitary** nucleus of the medulla receives taste sensation via the solitary tract from three sources:
   1. The anterior two thirds of the tongue via the **chorda tympani** nerve of the facial nerve (CN VII)
   2. The posterior third of the tongue via the **glossopharyngeal** nerve (CN IX)
   3. The epiglottic region of the pharynx via the **vagus** nerve (CN X)

B. Neurons carrying taste sensations ascend in the ventral tegmental tract to the VPM nucleus of the thalamus.

C. The VPM nucleus of the thalamus sends fibers to the parietal lobe.

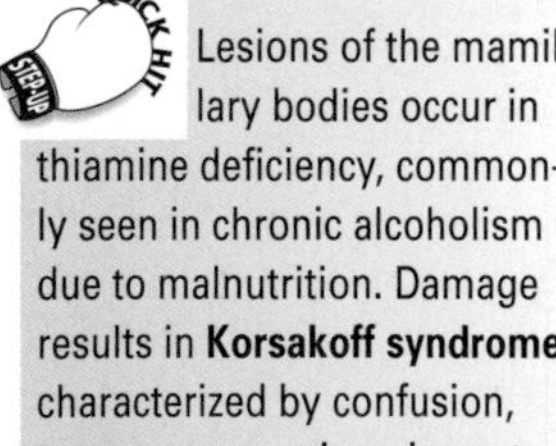

Lesions of the mamillary bodies occur in thiamine deficiency, commonly seen in chronic alcoholism due to malnutrition. Damage results in **Korsakoff syndrome**, characterized by confusion, severe memory impairment, and confabulation, which is **irreversible**.

VII. Limbic system

A. Mediates behavior and emotion, specifically
   1. Feeding
   2. Feeling (emotions)
   3. Fighting
   4. Fleeing
   5. Sexual activity

B. Primarily controlled by the hypothalamus and autonomic nervous system

C. Other important areas include
   1. Anterior nucleus of thalamus
   2. Cingulate gyrus
   3. Mamillary bodies
   4. Septal area
   5. Hippocampus
   6. Amygdala

COMMON OCULAR PATHOLOGY (Table 2-5) (Figures 2-11 AND 2-12)

TABLE 2-5 Common Ocular Pathology

Disorder	Etiology	Pathology	Clinical Features
Diabetic retinopathy	Proposed mechanism: accumulation of sorbitol in capillary pericytes results in loss of function leading to retinal ischemia	Nonproliferative type observes microaneurysms, flame hemorrhages, dot and blot hemorrhages, soft exudates (cotton-wool spots), hard exudates (deposits of protein that have leaked from damaged capillaries), venous beading; proliferative type also observes neovascularization and fibrosis	Loss of visual acuity; advanced disease major cause of blindness
Age-related macular degeneration	Proposed mechanism: genetic	Pigmentary changes (drusen), macular hemorrhage or edema	Loss of central vision
Cataract	Aging; diabetes; galactosemia, Hurler disease; congenital causes (trisomy, myotonic dystrophy, hypoglycemia, TORCH infections)	Opacity of lens as a result of precipitation of sorbitol (diabetes), galactitol (galactosemia), mucopolysaccharide (Hurler disease), lens proteins (senile)	Decreased visual acuity, glare
Hypertensive retinopathy	High blood pressure → damages capillary walls	Copper wiring, flame hemorrhages, arteriovenous nicking, optic disc swelling (acute rise in blood pressure)	
Atherosclerosis	Atherosclerotic plaque from carotid artery embolizes into ipsilateral retinal artery	Hollenhorst plaque; copper wiring, flame hemorrhages, arteriovenous nicking	Amaurosis fugax (transient loss in vision, classically described as "shade falling over eye")
Papilledema	Increased intracranial pressure	Optic disc swelling (bilateral)	Headache; no changes in visual acuity until advanced disease

TORCH, toxoplasmosis, other infections, rubella, cytomegalovirus, and herpes simplex virus.

FIGURE 2-11 Age-related macular degeneration
(Reproduced from Tasman W, Jaeger E. The Wills Eye Hospital Atlas of Ophthalmology. 2nd Ed. Baltimore, MD: Lippincott Williams & Wilkins, 2001, with permission.)

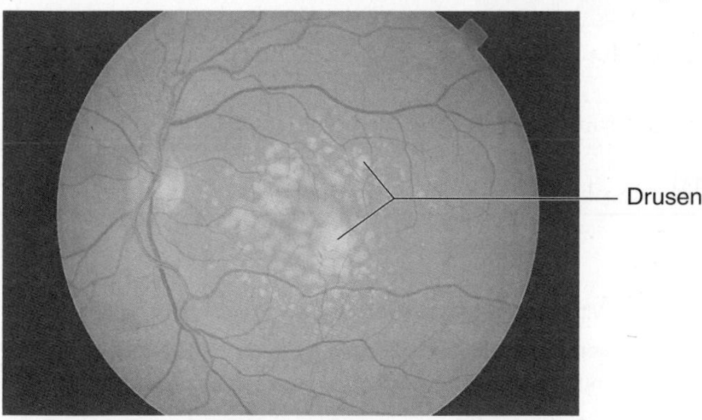

FIGURE 2-12 Diabetic retinopathy
(Reproduced from Tasman W, Jaeger E. The Wills Eye Hospital Atlas of Ophthalmology. 2nd Ed. Baltimore, MD: Lippincott Williams & Wilkins, 2001, with permission.)

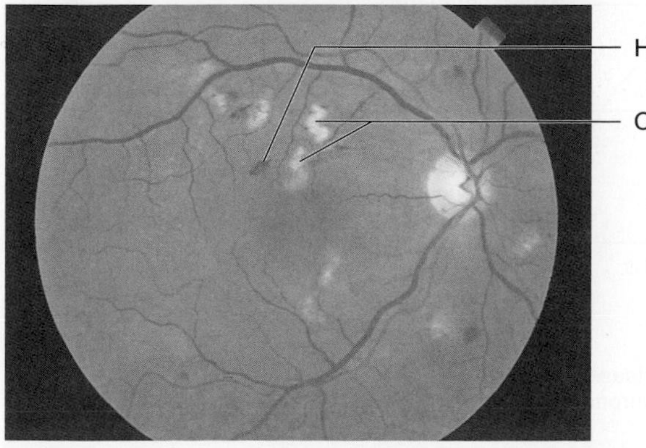

CLASSIC LESIONS OF THE SPINAL CORD (Figure 2-13)

FIGURE 2-13 Classic lesions of the spinal cord

A

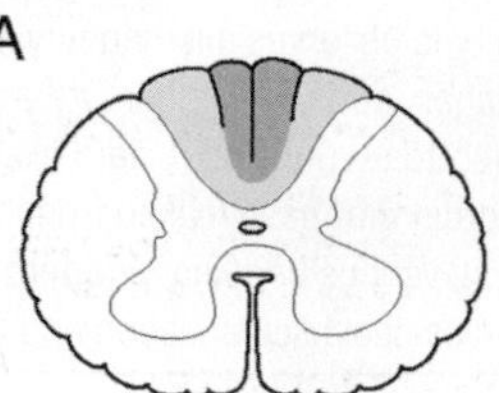

Tabes dorsalis

- Seen in tertiary syphilis
- Bilateral loss of touch, vibration and tactile sense from lower limbs due to lesion of fasciculus gracilis

B

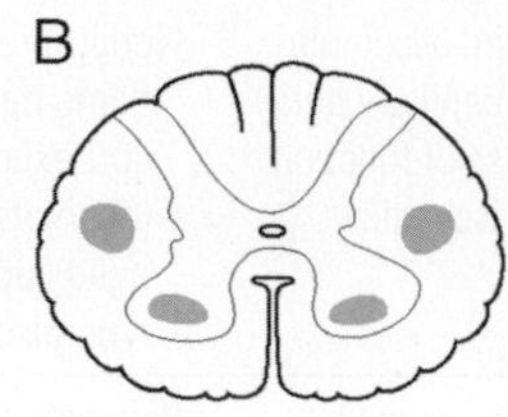

Amyotrophic lateral sclerosis

- Combined UMN and LMN lesion of corticospinal tract
- Spastic paresis (UMN sign)
- Flaccid paralysis with fasciculations (LMN)

C

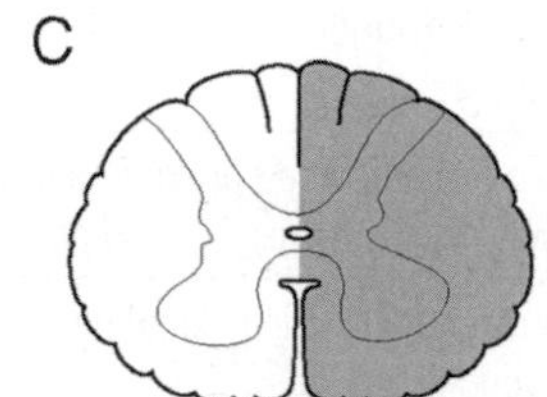

Brown-Séquard syndrome

- Ipsilateral loss of touch and vibration and tactile sense below lesion due to posterior white column lesion
- Contralateral loss of pain and touch due to loss of spinothalamic tract
- Ipsilateral spastic paresis below lesion due to lesion of corticospinal tract
- Ipsilateral flaccid paralysis at level of lesion due to loss of LMN
- If lesion occurs above T1, Horner's syndrome on side of lesion will result

D

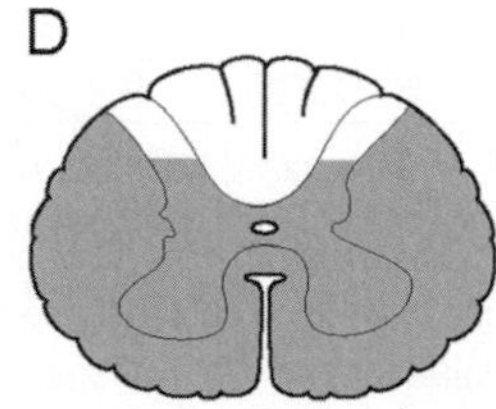

Spinal artery infarct

- Bilateral loss of pain and temperature one level below lesion due to loss of spinothalamic tract
- Bilateral spastic paresis below lesion due to lesion of corticospinal tract
- Bilateral flaccid paralysis at level of lesion due to loss of LMN
- Loss of bladder control due to lesion of corticospinal tract innervation of S2–S4 parasympathetics
- Bilateral Horner's syndrome if above T2

E

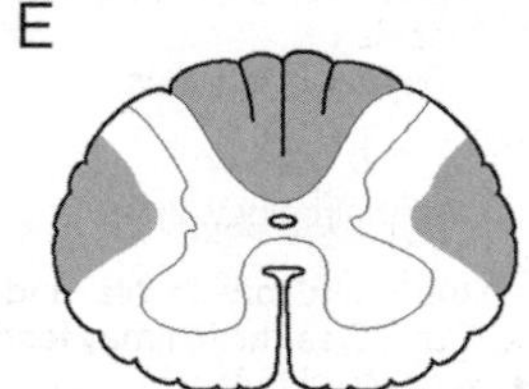

Subacute combined degeneration (Vitamin B_{12} deficiency)

- Bilateral loss of touch, vibration and tactile sense due to posterior white column lesion
- Bilateral spastic paresis below lesion due to lesion of corticospinal tracts

F

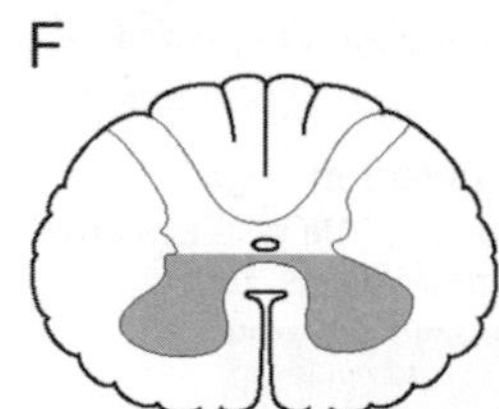

Syringomyelia

- Bilateral loss of pain and temperature one level below due to lesion of ventral white commissure (spinothalamic tract)
- Bilateral flaccid paralysis of level of lesion due to loss of LMN

HYPOTHALAMUS (Figure 2-14)

FIGURE 2-14 Hypothalamus

(Redrawn from Fix JD. High-Yield Neuroanatomy. Baltimore, MD: Williams & Wilkins, 1995:84, with permission.)

Paraventricular and supraoptic nuclei
- Regulate water balance
- Produce ADH and oxytocin
- Destruction causes diabetes insipidus

Anterior commissure

Anterior nucleus
- Thermal regulation (dissipation of heat)
- Stimulates parasympathetic NS
- Destruction results in hyperthermia

Preoptic area
- Contains sexual dimorphic nucleus
- Regulates release of gonadotropic hormones

Suprachiasmatic nucleus
- Receives input from retina
- Controls circadian rhythms

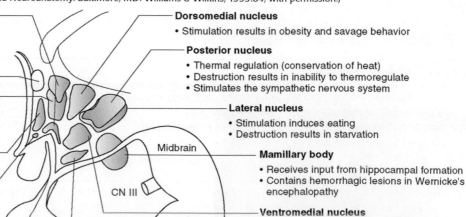

Dorsomedial nucleus
- Stimulation results in obesity and savage behavior

Posterior nucleus
- Thermal regulation (conservation of heat)
- Destruction results in inability to thermoregulate
- Stimulates the sympathetic nervous system

Lateral nucleus
- Stimulation induces eating
- Destruction results in starvation

Midbrain

Mamillary body
- Receives input from hippocampal formation
- Contains hemorrhagic lesions in Wernicke's encephalopathy

CN III

Pons

Ventromedial nucleus
- Satiety center
- Destruction results in obesity and savage behavior

Arcuate nucleus
- Produces hypothalamic releasing factors
- Contains DOPA-nergic neurons that inhibit prolactin release

THALAMUS (Figure 2-15)

FIGURE 2-15 Thalamus

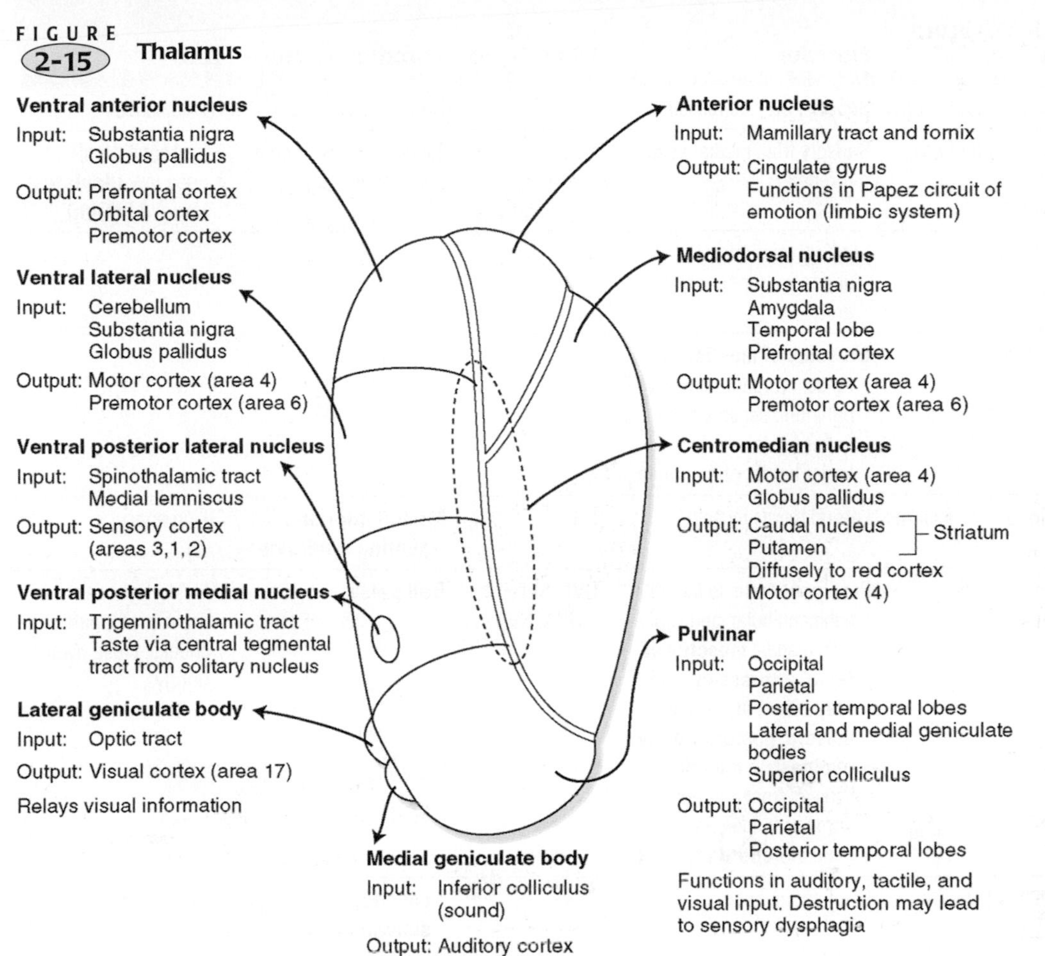

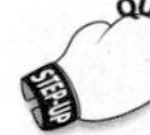

QUICK HIT: The olfactory neurons are the only neurons in the adult that actively divide.

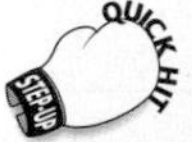

QUICK HIT: **Injury to CN III** (oculomotor) results in **ptosis** because of loss of the levator palpebrae superioris muscle, **exotropia** because of the unopposed pull of the lateral rectus, **dilation** of the pupil because of unopposed pull of the dilator pupillae muscle, and **impairment of near vision** as a result of loss of accommodation of the ciliary muscle.

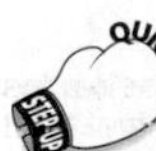

QUICK HIT: Weber syndrome is caused by a medial midbrain injury and results in ipsilateral CN III paralysis with contralateral spastic hemiparesis.

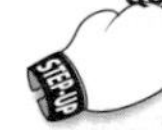

QUICK HIT: The trochlear nerve is particularly susceptible to head trauma owing to its course around the midbrain.

QUICK HIT: Tic douloureux (trigeminal neuralgia) is marked by severe stabbing bursts of pain in the distribution of CN V.

CRANIAL NERVES

The 12 cranial nerves arise from various nuclei within the brain stem and cortex and serve multiple functions in the body. Their extracranial course is important for locating lesions, which can be tested by asking the patient to perform simple tasks. Table 2-6 outlines important information about cranial nerves I to XII.

TABLE 2-6 Cranial Nerves

Nerve	Site of Exit From Skull	Function	Fiber Types	Common Lesions	Test
I—Olfactory	Cribriform	Smell	SVA	Cribriform plate fracture; Kallmann syndrome	Smell
II—Optic	Optic canal	Sight	SSA	Figure 2-9	Snellen chart; peripheral vision
III—Oculomotor	Superior orbital fissure	**Parasympathetic** to **ciliary** and **sphincter muscles;** medial rectus, superior rectus, inferior rectus, inferior oblique	GVE, GSE	Transtentorial (uncal) herniation; **diabetes;** Weber syndrome	"H" in space; pupillary light reflexes; convergence

(continued)

TABLE 2-6 Cranial Nerves *(Continued)*

Nerve	Site of Exit From Skull	Function	Fiber Types	Common Lesions	Test
IV—Trochlear	Superior orbital fissure	Superior oblique muscle	GSE	Head trauma	"H" in space
V—Trigeminal V1—Ophthalmic	Superior orbital fissure	Sensory from medial nose, forehead	SVE, GSA	Tic douloureux (trigeminal neuralgia)	Facial sensation; open jaw **(deviates toward lesion)**
V2—Maxillary	Foramen rotundum	Sensory from lateral nose, upper lip, superior buccal area			
V3—Mandibular	Foramen ovale	**Muscles of mastication,** tensor tympani, tensor veli palantini; sensory from lower lip, lateral face to lower border of mandible			
VI—Abducens	Superior orbital fissure	Lateral rectus muscle	GSE	**Medial inferior pontine syndrome**	"H" in space
VII—Facial	Internal acoustic meatus	Parasympathetic to lacrimal, submandibular, and sublingual glands; **muscles of facial expression and stapedius, stylohyoid muscle, posterior belly of digastric muscle;** sensory from anterior two thirds of tongue (including taste **via chorda tympani**)	GVE, SVE, GSA, SVA	**Bell palsy**	Wrinkle forehead; show teeth; puff out cheeks; close eyes tightly
VIII—Vestibulocochlear	Internal acoustic meatus	Equilibrium; hearing	SSA	**Acoustic schwannoma**	Hearing; nystagmus (slow phase toward lesion)
IX—Glossopharyngeal	Jugular foramen	Parasympathetic to parotid gland; stylopharyngeus muscle; sensory from pharynx, middle ear, auditory tube, carotid body and sinus, external ear, posterior third of tongue (including taste)	GVE, SVE, GSA, GVA, SVA	Posterior inferior cerebellar artery **(PICA)** infarct	Gag reflex (no response ipsilateral to lesion)
X—Vagus	Jugular foramen	Parasympathetic to body viscera; laryngeal and pharyngeal muscles; sensory from trachea, esophagus, viscera, external ear, epiglottis (including taste)	GVE, SVE, GSA, GVA, SVA	Thyroidectomy, **PICA** infarct	Gag reflex **(uvula deviates away from lesion)**
XI—Accessory	Jugular foramen	Sternocleidomastoid and trapezius muscles	SVE	**PICA** infarct	Turning head (weakness turning away from lesion); raising shoulder against resistance (ipsilateral)
XII—Hypoglossal	Hypoglossal canal	Intrinsic tongue muscles	GSE	Anterior spinal artery infarct	Tongue protrusion **(deviates toward lesion)**

GSA, general somatic afferent; GSE, general somatic efferent; GVA, general visceral afferent; GVE, general visceral efferent; SSA, special somatic afferent; SVA, special visceral afferent; SVE, special visceral efferent.

CONTENTS OF THE CAVERNOUS SINUS (Figure 2-16)

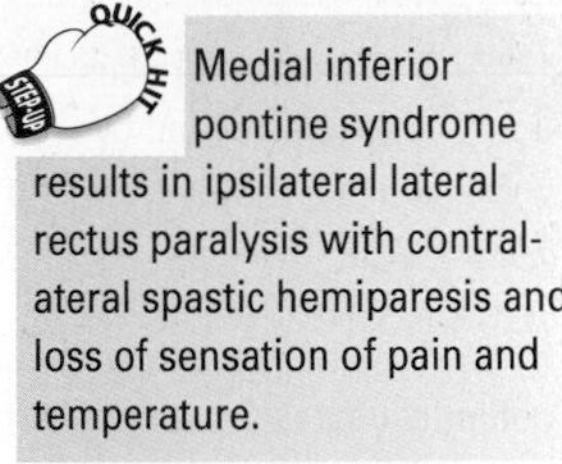

Medial inferior pontine syndrome results in ipsilateral lateral rectus paralysis with contralateral spastic hemiparesis and loss of sensation of pain and temperature.

FIGURE 2-16 **Contents of the cavernous sinus**

(Adapted from Bushan V, Le T, Amin C. First Aid for the USMLE Step 1. Stamford, CT: Appleton & Lange, 1999:110, with permission.)

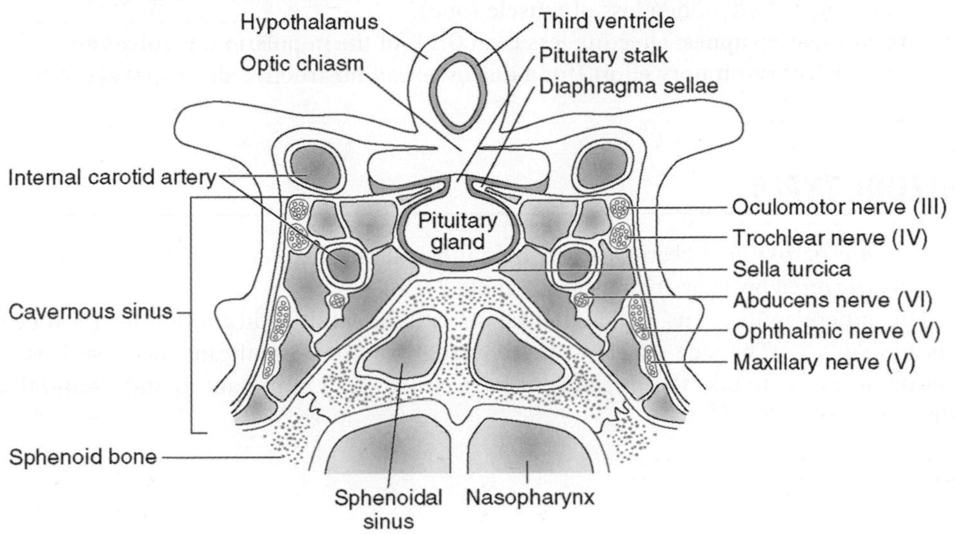

SLEEP (Figure 2-17)

FIGURE 2-17 **The sleep cycle**

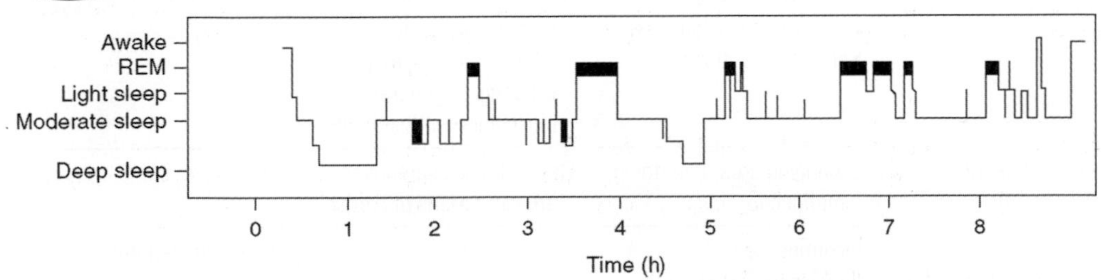

Stages of REM sleep in the young adult. As sleep progresses, slow wave sleep decreases and REM sleep episodes increase in duration and frequency. In the elderly, there is decreased slow wave sleep, increased awakenings, early sleep onset, and early morning awakenings. Solid bars indicate REM sleep.

I. Sleep–wake cycles

A. Based on circadian rhythms controlled by the suprachiasmatic nucleus of the hypothalamus.
B. **Serotonin** released from the raphe nuclei of the brain stem is important in initiating sleep, whereas the **reticular activating system** maintains alertness.
C. **Stage 1** of sleep (when an individual is alert and relaxed) shows **alpha waves** on electroencephalograph (EEG).
D. **Stages 3 and 4** of sleep are called delta sleep and show **slow waves** on EEG.
E. Dreaming occurs during rapid eye movement (REM) sleep, which normally occurs at 90-min intervals. During this period of "paradoxical sleep" the EEG registers beta waves, which mirror those seen in the alert individual in the waking state.

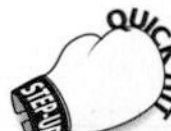

The time spent in stage 4 sleep decreases with age and with the use of some drugs (e.g., benzodiazepines).

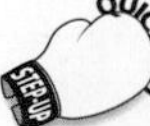

Slow-wave sleep, which is the deepest, most relaxed sleep, is the sleep stage in which night terrors, bed-wetting, and sleepwalking occur.

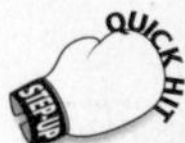

Status epilepticus (characterized by continuous or rapidly recurring seizures with no return of consciousness) can be caused by any type of seizure and is potentially fatal. Treatment is intravenous diazepam.

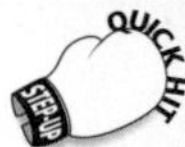

Barbiturates and benzodiazepines are **sedative-hypnotics** that are often used to treat seizure activity. The more common examples are flurazepam, phenobarbital, temazepam, triazolam, and zolpidem.

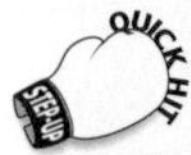

Narcolepsy can be associated with hypnagogic hallucinations upon going to sleep, and hypnapompic hallucinations upon awakening.

II. Common sleep disorders

A. Insomnia affects 30% of the US population. It is associated with anxiety and leads to daytime sleepiness.

B. Narcolepsy is seen in 0.04% of the population and is characterized by sudden onset of sleep with rapid onset of REM sleep. It may be associated with hallucinations and cataplexy (sudden loss of muscle tone).

C. Central sleep apnea, affecting less than 0.5% of the population, involves an absence of respiratory effort (for a discussion of obstructive sleep apnea, see System 4.)

SEIZURE TYPES

Seizures are paroxysmal events caused by abnormal and excessive discharges from CNS neurons triggered by a variety of causes (Table 2-7).

The antiepileptic agents, which include several different medications, affect **ion channels** (Table 2-8). The side effects of these agents are often significant. Because it is frequently necessary to take these agents for long periods, it is important to understand these side effects.

TABLE 2-7 Seizure Types

Type	Patient	Presentation	Pathology	Treatment
Simple partial seizures	All ages	Malfunction of one muscle or muscle group No loss of consciousness Sensory distortions	Single focus in brain No spread, localized muscular manifestations With chronicity, may progress to generalized muscular manifestations	Phenytoin; carbamazepine
Jacksonian seizures	All ages (subtype of simple partial)	Expanding area of motor malfunction	Original focus spreads to adjacent areas of cortex	Carbamazepine
Complex partial seizures	First seizure during first two decades of life may be caused by fever in children 6 months to 5 years of age (febrile seizure)	Incontinence Jaw movements (or other automatisms) Loss of consciousness Elaborate sensory distortions	Single focus	Phenytoin; carbamazepine
Absence (petit mal) seizures	Begin at 2–3 years of age Often end with puberty	1–5 s loss of consciousness Several episodes per day Blank stare with rapid blinking	Original focus rapidly **spreads across both hemispheres**	Ethosuximide, valproic acid
Tonic–clonic (grand mal) seizures	Most common type Encountered in different clinical settings, often in patients with metabolic disorders	Sudden loss of consciousness Loss of postural control and continence Tonic phase (static extension) Clonic phase (jerking movements) Recovery period with exhaustion and disorientation	Original focus rapidly spreads across both hemispheres	Phenytoin; carbamazepine

TABLE 2-8 Antiepileptic Agents

Drug	Mechanism of Action	Type(s) of Seizure(s) Controlled	Side Effects	Notes
Carbamazepine	Blocks voltage-gated **sodium channels** by increasing the refractory period	Tonic–clonic (grand mal) Partial Jacksonian	Liver enzyme induction, ataxia, diplopia, blood dyscrasias (agranulocytosis, aplastic anemia), teratogenesis, **induction of cytochrome P450**	Can be used to treat trigeminal neuralgia
Ethosuximide	Inhibits certain **sodium channels,** particularly in certain parts of thalamus that produce cyclic cortical discharges	Absence	Headache, lethargy, diarrhea, urticaria, Stevens–Johnson syndrome	
Phenytoin	Blocks voltage-gated **sodium channels** by increasing refractory period	Tonic–clonic (grand mal) Partial	Liver enzyme induction, ataxia, diplopia, megaloblastic anemia, lupuslike syndrome, nystagmus, sedation, teratogenesis (fetal hydantoin syndrome), peripheral neuropathy, **hirsutism, gingival hyperplasia, induction of cytochrome P450,** malignant hyperthermia (rare)	
Valproic acid	May affect **potassium channels** to cause hyperpolarization of neuronal membranes	Absence Tonic–clonic (grand mal) Partial	Liver enzyme induction, diarrhea; rarely hepatotoxic, tremor, weight gain, neural tube defects in fetus (spina bifida)	Contraindicated in pregnancy
Phenobarbital (Barbiturate)	Increase inhibitory effects of γ-aminobutyric acid (GABA) by increasing **duration of chloride channel** opening	Tonic–clonic (grand mal) Partial	Liver enzyme induction, sedation, tolerance, dependence, induction of cytochrome P450	First line in pregnant women, children
Benzodiazepines (Diazepam, Lorazepam)	Increase inhibitory effects of γ-aminobutyric acid (GABA) by increasing **frequency of chloride channel** opening	First line for acute **status epilepticus**	Sedation, tolerance, dependence	Used for seizures of eclampsia
Lamotrigine	Blocks voltage-gated sodium channels	Tonic–clonic (grand mal) Partial	Stevens–Johnson syndrome	
Gabapentin	Increases GABA release	Tonic–clonic (grand mal) Partial	Sedation, ataxia	Used for peripheral neuropathy
Topiramate	Blocks sodium channels, increases $GABA_A$ action	Tonic–clonic (grand mal) Partial	Sedation, weight loss, nephrolithiasis	

DEGENERATIVE DISEASES

Degeneration in specific parts of the CNS can lead to focal or systemic loss of function. Many of the degenerative diseases affecting the CNS are irreversible, and are listed in Table 2-9.

Parkinson disease, a movement disorder, results from deterioration of the **basal ganglia. Dopamine** production decreases, which in turn increases the relative effects of **acetylcholine.** Treatment is symptomatic and is aimed at trying to restore the balance between the two hormones (Table 2-10).

QUICK HIT: CNS stimulants, which are at the other end of the spectrum from the sedative-hypnotics, usually cause sympathetic stimulation, resulting in increased alertness. They can also lower the seizure threshold. Common drugs of this type are amphetamine, caffeine, cocaine, dextroamphetamine, ephedrine, and methylphenidate.

(text continues on page 68)

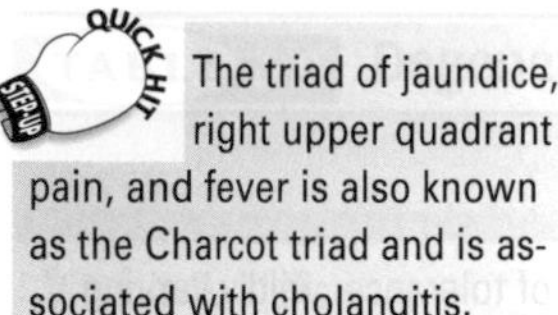

The triad of jaundice, right upper quadrant pain, and fever is also known as the Charcot triad and is associated with cholangitis.

Clinical Vignette 2-2 *(Continued)*

neuritis. Optic neuritis presents as monocular visual loss, pain on movement of eyes, central scotoma (black spot in center of vision), or decreased pupillary reaction to light. Also, be aware of the **Charcot triad:** intention tremor, nystagmus, and scanning speech.

Management: Treat this patient with **high-dose intravenous (IV) corticosteroids,** which can shorten an **acute** attack. After treatment of an acute attack, manage patient with **interferon therapy,** which should be started early in the course of disease. Treat symptoms of muscle spasticity with baclofen and carbamazepine or gabapentin for neuropathic pain.

DEMYELINATING DISEASES

Loss of the neuronal sheath can lead to impaired nerve conduction, which, in turn, causes deficits and disease (Table 2-11).

QUICK HIT: Werdnig–Hoffmann disease is an infantile, autosomal recessive, and lower motor neuron disease similar to ALS.

QUICK HIT: Progressive multifocal leukoencephalopathy is a demyelinating disease caused by JC virus infection of oligodendrocytes. It is seen in patients with immune deficiency.

QUICK HIT: Subacute sclerosing panencephalitis is a demyelinating disease caused by the measles virus. Infection is chronic but progressive and ultimately fatal.

TABLE 2-11 Demyelinating Diseases of the Nervous System

Disease	Etiology	Clinical Manifestation	Notes
Amyotrophic lateral sclerosis (ALS, Lou Gehrig disease)	No specific pattern of inheritance, although autosomal dominant in 5% of cases (similar symptoms with some heavy metal poisonings, infections, or tumors)	**Both upper and lower motor neuron signs;** loss of lateral corticospinal tracts and anterior motor neurons leading to muscle atrophy	Most common motor neuron disease; rapidly fatal course
Guillain–Barré syndrome	Postviral autoimmune reaction involving peripheral nerves	Muscle weakness and paralysis **ascending upward** from the lower extremities	Young adults; **albuminocytologic dissociation is** pathognomonic (high albumin, low cell count)
Huntington disease	Chromosome 4; **CAG triple-base repeat** with anticipation	Degeneration of **caudate nucleus**; onset at 30–40 years of age; athetoid movements; muscular deterioration; dementia	Usually involves acetylcholine (ACh) and γ-aminobutyric acid (GABA) neurons
Krabbe disease	Autosomal recessive; decrease in β-galactocerebrosidase	Loss of myelin from globoid cells and peripheral nerves; mental retardation; blindness; paralysis; **globoid-bodies** in white matter	Usually affects infants; **rapidly fatal**
Metachromatic leukodystrophy	Autosomal recessive defect of arylsulfatase A	Progressive paralysis and dementia; loss of myelin; accumulation of sulfatides; nerves stain **yellow-brown** in color; ataxia	Fatal in first decade
Multiple sclerosis	Unknown; more common in northern Europe; more common in women	Multiple focal areas of demyelination; variable course; **Triad of MS:** intention tremor, scanning speech, nystagmus	Most common demyelinating disease; increased cerebrospinal fluid (CSF) immunoglobulin

DISEASES THAT CAUSE DEMENTIA

Dementia is a chronic progressive deterioration in cognitive ability in which mental faculties, such as executive function, attention span, judgment, memory, mood, and behavior are affected (Table 2-12).

TABLE 2-12 Diseases that Cause Dementia

Disease	Etiology	Clinical Manifestation	Notes
Alzheimer dementia	Unknown; possibly **chromosome 21**; degeneration of nucleus basalis of Meynert; decreased choline acetyltransferase	Progressively worsening memory loss; **neurofibrillary tangles; senile plaques** (amyloid **β/A4** protein); Hirano bodies	**Most common cause of dementia;** age of onset is usually 65 years (younger in Down syndrome patients)
Multi-infarct dementia	Cerebral atherosclerosis	Stepwise decline of function; signs of dementia and motor deficits	**Second most common cause of dementia**
Primary HIV dementia	Macrophages, infected with HIV, enter CNS	Onset before immunodeficiency; slow thinking; ataxia; Toxoplasma gondii on autopsy	**Most common CNS manifestation of HIV**

CNS, central nervous system.

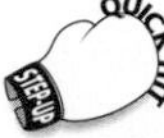

Dementia is a chronic loss of cognitive function without an altered level of consciousness. Delirium is an acute altered level of consciousness accompanied by disordered cognition.

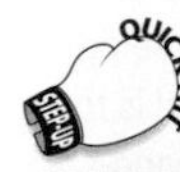

Toxoplasma gondii can infect the immunocompromised individual via three routes: undercooked meat, cat feces, or in utero. It is the most common CNS infection in AIDS patients.

MNEMONIC

To recall the features of Alzheimer disease, remember **RONALD** Reagan:
Reduced acetylcholine
Old age
Neurofibrillary tangles
Amyloid plaques; **A**trophy of cerebral cortex
Language impairment
Dementia/**D**own syndrome

ACUTE MENINGITIS

Meningitis is an infection of the meninges resulting in an inflammatory reaction characterized by severe headache, fever, photophobia, and positive **Kernig** and **Brudzinski** signs. **Meningitis in** immunocompetent adults is generally caused by *Streptococcus pneumoniae* or *Neisseria meningitidis*. Conditions predisposing an individual to acute bacterial meningitis as a result of pneumococcus include distant foci of infection (such as otitis, sinusitis, or pneumonia), sickle cell disease (secondary to splenic autoinfarction), alcoholism, or trauma with loss of meningeal integrity. Patients with a deficiency of complement components C5–C8 are at a greater risk of developing meningococcal meningitis. *Haemophilus influenzae*, type B, is a common cause of meningitis in children, although these numbers are decreasing because of widespread use of a capsular polyribitol phosphate vaccine conjugated to diphtheria toxoid (Table 2-13).

TABLE 2-13 Common Causes of Meningitis in Various Age Groups

Age Group	Causes
Newborns	Group B streptococci *Escherichia coli* Listeria
Children	*Haemophilus influenzae* b (declining since Hib vaccine introduced) *Streptococcus pneumoniae* *Neisseria meningitidis* Enteroviruses
Adolescents and young adults	Enteroviruses *Neisseria meningitidis* *Streptococcus pneumoniae* Herpes simplex virus
Elderly	*Streptococcus pneumoniae* Gram-negative rods *Listeria*

TABLE 2-14 Evaluation of Cerebrospinal Fluid to Determine Cause of Meningitis

Laboratory Test	Bacterial	Viral	Fungal
Opening CSF pressure	↑	N	↑
Lymphocytes	N	↑	↑
Neutrophils	↑	N	N
Glucose	↓	N	↓
Protein	↑	N	↑

↑, Increased; ↓, decreased; CSF, cerebrospinal fluid; N, normal.

QUICK HIT: **Prevnar** is a heptavalent pneumococcal conjugate vaccine that is being given to children. The goal is to prevent invasive pneumococcal infections. The 23 serotypes used to make the immunization are thought to be responsible for the majority of severe, invasive pneumococcal infections. Common, less-invasive infections, such as otitis media, are unlikely to be affected because many other serotypes are not included in the vaccine.

Lumbar puncture (LP) is often performed to confirm a suspected diagnosis of meningitis. The LP usually shows increased neutrophils, increased protein, and decreased glucose if bacterial in origin. Also, organisms may be seen on Gram stain. However, if the CSF contains increased lymphocytes and a normal glucose level, viral agents such as **enterovirus**, HIV, and herpes simplex virus should be considered (Table 2-14). If the LP shows organisms with a thick capsule when stained with India ink, this suggests *Cryptococcus neoformans*, and the infected individual is most likely immunocompromised as a result of HIV infection. Immunocompromised adults are also at risk for developing meningitis caused by *Listeria monocytogenes*.

NERVOUS SYSTEM TUMORS

Nearly 50% of the tumors occurring within the nervous system are primary tumors. The other 50% are metastases to the brain from tumors elsewhere in the body. Table 2-15 lists nervous system tumors in order of clinical significance.

TABLE 2-15 Nervous System Tumors

Tumor	Presentation	Significant Features
Glioblastoma multiforme (grade IV astrocytoma)	Cerebral hemisphere tumor; irregular mass with necrotic center surrounded by edema seen on CT; **pseudopalisading** arrangement of cells	**Most common primary intracranial neoplasm;** poor prognosis; neural tube origin
Meningioma	**Psammoma bodies;** slowly growing; originates in arachnoid cells; follows sinuses	Second most common primary CNS tumor; usually occurs in women; resectable; neural crest origin
Medulloblastoma	Ataxic gait; projectile vomiting; cerebellar mass; highly malignant; tightly packed cells in rosette pattern	**Most common intracranial tumor of childhood;** neural tube origin
Craniopharyngioma	Papilledema; endocrine abnormalities; **bitemporal hemianopsia**	Enlarged sella turcica; **most common supratentorial brain tumor in children; ectodermal origin** (Rathke pouch)
Schwannoma	Hearing loss; ataxic gait; positive Romberg sign; increased intracranial pressure; hydrocephalus; benign	Usually occurs in the cerebellopontine angle and involves CN VIII; seen **bilaterally in neurofibromatosis type 2 (NF-2)**; third most common primary intracranial tumor; neural crest origin
Neuroblastoma	Occurs in cerebral hemispheres; related to neuroblastoma of adrenal gland	Increasing **N-myc amplification** directly proportional to worsening prognosis; seen in children; neural crest origin
Ependymoma	Hydrocephalus; blocked fourth ventricle; rosettes surround fourth ventricle	Seen in children; neural tube origin
Metastatic neoplasms	Headache; focal defects; formation of discrete nodules in brain	Nearly half of all intracranial neoplasm; usually bloodborne; commonly from lung, breast, gastrointestinal, thyroid, kidney, genitourinary, and melanoma

HEADACHE (Table 2-16)

TABLE 2-16 Primary Headache Syndromes

Type	General Characteristics	Clinical Features	Treatment
Tension	Worsens throughout the day; precipitated by stress, anxiety, and depression; more frequent in women	Tight, **bandlike** pain encircling the entire head; most intense around the neck or back of head; tenderness in posterior neck muscles	Stress reduction, NSAIDs, acetaminophen, and aspirin if mild/moderate; if severe, TCAs or SSRIs
Cluster	Usually occurs in **middle-age men; episodic**—lasts 2–3 months, with remissions of months to years; occurs around bedtime and lasts 30–90 min	Excruciating periorbital pain **("behind the eye"), unilateral; stabbing or deep, burning pain;** accompanied by ipsilateral lacrimation, nasal congestion or discharge, facial flushing	Acute: **sumatriptan, O_2 inhalation** Prophylaxis: **verapamil** taken daily —drug of choice (alternatives: ergotamine, methylithium, sergide, corticosteroids)
Migraine	**Inherited;** caused by serotonin depletion; women > men; family history Subtypes: 1. **classic:** migraine with **aura** (aura usually visual such as flashing lights, scotoma, visual distortions) 2. **common:** migraine without aura 3. **menstrual**	Prodromal phase; severe **throbbing or dull achy unilateral headaches**, may be generalized; lasts for 4–72 h; pain is **aggravated by coughing, physical activity, and bending down;** other symptoms include nausea and vomiting, photophobia, and increased sensitivity to smell	Acute: NSAIDs, dihydroergotamine, sumatriptan Prophylaxis: first-line—TCAs and propranolol; second-line—verapamil, valproic acid, and methysergide

cAMP, cyclic adenosine monophosphate; cGMP, cyclic guanosine monophosphate; NSAID, nonsteroidal anti-inflammatory drug; SSRI, selective serotonin reuptake inhibitor; TCA, tricyclic antidepressant.

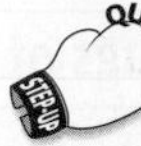

Tumors of the CNS are usually intracranial, with **adult tumors** commonly **supratentorial** and **childhood** tumors usually **infratentorial.**

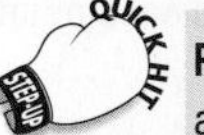

Psammoma bodies are also seen in papillary adenocarcinoma of the thyroid, serous papillary cystadenocarcinoma of the ovary, and malignant mesothelioma.

MNEMONIC

ClAssic migraines have an **A**ura, common migraines are without aura.

PSYCHIATRY AND BEHAVIORAL SCIENCE

I. Drugs of abuse and dependence (Table 2-17)

II. Defense mechanisms (Table 2-18)

III. Personality disorders (Table 2-19)

IV. Psychoses and other neuropsychiatric disorders (Table 2-20)

V. Antidepressants (Table 2-21)

The "**amine theory**" attributes mood to levels of certain amines such as norepinephrine (NE) and serotonin (5-HT). It is theorized that low levels of these hormones lead to depression, and many of the antidepressants **boost amine levels**. Originally, the agents used as antidepressants boosted both NE and 5-HT levels. Today, however, drugs that selectively increase 5-HT levels are preferred because they have fewer side effects. The sites of action of the antidepressants are represented graphically (Figure 2-18).

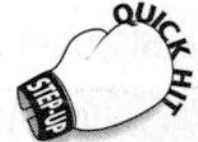

Substance abuse is defined as use of psychoactive substances for at least 1 month with interference in the user's life, but without meeting the criteria for dependence. Substance dependence involves craving, withdrawal, and tolerance.

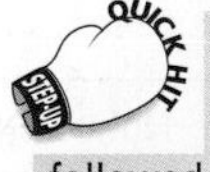

Alcohol is the most widely used drug, followed by nicotine. Caffeine is the most often used psychoactive substance, followed by nicotine.

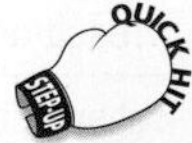

Dependence is mediated by **Dopamine**, the neurotransmitter linked to the pleasure and reward center.

(text continues on page 76)

TABLE 2-17 Drugs of Abuse and Dependence

Drug	Mechanism	Intoxication Effect	Withdrawal Effects
Alcohol	Unknown; possible effect at GABA receptor directly on membranes	Sedation; hypnosis; slurred speech; ataxia; loss of motor coordination; Wernicke–Korsakoff syndrome	Malaise; tachycardia; tremors; seizures; **delirium tremens;** death
Amphetamine	Release of intracellular stores of catecholamines	Insomnia; irritability; tremor; hyperactive reflexes; arrhythmias; anorexia; psychosis	Lethargy; depression; hunger; craving for drug resulting in bizarre psychological behavior; anxiety
Barbiturates	**Potentiation of GABA** action on chloride by **increase of duration** of chloride channel opening	Mental sluggishness; anesthesia; hypnosis	Restlessness; anxiety; tremor; death
Caffeine	Translocation of Ca^{2+}; inhibition of phosphodiesterase (increase in cAMP, cGMP)	Insomnia; anxiety; agitation	Lethargy; irritability; headache
Cocaine	Blockade of norepinephrine, serotonin, and dopamine reuptake	Hallucinations; anxiety; arrhythmias; nasal problems; sudden death	Craving; depression; excessive sleeping; fatigue
Lysergic acid diethylamide (LSD)	5-HT agonist action in the midbrain	Pupillary dilation; increased blood pressure and body temperature; piloerection; hallucinations	Flashbacks
Marijuana	Unknown; tetrahydro cannabinol (THC) is active compound; possible endogenous receptors in brain	Increased appetite; visual hallucinations; increased heart rate; decreased blood pressure Impairment of short-term memory and mental activity	
Nicotine	Low doses—ganglionic stimulation; high doses—ganglionic blockade	**Increased heart rate and blood pressure;** irritability; tremors; intestinal cramps	Irritability; anxiety; restlessness; headaches; insomnia; difficulty in concentrating
Opioids (heroin)	Inhibition of adenylate cyclase by opioid receptors within the CNS	Constipation; **pinpoint pupils;** potentially lethal via **respiratory depression;** sedation	Insomnia; diarrhea; sweating; fever; piloerection
Phencyclidine (PCP)	Inhibition of dopamine, serotonin, and norepinephrine reuptake	Hostile, bizarre behavior; hypersalivation; anesthesia	Sudden onset of violent behavior

cAMP, cyclic adenosine monophosphate; cGMP, cyclic guanosine monophosphate; CNS, central nervous system; GABA, γ-aminobutyric acid; 5-HT, 5-hydroxytryptamine (serotonin).

TABLE 2-18 Defense Mechanisms

Mechanism	Characteristics	Example
Acting out	Stress is dealt with through actions; immature	After the death of his brother, a priest breaks all the windows in his church
Denial	Not accepting the reality of a situation; immature	A woman refuses to consider the possibility of pregnancy after having unprotected intercourse and missing two periods
Displacement	Feelings for causal source are transferred to another object; immature	A man kicks his dog after getting fired from his job
Dissociation	Loss of memory or change in personality as a result of stressor; immature	A woman who was sexually abused as a child develops another personality
Identification	Behavior patterned after another; immature	A teenager smokes pot because his favorite rock star does
Intellectualization	Reason is used to cope with anxiety; immature	A physician starts reading textbooks and journal articles about her father's cancer
Isolation of affect	Events are separated from emotion; immature	An airline passenger describes an emergency landing to his family without any emotion
Projection	One's own characteristics are applied to another; immature	A flirtatious man accuses his wife of cheating

(continued)

TABLE 2-18 Defense Mechanisms *(Continued)*

Mechanism	Characteristics	Example
Rationalization	Analytical reason is used to justify unacceptable feelings; immature	A man claims that his driving under the influence arrest would never have happened if his softball team had won
Reaction formation	Feelings are denied and opposite actions are performed; immature	A woman who wants to cheat on her husband instead buys him a new car
Regression	Stress-induced behavior that involves returning to a childlike state; immature	Medical students have a food fight during their lunch break on the day of board examinations
Repression	Holding back an unacceptable feeling or idea from reaching consciousness; immature	A recent widower feels no sense of loss
Splitting	Feelings or stressors are placed in distinct, opposite compartments (i.e., either all good or all bad); immature	A man in a doctor's office describes how much he hates the nurses, but loves the receptionist
Altruism	One unselfishly assists others; mature	A woman donates her entire estate to her favorite charities upon her death
Humor	Humor is used to reduce stress; mature	While stuck in an elevator, a young man makes jokes to ease the tension
Sublimation	Unacceptable impulse is directed into a socially accepted action; mature	A boy who got into a lot of fights as a kid decides to become a professional boxer
Suppression	Conscious effort to suppress thoughts or feelings; mature	A recent widower actively refuses to think about his deceased wife while packing her things away

TABLE 2-19 Personality Disorders

Disorder	Characteristics	Example
CLUSTER A		
Paranoid	Hostile; suspicious; mistrustful; usually male	A patient being prepared for surgery yells at the doctors on rounds because he feels they are gossiping about him
Schizoid	**Voluntarily** socially withdrawn without psychological problems; usually male	A 52-year-old computer programmer lives alone, is not married, has no friends, and is content
Schizotypal	Odd behavior, thoughts, and appearance without psychosis	A woman wears many-layered clothing and inappropriately applied makeup, and only talks to people with brown-colored hair
CLUSTER B		
Histrionic	Dramatic; overemotional; sexually provocative; unable to maintain close friendships; usually female	A woman exaggerates her suffering over a mild cold, and behaves seductively toward the physician
Narcissistic	Grandiosity, hypersensitivity to criticism, and lack of empathy	A resident refuses to operate with anyone but the best surgeon in the hospital because he feels it is beneath his talent
Antisocial	Inability to conform to societal rules; criminal behavior; more often males, requires diagnosis of conduct disorder as child	A multiple rapist has no concern for his victims or the law
Borderline	Unstable; impulsive; suicide attempts, vulnerable to abandonment; usually female; uses splitting	After an argument with her boyfriend, a woman chases him out of her home and later calls him and tells him she cannot live without him
CLUSTER C		
Avoidant	Shy; **involuntarily** (compare to schizoid) withdrawn because fears rejection; usually female	A businesswoman defers speaking during presentations to her project partner and has few friends
Obsessive–compulsive	Rigid; perfectionist; stubborn; orderly. Found twice as often in males	A businessman works long hours on a project, holding up both the project deadline and his personal life in vain attempts to make it perfect
Dependent	Defers decision making; not comfortable with an authority position; insecure; has the ability to make long-lasting relationships (unlike avoidant); usually female	A third-year resident often accepts on-call duty for other residents, never speaks up when talked down to by the junior residents, and has trouble writing orders
Passive–aggressive	Obstinate; inefficient; procrastinating; noncompliant	School student intentionally does poorly on homework because he does not like his teacher

TABLE 2-20 Psychoses and Other Neuropsychiatric Disorders

Disorder	Characteristics	Neurotransmitter(s) Involved	Treatment	Notes
Anorexia nervosa	Body weight < 85% of predicted		Antidepressants; cyproheptadine; family therapy	Higher incidence in females and **upper-middle socioeconomic classes**; amenorrhea; decreased libido
Attention deficit hyperactivity disorder (ADHD)	Hyperactive; poor attention span; highly sensitive to stimuli		Amphetamines (methylphenidate)	More common in **male children**
Bipolar disorder	Rapid speech, decreased need for sleep, hyperenergetic state, impaired judgment followed by a state of depression	Decreased serotonin	**Lithium**	
Bulimia nervosa	Purging after binge eating; **normal weight;** abuse of laxatives		Behavioral therapy; psychotherapy fluoxetine; MAOI	Normal libido; no amenorrhea (unlike anorexics); erosion of tooth enamel
Delirium	Impaired cognitive processes; diurnal variation in mood (worse at night—**"sundowning"**); illusions and hallucinations	Autonomic dysfunction	Treat the underlying cause	**Most common** problem in hospitalized psychiatric patients
Dissociative disorders	Psychological factors resulting in memory loss and loss of function		Psychotherapy; hypnotherapy; medication for associated symptoms	Includes amnesia, fugue, identity disorder, depersonalization
Generalized anxiety disorder	Generalized, persistent anxiety; tension; insomnia; irritability	Decreased serotonin, norepinephrine, GABA	Buspirone; benzodiazepines; **SSRIs**	Anxiety for more than **6 months**
Major depressive disorder	**Early morning waking;** anhedonia; depressed mood; suicidal thoughts	Decreased norepinephrine and serotonin	SSRIs; TCAs, or MAOIs; electroconvulsive therapy; hospitalization	Decreased REM latency and slow-wave sleep; more common in women. Refer to Table 2-21 for pharmacologic treatment options
Obesity	BMI > 30		Dieting and exercise; strict fad dieting ineffective; surgery not useful	Lower socioeconomic groups; genetics plays a role; increased risk of disease
Obsessive–compulsive disorder	Recurrent thoughts and actions; patients are distressed by repetitive actions	Decreased serotonin	Behavioral therapy; clomipramine; trazodone; SSRIs	EEG changes
Panic disorder	Discrete, episodic periods of intense anxiety or discomfort; palpitations; chest pain; sweating; fear of dying	Decreased serotonin, norepinephrine, GABA	Imipramine; behavior therapy	Associated with mitral valve prolapse; young women predominantly affected; genetic component
Phobias	Irrational, situational fear	Decreased serotonin, norepinephrine, and GABA	Systemic desensitization; propranolol useful for physiologic manifestations	
Post-traumatic stress disorder (PTSD)	Result of trauma; hypervigilance; nightmares; flashbacks	Decreased serotonin, norepinephrine, and GABA	Counseling; group therapy; benzodiazepines for symptoms	The first 3 months after the trauma disorder is acute PTSD; symptoms lasting longer than 3 months after the trauma is chronic PTSD

(continued)

TABLE 2-20 Psychoses and Other Neuropsychiatric Disorders *(Continued)*

Disorder	Characteristics	Neurotransmitter(s) Involved	Treatment	Notes
Schizophrenia	Autism; blunted affect; loose associations; ambivalence; auditory hallucinations; **negative symptoms** (i.e., flattened affect, lack of motivation, withdrawal); **positive symptoms** (i.e., hallucinations, hyperexcitability	Increased dopamine; increased norepinephrine in paranoid schizophrenia	Antipsychotics with a trial period of 3–5 weeks; clozapine has decreased extrapyramidal side effects (as opposed to haloperidol)	Occurs in young adults; enlarged lateral and third ventricles; patients oriented 4' 3 (person, place, and time); types include disorganized, catatonic, and paranoid
Somatoform disorders	Symptoms of disease occur without related pathology	Psychotherapy and therapeutics may help; variable response		Patients truly believe in having illness whereas factitious disorders are the result of faking illness
Tourette syndrome	Involuntary **motor and vocal** movements (need both)	Improper dopamine regulation	Haloperidol, clonidine	Onset occurs in childhood

EEG, electroencephalograph; GABA, γ-aminobutyric acid; MAOI, monoamine oxidase inhibitor; SSRI, selective serotonin reuptake inhibitor; REM, rapid eye movement; TCA, tricyclic antidepressant.

TABLE 2-21 Antidepressants

Class of Antidepressant (Specific Agent)	Mechanism of Action	Clinical uses	Side Effects	Notes
Tricyclic antidepressants (TCAs) (e.g., amitriptyline, imipramine, nortriptyline, desipramine, clomipramine, doxepin, amoxapine)	Inhibit **reuptake** of NE and 5-HT at neuronal synapses	Major depression, nocturnal enuresis (imipramine), OCD (clomipramine), panic disorder	Sedation, **α-blocking effects** (orthostatic hypotension), **anticholinergic** (tachycardia, dry mouth, urinary retention), hallucinations (in elderly), confusion (elderly). Overdose toxicity results in **convulsions, coma, cardiotoxicity** (arrhythmias), respiratory depression, hyperpyrexia	Desipramine is the least sedating
Monoamine oxidase inhibitors (MAOI) (e.g., isocarboxazid, phenelzine, tranylcypromine)	Inhibit **degradation** of NE and 5-HT at neuronal synapses	**Atypical depression** (with hypersomnia, anxiety, sensitivity to rejection, hypochondriasis)	**Hypertensive episodes** with ingestion of tyramine-containing foods or beta agonists, hyperthermia, convulsions	Contraindicated with **SSRIs** and **meperidine** secondary to **serotonin syndrome** (hyperthermia, muscle rigidity, cardiovascular collapse)
Selective serotonin reuptake inhibitors (SSRIs) (e.g., fluoxetine, paroxetine, sertraline, citalopram)	Inhibit **reuptake** of 5-HT at neuronal synapses	Major depression, OCD, anorexia, bulimia	Inhibits liver enzymes, nausea, agitation, **sexual dysfunction** (anorgasmia), dystonic reactions	Contraindicated with **MAOIs** secondary to **serotonin syndrome** (hyperthermia, muscle rigidity, cardiovascular collapse). Allow time for antidepressant effect, usually takes 2–3 weeks

(continued)

TABLE 2-21 Antidepressants *(Continued)*

Class of Antidepressant (Specific Agent)	Mechanism of Action	Clinical uses	Side Effects	Notes
Other antidepressants				
Buproprion (Wellbutrin)	Unknown	Major depression, smoking cessation	Tachycardia, insomnia, headache, seizure (especially bulimic patients)	Does not have sexual side effects
Venlafaxine	Inhibits 5-HT, NE, dopamine reuptake	Generalized anxiety disorder	Sedation, nausea, constipation, hypertension	
Mirtazapine	α_2-antagonist → increases release of NE and 5-HT	Major depression (especially with insomnia)	**Weight gain,** dry mouth, increased appetite, sedation	
Maprotiline	Blocks NE uptake	Major depression	Sedation, orthostatic hypotension	
Trazodone	Inhibits 5-HT reuptake	Major depression (especially with insomnia), insomnia	Sedation, nausea, **priapism**, postural hypotension	

5-HT, serotonin; NE, norepinephrine.

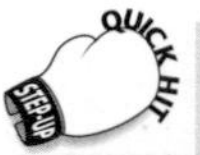

Dissociative disorders result in retrograde amnesia, whereas head trauma results in anterograde amnesia.

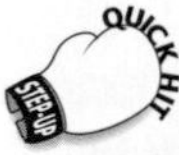

Münchhausen syndrome is a factitious disorder in which the patient fakes illness in order to receive medical attention such as a nurse purposely injecting himself or herself with insulin to receive medical attention. **Münchhausen syndrome by proxy** is a syndrome wherein the attention seeker feigns or creates illness in another, usually his or her child, to gain medical attention. It is considered a form of abuse

An **overdose** of a tricyclic antidepressant (TCA) causes delirium, coma, seizures, respiratory depression, and arrhythmias, and is potentially fatal and difficult to treat. The large volume of distribution of a TCA makes dialysis relatively ineffective.

FIGURE 2-18 **Antidepressant sites of action**
5-HT, 5-hydroxytryptamine (serotonin); MAO, monoamine oxidase; MOAI, monoamine oxidase inhibitor; NE, norepinephrine; SSRIs, selective serotonin reuptake inhibitors; TCAs, tricyclic antidepressants.

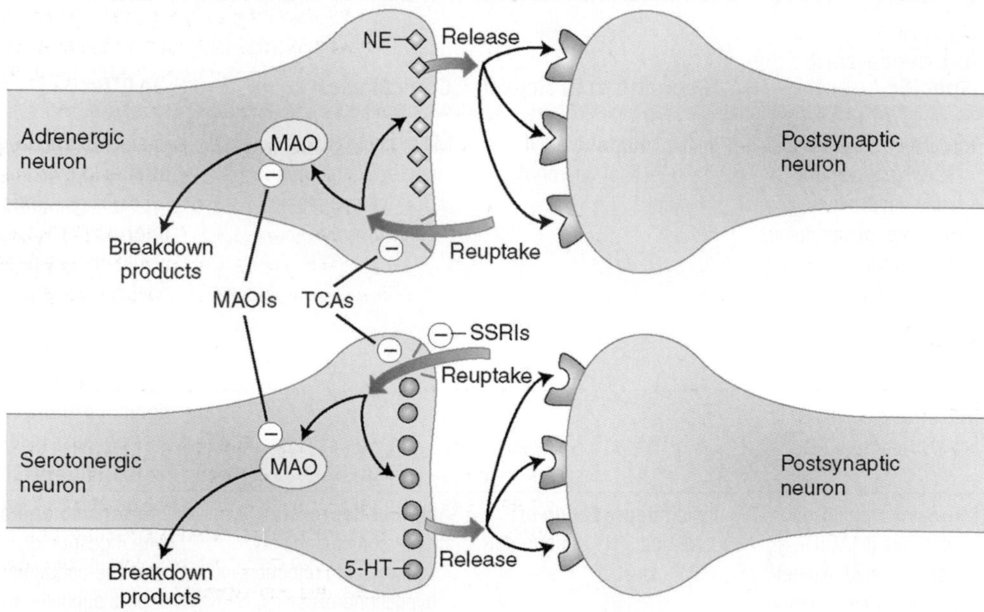

VI. Antipsychotics (Table 2-22)

Experts theorize that an excess of **dopamine** in certain areas of the brain is in some way responsible for psychosis. The development of psychosis as a common side effect of treatment of Parkinson disease with dopamine and dopamine agonists supports this theory. It is thought that most antipsychotics exert their effect by blocking **dopamine receptors.**

As a group, antipsychotics (excluding lithium) have several particular side effects in common. The side effects may be grouped into the following categories: (1) **extrapyradmidal**, (2) **anticholinergic**, (3) **alpha blocking effect**, and (4) **histamine receptor effects**. Extrapyradmidal side effects refer to acute dystonia, akinesia, and akathisia. **Dystonia** presents acutely within a few hours of starting the medication as a muscular spasm, stiff-

TABLE 2-22 Antipsychotics

Class/Drug	Targeted Receptors (Strongest to Weakest)	Clinical uses	Side effects	Notes
Typical Antipsychotics				
Butyrophenone: Haloperidol	D_2, α_1	**Schizophrenia, psychosis, acute mania, Tourette syndrome**	**Extrapyramidal** (dystonia, akinesia, akathisia, tardive dyskinesia), **endocrine** (galactorrhea), **anticholinergic** (dry mouth, constipation), **alpha blockade** (hypotension), **histamine** (sedation); prolonged QT syndrome; toxicity results in neuroleptic malignant syndrome (rigidity, myoglobinuria, autonomic instability, hyperpyrexia)	Extrapyramidal side effects are more common. Neuroleptic malignant syndrome is treated with dantrolene and dopamine agonists
Lithium	Unclear; inhibits regeneration of IP_3 and DAG; important for many second-messenger systems	Bipolar disorder, acute manic events	Tremor, hypothyroidism, polyuria, teratogenesis	Close monitoring of serum levels required due to narrow therapeutic window
Phenothiazines: Chlorpromazine	D_2, α_1, H_1		**Extrapyramidal** (dystonia, akinesia, akathisia, tardive dyskinesia), **anticholinergic** (dry mouth, constipation), **alpha blockade** (hypotension), **histamine** (sedation); Toxicity results in neuroleptic malignant syndrome (rigidity, myoglobinuria, autonomic instability, hyperpyrexia)	Atropine-like effects fairly common
Fluphenazine	D_2, α_1, H_1		**Extrapyramidal** (dystonia, akinesia, akathisia, tardive dyskinesia), **anticholinergic** (dry mouth, constipation), **alpha blockade** (hypotension), **histamine** (sedation); Toxicity results in neuroleptic malignant syndrome (rigidity, myoglobinuria, autonomic instability, hyperpyrexia)	**Extrapyramidal** side effects are more common
Thioridazine	Muscarinic, D_2, α_1		**Extrapyramidal** (dystonia, akinesia, akathisia, tardive dyskinesia), **anticholinergic** (dry mouth, constipation), **alpha blockade** (hypotension), **histamine** (sedation); Toxicity results in neuroleptic malignant syndrome (rigidity, myoglobinuria, autonomic instability, hyperpyrexia)	**Atropine-like effects** are very common; antimuscarinic effects exacerbate tardive dyskinesia, visual impairment has been reported
Thioxanthene: Thiothixene	D_2, α_1, H_1			No unique side effects or uses
Atypical Antipsychotics				
Clozapine	D_4, α_1, 5-HT, muscarinic	Schizophrenia, useful for positive and negative symptoms	Agranulocytosis, **Extrapyramidal** (occurs at a lower rate than typicals), **anticholinergic** (dry mouth, constipation), **alpha blockade** (hypotension), **histamine** (sedation); Toxicity results in neuroleptic malignant syndrome (occurs at a lower rate than typicals)	Second-line agent used for refractory schizophrenia; weekly blood counts for patients on this agent due to agranulocytosis.
Olanzapine	D_4, α_1, 5-HT, muscarinic	Schizophrenia, OCD, anxiety disorder, depression, mania, Tourette's syndrome	Agranulocytosis, **Extrapyramidal** (occurs at a lower rate than typicals), **anticholinergic** (dry mouth, constipation), **alpha blockade** (hypotension), **histamine** (sedation); Toxicity results in neuroleptic malignant syndrome (occurs at a lower rate than typicals)	

(continued)

TABLE 2-22 Antipsychotics *(Continued)*

Class/Drug	Targeted Receptors (Strongest to Weakest)	Clinical uses	Side effects	Notes
Risperidone	D_2, 5-HT, α_1, H_1	Schizophrenia, useful for positive and negative symptoms	Agranulocytosis, **Extrapyramidal** (occurs at a lower rate than typicals), **anticholinergic** (occurs at lower rate than other agents), **α-blockade** (hypotension), **histamine** (sedation); Toxicity results in neuroleptic malignant syndrome (occurs at a lower rate than typicals)	Second-line agent used for refractory schizophrenia
Quetiapine	D_2, 5-HT, α_1, H_1	Schizophrenia, acute mania,	Suicide attempt in major depression, arrhythmia, **extrapyramidal** (occurs at a lower rate than typicals), **anticholinergic** (occurs at lower rate than other agents), **α-blockade** (hypotension), **histamine** (sedation); Toxicity results in neuroleptic malignant syndrome (occur at a lower rate than typicals)	

α_1, α_1-adrenergic; D_2, dopamine D_2; D_4, dopamine D_4; DAG, diacylglycerol; H_1, histamine H_1; 5-HT, serotonin; IP_3, inositol triphosphate.

MNEMONIC

Remember the four A's as the negative features of schizophrenia:
- **A**ffect (blunted)
- **A**utism
- **A**mbivalence
- **A**ssociations (loose)

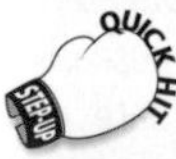

The timeline for extrapyramidal side effects is:
4 h—acute dystonia
4 days—akinesia
4 weeks—akathisia
4 months—tardive dyskinesia.

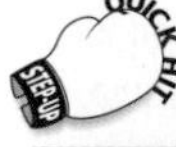

Amitriptyline is somewhat more potent than imipramine and nortriptyline, which means that it often has more significant side effects.

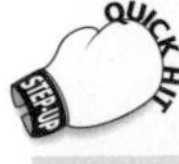

The use of the combination of selective serotonin reuptake inhibitors (SSRIs) and monoamine oxidase inhibitors (MAOIs) may produce a **"serotonin syndrome."** This constellation of hyperpyrexia, muscle spasm, and mental status changes can be fatal.

ness, and oculogyric crisis. **Akinesia** presents within a few days of starting the medication as parkinsonian symptoms. **Akathisia** presents within a few weeks of starting the medication as restlessness. **Tardive dyskinesia** presents after a few months of starting the medication with stereotypic oral facial movements likely due to dopamine receptor sensitization. Tardive dyskinesia is often irreversible, and is most common in older women who have received long term treatment with high doses. **Anticholinergic side effects** include dry mouth and constipation. **Alpha blocking effects** include hypotension. **Histamine receptor effects** include sedation. **Atypical antipsychotics** such as clozapine, olanzapine, risperidone, quetiapine, aripiprazole, and ziprasidone have a lower incidence of extrapyramidal and anticholinergic side effects. Finally, antipsychotics also may be **antiemetic** and have a tendency to **lower the seizure threshold.**

VII. Nonpharmacologic therapeutic modalities (Table 2-23)

ETHICS AND THE ROLE OF THE PHYSICIAN

The role of the nervous system in the manifestation of psychological problems is under debate. The occurrence of certain psychopathology has been linked to neurotransmitters and the lack of regulation in certain parts of the CNS.

Communication skills are essential to determine a patient's physical and psychological problems. Establishing trust and confidence via facilitation, reflection, and an open-ended clinical interview allows the physician to gather physical, psychological, and social information. If an individual suffers from psychopathology, proper steps must be taken not to alienate, offend, or judge the patient. On the other hand, the individual's problems must be dealt with directly.

When presenting therapeutic options or advice, the physician should be forthright, direct, and honest. In making an assessment of any patient, the physician needs to be sensitive to problems affecting certain populations. For instance, it is important to remember that in elderly patients, sexual changes occur (i.e., men may have slower erections and women may have increased vaginal dryness and decreased vaginal length, though libido is not necessarily affected), sleep may decrease, suicide rate may increase, and depression becomes more prevalent.

Although the physician must be **nonmaleficent** (not intending to do harm) and **beneficent** (doing what is best for the patient), **patient autonomy** ultimately prevails in making

TABLE 2-23 Nonpharmacologic Therapeutic Modalities

Therapy	Characteristics	Notes
Biofeedback	Gaining control over physiology via continuous information; motivation and practice required	Used for hypertension, migraine headaches, and tension headaches
Classical conditioning	A **reflexive, natural behavior** is elicited in **response to a learned stimulus** (e.g., ringing of a bell causing salivation)	**Aversive conditioning** pairs an unwanted response to a painful stimulus; stages include acquisition, extinction, and recovery
Cognitive therapy	**Negative thinking** is reorganized into self-affirming, positive thoughts	Short-term psychotherapy used to treat depression and anxiety
Electroconvulsive therapy (ECT)	Electric current introduced into brain to alter neurotransmitter function; improvement seen faster than with pharmacologic regimens	Used for **major depression**; safe; effective; retrograde amnesia is a major side effect
Operant conditioning	Behavior that is not part of the natural repertoire is learned by altering the reward **(reinforcement)**	Reinforcement can be positive or negative; reward schedule includes continuous, fixed, or variable
Psychoanalysis	Intensive treatment based on recovering and integrating past experiences from the unconscious via free association; based on **Freud's theories**	**Id**—sexual drives and aggression; **ego**—controls instinct and interacts with the world; **superego**—morality and conscience
Systemic desensitization	Classical conditioning technique in which relaxation procedures are combined with increasing doses of anxiety-provoking stimuli	Used to **eliminate** phobias
Token economy	Positive reinforcement in which a reward is used to elicit a desired response	Seen often in mental hospitals or parents dealing with children

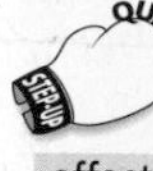

In its most severe form, extrapyramidal effects may develop into **neuroleptic malignant syndrome,** a potentially fatal combination of severe rigidity, decreased perspiration, hyperpyrexia, and autonomic instability. Treatment involves immediate discontinuation of antipsychotic medications, supportive measures, and administration of **dantrolene.**

Behavior learned through a variable interval schedule of reinforcement is most difficult to extinguish. Behavior learned through a fixed schedule is easiest to extinguish.

the final decision about treatment. The physician must consider the patient's ability to make decisions based on communication skills, level of understanding about medicine, stability, consistency, and soundness of mind. Physicians have a **duty** to provide medical care to their patients, and if **breach** of this duty directly leads to **damage**, the physician has been **negligent** and therefore is **liable** for malpractice. The breach of duty owing to negligence and the damages caused by it represent a **tort**.

Before making a final decision regarding patient care, physicians should make an effort to obtain an **informed consent**, which indicates that the patient understands the risks and benefits of therapy. Disheartening as it may be, terminal disease may require the physician to explain to the patient and his family that further intervention is inappropriate inasmuch as maximal treatment has failed and it seems to be a reasonable conclusion that the goals of care will not be reached. **Advance directives** from the patient, either written or oral, may assist the physician in coming to a conclusion about when to terminate treatment measures.

Information about the patient must remain **confidential** unless the patient poses a risk to self or to others; information concerning the patient's own disease, diagnosis, or prognosis cannot be withheld from the patient, despite the wishes of the family.

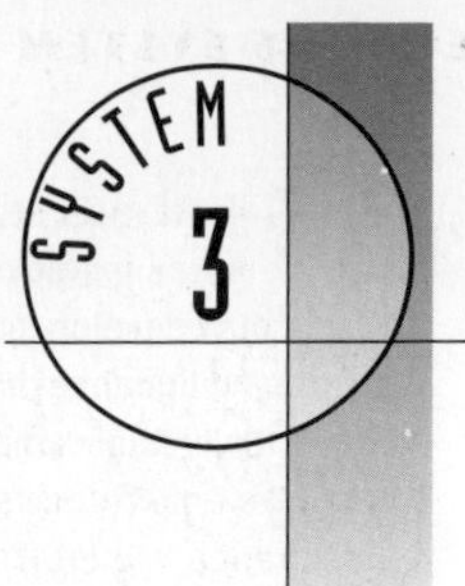

The Cardiovascular System

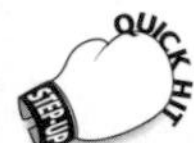

The umbilical circulation is one of the only places in the body (along with the pulmonary circulation) where an artery does not carry oxygenated blood. The paired umbilical arteries carry deoxygenated blood to the placenta while the umbilical vein brings oxygenated blood back to the fetus.

DEVELOPMENT

I. Heart

A. The cardiovascular system is derived from the **mesoderm**.

B. Paired endocardial heart tubes form in the **cephalic region** of the embryo.

C. Lateral and cephalocaudal folding causes the heart tubes to join together and lie in a **ventral location** between the primitive mouth and the foregut.

D. The **primitive heart** dilates into five areas, shown in Figure 3-1. The five embryologic regions and their adult derivatives are as follows:

1. **Truncus arteriosus** → proximal aorta and proximal pulmonary artery
2. **Bulbus cordis** → smooth parts of the right ventricle (conus arteriosus) and left ventricles
3. **Primitive ventricle** → right and left ventricles (trabeculated parts)
4. **Primitive atrium** → right and left atria
5. **Sinus venosus** → smooth part of right atrium, the coronary sinus, and oblique vein

FIGURE 3-1 **Embryologic development of the heart**

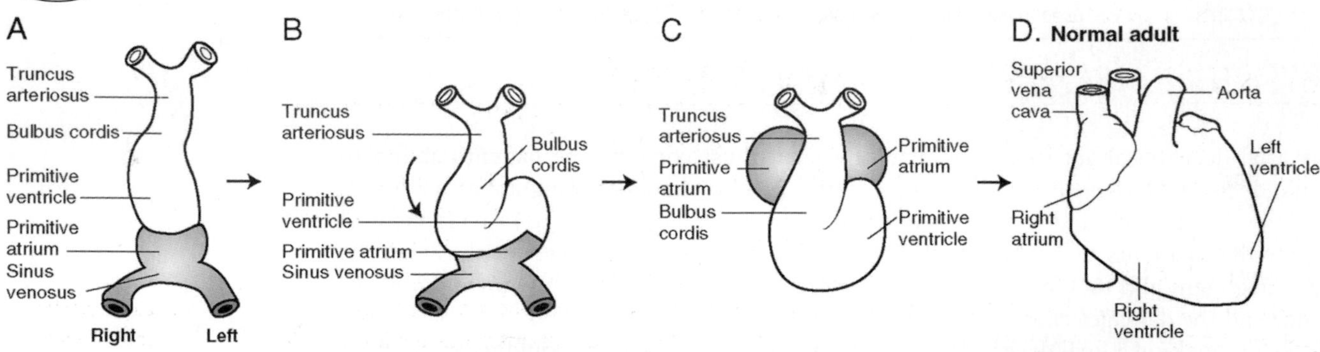

Folding of the developing heart **(A-C)** during weeks 5–8 into the normal adult heart **(D)**.

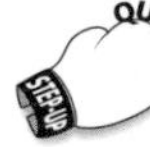

Down syndrome is associated with endocardial cushion defects, which may manifest as ASD or ventral septal defect (VSD).

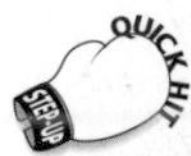

Paradoxical emboli are emboli that originate in the venous circulation and pass through a patent foramen ovale or ASD to produce symptoms on the arterial side.

E. The lumen of the truncus arteriosus and bulbus cordis is divided into the **aorta** and **pulmonary trunk** by the aorticopulmonary septum.

F. The septum primum, septum secundum, and atriovenous (AV) cushion form the **atrial septum**.

G. The **foramen ovale** is a communication between the right and left atria, which is formed by the walls of the septum primum and septum secundum

1. It allows blood to flow from the venous side of the circulation to the arterial side without passing through the lungs as a result of **higher pressure on the venous side during gestation**.
2. **After birth**, the foramen ovale closes because of **increased arterial pressure** that pushes the septum primum against the atrial septum.

H. The aorticopulmonary septum, the right and left bulbar ridges, and the AV cushion form the **interventricular septum**.

II. Arterial vessels

A. **Aortic (pharyngeal) arches**. Initially, there are six paired aortic arches. Arches 3, 4, and 6 play a significant role in the adult. Arch 5 degenerates early in fetal development
   1. **Arches 1 and 2** give rise to the maxillary artery and stapedial artery, respectively.
   2. **Arch 3** helps form the adult common carotid arteries bilaterally.
   3. **Arch 4** helps form the aorta on the left and the proximal subclavian artery on the right.
   4. **Arch 6** helps form the ductus arteriosus and part of the pulmonary trunk.

B. Paired dorsal aortae are paired vessels that run along the length of the embryo. They coalesce to form the **descending aorta**.

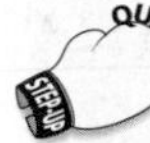

In dextrocardia, the heart is located on the right side in the thorax. An isolated misplaced heart is often accompanied by multiple anomalies. If all of the body's organs are transposed (situs inversus-associated with Kartagener syndrome; immotile cilia caused by a defect in the dynein arms resulting in lung disease and male sterility), the heart is often normal.

III. Venous vessels

A. The paired vitelline, umbilical, and cardinal veins form the definitive adult structures.

B. The **vitelline veins** help form the ductus venosus and hepatic sinusoids, the inferior vena cava, the portal vein, and the superior and inferior mesenteric veins.

C. **Umbilical veins**
   1. No adult vascular structures are formed by these veins.
   2. The left umbilical vein connects to the ductus venosus and carries oxygenated blood from the placenta to the fetus.
   3. **Left umbilical vein** gives rise to ligamentum teres hepatis.
   4. **Right umbilical vein** regresses.

D. **Cardinal veins**
   1. The **anterior cardinal veins** help form the internal jugular vein and the superior vena cava.
   2. The **posterior cardinal veins** help form the inferior vena cava, common iliac veins, azygos vein, and renal veins.

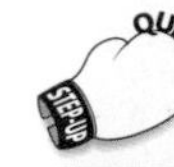

The ductus arteriosus closes in the first days of life. Exposure to oxygenated blood alters the production of prostaglandins (PGs). Indomethacin (PG synthesis inhibitor) induces closure of a patent ductus arteriosus (PDA), whereas alprostadil (PGE1) therapy maintains patency.

IV. Fetal circulation (Figure 3-2)

V. Congenital defects of the heart and great vessels (Table 3-1)

PHYSIOLOGY AND PATHOLOGY OF HEART FUNCTION

Properly timed and integrated myocyte contraction is essential to normal heart function. Cardiac myocytes (Figure 3-3) have gap junctions that allow for rapid relay of electrical signals between them. Electrical impulses are transmitted via the electrical conduction system composed of the sinoatrial (SA) node, AV node, and His-Purkinje cells (Figure 3-4). Normally, the SA node is the pacemaker of the heart. The node exhibits automaticity in which spontaneous phase 4 depolarization generates rhythmic action potentials (APs). These electrical signals propagate from the SA node through the atrial tissue and cause it to contract. Further propagation leads to excitation of the AV node, the ventricular bundles, and, lastly, the ventricular tissue. The nodal tissues are dependent on Ca^{2+} for their phase 0 depolarization whereas the cardiac muscular tissue uses Na^{+} for phase 0 depolarization. The AV node transmits APs more slowly than do the other cardiac tissues. This feature allows the atria to contract before the ventricles, with time for the ventricles to repolarize, fill with blood, and prepare to receive their next electrical signal. Furthermore, it also prevents excessively rapid beats from reaching and damaging the ventricular tissue. The conduction system of the heart can best be visualized on an electrocardiogram (ECG). ECG plots can determine disturbances, such as arrhythmias, along the cardiac conduction path.

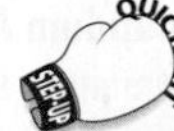

Conduction velocity depends on the rate of depolarization (represented by upstroke of the action potential), not on action potential duration.

Drugs that are used to treat arrhythmias may also cause them, especially when their use is stopped suddenly. This is an important consideration for digoxin, class IA (quinidine, disopyramide, and procainamide), class IC (propafenone, flecainide, and encainide), and class II (propranolol) drugs.

Multiple mechanisms can affect the intrinsic mechanical properties of the heart. Chronotropic effects on the heart cause a change in heart rate by affecting the rate of depolarization of the SA node. Inotropic effects cause a change in contractility of the heart. Greater contractility allows the heart to squeeze harder and increase cardiac output. Increased intracellular Ca^{2+}, either drug-mediated (e.g., cardiac glycosides, diltiazem, verapamil, and nifedipine) or as a result of sympathetic β-receptor stimulation, allows for an increased inotropic effect. The preload and afterload also affect the function of the heart. Increased preload as a result of

(text continues on page 84)

FIGURE 3-2 Fetal circulation

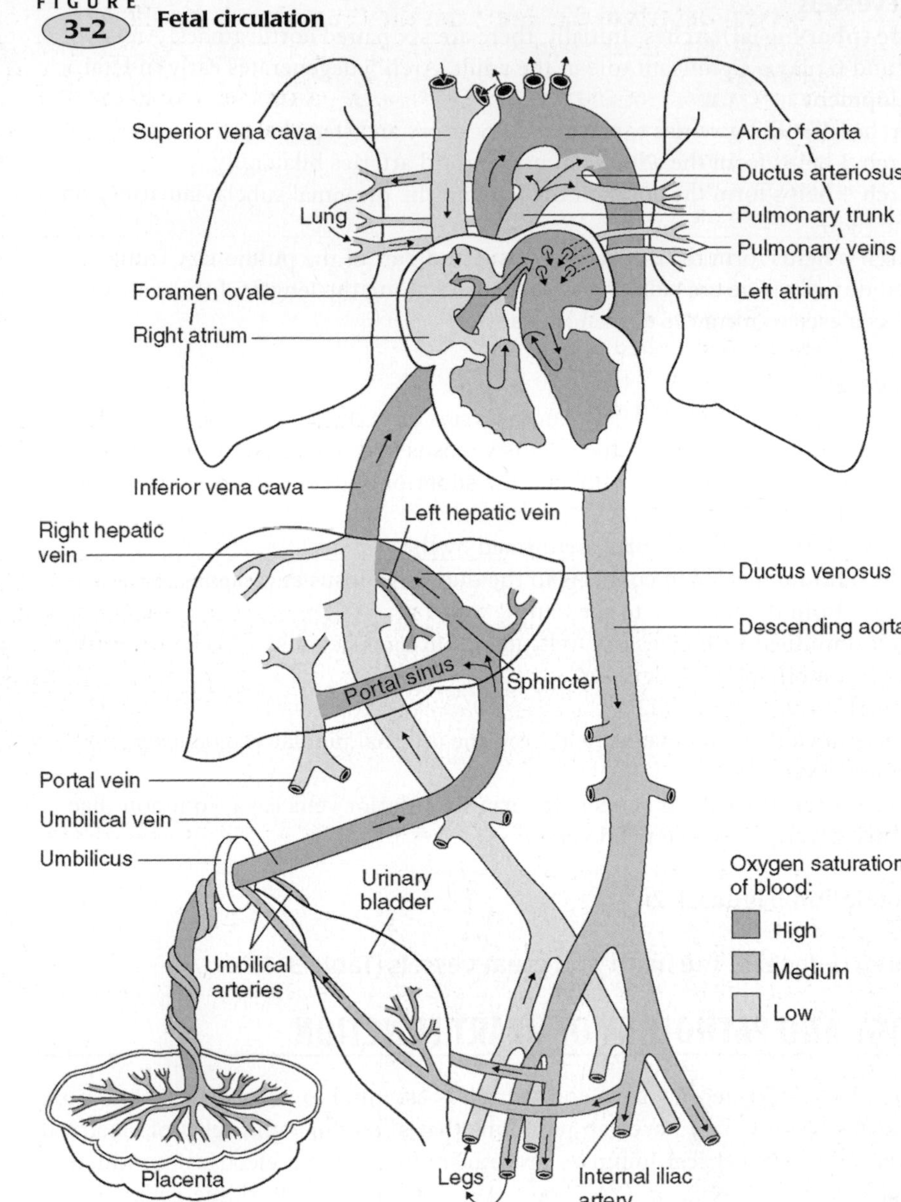

QUICK HIT: Aberrant development of the aorticopulmonary septum is responsible for tetralogy of Fallot, transposition of the great vessels, and persistent truncus arteriosus.

QUICK HIT: The most common type of atrial septal defect (ASD) is a patent foramen ovale.

QUICK HIT: Eisenmenger syndrome is the change from a left-to-right shunt to a right-to-left shunt secondary to increasing pulmonary hypertension; it usually occurs as a result of a chronic, adaptive response to pre-existing left-to-right shunts, such as a VSD.

TABLE 3-1 Congenital Defects of the Heart and the Great Vessels

Anomaly	Pathology	Clinical Presentation	Notes
ASD	**Secundum ASD** (defect of septum primum or septum secundum) Primum ASD (low) Sinus venosus ASD (high)	**Left-to-right shunt;** asymptomatic into the 4th decade; murmur; right ventricular hypertrophy	Much higher incidence in females (3:1); 75–80% are secundum type
Coarctation of the aorta	Infantile (proximal to PDA); adult (constriction at closed ductus arteriosus, distal to the origin of left subclavian artery)	Symptoms depend on the extent of narrowing; infant presents with lower-limb cyanosis and right-heart failure at birth; adult asymptomatic with upper-limb hypertension, rib notching on radiograph from collateral circulation through intercostal arteries, and **weak pulses in lower limbs**	Much higher incidence in males (3:1) and females with **Turner syndrome**

(continued)

TABLE 3-1 Congenital Defects of the Heart and the Great Vessels *(Continued)*

Anomaly	Pathology	Clinical Presentation	Notes
PDA	Failure of closure of the ductus arteriosus; may be caused by premature birth with **hypoxemia** or structural defects	Continuous **machinery murmur**	Second most common congenital heart defect
Tetralogy of Fallot	Defective development of the infundibular septum; results in **overriding aorta, ventricular septal defect (VSD), pulmonary stenosis, and hypertrophy of the right ventricle**	Cyanosis (may not be present at birth); right-to-left shunt; **"boot-shaped heart"**	Survival to adulthood possible; patient assumes squatting position to relieve symptoms
Transposition of the great vessels	Aorta drains right ventricle; pulmonary artery from left ventricle; **separate pulmonary and systemic circuits**	Incompatible with life unless shunt present; cyanosis (present at birth)	Diabetic mother
VSD	Membranous VSD; Single muscular VSD	Left-to-right shunt; **loud holosystolic murmur means small defect;** large defects can present as heart failure at birth; small defects can close spontaneously	Much higher incidence in males; most common congenital heart defect (33%); 90% are membranous type

FIGURE 3-3 Histology of cardiac myocyte; A longitudinal section of cardiac muscle cells is shown

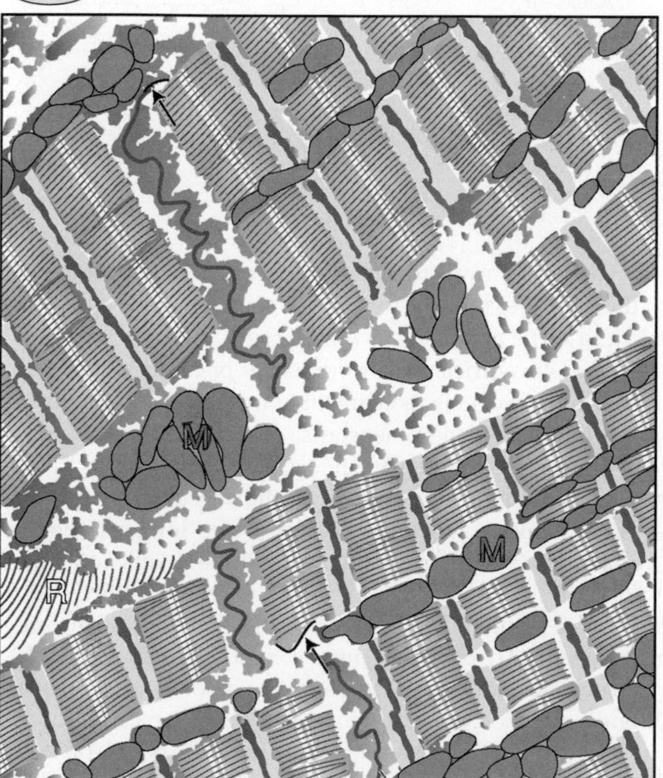

QUICK HIT: Cyanosis occurs in right-to-left shunts: tetralogy of Fallot and transposition of the great vessels (TGA). Cyanosis can lead to clubbing, hypertrophic osteoarthropathy, and polycythemia. Initial left-to-right shunts are not cyanotic: ASD, VSD, PDA, and atrioventricular septal defect (AVSD).

QUICK HIT: Congenital cardiac defects with the **letter D** are initially **left-to-right shunts** (PDA, VSD, AVSD, and ASD) whereas those cardiac defects without the letter D are right-to-left shunts.

FIGURE 3-4 Heart anatomy and signal conduction

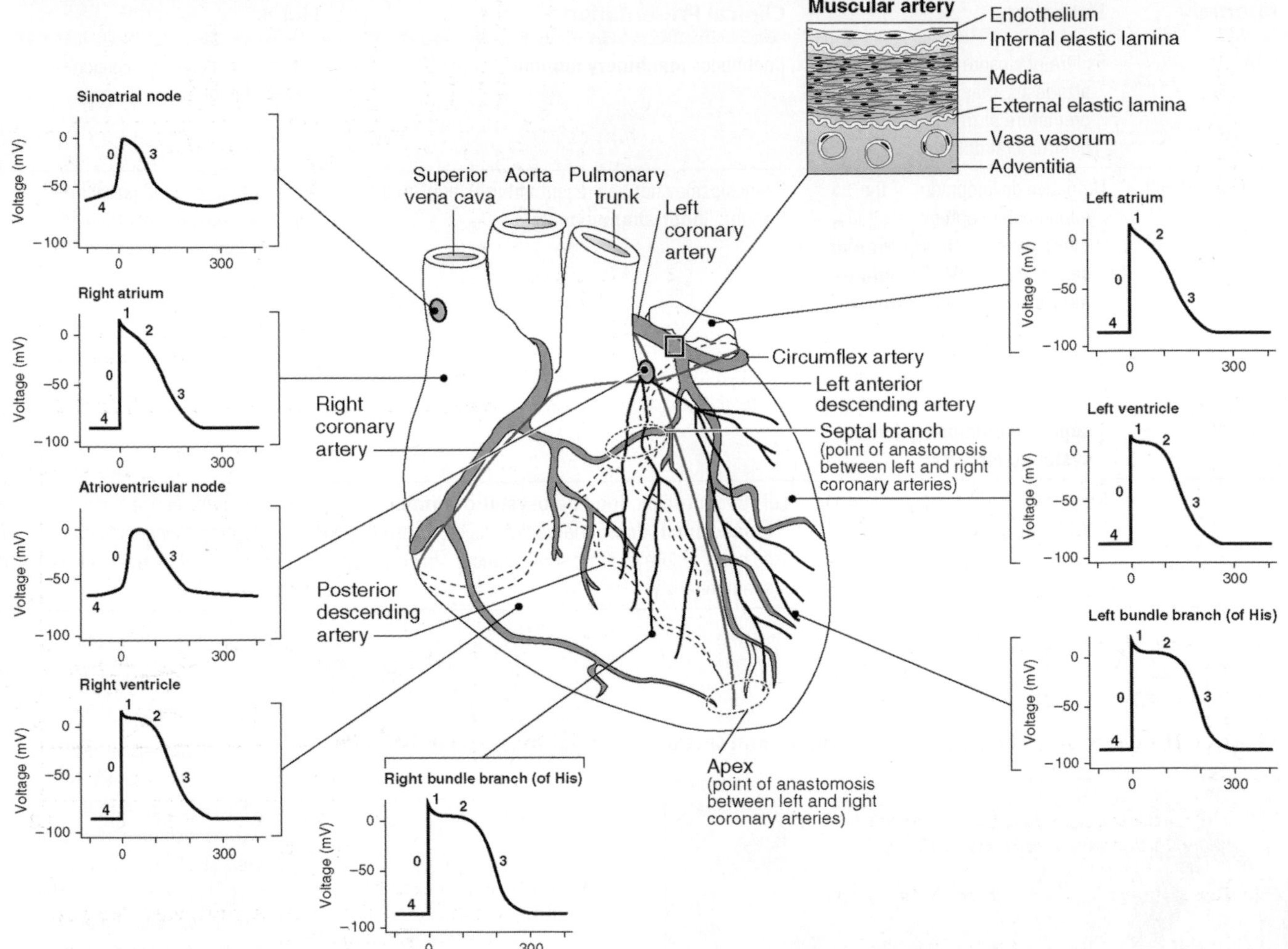

increased filling of the ventricles lengthens the myocytes, which induces stronger contraction, up to a certain point, after which the myocytes are too stretched to contract effectively. Afterload of the left ventricle is equivalent to aortic pressure. It is influenced by the total peripheral resistance. A higher afterload means the left ventricle must work harder or cardiac output will fall. The cardiovascular system is constantly working to maintain homeostatic equilibrium.

QUICK HIT: The baroreceptor reflex greatly affects total peripheral resistance. The carotid sinus baroreceptors, located at the bifurcation of the carotid arteries, sense arterial pressure. Afferent signals via cranial nerve (CN) IX induce efferent signals via CN X to influence heart rate. Increased arterial pressure causes an increase in vagal output and a reduction of heart rate and blood pressure. A decrease in arterial pressure causes a decrease in vagal output, resulting in an increase in heart rate and blood pressure.

Hormonal systems also respond to changes in homeostasis. A major influence on the cardiovascular system is exerted by the renin–angiotensin–aldosterone (RAA) axis. Whereas the baroreceptors attempt to maintain adequate pressures in the vascular system over a short-term period, the RAA system helps to regulate pressure over a longer period of time. The RAA axis responds to changes in arterial pressure by altering salt and water retention by the kidneys. Low blood pressure causes an increased release of renin, which converts angiotensinogen from the liver to angiotensin I. Angiotensin I travels to the lung where it is cleaved to angiotensin II (Ang II) by angiotensin-converting enzyme (ACE). Ang II stimulates constriction of arterioles and increases release of aldosterone (salt and water retention; see System 6), both of which increase blood pressure. Atrial natriuretic peptide (ANP) also responds to blood pressure changes. An increase in blood pressure causes stretch of atrial myocytes, which then release ANP. ANP lowers blood pressure by relaxing smooth muscle, increasing salt and water excretion, and inhibiting renin release. Antidiuretic hormone (ADH), also known as arginine vasopressin (AVP), is involved in the response to changes in blood pressure. When released from the pituitary, it acts on the kidney to reduce urine output and retain water while simultaneously constricting arterioles to increase total peripheral resistance (Figure 3-5).

FIGURE 3-5 **Blood pressure control mechanisms**

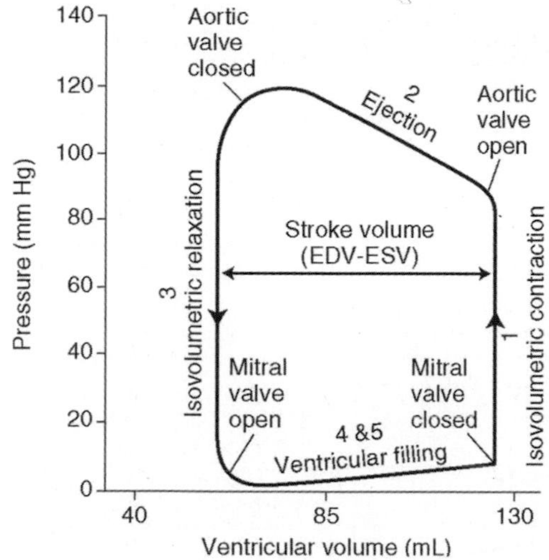

1. **Isovolumetric contraction:** Time between mitral valve closure and aortic valve opening, time of highest oxygen consumption
2. **Systolic ejection:** Time between aortic valve opening and closing
3. **Isovolumetric relaxation:** Time between aortic valve closing and mitral valve opening
4. **Rapid filling:** Time after mitral valve opening
5. **Reduced filling:** Time right before mitral valve closing

A. **Pressure–volume loop**

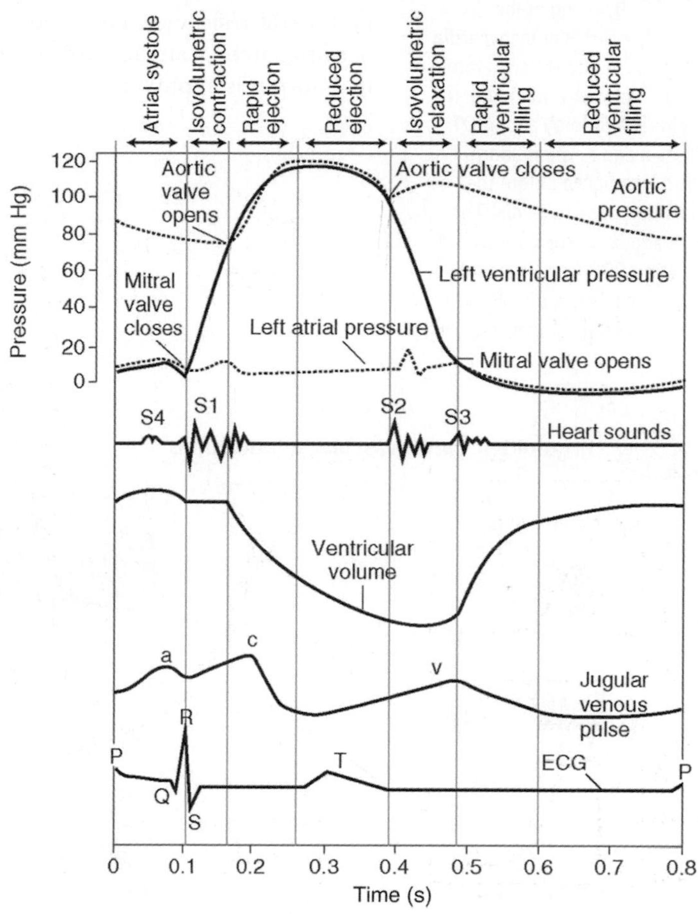

a wave – atrial contraction
c wave – contraction of right ventricle, peak due to tricupsid valve bulging into atrium
v wave – increased atrial pressure secondary to filling against closed tricuspid valve

B. **The Cardiac cycle**

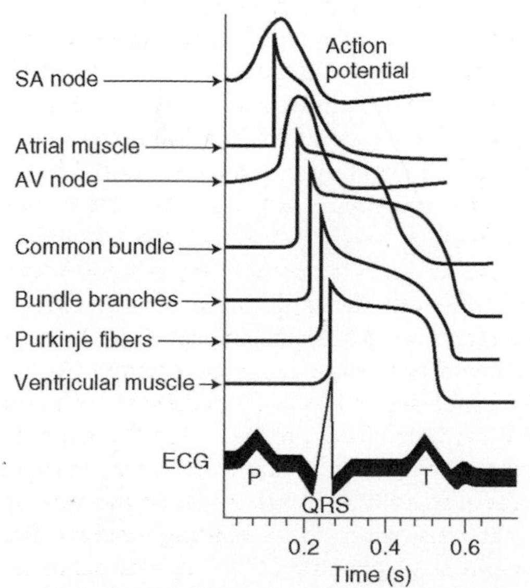

C. **Progression of the action potential through cardiac muscle cells**

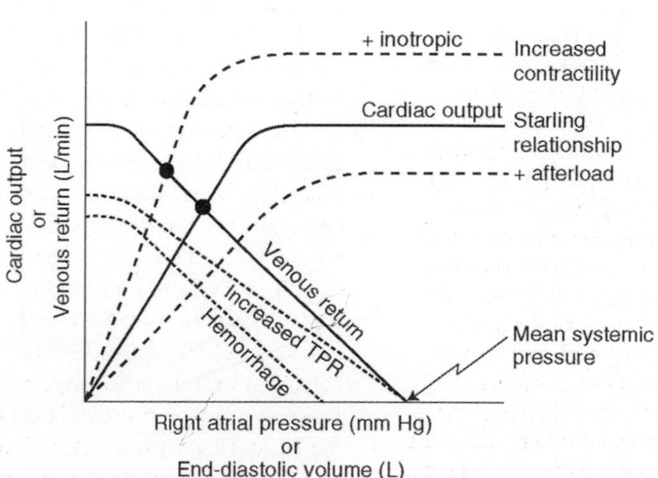

D. **Frank-Starling relationship**

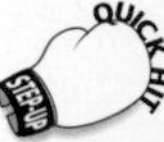

Torsade de pointes (twisting of the points): ventricular tachycardia often caused by antiarrhythmic drugs, especially quinidine. It is characterized by a long QT interval and a "short–long–short" sequence before the inception of tachycardia. The ECG shows a series of upward-pointing QRS complexes followed by a series of downward-pointing complexes.

The physiologic function of the heart can be represented in several ways (e.g., pressure–volume loops and the cardiac cycle) (Figure 3-6). The effects of cardiac output, total peripheral resistance, contractility, preload, and afterload are represented on the Frank–Starling curve. Cardiac output is measured using the Fick principle (Figure 3-7) and normal output is approximately 5 L/min.

FIGURE 3-6 **Physiologic cardiovascular relationships**

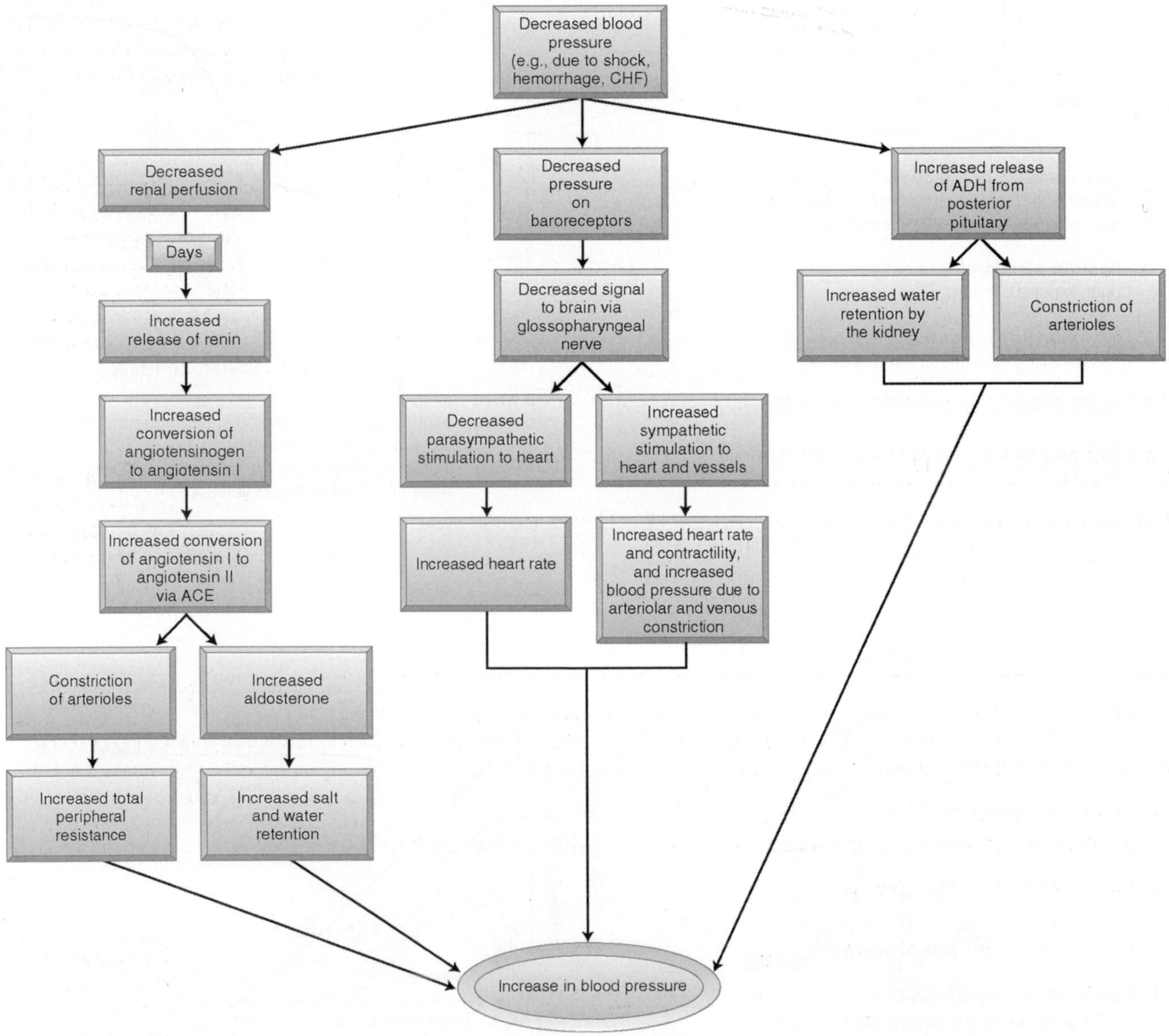

Decreased blood pressure (e.g., due to shock, hemorrhage, CHF)

Decreased renal perfusion
Days
Increased release of renin
Increased conversion of angiotensinogen to angiotensin I
Increased conversion of angiotensin I to angiotensin II via ACE
Constriction of arterioles
Increased total peripheral resistance
Increased aldosterone
Increased salt and water retention

Decreased pressure on baroreceptors
Decreased signal to brain via glossopharyngeal nerve
Decreased parasympathetic stimulation to heart
Increased heart rate
Increased sympathetic stimulation to heart and vessels
Increased heart rate and contractility, and increased blood pressure due to arteriolar and venous constriction

Increased release of ADH from posterior pituitary
Increased water retention by the kidney
Constriction of arterioles

Increase in blood pressure

FIGURE 3-7 **Important cardiovascular equations**

$CO = \frac{O_2 \text{ consumption}}{([O_2] \text{ pulmonary vein} - [O_2] \text{ pulmonary artery})}$	**The Fick equation** is used to calculate either cardiac output (CO) or oxygen (O_2) consumption
$CO = SV \times HR$	CO = cardiac output SV = stroke volume HR = heart rate
$R \propto \frac{1}{r^4}$	This relationship shows how arteriolar diameter can effectively control systemic resistance. For instance, if the radius (r) is increased by 2, the resistance (R) drops 16-fold.
$\dot{Q} = \frac{\Delta P}{R}$	$\dot{Q}$ = flow ΔP = Aortic pressure–right atrial pressure or pressure difference R = resistance
$MBP = CO \times TPR$	MBP = mean blood pressure (equivalent to ΔP) CO = cardiac output (equivalent to $\dot{Q}$) TPR = total peripheral resistance (equivalent to R)
Series resistance: $R_{total} = R_1 + R_2 + R_3 + R_4 \cdots$	R_1 R_2 R_3 R_4 R_{total}
Parallel resistance: $\frac{1}{R_{total}} = \frac{1}{R_1} + \frac{1}{R_2} + \frac{1}{R_3} + \frac{1}{R_4} \cdots$	This relationship lowers resistance when the body recruits unused parallel vessels (especially in capillary beds) R_{total} R_1 R_2 R_3 R_4

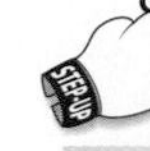

Myocardial infarctions (MI) can cause both second-degree and third-degree heart block.

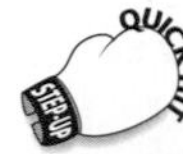

Because of state-dependent block, lidocaine works on slightly depolarized or ischemic tissue more so than normal tissue. Therefore, use lidocaine (IV) to suppress acute MI-associated ventricular arrhythmias.

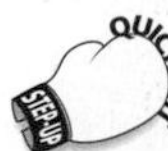

Class IB agents (lidocaine, tocainide, mexiletine, and phenytoin) all have central nervous system (CNS) side effects. Long-term control using tocainide can also cause neutropenia and thrombocytopenia.

ARRHYTHMIAS (Figure 3-8) (Table 3-2)

Arrhythmias can be organized into tachycardias and bradycardias. The ECGs of important arrhythmias as seen in Figure 3-8 and features of the heart blocks are described in Table 3-2.

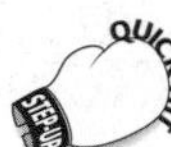

Diltiazem can be used to control the ventricular response rate in atrial fibrillation because it slows AV nodal conduction.

ANTIARRHYTHMICS (Figure 3-9) (Table 3-3)

Antiarrhythmics work to change different phases of depolarization and repolarization. They also alter the conduction velocity, change the effective refractory period (ERP), and alter the AP duration. The treatment options for arrhythmias are as follows:

Chronic atrial fibrillation can lead to clots in the atrium that may embolize to the systemic circulation. Treatment is to prevent emboli with anticoagulation such as warfarin.

I. Atrial fibrillation
   A. **Verapamil**, β-blockers, or diltiazem for conversion back to sinus rhythm.

II. Supraventricular tachycardia
   A. Adenosine (diagnostic purposes)
   B. Verapamil (long-term control)

III. Ventricular fibrillation
   A. Lidocaine or amiodarone

IV. Ventricular tachycardia
   A. Digoxin

(text continues on page 91)

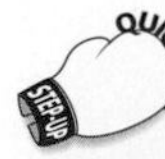

Of the antiarrhythmics, class II and class III agents decrease mortality, whereas other antiarrhythmics can be proarrhythmics, so carefully monitor a patient.

FIGURE 3-8 **ECGs of important arrhythmias**

Normal ECG

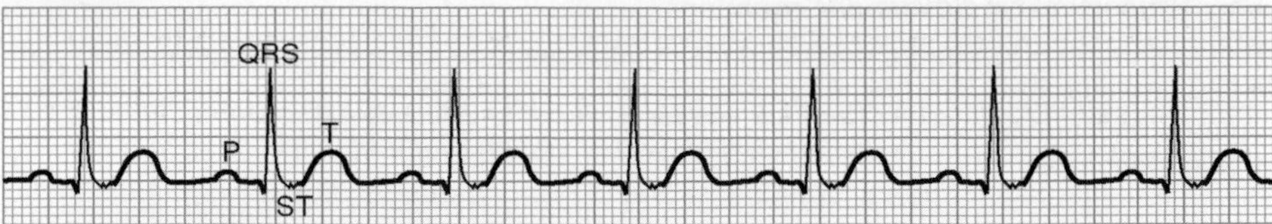

- P wave is atrial depolarization (atrial repolarization usually occurs during the QRS and remains unseen in ECG)
- PR interval (0.12–0.2 s) measures time between atrial and ventricular depolarization
- QRS interval (normally less than 0.1 s) reflects the duration of ventricular depolarization
- T wave is ventricular repolarization

Sustained ventricular tachycardia

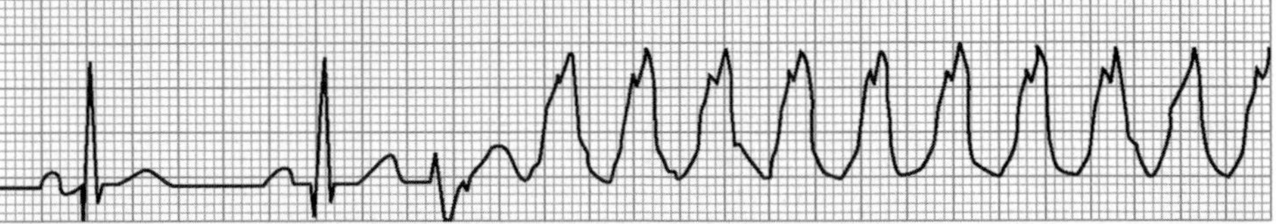

- Constant QRS morphology and fairly regular cycle length
- Initiating beat morphology may differ from ongoing VT
- AV dissociation a hallmark but not always present, nor easy to identify when present

Ventricular fibrillation

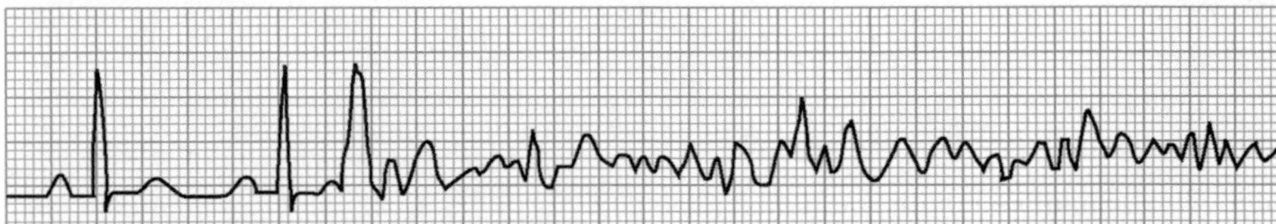

- Undulating baseline, no organized electrical activity
- Incompatible with life
- Atria may be dissociated, still in sinus rhythm

Atrial flutter

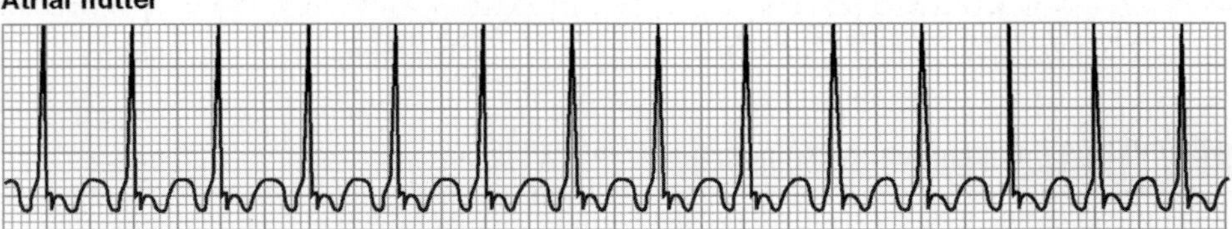

- A regular, saw-toothed pattern of atrial activity, usually very near 300/min
- Discrete, organized atrial activity on intracardiac electrograms
- Usually even-numbered AV conduction ratio (2:1, 4:1)

Atrial fibrillation

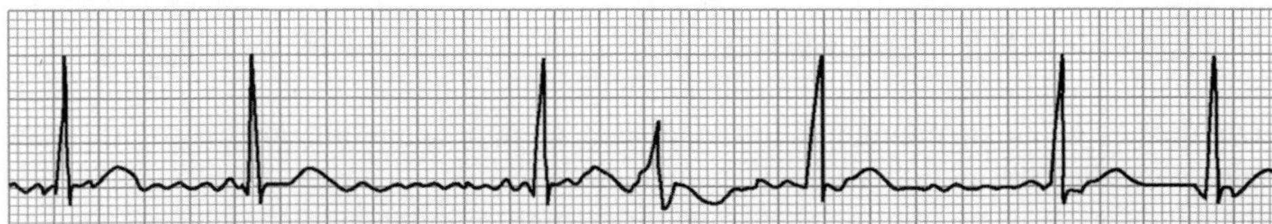

- Undulating, low amplitude atrial activity on ECG
- Intracardiac electrogram shows chaotic rapid spikes
- Variable conduction pattern as AV node is constantly bombarded with impulses; "long-short" sequences yield wide QRS complexes (aberrant, "Ashman" beats)

Wolff–Parkinson–White syndrome

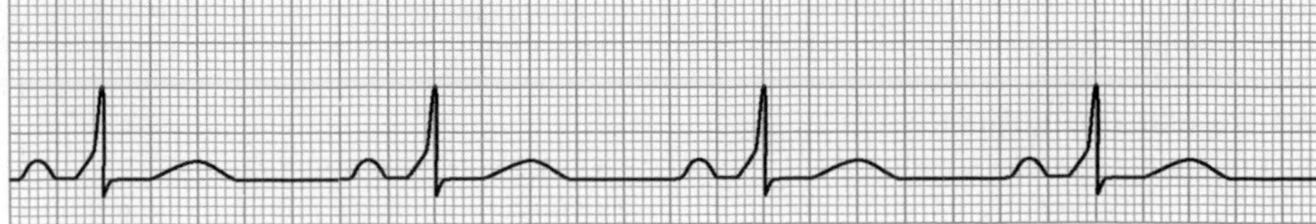

- Accessory atrioventricular conductions
- Anterograde or retrograde conduction
- Tachyarrhythmias
- Blurred QRS (referred to as δ-wave)

TABLE 3-2 Conduction Anomalies

Anomaly	Pathology	Notes	ECG
First-degree heart block	AV nodal anomaly **lengthens PR interval** (greater than 0.2)	May be caused by drugs (e.g., β-blockers, digitalis, and calcium-channel blockers)	
Second-degree heart block: Mobitz type 1 (Wenckebach)	Defect in atrioventricular node; progressively **increasing PR interval until QRS wave is lost**	Relatively common; usually **does not require treatment**	
Second-degree heart block: Mobitz type 2	**Defect in His-Purkinje system;** constant PR interval with random dropped QRS complexes	Less common and more dangerous than Mobitz type 1; **pacemaker**	
Third-degree heart block	No electrical connection between atria and ventricles; **atria and ventricles contract independently**	His-Purkinje system sets the rate of ventricular contraction; pacemaker may be necessary	

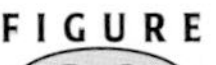

Antiarrhythmic drugs

Class IA (slows phase 0, prolongs phase 3); Class IB (shortens phase 3); Class IC (markedly slows phase 0); Class II (suppresses phase 4 depolarization rate); Class III (prolongs phase 3); Class IV (slows the action potential)

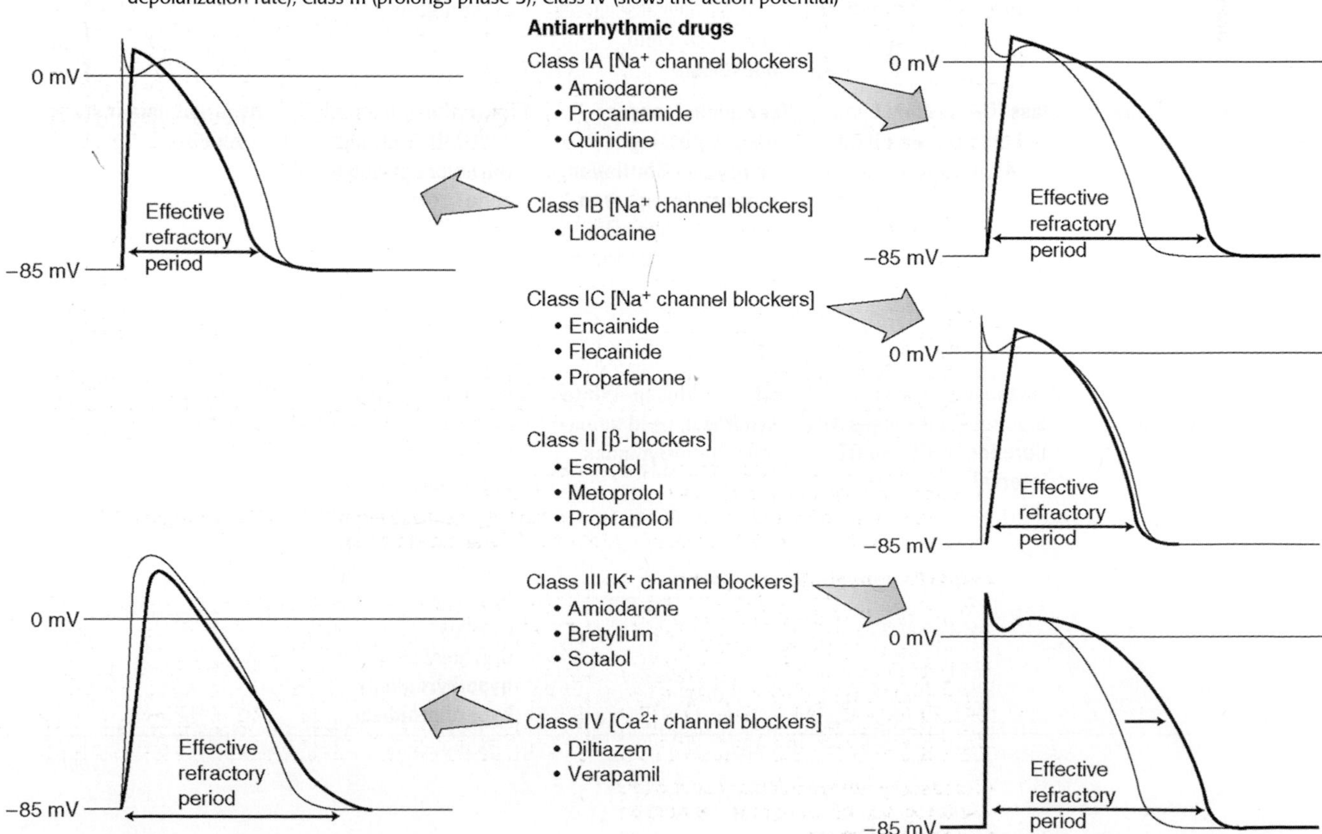

TABLE 3-3 Antiarrhythmics

Therapeutic Agent (common name, if relevant) [trade name, where appropriate]	Class—Pharmacology and Pharmacokinetics	Indications	Side or Adverse Effects	Contraindications or Precautions to Consider; Notes
Digoxin	**Inotropic agent—cardiac glycoside; inhibits Na/K/ATPase → indirect inhibition of Na^+/Ca^{2+} exchanger → increases Ca^{2+} → increases cardiac contractility**	**Severe left ventricular systolic dysfunction** (increases contractility); **atrial fibrillation** (decreases conduction at AV node and depresses SA node)	**Progressive dysrhythmia;** anorexia; nausea; vomiting; headache; fatigue; **confusion; blurred vision; altered color perception; halos around dark objects**	Contraindicated in patients with right-sided heart failure, diastolic failure; **ECG changes: increases PR, decreases QT, depresses ST, and inverts T; Toxicities of digoxin are increased by renal failure** (decreases excretion), **hypokalemia** (potentiates the drug's effects), and **quinidine** (decreases clearance and displaces digoxin)
Sodium channel blockers (Class I)				
Quinidine, amiodarone, -procainamide, disopyramide	**Class IA—sodium channel blocker → increases AP duration, ERP, QT interval**	**Atrial and ventricular arrhythmia** (especially re-entrant and ectopic supraventricular and ventricular tachycardia)	**Torsades de pointers**; reversible lupus like syndrome (procainamide); **Cinchonism**—headache, tinnitus, thrombocytopenia (quinidine)	Hyperkalemia increases toxicity
Lidocaine, mexiletine, tocainide	**Class IB—sodium channel blocker → decreases AP duration**	**Acute ventricular arrhythmias** (especially post-MI), digitalis-induced arrhythmia; **local anesthesia**	**CNS stimulation and depression; cardiovascular depression**	**Hyperkalemia increases toxicity**
Flecainide, encainide, propafenone	**Class IC—sodium channel blocker; no effect on AP duration**	**Ventricular tachycardia progressing to ventricular fibrillation, intractable supraventricular tachycardia,** last resort in ventricular arrhythmias	**Proarrythmic (especially post-MI), prolongs refractory period in AV node**	**Hyperkalemia increases toxicity**
Potassium channel blocker				
Sotalol, ibutilide, bretylium, amiodarone	**Potassium channel blocker—increases AP duration, ERP, and QT interval**	**Wolff–Parkinson–White syndrome; used when other antiarrythmics fail**	**Torasades de pointes**, excessive beta block, and hypotension; amiodarone-**pulmonary fibrosis**, corneal deposits, **hepatotoxicity**, skin deposits, photodermatitis, neurologic effects, constipation, bradycardia, CHF, heart block, and **hypothyroidism/ hyperthyroidism**	

(continued)

TABLE 3-3 Antiarrhythmics *(Continued)*

Therapeutic Agent (common name, if relevant) [trade name, where appropriate]	Class–Pharmacology and Pharmacokinetics	Indications	Side or Adverse Effects	Contraindications or Precautions to Consider; Notes
Calcium-channel blockers				
Verapamil, diltiazem	**Calcium-channel blocker—decreases conduction velocity of AV nodal cells, increases ERP, PR interval**	**Prevent nodal arrhythmias (supraventricular tachycardia)**	Constipation, **flushing, edema**, CHF, AV block, sinus node depression, torsades de pointes	
β-blockers				
Propranolol, esmolol, metoprolol, atenolol, timolol	β-blocker—decreases cAMP and calcium currents → increases PR interval, suppresses abnormal pacemakers, especially in AV node	**Ventricular tachycardia, supraventricular tachycardia**, slowing the ventricular rate during **atrial fibrillation and atrial flutter**	**Impotence, exacerbation of asthma, bradycardia**, AV block, CHF, sedation, sleep alteration, dyslipidemia (metoprolol)	Esmolol very short acting.
Other				
Adenosine	**Increases potassium efflux → hyperpolarizes the cell**	**Diagnosis and treatment of AV nodal arrhythmias**	**Flushing, hypotension, and chest pain**	Very short acting
Potassium	**Depresses ectopic pacemaker in hypokalemia**	**Digoxin toxicity**		

AP, action potential; ERP, effective refractory period.

V. Digitalis toxicity

A. Anti-Fab Fragments

VI. Torsade de pointes

A. Mg^{2+}

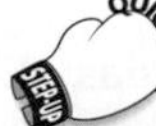

Class II agents (β-blockers) work at nodal tissue, so use these to control ventricular rate affected by atrial fibrillation, atrial flutter, and excess catecholamines.

ATHEROSCLEROSIS

I. Atherosclerosis is a disease of large-size and medium-size vessels and is characterized by the formation of atheromas (i.e., lesions that have a central lipid rich core surrounded by fibrous tissue) deposited in the intima of arteries.

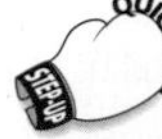

Although amiodarone has class I, II, III, and IV activity, it has a number of side effects: pulmonary fibrosis, photodermatitis, thyroid changes (mostly hypothyroid), CNS effects (rare), and decreased liver function (rare).

II. It is the leading cause of mortality in the United States.

III. Risk factors

A. Major risk factors
1. Hyperlipidemia: high blood cholesterol, high triglycerides, and decreased high-density lipoproteins (HDLs; <45) (Table 3-4 later in the chapter)
2. Diabetes mellitus
3. Cigarette smoking
4. Hypertension
5. Obesity

B. Minor risk factors
1. Lack of physical activity
2. Male sex

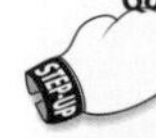

Adenosine terminates reentry pathways, so it is the drug of choice for acute paroxysmal supraventricular tachycardia (PSVT). It can also help diagnose whether ventricular tachycardia was induced supraventricularly or ventricularly.

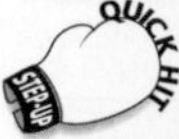

Frequency of fibrous plaques: abdominal aorta > proximal coronary artery > popliteal artery > descending thoracic aorta > internal carotid artery > renal artery.

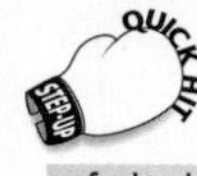

A low-fat diet with limited consumption of alcohol is beneficial for all patients with hyperlipidemia.

Type IIB and type IV are the two most common dyslipidemias.

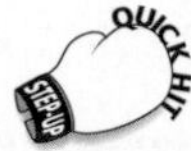

Vitamin E inhibits the oxidation of LDL and its subsequent absorption by macrophages. Compounds such as superoxide, nitric oxide, and hydrogen peroxide promote oxidation of LDL and blood vessel injury.

3. Increased age
4. Family history
5. Oral contraceptives, decreased estrogens, or premature menopause
6. Type A personality
7. Elevated homocysteine level

IV. Pathogenesis

A. Atheroma formation
   1. Monocytes adhere to vessel walls, enter tissue, and become macrophages.
   2. Macrophages are transformed into foam cells after engulfing oxidized low-density lipoproteins (LDLs).
   3. Foam cells accumulate in the intima.
   4. Foam cells release factors that cause the aggregation of platelets, the release of fibroblast growth factor, and the accumulation of smooth muscle.
   5. After formation of plaque, calcification occurs.
   6. The central core of the plaque consists mainly of cholesterol.

B. Complications
   1. Plaque rupture
   2. Ischemic heart disease or MI
   3. Stroke
   4. Renal arterial ischemia
   5. Death

FAMILIAL DYSLIPIDEMIAS (Table 3-4)

TABLE 3-4 Familial Dyslipidemia

Familial Dyslipidemias	Elevated	Blood Lipid Levels	Pathology (see System 5: The Gastrointestinal System)	Clinical Picture	Treatment
Hyperchylomicronemia I	Chylomicrons	↑↑TG	Lipoprotein lipase deficiency	Increased vascular and heart disease	Low-fat diet
Hypercholesterolemia IIa	LDL	↑Cholesterol	**Decreased LDL receptors**	Greatly increased vascular and heart disease; **xanthomas**	Cholestyramine/colestipol, lovastatin (and niacin for homozygotes)
Combined hyperlipidemia IIb	LDL, VLDL	↑TG, ↑cholesterol	Hepatic overproduction of VLDL	Increased vascular and heart disease	Cholestyramine/colestipol, lovastatin (and niacin for homozygotes)
Dysbetalipoproteinemia III	VLDL	↑TG, ↑cholesterol	Altered apolipoprotein E	Increased vascular and heart disease; xanthomas	Niacin and clofibrate or lovastatin
Hypertriglyceridemia IV	VLDL	↑↑TG, normal to ↑cholesterol	Hepatic overproduction (with possible decreased clearance) of VLDL	Increased vascular and heart disease; obese, **diabetic, pregnant,** and **alcoholic** patients	Weight loss; low-fat diet; niacin and clofibrate or lovastatin (if necessary)
Mixed hypertriglyceridemia V	VLDL, chylomicrons	↑↑TG, ↑cholesterol	Overproduction or decreased clearance of VLDL and chylomicrons	Obese and diabetic patients	Diet modification; niacin and clofibrate or lovastatin (if necessary)

LDL, low-density lipoproteins; TG, triglycerides; VLDL, very-low-density lipoproteins.

LIPID-LOWERING AGENTS (Table 3-5)

TABLE 3-5 Lipid Lowering Agents

Therapeutic Agent (common name, if relevant) [trade name, where appropriate]	Class–Pharmacology and Pharmacokinetics	Indications	Side or Adverse Effects	Contraindications or Precautions to Consider; Notes
Lovastatin, pravastatin, simvastatin, atorvastatin	**HMG-CoA reductase inhibitors**—inhibits the synthesis of cholesterol precursor mevalonate; **decreases LDL, increases HDL, and decreases TG**	**High LDL, preventative after thrombotic event (e.g., MI, stroke)**	Reversible increase in LFTs, myositis	
Niacin	**Inhibits lipolysis** in fat tissue, **reduces hepatic VLDL secretion** into circulation; **decreases LDL, increases HDL, and decreases TG**	**Increased LDL**	Flushing (decreased by aspirin or long-term use)	
Cholestyramine, colestipol	**Bile acid resin/Cholesterol absorption blocker**—binds bile acids → prevents intestinal reabsorption of bile acid and therefore cholesterol; **decreases LDL and increases HDL**	**Increased LDL**	**Tastes like sand, GI irritation**, and decreased absorption of fat soluble vitamins	
Ezetimibe	**Cholesterol absorption blocker**—Prevents cholesterol reabsorption at brush border in the small intestine; **decreases LDL; no effect on HDL or TG**	**Increased LDL**	Increases LFT (rarely)	
Gemfibrozil, clofibrate, bezafibrate, fenofibrate	**Upregulates lipoprotein lipase (periphery) → increases TG clearance; decreases LDL, increases HDL, and decreases TG**	**Increased TG, increased LDL**	Myositis, increased LFTs	Reduces TG more than other agents

LDL, low-density lipoprotein; HDL, high-density lipoprotein; HMG CoA reductase, 3-hydroxy-3-methylglutaryl-coenzyme A reductase; TG, triglycerides.

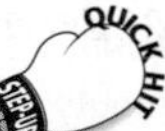

HDL works to remove cholesterol from tissues and plaques, thereby exerting a protective effect. HDL is increased by exercise.

HYPERTENSION

I. Essential
- A. Most common type (95% of cases)
- B. Unknown etiology
- C. Risk factors
  1. Family history
  2. Race (more common in Blacks)
  3. Obesity
  4. Cigarette smoking
  5. Physical inactivity
- D. Characteristics
  1. Blood pressure greater than 140/90 mm Hg on two separate occasions with the patient comfortably sitting and arm at the level of the patient's heart.
- E. Chronic complications
  1. Hypertrophy of left ventricle
  2. Onion-skinning of vessel walls
  3. Retinal hemorrhages
- F. Essential hypertension predisposes to ischemic heart disease (see next section)

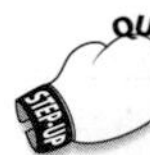

Metabolic syndrome includes hypertriglyceridemia, low HDL, central obesity, hypertension, and poorly controlled type II diabetes mellitus. Risk factors for this syndrome correlate to the state of insulin resistance.

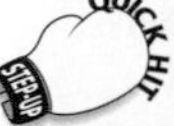

Hypertrophy of the left ventricle is also caused by left-sided valvular disease such as aortic stenosis and mitral regurgitation.

II. Secondary hypertension refers to elevated systemic arterial pressure associated with a condition known to cause hypertension
- A. Renal diseases are the most common cause of secondary hypertension:
  1. Renal parenchymal disorders

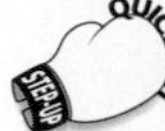

Fibromuscular dysplasia of the renal artery causes a "beads-on-a-string" sign on radiograph.

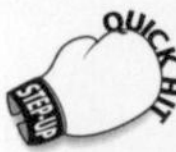

Treatment for emergent (malignant) hypertension (systolic blood pressure greater than 220 mm Hg or diastolic pressure greater than 120 mm Hg) includes IV sodium nitroprusside. It is dangerous to give pure β-blockers because of unopposed α stimulation. Therefore, an α/β blocker such as labetalol can be given.

MNEMONIC

To remember the side effects of ACE inhibitors, think **CAPTOPRIL:**
C–cough, persistent dry
A–angioedema
P–postural hypotension
T–teratogenic
O–oh, it makes me dizzy
P–proteinuria
R–renal failure in bilateral renal artery stenosis
I–increased K⁺
L–low neutrophils (neutropenia)

β-Blockers mask many of the symptoms of hypoglycemia (tremors, sweating, palpitations, etc.) that are mediated by epinephrine. This, as well as the endocrine effects, puts individuals with insulin-dependent diabetes taking β-blockers at increased risk for profound hypoglycemia.

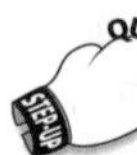

Cocaine use can also result in coronary vasospasm resulting in myocardial ischemia. In general, cocaine works by inhibiting the reuptake of endogenous catecholamines (dopamine, norepinephrine, epinephrine, and serotonin). Conversely, amphetamines stimulate the release of endogenous catecholamines.

2. Unilateral renal artery stenosis
    a. Atherosclerosis (more common in Black males and older individuals)
    b. Fibromuscular dysplasia (more common in White females and young people)
3. Renin–angiotensin axis activated

B. Endocrine causes
1. Primary aldosteronism
2. Pheochromocytoma
3. Hyperthyroidism
4. Acromegaly
5. Cushing syndrome

C. Coarctation of the aorta

III. Malignant (emergent) hypertension

A. Accelerated course results in end-organ damage in days.

B. End-organ damage occurs to the following organ systems:
1. Cardiovascular—vascular damage, aortic dissection
2. Pulmonary—pulmonary edema
3. Renal—"flea-bitten kidneys," azotemia
4. Ocular—fundal hemorrhages, papilledema
5. CNS—encephalopathy, seizures, coma

C. This type of hypertension causes early death because of cerebrovascular accident (CVA).

D. Young Black males are the usual victims of this type of hypertension.

ANTIHYPERTENSIVE AGENTS (Table 3-6)

I. α-Blockers

A. α-Adrenergic receptors are the primary controllers of vascular tone, blockers used primarily to lower blood pressure.
1. α_1-Selective agents commonly used in the treatment of hypertension include prazosin, doxazosin, and terazosin.
2. They have little impact on the heart, but they do have selective effects that allow them to have other clinical uses (such as treatment for benign prostatic hypertrophy).

B. Side effects
1. Postural hypotension with reflex tachycardia (most common)
2. Nasal congestion and headache
3. Rebound hypertension if stopped abruptly

C. Phenoxybenzamine and phentolamine are nonselective α-blockers that can be used in the diagnosis and treatment of the symptoms of pheochromocytoma.

II. β-Blockers

A. β-Blockers can be divided into four subgroups:
1. Nonselective β-blockers (β_1 and β_2): propranolol, timolol, and nadolol
2. β_1-Selective agents: metoprolol, atenolol, acebutolol, and esmolol
3. β_2-Selective agents (discussed in System 4)
4. α/β Blockers (carvediolol, labetalol)

B. This important class of drugs has many clinical uses:
1. Cardiac uses (most common)
    a. Hypertension
    b. Stable angina
    c. Prophylaxis after a myocardial infarction
2. Less common uses
    a. Symptomatic treatment of hyperthyroidism
    b. Prophylaxis against migraine headaches
    c. Anxiety disorder

C. Therapeutic effects of β-blockers on various organ systems are listed in Table 3-7.

(text continues on page 97)

TABLE 3-6 Antihypertensive Agents

Therapeutic Agent (common name, if relevant) [trade name, where appropriate]	Class–Pharmacology and Pharmacokinetics	Indications	Side or Adverse Effects	Contraindications or Precautions to Consider; Notes
Diuretics				
Hydrochlorothiazide	Thiazide diuretic—Inhibits transport of Na^+ and Cl^- into the cells of DCT	**Hypertension, CHF,** iciopathic hypercalciuria, nephrogenic diabetes insipidus	**Hypokalemia, metabolic alkalosis, mild hyperlipidemia, hyperuricemia,** malaise, **hypercalcemia,** hyperglycemia, hyponatremia	Do not give in patients with sulfa drug allergy
Furosemide	Loop diuretic—Prevents cotransport of Na^+, K^+, and Cl^- in **thick ascending limb**	**Hypertension; CHF;** cirrhosis, nephrotic syndrome, **Pulmonary edema,** and hypercalcemia	**Potassium wasting, metabolic alkalosis,** hypotension, dehydration, **ototoxicity,** nephritis, and gout	Do not give in patients with **sulfa drug allergy**
RAA system				
Captopril, enalapril, fosinopril	ACE inhibitor → inhibits conversion of angiotensin I to II → decreases ang II levels → prevents vasoconstriction from ang II	Hypertension, CHF, post-MI agent, and vasodilator	**Hyperkalemia, cough** (persistent dry), **angioedema,** taste changes, orthostatic hypotension, proteinuria, renal failure (in bilateral renal artery stenosis), neutropenia, and rash	Contraindicated in pregnancy (fetal renal malformation)
Losartan	ARBs → prevents vasoconstriction from ang II	**Hypertension**	Fetal renal toxicity, **hyperkalemia**	
Sympathoplegics				
Metoprolol, atenolol, acebutolol, esmolol, propranolol, Timolol, carvedilol	β_1-blocker (metoprolol, atenolol, acebutolol, esmolol), β_1- and β_2-blocker (propanolol, timolol), carvedilol (α and β blocker)	**Hypertension, angina, MI, antiarrythmic**	**Impotence, asthma, bradycardia,** AV block, heart failure, sedation, and sleep alterations	
Prazosin	**α_1-blocker** → vasodilation → decreases total peripheral resistance	**Pheochromocytoma; hypertension**	**Orthostatic hypotension;** dizziness and headache	First dose orthostatic hypotension
Clonidine	Centrally acting sympathetic agent (α_2-agonist) → decreases sympathetic outflow from CNS → decreases peripheral resistance	**Hypertension, smoking withdrawal, and heroin and cocaine withdrawal**	Drowsiness; **dry mouth; and rebound hypertension after abrupt withdrawal**	
Methyldopa	Centrally acting sympathetic agent (α-agonist) → decreases sympathetic outflow from CNS	**Hypertension**	Sedation and hemolytic anemia	**Positive Coombs test**

(continued)

TABLE 3-6 Antihypertensive Agents *(Continued)*

Therapeutic Agent (common name, if relevant) [trade name, where appropriate]	Class–Pharmacology and Pharmacokinetics	Indications	Side or Adverse Effects	Contraindications or Precautions to Consider; Notes
Hexamethonium	Nicotinic ganglionic blocker	Hypertensive emergency	Severe orthostatic hypotension, blurred vision, constipation, and sexual dysfunction	
Reserpine	Prevents the storage of monoamines in synaptic vesicle	Hypertension	**Mental depression,** sedation, nasal stuffiness, and diarrhea	
Guanethidine	Interferes with norepinephrine release	**Severe hypertension**	Orthostatic hypotension, exercise hypotension, impotence, and diarrhea	**Contraindicated in patients taking TCAs**
Vasodilators				
Hydralazine	Increases cGMP → smooth muscle relaxation → vasodilates arterioles → afterload reduction	**Severe hypertension, CHF**	**Compensatory tachycardia**, fluid retention, and **lupus like syndrome.**	**First line therapy for hypertension in pregnancy,** used with methyldopa; contraindicated in angina/CAD because of compensatory tachycardia
Minoxidil	**K^+ channel opener** → hyperpolarizes and relaxes vascular smooth muscle	**Severe hypertension**	**Hypertrichosis** and pericardial effusion	
Nifedipine, verapamil	**Calcium channel antagonists**—block voltage dependent calcium channels of **cardiac (verapamil > diltiazem > nifedipine) and vascular smooth muscle (nifedipine > diltiazem > verapamil)**	**Hypertension, angina, arrhythmia** (not nifedipine), **Prinzmetal angina, Raynaud's**	Cardiac depression, peripheral edema, **flushing, dizziness,** and constipation	
Nitroprusside	Direct release of NO → increases cGMP → vasodilator (arterial dilation)	**Hypertensive emergency, CHF, and angina**	Cyanide toxicity; hypotension	Short acting
Diazoxide	**K^+ channel opener**—hyperpolarizes and relaxes vascular smooth muscle	**Hypertension**	Hypoglycemia (reduces insulin release) and hypotension	

ACE, angiotensin-converting enzyme; ARB, angiotensin II receptor blocker; cGMP, cyclic guanosine monophosphate; CHF, congestive heart failure; MI, myocardial infarction.

TABLE 3-7 Therapeutic Effects of β-Blockers

Organ System	Effect	Clinical Implication
Cardiac (β_1)	Negative inotropic and chronotropic effects; slowing of SA and atrioventricular nodes	Decreases cardiac output; bradycardia can limit dosing; atrioventricular nodal slowing is useful in supraventricular tachycardia
Pulmonary (β_2)	Constriction of airway smooth muscle	β-Blockers are contraindicated in patients with chronic obstructive pulmonary disease
Endocrine	Decreased glycogenolysis; decreased glucagon release	β-Blockers must be used with caution in diabetic patients taking insulin who are at a risk for hypoglycemia
Ocular	Decreased aqueous humor production by processes of ciliary body	β-Blockers, such as timolol, can be used topically for glaucoma

Note: Those effects known to be predominantly caused by either β_1- or β_2-blockers are listed as such.

D. Adverse effects
   1. Sexual dysfunction in males
   2. Arrhythmias if the drug is stopped abruptly
   3. Bronchoconstriction
   4. Blocking hypoglycemic response in a diabetic

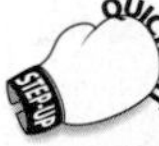

α_1-Blockers can also be used to treat the symptoms of benign prostatic hyperplasia.

III. Calcium-channel blockers

A. Second-line antihypertensive agents.
B. Act by binding to the L-type calcium channel of vascular smooth muscle cells and myocytes.
C. Block the entry of calcium into these cells.
D. These agents affect both vascular tone and the heart itself. Effects on the heart include negative inotropy and slowing of the conduction system.
E. Calcium-channel blockers are often divided into two groups:
   1. Dihydropyridines
      a. Examples: nifedipine and amlodipine
      b. Greater effect on vascular smooth muscle than on the heart
   2. Nondihydropyridines
      a. Examples: diltiazem and verapamil
      b. Increasingly greater effects on the myocardium
F. Adverse effects include hypotension, headache, constipation, and exacerbation of gastroesophageal reflux and bradycardia.

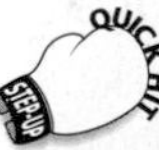

Berry aneurysms are commonly associated with adult polycystic kidney disease, an autosomal dominant disease; the gene is located on chromosome 16.

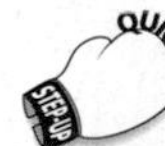

Syphilis is a sexually transmitted disease caused by *Treponema pallidum* (a spirochete) that is characterized initially (primary stage) by a painless, hard chancre. Untreated syphilis progresses to secondary and tertiary stages which are characterized by rashes, lymphadenopathy, condylomata lata, Argyll Robertson pupils (pupils constrict with accommodation but not with light), and aortic root aneurysms.

IV. Other antihypertensive agents

A. Clonidine
   1. Along with α-methyldopa, a centrally acting antihypertensive agent.
   2. This agent acts as an agonist at presynaptic α_2 receptors, thereby decreasing central sympathetic tone.
   3. Adverse effects include sedation and rebound hypertension if the drug is stopped abruptly.
B. Sodium nitroprusside
   1. Given intravenously, this agent is the drug of choice for hypertensive emergencies.
   2. Given orally, this drug is toxic because it results in cyanide production.
   3. It affects both arterial and venous smooth muscle.
C. Vasodilators (hydralazine, minoxidil)
   1. Dilate both arteries and veins (predominantly arteries), lowering blood pressure
      a. Reflex tachycardia that results can actually precipitate attacks of angina.
      b. These agents are not first-line agents for hypertension.
      c. These are often used along with β-blockers and diuretics.
   2. Adverse reactions to hydralazine include headache, arrhythmias, and a lupuslike reaction.
   3. Adverse effects of minoxidil include sodium retention and hypertrichosis.

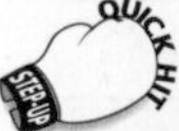
The most common location for an abdominal aorta aneurysm (AAA) is infrarenal. Therefore, an AAA is palpated superior to the umbilicus because the aorta bifurcates at the level of the umbilicus.

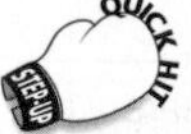
Although hypertension is not a risk factor for the presence of AAA, it increases the risk of rupture of an AAA. The triad for ruptured AAA is hypotension, abdominal pain, and pulsatile mass in the abdomen.

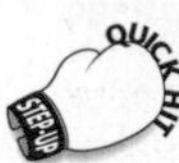
Emphysema is associated with AAA because increased matrix metalloprotein proteinase (MMP) activity leads to decreased collagen levels, weakening the vessel wall and predisposing to aneurysmal formation.

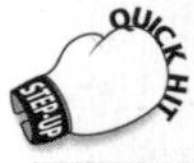
The most common diagnosis mistaken for AAA in the emergency setting is kidney stones.

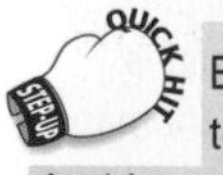
Exercise tolerance testing (stress testing) is a good way to diagnose subacute coronary occlusion. Thallium-201 scans reveal perfusion defects. Technetium (^{99m}Tc) scans are useful for imaging MIs.

Risk factors for coronary artery disease: smoking; diabetes; ↑ LDL, ↓ HDL; family history; men or postmenopausal women; sedentary lifestyle; hypertension; ↑ age; ↑ homocysteine; obesity.

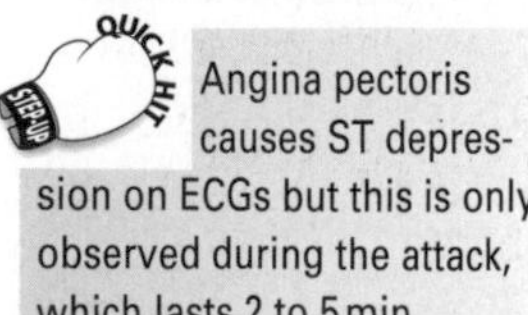
Angina pectoris causes ST depression on ECGs but this is only observed during the attack, which lasts 2 to 5 min.

ANEURYSMS (Table 3-8)

TABLE 3-8 Aneurysms

Type of Aneurysm	Etiology	Characteristics
Arteriovenous fistula	Abnormal communication between arteries and veins; usually secondary to **trauma**	Ischemic changes; aneurysm formation; **high-output cardiac failure**
Atherosclerotic	**Atherosclerotic** disease; coronary artery disease	Usually in the **abdominal** aorta; located between renal arteries and iliac bifurcation
Berry	Congenital medial weakness at the bifurcations of the cerebral arteries	Saccular lesions in cerebral vessels (especially at the **circle of Willis**); hemorrhage into the **subarachnoid** space
Dissecting	**Hypertension;** cystic medial necrosis; **Marfan syndrome**	**Tearing pain;** longitudinal separation of tunica media of aortic wall
Syphilitic	Tertiary syphilis; obliteration of the vasa vasorum; necrosis of the media	Involves **ascending** aorta and aortic root; aortic valve insufficiency
Mycotic (infectious)	Inflammation secondary to bacterial infection; usually salmonella	Involves abdominal aorta

Clinical Vignette 3-1

Clinical Presentation: A 59-year-old male presents to the emergency room with **sudden, severe, and constant low back pain.** Past medical history is significant for **hypertension, hyperlipidemia, emphysema,** coronary artery disease, stable angina, and 25 pack-years of **smoking.** The patient was hospitalized for a CVA 7 years ago. Physical examination revealed a 5.8 cm **pulsatile mass** superior to the umbilicus in the abdomen. T = 98.5°F, **BP = 150/90 mm Hg,** HR = 80 bpm, and RR = 23 breaths/min.

Differentials: AAA, aortic dissection, pyelonephritis/nephrolithiasis, prostatitis, and pancreatitis. Given that this pain developed suddenly and the presence of an abdominal pulsatile mass, this patient most likely has an AAA.

Laboratory Studies: Proper follow-up for this patient would include an **abdominal ultrasound** and/or **computerized tomography (CT) scan with contrast.** The typical diameter for abdominal aorta is **2 cm;** therefore, any size greater than this indicates presence of an aneurysm. Advantages of an ultrasound are that it is quick, easy, and inexpensive; however, it is very operator dependent, less useful in obese individuals, and does not provide information about the iliac arteries, which could also be aneurysmal. **CT angiogram** can also be helpful in describing the anatomy of the aorta prior to surgery but is not commonly done in clinical practice. All patients with AAA should also undergo cardiac evaluation because patients with AAA often have underlying vascular pathology. In these patients, **cardiac catheterization** should also be performed to assess cardiac risk and potentially revascularize the patients prior to operation.

Management: As an aneurysm becomes larger than 5.5 cm, the risk of rupture increases exponentially; an aneurysm smaller than 5.5 cm in diameter is less likely to rupture and risk-to-benefit ratio of surgery is less supportive. Therefore, if an AAA is **smaller than 5.5 cm** in diameter and asymptomatic, the patient can be followed with ultrasound or CT surveillance every 6 months. If the aneurysm is **larger than 5.5 cm** in diameter and symptomatic, the patient should be taken to the operating room. A patient with a ruptured AAA is taken to the operating room.

ISCHEMIC HEART DISEASE

I. It is defined as an inadequate supply of oxygen relative to demand.

II. Ischemic heart disease is most often caused by atherosclerosis.

III. There are four types of ischemic heart diseases.

A. Angina pectoris
1. Paroxysmal attacks of retrosternal pain, heaviness, and pressurelike or squeezing chest pain occur and may radiate to the neck, jaw, left shoulder, or arm. Angina pectoris is often associated with diaphoresis and nausea.
2. Imbalance between cardiac perfusion and cardiac demand is characteristic. Ninety percent occlusion of coronary vessel produces symptoms.
3. Three types of angina pectoris
   a. Stable angina
      - Most common form
      - Induced by exercise
      - Relieved by rest
      - Results from chronic stenosis of coronary arteries

   b. Prinzmetal (variant) angina
      - Episodic pain occurs at rest.
      - Attacks are unrelated to activity, blood pressure, or heart rate but are related to coronary artery vasospasm.
      - Significant artery stenosis is often present.

   c. Unstable angina
      - This type occurs at both rest and activity.
      - It is usually preceded by decreasing physical activity or gradual increase in stable anginal symptoms.
      - It produces pain of increasing duration.
      - It is induced by ruptured atherosclerotic plaque with subsequent thrombosis and embolization.
      - Activated platelets help cause thrombosis and vasospasm.
      - Microinfarcts may be caused.
4. Treatment of stable angina
   a. Nitrates
      - These drugs are converted within the cell to nitric oxide, a smooth muscle relaxant
        (1) The relaxation of vascular smooth muscle causes widespread venous dilation.
        (2) This lowers preload and therefore reduces the workload and oxygen demand of the heart.
        (3) To a lesser extent, the relaxation of coronary arteries provides ischemic myocardium with increased oxygen.
      - Sublingual nitroglycerin is the treatment of choice for acute episodes of angina.
      - A long-acting nitrate such as isosorbide dinitrate can be used for angina prophylaxis.
      - Unwanted side effects of nitrate therapy include headache and tachyphylaxis, postural hypotension, and facial flushing.
        (1) Calcium-channel blockers
        (2) β-Blockers

B. Myocardial infarction
1. Lack of adequate perfusion to cardiac tissue leads to myocyte death in affected area.
2. MI is most often caused by atherosclerosis with plaque rupture and thrombus.
3. The subendocardium is most vulnerable to ischemia (because of decreased blood flow during systole) and thus most likely to infarct.
4. In a transmural infarct (see below), the full thickness of the ventricular wall is affected within 35 h.

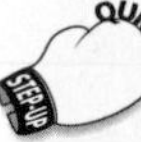

Anticoagulants (heparin, low-molecular weight heparin, and aspirin), nitrates, and β-blockers can be used to treat unstable angina. Do *not* use calcium-channel blockers or tissue plasminogen activator to treat unstable angina.

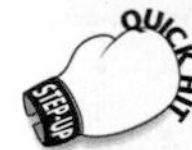

Dressler syndrome is a post-MI syndrome that presents with fever and pericarditis 6 weeks after an MI.

MNEMONIC

When remembering the sequence of histopathologic changes after an MI, think of the 1-3-1-3 rule:

1 day (**neutrophils** predominate), 3 days (**macrophages** infiltrate), 1 week (**fibroblasts** infiltrate), and 3 weeks (**granulation tissue** most prominent).

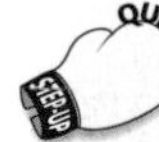

The left anterior descending artery is the most common artery involved in acute MI. Infarcts of this artery affect the left ventricle near its apex or the anterior portion of the interventricular septum.

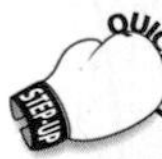

ST elevation is pathognomonic for transmural (Q-wave) infarcts. However, ST depression is not pathognomonic for nontransmural (non-Q-wave) infarcts as it can also be produced by digitalis drugs and also in stable/unstable angina.

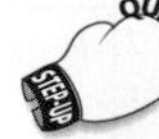

Reentry is the most common cause of arrhythmias. Reentry requires a circuit, refractory tissue (unidirectional block), slow conduction velocity, and an initiating event (usually a premature beat).

MNEMONIC

For the acute management of an MI, think **MONA B** (**m**orphine, **o**xygen, **n**itrates, **a**spirin, and **b**eta-blockers). To remember maintenance therapy (i.e., when discharging an MI patient from the hospital), think **ABC²: a**spirin, **β**-blockers, ACE inhibitor, and **c**holesterol-lowering drugs.

5. Two types of MI are possible:
   a. Nontransmural (non-Q-wave) infarcts (circumferential)
      - Diffuse coronary atherosclerosis is found.
      - This causes overall reduction of coronary flow.
      - Rupture or thrombosis eventually results, followed quickly by clot lysis.
      - Loss of perfusion to inner one-third of muscular wall of ventricle occurs.
      - ST-segment depression is seen on ECG.
   b. Transmural infarct (Q-wave infarct)
      - Atherosclerotic plaques rupture.
      - Platelet-mediated thrombosis occludes vessel.
      - Occluded vessel stops the flow of blood to the entire muscular wall.
      - ST-segment elevation is seen on ECG.
6. Cardiac enzymes are released when myocytes are damaged (Figure 3-10).
7. Complications
   a. Arrhythmia
   b. Heart block
   c. Myocardial rupture occurring most commonly during the first week post-MI
   d. Papillary muscle rupture
   e. Mural thrombus with possible embolization
   f. Aneurysm
   g. Death
8. Remodeling and scar formation occur over a period of 36 months after an infarct (Figure 3-10).

FIGURE 3-10 **Myocardial infarction enzyme release and timeline of histologic changes**

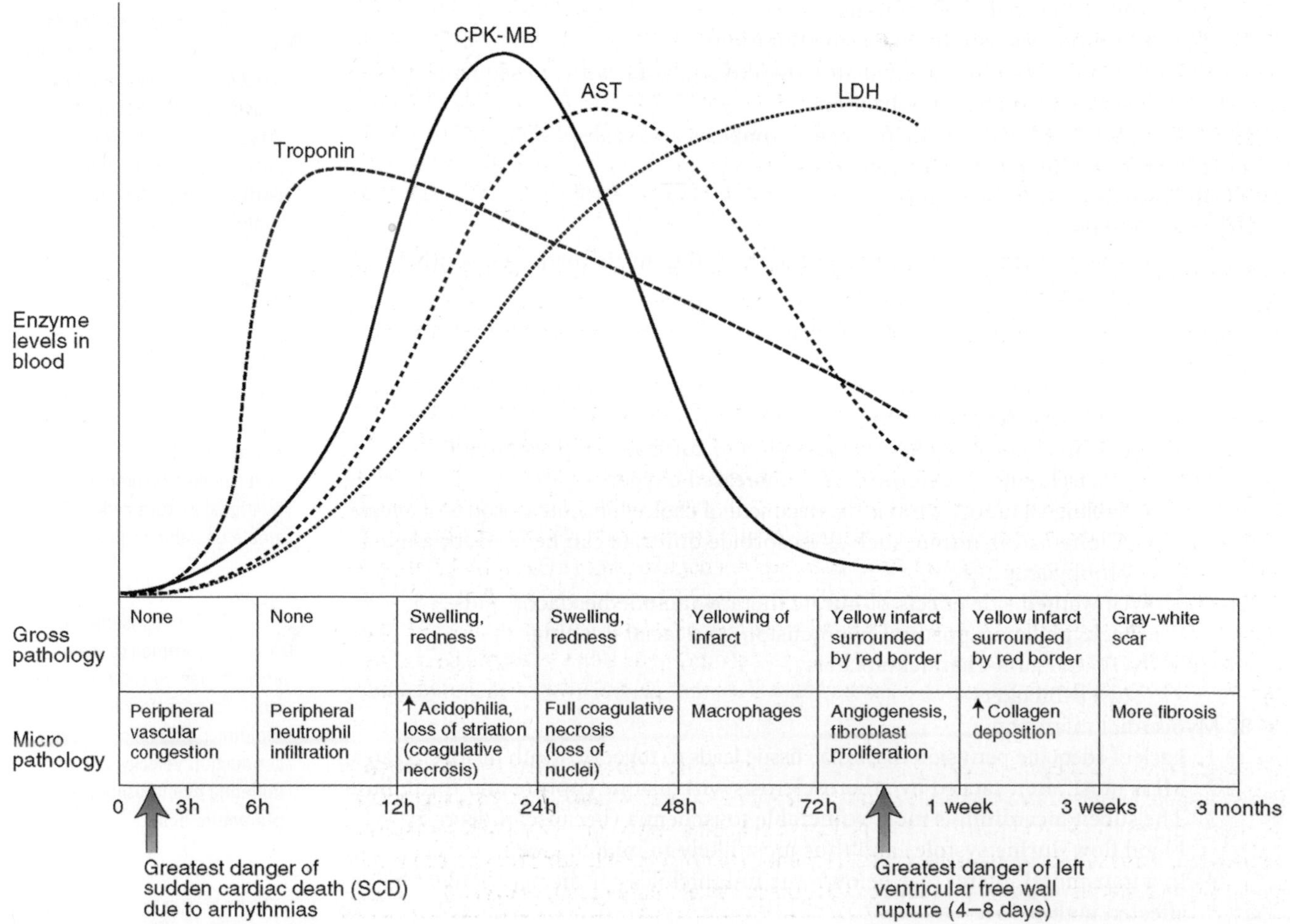

C. Chronic ischemic heart disease (CIHD)
   1. Congestive heart failure (CHF) that results from ischemic cardiac damage leads to CIHD.
   2. Hypertrophy of the heart and cardiac decompensation occur as a result of infarction.
   3. CIHD is most often found in the elderly.

D. Sudden cardiac death
   1. This is unexpected death from cardiac failure occurring within 2 h post-MI.
   2. This is caused less commonly by a congenital anomaly.
   3. Marked atherosclerosis is usually present.
   4. The mechanism of death is almost always because of arrhythmia.

CONGESTIVE HEART FAILURE (Table 3-9 and Figures 3-10 to 3-12)

CHF is a clinical diagnosis in which the heart is unable to pump an adequate amount of blood to meet the metabolic needs of the body. A number of factors play a role in CHF, including hormonal changes (RAA and sympathetic activation), peripheral vasoconstriction, and myocardial dysfunction. One of the final common pathways in CHF is hypoperfusion of the kidneys and activation of the RAA axis, which leads to sodium and water

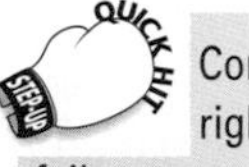

Cor pulmonale is right-sided heart failure secondary to lung disorders that lead to pulmonary arterial hypertension.

Idiopathic dilated cardiomyopathy is the most common form of cardiomyopathy. Treatment includes digitalis, ACE inhibitors, heart transplant, and sometimes chronic anticoagulation.

Clinical Vignette 3-2

Clinical Presentation: A 45-year-old male was brought to the emergency department complaining of **crushing chest pain of 1 h duration,** which he described as "a belt closed **tightly** around my chest." He indicated the location of the pain with a closed fist in the substernal region. The morning of admission, the patient was feeling ill and then experienced pain in the chest, which **radiated to his jaw, left shoulder, and down the left arm.** The pain was associated with **nausea;** the patient denied conditions that improved or worsened the pain. The patient's past medical history was significant for **hyperlipidemia** and **hypertension.** The patient stated that **his father recently underwent coronary artery bypass.** Past social history was significant for a 35-pack-year history of **smoking** and social drinking. On physical examination, the patient was found to be in acute distress and diaphoretic. *T* = 97.6 °F; BP = 145/90 mm Hg; **HR = 101 bpm; and** RR = 23 breaths/min.

Differentials: Acute MI, angina pectoris, aortic dissection, gastroesophageal reflux disease (GERD), pancreatitis and biliary tract disease, pericarditis, and pulmonary embolism (PE). Given the patient's description of pain and family history of coronary artery disease, he most likely has suffered from an acute MI.

Laboratory Studies: An acute MI would be diagnosed via (a) **blood chemistry** showing elevated cardiac enzymes or (b) **ECG** showing ST elevation if transmural or ST depression if subendocardial. With these changes, aortic dissection, GERD, and PE can be ruled out. In an aortic dissection, we would expect a widened mediastinum on **chest radiograph,** confirmed by **CT scan;** also, an **aortogram** showing a double lumen would be diagnostic. Stable angina can be ruled out because it typically lasts a few minutes, and although it can precede an MI, this pain is characteristically **relieved by rest or nitroglycerin.** Other laboratory studies that would be done in this patient include **amylase, lipase, alkaline phosphatase** (elevated in pancreatitis), and **echocardiography** (to rule out pericarditis). Interestingly, pericarditis presents with chest pain that radiates to the trapezoid region, worsens with inspiration, and is relieved by sitting up/leaning forward.

Management: Revascularization, if done early, is beneficial via **thrombolytics** or **angioplasty.** Patients should also receive **morphine** (reduces pain and is a vasodilator), **heparin** (to prevent formation of thrombus), and **nitrates.** This patient should be started and maintained on **aspirin** (shown to decrease mortality), **α-blockers** (prevent remodeling), **ACE inhibitors** (prevent remodeling), and **statins** (lower cholesterol and decrease risk of future coronary events).

TABLE 3-9 Congestive Heart Failure

	Etiology	Clinical Manifestations
Left-sided CHF	Ischemia (coronary artery disease) Systemic Hypertension Left-sided valvular disease Myocarditis Cardiomyopathy Congenital heart disease Pericardial disease	**Pulmonary edema** Dyspnea on exertion/fatigue **Orthopnea** Paroxysmal nocturnal dyspnea Hyperventilation Reduction in renal perfusion (activates renin–angiotensin–aldosterone axis) **S3**
Right-sided CHF	Left-sided heart failure Left-sided lesions **Cor pulmonale** Myocarditis Cardiomyopathy Right-sided valvular disease	Hepatomegaly/ascites (**nutmeg liver**) Splenomegaly **Peripheral edema** (especially pitting edema of the ankles) **Distention of neck veins** Renal hypoxia

FIGURE 3-11 Congestive heart failure

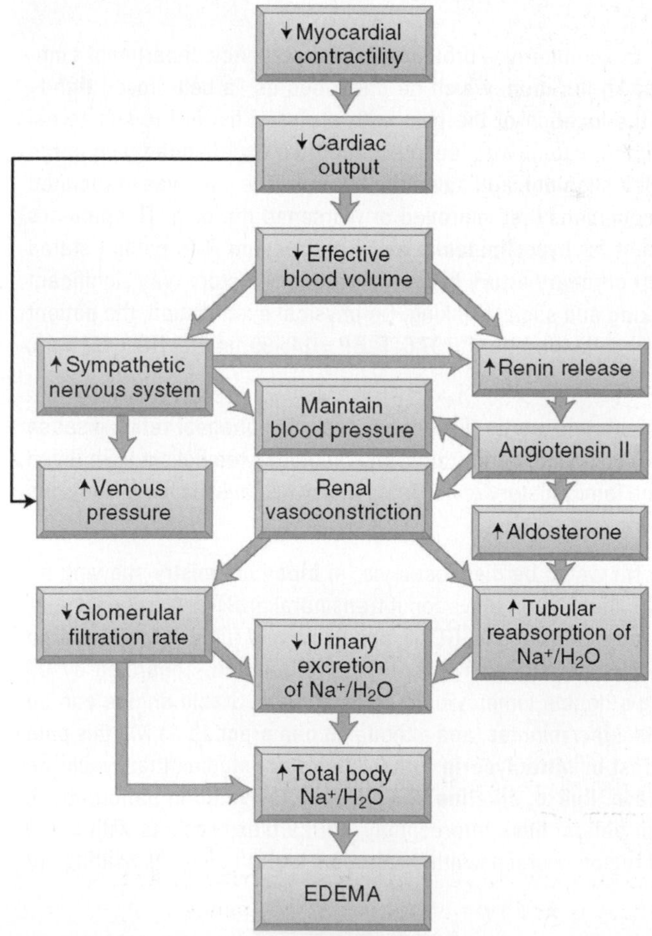

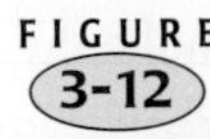
FIGURE 3-12 **A chest radiograph showing congestive heart failure and pulmonary edema**
(Reproduced with permission from Daffner RH. Clinical Radiology: The Essentials. 2nd Ed. Baltimore: Williams & Wilkins; 1999:204.)

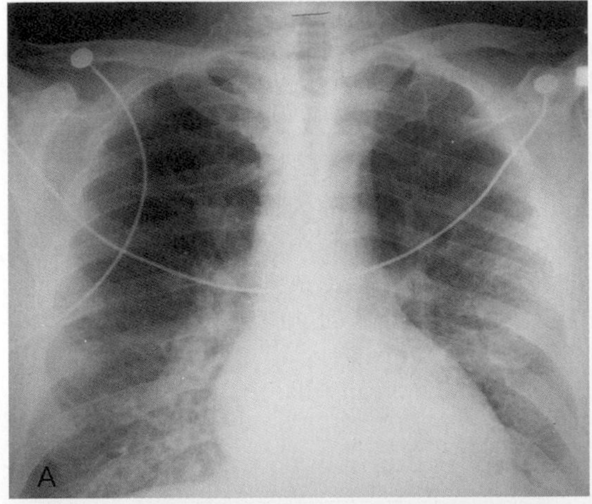

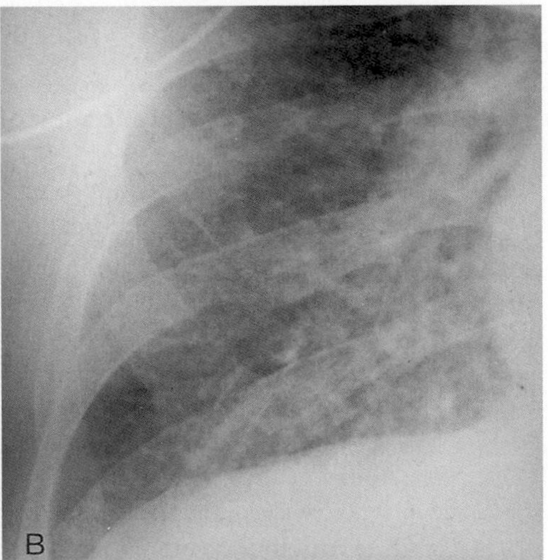

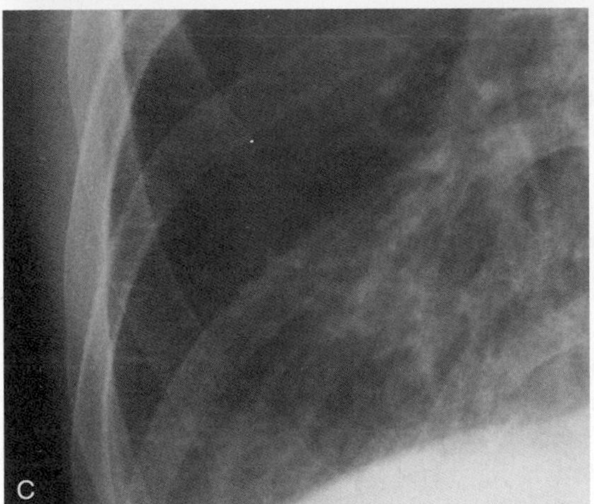

retention. Treatment is directed at either blocking the RAA axis or increasing the cardiac performance and, therefore, renal perfusion. Therapeutic agents in CHF treatment include ACE inhibitors, angiotensin II receptor blockers (ARBs), digitalis, diuretics, and dobutamine.

I. ACE inhibitors

A. First-line treatment for CHF.
B. ACE inhibitors are able to lower blood pressure (lower afterload), improve cardiac performance, and prevent the aldosterone-mediated salt and water retention typical of CHF.
C. Specific agents:
   1. Enalapril decreases mortality in CHF.
   2. Other ACE inhibitors include captopril and lisinopril.
D. Adverse effects of ACE inhibitors:
   1. Reversible renal failure
   2. Angioedema, hyperkalemia, dry cough, and orthostatic hypotension
   3. ACE inhibitors are fetotoxic and contraindicated in pregnancy

II. ARBs

A. These agents block the RAA axis at the Ang II receptor, producing the same benefits as ACE inhibitors.
B. Examples of ARBs are losartan and valsartan.

C. These drugs have all the same effects as the ACE inhibitors except that, unlike the ACE inhibitors, they do not increase levels of bradykinin and hence do not cause cough as a side effect.

III. Digitalis

A. Treats CHF by increasing cardiac performance; digitalis treats CHF by increasing the intracellular concentration of calcium in cardiac myocytes, thus increasing contractility.
B. Blocks sodium–potassium pump:
  1. This increases the intracellular sodium concentration.
  2. Activity of a sodium–calcium antiporter is decreased.
  3. Decreased activity of this antiporter raises intracellular calcium levels.
C. Digitalis improves the symptoms of CHF, but unlike ACE, it has not been shown to decrease mortality.
D. Digitalis also has a low therapeutic index, which means that the toxic dose is closer to the therapeutic dose.
E. Common adverse reactions:
  1. Nausea and headache
  2. Arrhythmias (more serious)

IV. Diuretics, the other major treatment modality for CHF, are not discussed here (see System 6).

Clinical Vignette 3-3

Clinical Presentation: A 67-year-old female complains to her primary care physician of **easy fatigue** and that each night she has to **wake up to urinate (nocturia).** She also mentions that each night her **ankles swell** and she **sleeps with her head elevated on two to three pillows (orthopnea),** otherwise she finds herself waking to **catch her breath (paroxysmal nocturnal dyspnea).** Her past medical history is significant for **hypertension;** however, the patient has been noncompliant with medication. Physical examination reveals congestion; **1+ pitting edema,** an **enlarged liver,** and **elevated JVP.** Other findings include **cold and clammy skin and S3 and S4 heart sounds.** *T* = 98.5°F; **BP = 165/100 mm Hg; HR = 92 bpm; and RR = 34 breaths/min.**

Differentials: CHF and renal failure. Given the patient's history and classic presentation, this patient likely has CHF secondary to chronic hypertension.

Laboratory Studies: Proper follow-up for suspect CHF would be (a) **chest radiograph** showing cardiomegaly (Figure 3-12), interstitial edema in the lungs, and pleural effusion; (b) **echocardiogram** (determines the cause of CHF, whether systolic or diastolic; quantifies ejection fraction [EF]); (c) **ECG** showing evidence of chamber enlargement or presence of ischemic disease; (d) **radionuclide ventriculography using technetium-99m** (quantifies EF when echo suboptimal as in chronic obstructive pulmonary disease [COPD]); (e) **cardiac catheterization;** (f) **stress testing;** (g) **urine analysis** (elevated protein would suggest renal failure); and (h) **blood chemistry** (blood urea nitrogen [BUN] and Creatinine [Cr] slightly elevated in CHF and markedly elevated in renal failure).

Management: Diastolic dysfunction is treated symptomatically. Systolic dysfunction should be managed by (a) **sodium restriction,** (b) **diuretics** (congestive symptoms), (c) **ACE inhibitors** (decrease preload, afterload, decrease mortality), and (d) **digitalis** (symptomatic relief; use in severe CHF). Note: If the patient cannot tolerate ACE inhibitors, use **ARBs, hydralazine,** and **isosorbide dinitrates.** Also, **α-blockers** have been proven to decrease mortality in post-MI CHF.

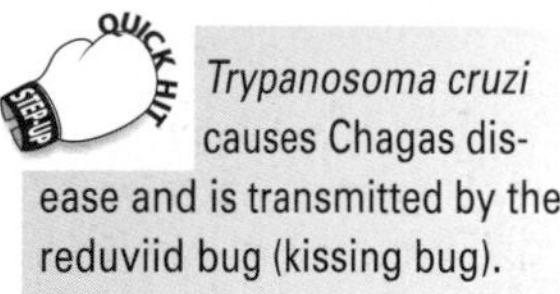

Trypanosoma cruzi causes Chagas disease and is transmitted by the reduviid bug (kissing bug).

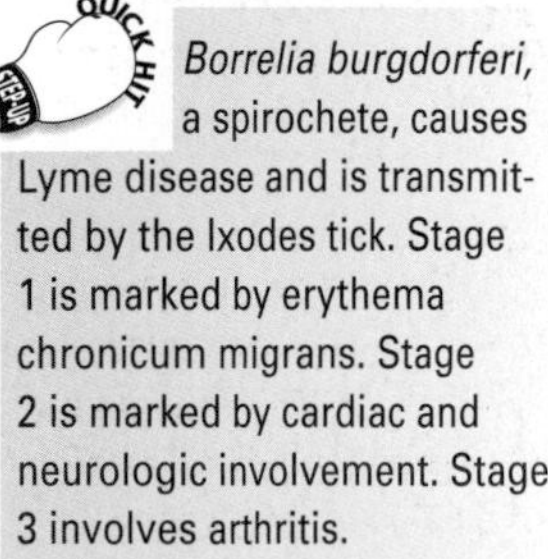

Borrelia burgdorferi, a spirochete, causes Lyme disease and is transmitted by the Ixodes tick. Stage 1 is marked by erythema chronicum migrans. Stage 2 is marked by cardiac and neurologic involvement. Stage 3 involves arthritis.

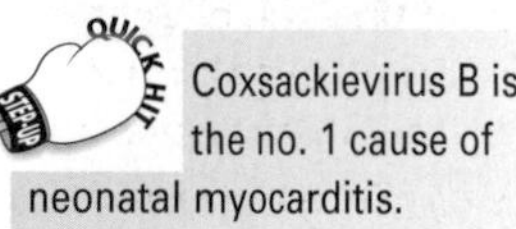

Coxsackievirus B is the no. 1 cause of neonatal myocarditis.

INTRINSIC DISEASES OF THE HEART

I. Myocarditis

A. This is defined as inflammation of the cardiac muscle
B. Etiology
 1. Viral etiology is the most common cause (usually coxsackie B virus).
 2. HIV (via toxoplasmosis and metastasis of Kaposi sarcoma) may cause myocarditis.
 3. Bacterial causes include *Staphylococcus aureus* and *Corynebacterium diphtheriae*.
 4. Chagas disease
 5. Lyme disease
 6. Hypersensitivity reactions
 7. Sarcoidosis
C. Physical examination
 1. Muffled S1
 2. Audible S3 heart sound
 3. Murmur of mitral regurgitation
 4. Cardiomegaly

II. Endocarditis

A. Inflammation of the heart lining and connective tissue
B. Causes
 1. Rheumatic heart disease—endocarditis may be caused by rheumatic fever (see below)
 2. Infective endocarditis
  a. Etiology
   - Bacteria, usually Gram-positive cocci, or fungi (Aspergillus and Candida) are the most common causes.
   - Damage, surgical repair, prosthetic heart valves, or congenital abnormalities are predisposing conditions.
   - Vegetative growth (usually on atrial surface of valves) can throw septic thrombi to brain or peripheral circulation.
   - Endocarditis is complicated by ulcerations of valves or rupture of chordae tendineae.
  b. Characteristics
   - Clinical features
    - Petechiae
    - Janeway lesions (peripheral hemorrhages with slight nodular character)
    - Osler nodes (small, tender nodules on fingers and toe pads)
    - Splinter hemorrhages (subungual linear streaks)
    - Roth spots (retinal hemorrhages)
    - Splenomegaly
   - The mitral and aortic valves are frequently involved.
   - The presence of right-sided valvular lesions, usually of the tricuspid, suggests intravenous (IV) drug abuse.
C. Types
 1. Acute endocarditis
  a. The cause is most often *S. aureus*.
  b. Onset is rapid.
  c. Clinical features include fever, anemia, embolic events, and heart murmur.
  d. Treatment is with IV antibiotics.
 2. Subacute endocarditis
  a. The cause is most often the viridans streptococci.
  b. It results from poor dentition or oral surgery in patients with preexisting heart disease (and pre-existing damage to heart valves).
  c. Onset is over a period of 6 months.
  d. Treatment is with IV antibiotics.

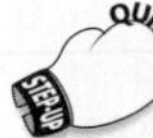

Associate native valve endocarditis or acute onset with Staphylococcus sp. and suspect *Streptococcus viridans* with prosthetic valve or late-onset endocarditis. Remember that *S. viridans* causes native valve endocarditis, more so than *Staphylococcus* sp. Associate endocarditis in intravenous drug abuse with *S. aureus*.

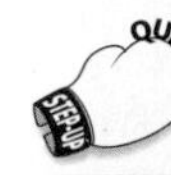

If an endocarditis is caused by *Streptococcus bovis*, look for signs and symptoms for gastrointestinal carcinoma in the patient.

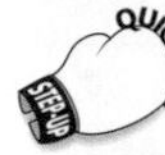

Culture-negative endocarditis can result from the HACEK group of organisms: *Haemophilus aphrophilus, Actinobacillus actinomycetemcomitans, Cardiobacterium hominis, Eikenella corrodens*, and *Kingella kingae*.

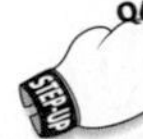

Prosthetic valves predispose individuals to endocarditis caused by *Staphylococcus epidermidis*.

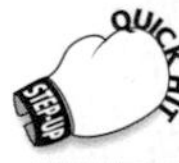

Primary tumors of the heart are very rare. Metastatic (secondary) tumors are more common. Atrial myxomas are the most frequently occurring primary tumors.

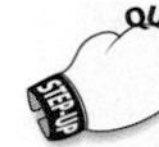

Systemic thromboembolism may develop in dilated cardiomyopathy, mitral valve prolapse, or from fragmented vegetations associated with infective endocarditis. Stasis of blood in the ventricle or atria leads to formation of mural thrombi as seen in dilated cardiomyopathy and mitral valve prolapse, respectively.

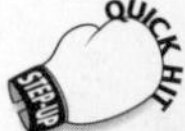
Antiphospholipid syndrome, common in SLE, results from antibodies to phospholipids primarily producing a hypercoagulable state leading to thrombotic disorders and multiple spontaneous abortions.

MNEMONIC

To remember the signs and symptoms of rheumatic heart disease, think **RHEUMATIC**: R = rheumatic; H = heart valve defects (long-term complication); E = erythema marginatum; U = under the skin nodules; M = migratory polyarthritis; A = Aschoff body; T = titer (antistreptolysin-O titer increased); I = infection (history of infection/pharyngitis); C = chorea.

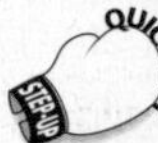
Senile amyloidosis is derived from transthyretin. Primary amyloidosis is caused by the amyloid light chain (AL) protein from immunoglobulin light chains. This is seen in plasma cell disorders (see System 10: The Hematopoietic and Lymphoreticular System).

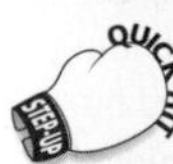
Mitral valve prolapse (MVP) is the most frequently occurring valvular lesion, often found in young women and in Marfan syndrome patients, and related to tissue laxity. Characteristics of the heart sound in MVP include midsystolic click followed by late systolic murmur.

A midsystolic click is often indicative of mitral prolapse.

3. Nonbacterial (marantic) endocarditis
    a. This type is associated with metastatic cancer.
    b. Sterile fibrin deposits appear on valves.
    c. Sterile emboli cause cerebral infarct.
4. Libman–Sacks endocarditis
    a. This is a manifestation of systemic lupus erythematosus (SLE).
    b. It is caused by autoantibody damage to valves.
    c. Vegetations form on both sides of the valve.
5. Carcinoid syndrome
    a. This syndrome is characterized by increased serotonin and other secretory products from a carcinoid tumor.
    b. Plaque builds on right-sided valves of the heart.

III. Rheumatic heart disease

A. This is a systemic inflammatory disorder with cardiac manifestations.

B. Pathogenesis
1. Rheumatic heart disease usually occurs 14 weeks after a bout of pharyngitis caused by group A β-hemolytic streptococci.
2. Antigenic mimicry occurs between streptococcal antigens and human antigens in the heart.
3. This results in immunologic origin for rheumatic heart disease.

C. Epidemiology
1. Children 5 to 15 years of age have the highest incidence of rheumatic fever.
2. Incidence is decreasing since the advent of penicillin.

D. Cardiac manifestations of rheumatic fever include the following conditions:
1. Pancarditis—inflammation of all structures of the heart
2. Pericarditis with effusions
3. Myocarditis
    a. Leads to cardiac failure
    b. Most common cause of early death in rheumatic fever
4. Endocarditis
    a. Usually afflicts the mitral and aortic valves (areas of high stress and turbulent flow).
    b. Mitral—aortic—tricuspid—pulmonary shows the order in which the valves become involved.
    c. Early nonembolic vegetations occur.
    d. With fibrosis and calcification, valvular damage leads to chronic rheumatic heart disease.

E. Other manifestations of rheumatic fever
1. Migratory polyarthritis
2. Sydenham chorea
3. Subcutaneous nodules
4. Erythema marginatum
5. Recent infection by group A streptococci (indicated by elevated antistreptolysin-O titers)
6. Aschoff body
    a. Lesion characterized by focal interstitial myocardial inflammation
    b. Fragmented collagen/fibrinoid material
    c. Anitschkow myocytes: large activated histiocytes
    d. Aschoff cells: granuloma with giant cells

IV. Cardiomyopathies (Table 3-10)

V. Valvular heart diseases (Table 3-11)

VI. Murmurs (Table 3-12)

VII. Peripheral vascular diseases (Table 3-13)

TABLE 3-10 Cardiomyopathies

	Pathology	Etiology	Clinical Manifestations	Notes
Dilated (systolic or contractile dysfunction)	Dilated ventricles; right and left heart failure; pulmonary edema	**Idiopathic;** alcoholics; thiamine deficiency; peripartum; **coxsackievirus** B; *Trypanosoma cruzi*; tricyclic antidepressants; lithium, doxorubicin; pregnancy associated	Premature ventricular contractions; **decreased ejection fraction;** JVP; cardiomegaly; hepatomegaly	**Most common** form
Restrictive (diastolic dysfunction or loss of compliance)	**Stiffened heart muscle;** may result in right and left heart failure; tricuspid regurgitation	Senile or primary amyloidosis; sarcoidosis; hemochromatosis (associated with systemic diseases)	Peripheral **edema;** ascites; jugular venous distention	Differentiate from hypertrophic cardiomyopathy
Hypertrophic (diastolic dysfunction or loss of compliance)	Ventricular and ventricular septal hypertrophy; mitral regurgitation	Usually **autosomal dominant** (the most common gene affected is β-myosin); young **athletes**	Dyspnea; syncope; **S4;** systolic murmur; cardiomegaly on chest radiograph	Relieved by **squatting; worsened by Valsalva,** exacerbated by physical exertion; sudden death

TABLE 3-11 Valvular Heart Disease

Valvular Disease	Etiology	Physical Examination	Clinical Manifestations
Mitral stenosis	Usually **rheumatic heart disease**	Cyanosis; **opening snap;** diastolic rumbling murmur	Dyspnea; orthopnea; left atrial enlargement; mid to late diastolic murmur
Mitral regurgitation	**Rheumatic heart disease** (50% of cases); mitral valve prolapse; hypertrophic cardiomyopathy; papillary muscle dysfunction (secondary to myocardial infarction)	Splitting of S2; **S3;** systolic murmur; radiation to the left axilla	Arrhythmias; infective endocarditis; dilated left atrium; holosystolic murmur
Aortic stenosis	Thickening and **calcification** of valve; bicuspid aortic valves	Delayed pulses; carotid thrill; **crescendo–decrescendo systolic ejection murmur; decreased intensity with Valsalva**	Syncope; angina; death; do not administer β-blockers
Aortic regurgitation	Rheumatic heart disease; syphilitic aortitis; nondissecting aortic aneurysm; Marfan syndrome	Wide pulse pressure; water-hammer pulse; **S3; blowing, decrescendo diastolic murmur**	Left ventricular enlargement; dyspnea; early diastolic murmur

TABLE 3-12 Murmurs

Systolic			Diastolic		
Ejection	**Holosystolic**	**Late**	**Early**	**Mid to Late**	**Continuous**
• Aortic valve stenosis	• Mitral regurgitation	• Mitral valve prolapse	• Aortic valve regurgitation	• Mitral stenosis	• PDA
• Hypertrophic cardiomyopathy	• Tricuspid regurgitation				
• Pulmonic valve stenosis	• Ventricular septal defect		• Pulmonic valve regurgitation		

THE CARDIOVASCULAR SYSTEM

TABLE 3-13 Peripheral Vascular Diseases

Disease	Pathology	Vessels Affected	Clinical Manifestations	Notes
Churg–Strauss	Eosinophils, vasculitis, p-ANCA	Small and medium sized arteries	**Asthma; elevated plasma eosinophils;** heart disease	May be associated with perinuclear antineutrophil cytoplasmic antibody (p-ANCA)
Henoch–Schönlein purpura	**IgA** immune complex-mediated acute vasculitis; renal deposits in mesangium	Arterioles; capillaries; venules	Hemorrhagic urticaria; palpable purpura; fever; red blood cell casts in urine; **atopic** patient	Often associated with an **upper respiratory infection; children**
Kaposi sarcoma	Viral origin; common malignancy in AIDS patients	Cutaneous and visceral vasculature	Malignant vascular tumor, especially in **homosexual** men	Probably results from reactivation of latent human herpesvirus 8 (HHV-8) infection
Kawasaki disease	Acute necrotizing inflammation	Large, medium, and small vessels	Fever; conjunctival lesions; lymphadenitis; coronary artery aneurysms	Affects **young children**
Rendu–Osler–Weber syndrome	**Autosomal dominant;** hereditary hemorrhagic telangiectasia	Dilation of venules and capillaries	Epistaxis; gastrointestinal (GI) bleeding	Increased occurrence in **Mormon** population
Polyarteritis nodosa (PAN)	Necrotizing degeneration of tunica media; aneurysms	Small and medium sized arteries	Fever; weight loss; abdominal pain (GI); hypertension (renal)	Associated with **hepatitis B infection**
Takayasu arteritis (pulseless disease)	Inflammation leading to stenosis; **aortic arch** and the origins of great vessels	Medium and large arteries	**Loss of carotid, radial, and ulnar pulses;** fever; night sweats; deficits arthritis; visual, low blood pressure in upper extremities, claudication caused by lack of blood reaching extremities	Pathology referred to as "aortic arch syndrome"; young **Asian females** Corkscrew, widened aorta on angiogram
Temporal arteritis (giant cell arteritis)	Nodular inflammation of branches of carotid (especially **temporal**)	Medium and large arteries	**Headache;** absence of pulse in affected vessels; **visual deficits;** polymyalgia rheumatica	Significant elevation of **sedimentation rate; usually population**
Thromboangiitis obliterans (Buerger disease)	Acute, full-thickness inflammation of vessels; may extend to nerves; occlusive lesions in extremities	Small and medium arteries and veins	Cold, pale limb; pain; **Raynaud phenomenon;** gangrene	Typical patient is a young **Jewish** man who **smokes heavily**
Wegener granulomatosis	Antineutrophil antibodies (cytoplasmic antineutrophil cytoplasmic antibody **[c-ANCA]** causes necrotizing, **granulomatous lesions** in **kidney, lung,** and upper respiratory tract	Small arteries; small veins of kidneys and respiratory tract	Cough; ulcers of sinuses and **nasal septum;** red blood cell casts in urine; classic triad: (a) necrotizing vasculitis (b) necrotizing granulomas of respiratory tract (c) necrotizing glomerulitis	More common in males

CARDIAC NEOPLASMS

I. Metastatic tumors to the heart are more common than primary tumors

II. Primary tumors

A. Myxomas
1. 90% found in atria
2. Left atrium > right atrium
3. Cause **ball-valve obstruction**, embolism, and fever

B. Rhabdomyoma
1. Most common primary cardiac tumor found in children
2. Often seen with tuberous sclerosis
3. Composed of "spider cells" and glycogen vacuoles

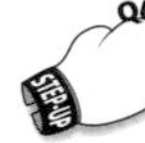

The pathophysiology of the vasculitides is thought to be mediated by immunopathology.

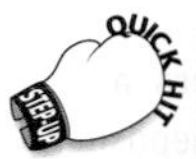

Temporal arteritis is the most common vasculitis in the United States.

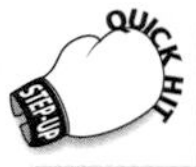

Carney syndrome is autosomal dominant and occurs in 10% of patients with myxomas. It also manifests with schwannomas, spotty pigmentation, and endocrine overreactivity.

DISEASES OF THE PERICARDIUM

I. Cardiac tamponade

A. This is an accumulation of fluid in the pericardial sac, which causes cardiac filling defects because of compression of the heart.
1. Blood is usually indicative of a traumatic perforation of the heart or aorta or rupture as a consequence of an MI.
2. Serous transudate may accumulate as a result of edema or CHF.

B. The most common causes are neoplasms, idiopathic pericarditis, and uremia.

C. Principal features of cardiac tamponade
1. Intracardiac pressure is elevated.
2. Ventricular filling is limited.
3. Cardiac output is reduced.
4. Decreased or absent heart sounds on auscultation.

D. Pulsus paradoxus is a greater than normal (10 mm Hg) decline in systolic arterial pressure on inspiration.

E. Treatment involves pericardiocentesis (removal of fluid from the pericardial cavity).

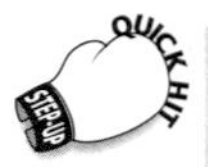

The needle for a pericardiocentesis passes through the skin, superficial fascia, pectoralis major muscle, external intercostal membrane, internal intercostal membrane, fibrous pericardium, and parietal layer of serous pericardium.

II. Pericarditis

A. Pericarditis is defined as an inflammation of the pericardium (fibroserous membrane) covering the heart.

B. Causes
1. Usually idiopathic
2. Coxsackievirus A or B (serous pericarditis)
3. Tuberculosis (hemorrhagic pericarditis)
4. Uremia (serofibrinous pericarditis)
5. SLE (serous pericarditis)
6. Scleroderma (serous pericarditis)
7. Post-MI (Dressler syndrome; fibrinous pericarditis)

C. Physical examination
1. Jugular venous distention (JVD)
2. Increase of jugular venous pressure (JVP) with inspiration (Kussmaul sign)
3. Pericardial friction rub
4. Distant heart sounds

D. Characteristics
1. Pain exacerbated by inspiration
2. Pain relieved by sitting
3. Cardiomegaly
4. Hypotension
5. Diffuse ST elevation on ECG

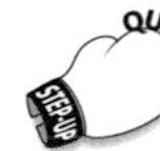

An MI also produces ST elevation. However, in an MI, ST elevation is limited to certain leads (corresponding to anatomical regions) and associated with possible QRS changes.

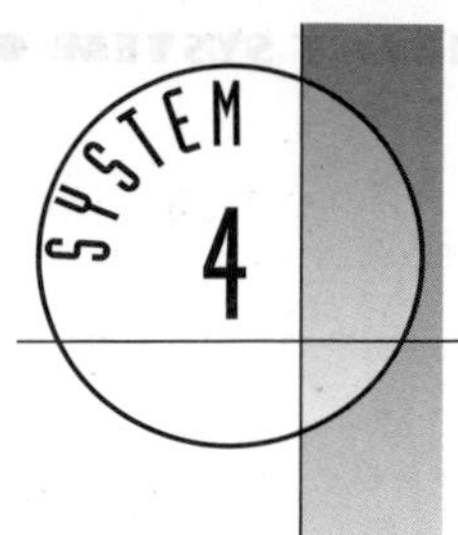

The Respiratory System

DEVELOPMENT

I. The lung bud forms from the foregut during week 4 of embryologic development.

II. The lining of the lower respiratory tract is derived from endoderm, whereas the connective tissue cartilage and muscle are derived from mesoderm.

III. Normal development causes the lung bud to completely separate from the esophagus at the level of the larynx.

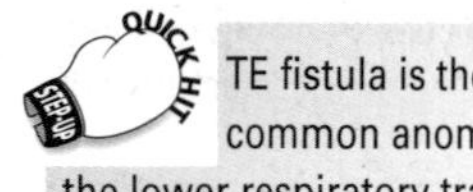

TE fistula is the most common anomaly of the lower respiratory tract.

Polyhydraminos is often associated with TE fistula due to the inability of excess amniotic fluid to pass through the stomach and intestine for absorption by the placenta into the mother's circulation.

IV. Incomplete separation causes a tracheoesophageal (TE) fistula (Figure 4-1).

A. In the most common form of TE fistula, the esophagus ends in a blind pouch (esophageal atresia) and air enters the stomach (gastric bubble on radiograph).

B. Signs and symptoms of esophageal atresia with a TE fistula:
1. Feeding difficulties within the first few days of life
2. Possible aspiration pneumonia with respiratory distress
3. Inability to pass nasogastric tube
4. Copious secretions

FIGURE 4-1 **Tracheoesophageal fistula**

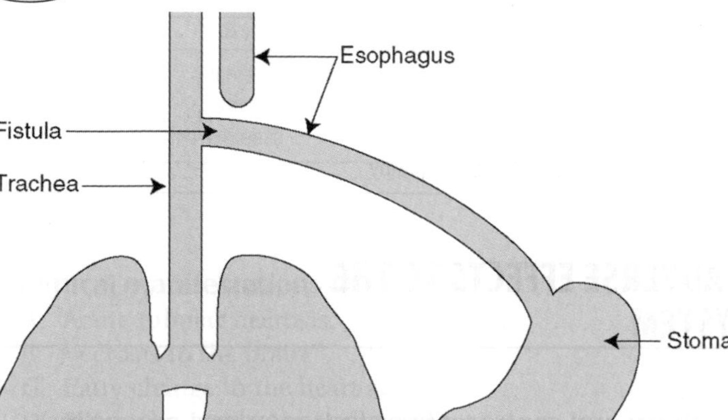

V. Stages of bronchial development

A. **Pseudoglandular period** (5 to 17 weeks)
  1. During this period, the primary bronchi are formed, followed by secondary, tertiary, and segmental bronchi.
  2. Bronchi appear as glandlike structures organized in tubules.
  3. Respiration is not yet possible in this stage.

B. **Canalicular period** (15 to 25 weeks)
  1. Respiratory bronchioles and terminal sacs begin to develop.
  2. Vascular structures begin to form around sacs.
  3. Respiration is possible only in the very latest weeks.

C. **Terminal sac period** (24 weeks to birth)
  1. Vascular structures and terminal sacs continue to proliferate.
  2. Cells differentiate into type I (blood–air barrier) and type II (surfactant producing) pneumocytes.
  3. Respiration is possible **after week 25.**
  4. The amount of surfactant is the primary determinant of survival.

D. **Alveolar period** (29 weeks to 8 years of age)
  1. The majority of alveoli develop after birth.
  2. As the child grows, the lung increases in size as a result of proliferation of respiratory bronchioles and terminal sacs.

QUICK HIT: The defect of CDH is also known as the foramen of Bochdalek and most commonly occurs on the left side in nearly 90% of cases due to the earlier closure of the right pleuroperitoneal opening.

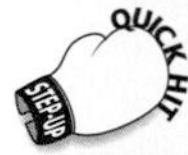

QUICK HIT: The primary molecule of surfactant is dipalmitoyl-phosphatidylcholine (lecithin). A lecithin-to-sphingomyelin ratio of 2:1 is the normal ratio of surfactant molecules in a newborn. A ratio below 2:1 can result in neonatal respiratory distress, especially in cesarean section delivery.

VI. Diaphragm muscle

A. This is the primary muscle used for breathing.

B. The diaphragm muscle separates the pleural and peritoneal cavities.

C. It is formed from fusion of the following structures:
  1. **Septum transversum**
  2. Paired **pleuroperitoneal membranes**
  3. **Dorsal mesentery** of the **esophagus**
  4. **Body wall**

D. It is innervated by the phrenic nerves (C3, C4, and C5).

E. Improper formation of the pleuroperitoneal membrane or its failure to fuse with the other three parts of the diaphragm can lead to a congenital **diaphragmatic hernia (CDH)**, a condition with serious complications.
  1. Abdominal contents are forced into the pleural cavity.
  2. Lung hypoplasia results from compression by abdominal viscera.
  3. Hernias appear most often on the **left side** (posterolateral).
  4. Diaphragmatic hernia is associated with polyhydramnios.
  5. Diaphragmatic hernia presents at birth as a flattened abdomen, cyanosis, and inability to breathe.

MNEMONIC

C3, C4, and C5 keep the diaphragm phrenically alive.

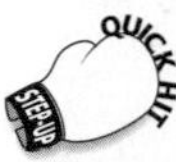

QUICK HIT: The sternocleidomastoid and the internal and external intercostals are accessory muscles of respiration. They are used when there is an increased demand for oxygen (such as in exercise) or in disease states.

PHYSICS AND FUNCTION OF THE LUNG

I. Lung volumes

A. **Capacities and volumes in the normal lung** (Figure 4-2)

B. Volumes and pressure during the breathing cycle (Figure 4-3)

C. Spirometry tracing—normal versus diseased (Figure 4-4)

D. Pulmonary function tests—obstructive versus restrictive (Figure 4-5)

II. Compliance

A. Defined as $\Delta V/\Delta P$, where V is volume and P is pressure, compliance describes the ability of the chest wall and lung to expand when stretched
  1. At functional residual capacity (FRC), the lungs have a tendency to collapse.
  2. This force is exactly balanced by the chest wall, which has a tendency to expand.
  3. Because these forces are in balance at FRC, the airway pressure is 0 mm Hg. Lung volumes above FRC create a positive airway pressure and volumes below FRC create a negative airway pressure.

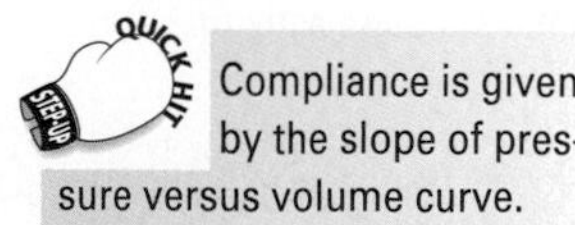

QUICK HIT: Compliance is given by the slope of pressure versus volume curve.

FIGURE 4-2 Lung volumes

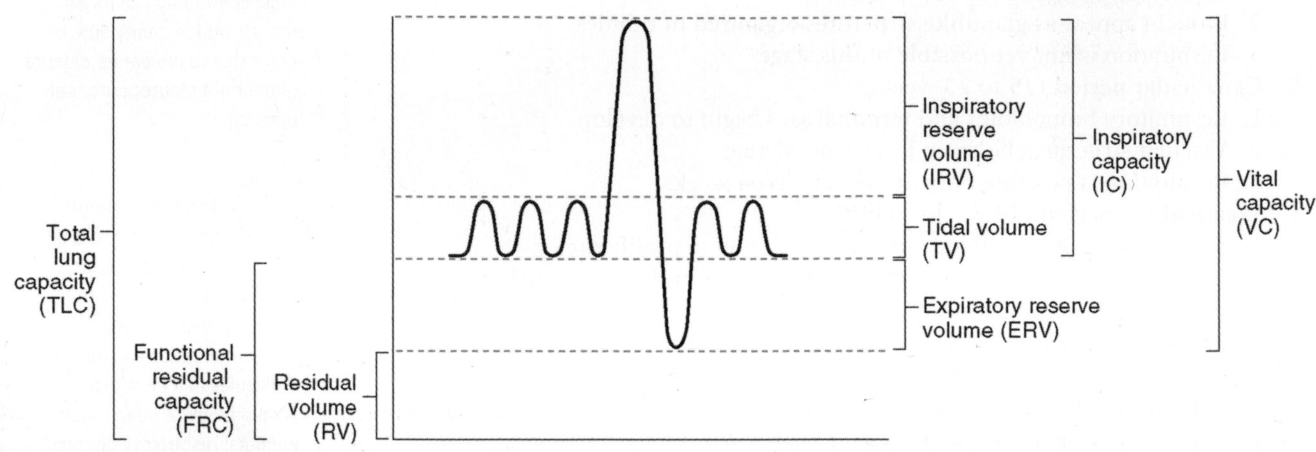

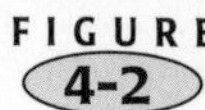

QUICK HIT: Residual volume or volumes containing residual volume (RV) cannot be directly measured by plethysmography or spirometry but are derived from helium dilution techniques.

FIGURE 4-3 Breathing cycle

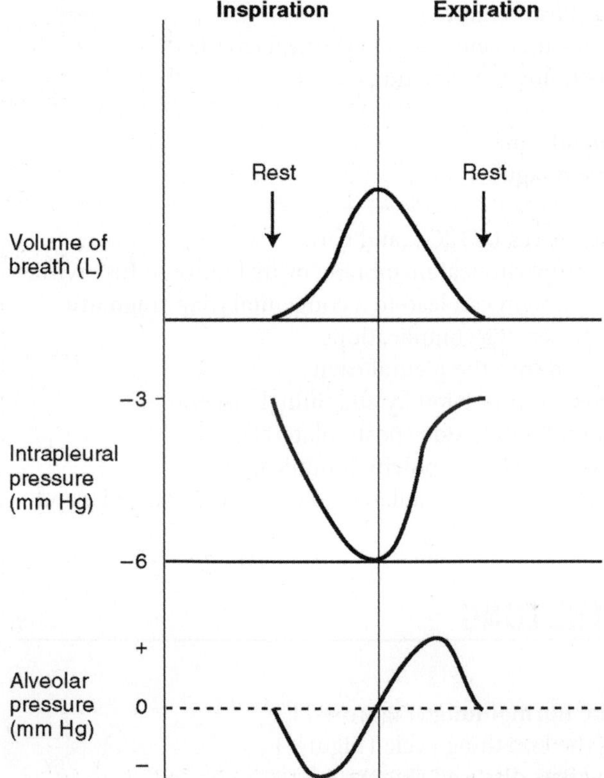

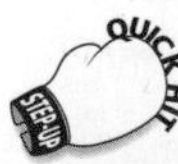

QUICK HIT: Type II pneumocytes are cuboidal cells with round nuclei, foamy cytoplasm (because of lipid content), and lamellar bodies (secreting granules) containing the surfactant.

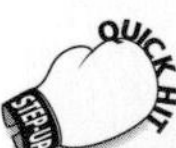

QUICK HIT: Glucocorticoids administered during pregnancy accelerate fetal lung development by stimulating the production of surfactant-associated proteins and increasing phospholipid synthesis by enhancing phosphatidylcholine activity.

QUICK HIT: Allergies and allergic asthma release histamine, which is a powerful constrictor of airway smooth muscle and causes increased airway resistance.

4. Low compliance implies a stiff chest wall or lung as seen in
   a. **Pulmonary fibrosis due to asbestosis, sarcoidosis, and adult respiratory distress syndrome (ARDS)**
   b. **Pulmonary edema**
   c. **Paralysis of the respiratory muscles**
5. High compliance implies a flaccid lung as a result of
   a. Decreased elastic recoil as seen in **emphysema** and **old age**
   b. **Bronchospasm** as in **asthma** (Figure 4-4)

FIGURE 4-4 **Spirometry tracings: normal versus diseased**

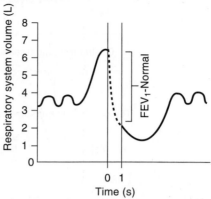

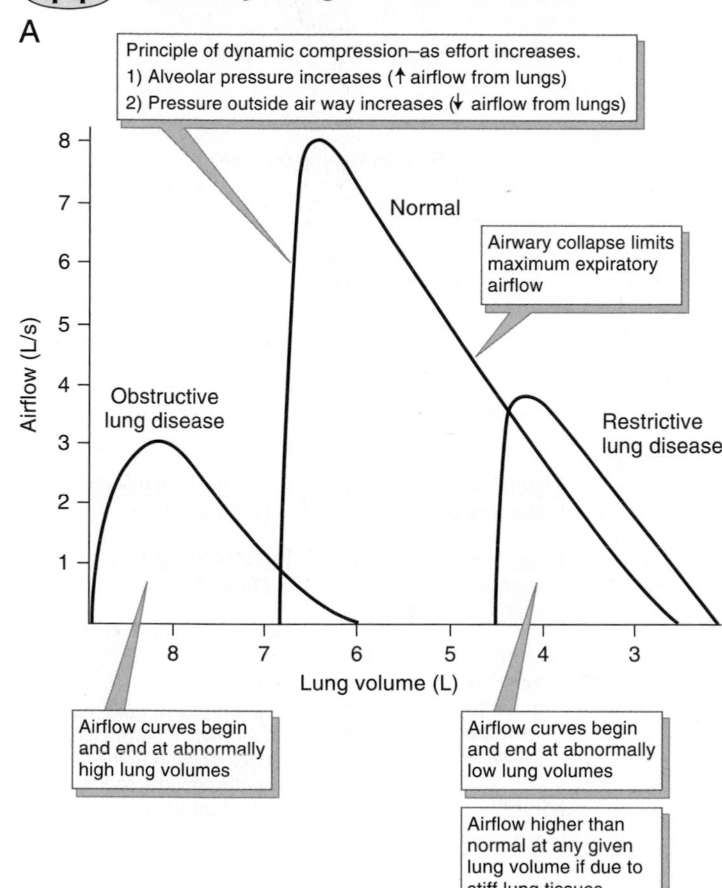

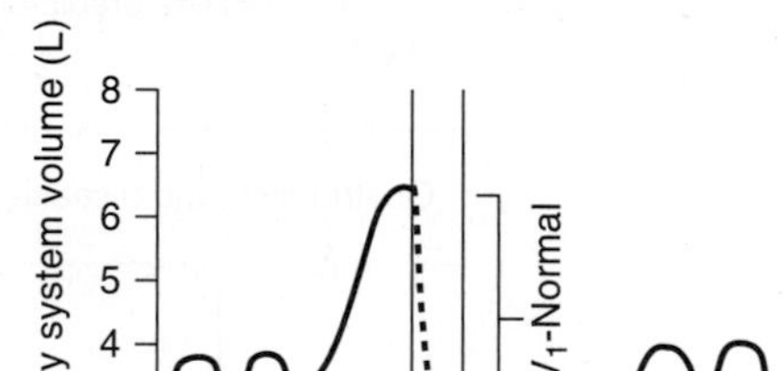

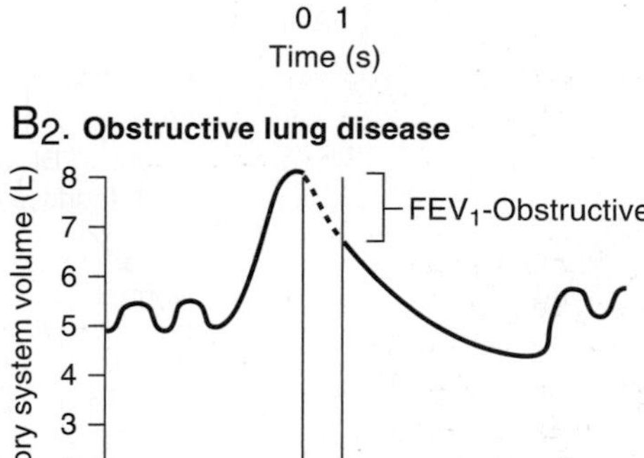

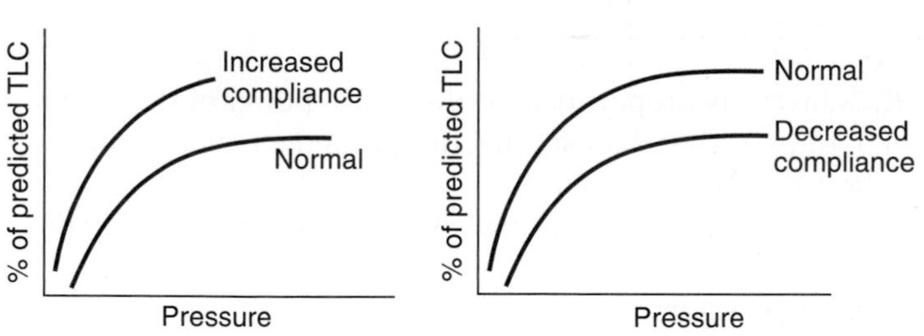

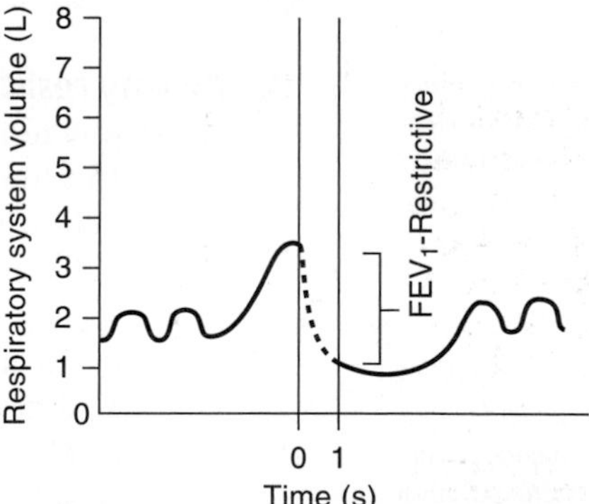

B. **Surfactant** plays an important role in lung compliance
   1. Alveoli have a tendency to collapse.
   2. An alveolus with a small radius has more collapsing pressure than an alveolus with a large radius, according to **Laplace law:**

      $P \propto T/r$

      where P is pressure required to prevent alveolar collapse; T is surface tension; and r is alveolar radius.
   3. Surfactant reduces the pressure and prevents collapse by reducing the intermolecular forces between water molecules lining the alveoli.
   4. Surfactant increases compliance and allows the alveoli to expand more easily.
   5. **Neonatal respiratory distress** occurs in premature infants (<37 weeks' gestation) because **type II** (surfactant-producing) **pneumocytes** are not yet fully developed and fail to produce sufficient surfactant or surfactant fast enough.

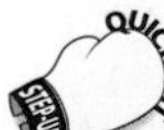

SRS-A is a combination of the leukotrienes C_4 and D_4 (LTC_4 and LTD_4). In the treatment of asthma, zileuton blocks production of leukotrienes by inhibiting the lipoxygenase enzyme, whereas zafirlukast blocks leukotriene receptors. Leukotriene (LTA_4) is a precursor to leukotriene B_4 (LTB_4), LTC_4, and LTD_4. LTB_4 is responsible for chemotaxis of neutrophils and adhesion of white blood cells.

FIGURE 4-5 Interpreting pulmonary function tests: obstructive versus restrictive

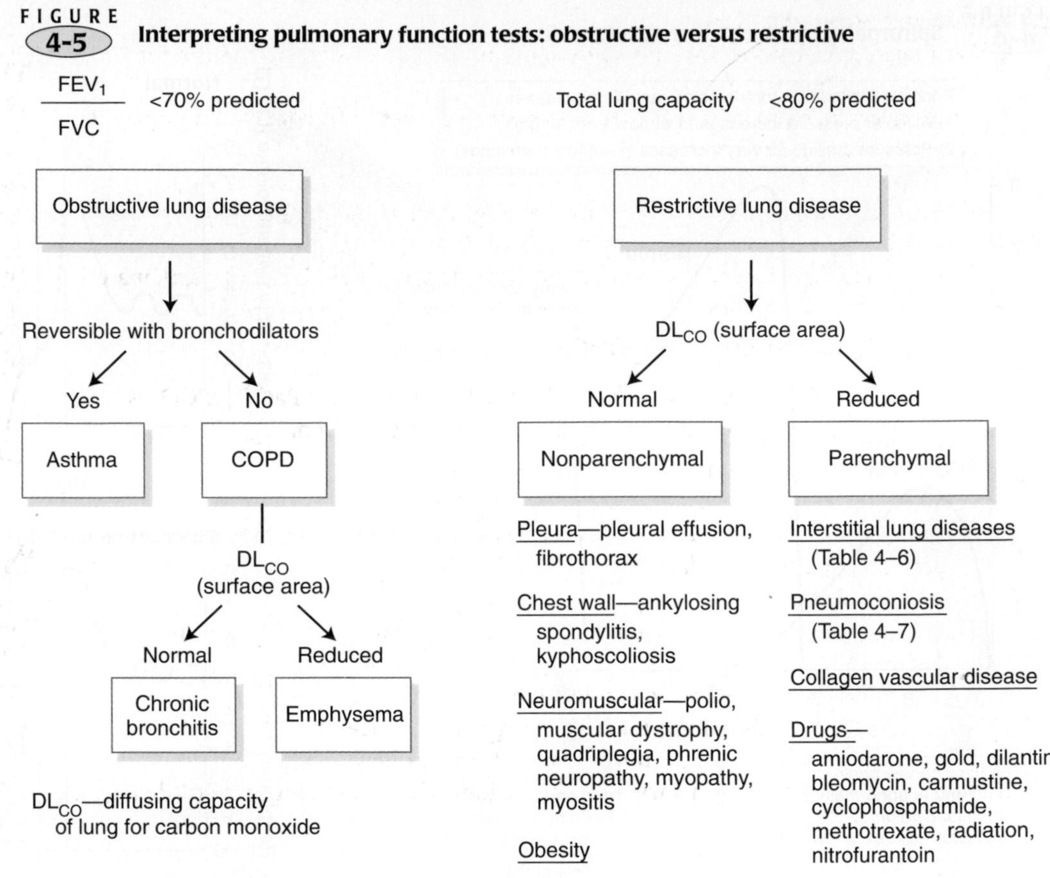

6. Atelectasis (collapsed alveoli) can result from neonatal respiratory distress syndrome (NRDS).

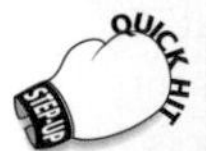

> QUICK HIT: Anatomic shunts are passageways of blood flow that go from the venous circulation to the arterial circulation without passing through the lungs. Normally approximately 2% of the cardiac output is shunted; however, it can be as much as 50% in certain congenital malformations (e.g., tetralogy of Fallot produces a right-to-left shunt).

> QUICK HIT: There are two types of dead space:
> (1) **Anatomic dead space,** measured by the **Fowler method,** is usually about 150 mL.
> (2) **Physiologic dead space,** measured by the Bohr-method, is considered to be the volume of the lung that does not eliminate CO_2.

III. Airway resistance

A. Airway resistance (*R*) is inversely proportional to the fourth power of the radius (*r*) (formula: $R \propto 1/r^4$); thus, any mechanism that decreases the radius of the bronchi will greatly affect the airway resistance.

B. **The airway radius** is under the control of the parasympathetic and sympathetic nervous systems

1. **Parasympathetic nervous system**
   a. Causes **constriction** of the airways
   b. Mediated by direct stimulation, airway irritation, and slow-reacting substance of anaphylaxis (SRS-A)
   c. Stimulates mucus secretion
2. **Sympathetic nervous system**
   a. Causes **dilation** of airways
   b. Used as treatment for allergy and asthma (β_2-agonists)
   c. Functions in fight-or-flight autonomic reflexes; dilates airways to help provide oxygen in times of stress
3. Airway radius is also affected by the lung parenchyma, which is bound to the airway and exerts radial traction on it
   a. In restrictive disorders such as interstitial fibrosis, radial traction of the airway increases → increasing airway diameter → decreasing airway resistance → increasing expiratory airflow and forced expiratory volume at 1 second/forced vital capacity (FEV_1/FVC) ratios.
   b. In obstructive disorder such as emphysema, destruction of elastic fibers → decreases radial traction → decreasing airway diameter → increasing resistance → decreasing expiratory airflow and FEV_1/FVC ratios.

IV. Ventilation and perfusion

A. **Ventilation/perfusion (*V/Q*) ratio:** the ratio of the rate of alveolar ventilation to the rate of pulmonary blood flow

B. Varies over the entire lung (higher in the apices, lower in the bases in an upright patient), but is 0.8 on average

C. Dead space

1. Anatomic dead space is regions of the lung, such as the conducting airways, which are incapable of exchanging O_2 and CO_2.
2. Physiologic dead space is the volume of the lungs which does not participate in the elimination of CO_2.

$$V_D = V_T \times [(PaCO_2 - PECO_2)/PaCo_2]$$

V_D, physiologic dead space (mL); V_T, tidal volume (mL); $PaCO_2$, PCO_2 of arterial blood (mm Hg); $PECO_2$, PCO_2 of expired air (mm Hg).

3. It causes a reduction in ventilation.
4. *V/Q* is reduced (to 0 in complete airway occlusion).
5. A *V/Q* of 0 is considered a shunt and no gas exchange will occur (areas are perfused, but not ventilated).

D. Blood flow obstruction

1. Blockage of a pulmonary artery or smaller vessel causes a reduction in perfusion.
2. A perfusion value of 0 yields an infinite *V/Q* ratio.
3. A *V/Q* of infinity is considered **physiologic dead space.**

E. Pulmonary embolism results in increased *V/Q* ratio (Table 4-1).

F. Blood flow and ventilation vary over the regions of the lung (Figure 4-6) due primarily to gravity.

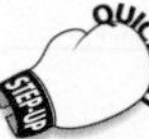

During exercise, pulmonary vascular resistance decreases as a result of dilation of the lung arterioles by metabolic products. The ratio becomes uniform over the entire lung. Conversely, during hypoxia, lack of oxygen constricts local lung vasculature, thus increasing pulmonary vascular resistance; this is opposite of what takes place in the systemic circulation, wherein lack of oxygen results in vasodilation.

The ventilation equation quantifies the relationship between alveolar ventilation and alveolar PCO_2: **alveolar ventilation = CO_2 production/alveolar PCO_2.** Therefore, a threefold increase in alveolar PCO_2 (expired PCO_2) indicates a threefold decrease in alveolar ventilation if CO_2 production is fixed.

TABLE 4-1 Causes of Hypoxemia

Cause	Associated Conditions	A–a Gradient	Lab Values	Notes
Right-to-left shunt	Congenital anomaly	Increased		Does not respond to oxygen
Ventilation/ perfusion mismatch	Pneumonia, COPD, atelectasis, pulmonary infarction, tumors, granulomatous disease, tumors		Increased	Responds to oxygen (A–a gradient corrects)
Decreased diffusion capacity	Thick blood–air barrier (diffuse interstitial fibrosis, sarcoidosis, asbestosis, respiratory distress syndrome), decreased surface area (pneumonec-tomy, emphysema), decreased hemoglobin (anemia, PE)	Increased	DL_{CO} decreased	Responds to oxygen but A–a gradient remains same
Decreased PO_2 in inspired air	High altitudes, erroneous setting on ventilator	Normal		Responds to oxygen
Hypoventilation of central origin	Opioid or barbiturate overdose	Normal	Elevated PCO_2	Responds to oxygen
Hypoventilation of peripheral origin	Polio, chest trauma (multiple rib fractures → pain with breathing), tetanus, obesity (pickwickian syndrome), suffocation, drowning, skeletal disease, phenic nerve paralysis	Normal	Elevated PCO_2	Responds to oxygen

COPD, chronic obstructive pulmonary disease; DL_{CO}, diffusing capacity of lung for carbon monoxide; PE, pulmonary embolus.

In determining the cause of hypoxemia in a patient, use a three-tier approach: (1) Check whether the A-a gradient is elevated; (2) check whether O_2 administration improved the condition and if the A–a gradient was corrected; and (3) look for other lab findings or associated conditions.

FIGURE 4-6 Pulmonary circulation

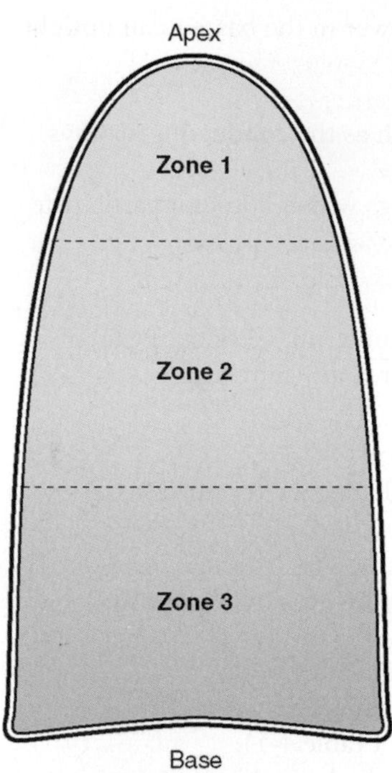

Zone 1
- Lowest blood flow
- Alveolar pressure > Arterial pressure > Venous pressure
- Capillaries collapse due to high alveolar pressure
- Ventilation ($\dot{V}$) is decreased less than blood flow [also called perfusion ($\dot{Q}$)]

so: $\frac{\dot{V}}{\dot{Q}} = \frac{\downarrow}{\downarrow\downarrow} = \uparrow$ (Ventilation in excess of perfusion)

Zone 2
- Blood flow is higher than Zone 1, but lower than Zone 3
- Arterial pressure > Alveolar pressure > Venous pressure
- Capillaries remain open because arterial pressure is greater than alveolar pressure
- Ventilation ($\dot{V}$) is approximately equivalent to perfusion ($\dot{Q}$)

so: $\frac{\dot{V}}{\dot{Q}} \approx 1$

Zone 3
- Highest blood flow
- Arterial pressure > Venous pressure > Alveolar pressure
- Capillaries remain open because arterial pressure is higher than both alveolar and venous pressure
- Ventilation ($\dot{V}$) is increased less than perfusion ($\dot{Q}$)

so: $\frac{\dot{V}}{\dot{Q}} = \frac{\uparrow}{\uparrow\uparrow} = \downarrow$ (Perfusion in excess of ventilation)

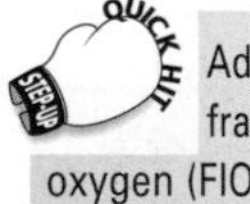

Administering high fraction of inspired oxygen (FIO_2) to chronically hypercapnic patients (i.e., COPD patients) can lead to respiratory failure because hypoxia is the only stimulus for respiration.

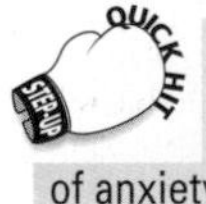

Hyperventilation associated with states of anxiety leads to decreased arterial PCO_2 that causes constriction of cerebral vasculature decreasing blood flow to the brain and producing feelings of faintness, suffocation, blurred vision, and chest tightness.

CONTROL OF BREATHING

I. Medulla

A. Mediates inspiration and expiration.
B. Generates the basic breathing rhythm.
C. Receives input via the vagus and glossopharyngeal nerves.
D. Sends output via the phrenic nerve to the diaphragm and via the spinal nerve to the intercostals and abdominal wall.
E. The cerebral cortex can override the medulla and provide voluntary control of breathing if desired.

II. The central nervous system (CNS) seeks to keep $PaCO_2$ (partial pressure of arterial CO_2) within a narrow range. On the other hand, in the case of oxygen, the nervous system responds only to very low levels of PaO_2 (partial pressure of arterial oxygen).

III. Depth and rate of respiration control these variables.

A. Central control
1. Chemoreceptors in the **medulla** sense the pH of the cerebrospinal fluid (CSF).
2. CO_2 crosses the blood–brain barrier where it binds with H_2O to form H_2CO_3. H_2CO_3 dissociates to H^+ and HCO_3, causing an increase in H^+ (decreasing the pH of the CSF).
3. Increases in $[H^+]$ (hydrogen ion concentration) directly stimulate the central chemoreceptors, which stimulate breathing.
4. Decreases in $[H^+]$ reduce stimulation of the receptors and slow respiration.

B. **Peripheral control**

1. Chemoreceptors in the **carotid bodies** and at the aortic arch bifurcation sense changes in PaO_2, $PaCO_2$, and $[H^+]$.
2. Decreases in **PaO_2** below 60 mm Hg stimulate the peripheral chemoreceptors to increase rate and depth of breathing (in the absence of lung disease, decreased PaO_2 is rarely the driving force for respiration).
3. Increases in **$PaCO_2$** potentiate peripheral chemoreceptor response to PaO_2 (major direct effect of changes in $PaCO_2$ is on the central chemoreceptors).
4. Increases in arterial $[H^+]$ directly stimulate the chemoreceptors, independent of the $PaCO_2$ (causes increased respiration in metabolic acidosis).
5. Stimulation of irritant receptors in large airways and stretch receptors in small airways inhibits inspiration.

C. **Abnormal breathing**

1. **Cheyne–Stokes breathing**
   a. Tidal volumes variably increase and decrease and are separated by a period of apnea.
   b. This breathing abnormality is a result of pontine dysfunction and is associated with drug overdose, hypoxia, CNS depression, congestive heart failure (CHF), and increased intracerebral pressure.
2. **Kussmaul breathing**
   a. Rate an metabolic acidosis.
3. **Sleep apnea**
   a. **Obstructive sleep apnea**
   - Risk factors
     (1) Middle age
     (2) Male sex
     (3) Obesity
     (4) Smoker
     (5) History of hypertension
     (6) History of pharyngeal malformations
     (7) Use of alcohol and other drugs
   - **Characteristics**
     (1) Ventilatory effort exists.
     (2) Airway is obstructed.
     (3) Apnea is terminated by self-arousal.
     (4) Apnea usually occurs in the nasopharynx or oropharynx when muscles relax during rapid eye movement (REM) sleep.

   b. **Central sleep apnea**
   - Ventilatory effort does not exist.
   - Airway is not obstructed.
   - Patient does not arouse self.
   - Central sleep apnea, like obstructive sleep apnea, occurs in the REM stage of sleep.
   - It is carbon dioxide threshold-dependent; that is, there is decreased chemoreceptor sensitivity to O_2 and CO_2 concentrations.

   c. **Therapy** includes weight loss (for obstructive sleep apnea), continuous positive airway pressure (CPAP), and, in some cases, tricyclic antidepressants.

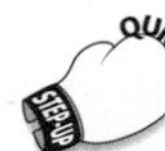

Obstructive sleep apnea causes CO_2 retention, leading to respiratory acidosis and hypoxemia.

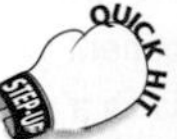

Patients with unexplained daytime sleepiness, arrhythmias, and mood changes should be evaluated for sleep apnea.

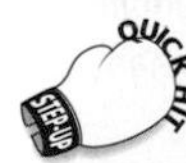

Remember that air contains higher oxygen (PO_2 = 160 mm Hg) and virtually no CO_2 (PCO_2 = 0 mm Hg) as compared to arterial gas levels (PO_2 = 100 mm Hg, PCO_2 = 40 mm Hg).

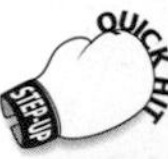

The blood–air barrier is made up of
(1) Membrane and cytoplasm of type I pneumocytes.
(2) Fused basement membrane of type I pneumocytes and endothelial cells.
(3) Membrane and cytoplasm of endothelial cells.

IV. Gas exchange

A. Diffusion of gas depends on the **partial pressure difference** between the gas in the alveolus and the gas in the blood (i.e., the difference in pressure across the blood–air barrier).

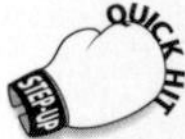

The **right main bronchus** is more vertically oriented than the left main bronchus and is therefore the path commonly taken by aspirated particles. If a patient is supine, the object is most likely to enter the **lower lobe.**

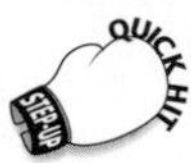

Karatanger syndrome is an autorecessive disorder causing a defect in the dynein arms of cilia resulting in infertility, situs inversus, chronic sinusitis, and bronchiectasis.

B. Partial pressure
   1. The alveolar partial pressure of oxygen (PaO_2) can be calculated as follows:
      $$PaO_2 = (760–47 \text{ mm Hg})\ FIO_2 – (PaCO_2/0.8)$$
      where 760 mm Hg = total atmospheric pressure (at sea level);
      47 mm Hg = partial pressure of completely humidified air as found in the alveoli;
      FIO_2 = percent of air that is oxygen (normally 0.21);
      $PaCO_2$ = partial pressure of CO_2 in the alveoli (normally 40);
      and 0.8 = the ratio of volume of CO_2 produced to the volume of O_2 consumed (respiratory quotient).
   2. For O_2, higher pressures will force more oxygen into the blood and allow it to equilibrate more readily.
   3. For CO_2, higher partial pressures in the blood (or lower in the alveoli) will force more CO_2 out of the blood and into the lungs, where it can be expired.
   4. The amount of O_2 delivered to the tissues is also determined by hemoglobin concentration and red blood cell number (hematocrit) (see System 10).

C. Disease affects diffusion capacity of the lung.
   1. Fibrosis causes a thickening of the interstitium, which hinders diffusion across the blood–air barrier.
   2. Emphysema destroys the alveolar walls and decreases the area available for gas exchange.

The most likely cause for lung abscess formation in a comatose patient is aspiration pneumonia as a consequence of a depressed cough reflex. Other causes of lung abscess formation are septic emboli (from infective endocarditis), spread from adjacent organs, and malignant tumors.

LUNG DEFENSES

I. Anatomic barriers

A. Impaction
   1. Large particles—**greater than 10 µm in diameter**—fail to turn the corners of respiratory tract.
   2. Common site: **nasopharynx.**

B. Sedimentation
   1. Medium particles—between **2 and 10 µm in diameter**—settle as a result of weight.
   2. Common site: **small airways.**

C. Diffusion
   1. Small particles—between **0.5 and 2 µm in diameter**—are engulfed by alveolar macrophages (dust cells).
   2. Common site: **alveoli.**

D. Suspension: particles **less than 0.5 µm in diameter** remain suspended in air.

Slow, deep breaths increase the deposition of dust by sedimentation and diffusion, whereas exercise results in higher rates of airflow and increased deposition by impaction.

II. Nonspecific

A. **Mucociliary escalator**
   1. Particles are trapped in gel layer of upper airway.
   2. Ciliary motion removes particles.

B. **Cough**
   1. Cough is a bronchoconstriction that occurs to prevent penetration of particles.
   2. It is also defined as deep inspiration followed by forced expiration.
   3. The cough reflex can be suppressed by antitussive agents such as opioids (see System 9).
   4. Specific mechanisms include **secretory IgA** and complement.

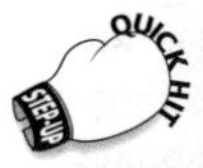

Hyaline membrane refers to eosinophilic membranous structures lining the alveolar wall.

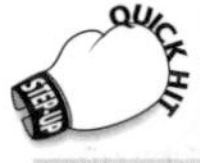

Hyaline membrane disease is associated with diabetes of the mother.

Hyaline membranes are characteristic of both ARDS and NRDS but are caused by distinctly different pathologic mechanisms.

ADULT RESPIRATORY DISTRESS SYNDROME AND NEONATAL RESPIRATORY DISTRESS SYNDROME

This group of diseases often leads to respiratory failure and death (Table 4-2).

TABLE 4-2 ARDS and NRDS

	ARDS (Diffuse Alveolar Damage)	NRDS (Hyaline Membrane Disease)
Age group	Adults	Premature infants
Causes	**Shock, infection, trauma, or aspiration** resulting in **neutrophil** recruitment and free radical production (oxygen toxicity)	**Lack of surfactant** production
Pathophysiology	Impaired gas exchange caused by pulmonary hemorrhage, pulmonary edema, or atelectasis	Increased work to expand lungs; infant can clear lungs of fluids, but cannot fill lungs with air; atelectasis
Features	Respiratory insufficiency; cyanosis; hypoxemia; heavy, wet lungs; diffuse pulmonary infiltrates on radiograph; hyaline membranes in alveoli; pneumothorax may result—may be rapid and fatal	Respiratory insufficiency; cyanosis; hypoxemia; heavy, wet lungs; diffuse pulmonary infiltrates on radiograph; hyaline membranes in alveoli

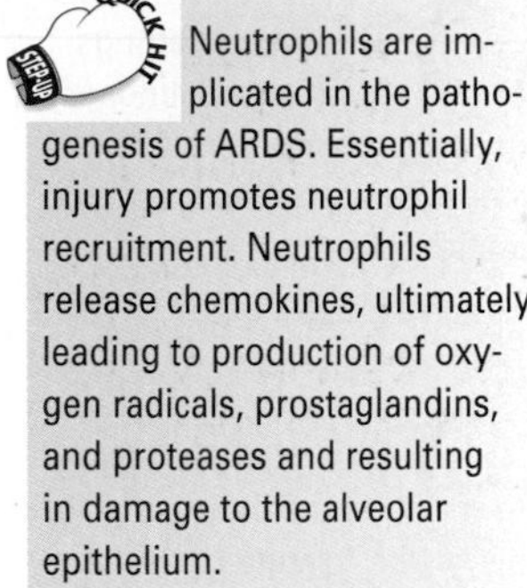

Neutrophils are implicated in the pathogenesis of ARDS. Essentially, injury promotes neutrophil recruitment. Neutrophils release chemokines, ultimately leading to production of oxygen radicals, prostaglandins, and proteases and resulting in damage to the alveolar epithelium.

PNEUMOTHORAX

I. Simple pneumothorax

A. May be caused by **spontaneous** rupture of a bleb (congenital or secondary to paraseptal emphysema) or penetrating trauma causing a loss of negative intrathoracic pressure.

B. Is most commonly seen in tall, slender **men 20 to 40 years of age.**

C. Presents as sudden chest pain, shortness of breath (SOB), **cough, hyperresonance** and **decreased breath sounds** over affected lung; chest radiograph shows **radiolucency** and in the case of a **tension pneumothorax** the **trachea deviates to the side of the pneumothorax.**

D. Has a 50% recurrence rate.

E. Treatment includes the insertion of a chest tube with suction to create a vacuum for larger defects, as well as monitoring for small defects such as air leaks.

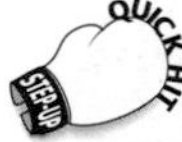

Decreased breath sounds and hyporesonance indicate pleural effusion.

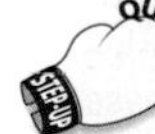

Lab values expected in a pneumothorax include increased PCO_2, depressed PO_2, acidotic pH, and compensatory increase in bicarbonate.

II. Tension pneumothorax

A. A flap of tissue allows air to enter pleural space but not to escape, causing an increase in pleural cavity pressure.

B. Pressure builds; the mediastinum is displaced; the **trachea deviates away from the lesion**; jugular venous distention (JVD) occurs; and breath sounds are uneven.

C. Cardiovascular and respiratory compromise may be rapidly **fatal.**

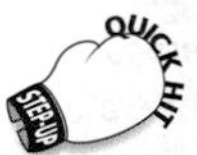

Bronchial obstruction can also lead to tracheal deviation with decreased breath sounds; however, in this case, the tracheal deviation is toward the side of the lesion because of the loss of volume. Decreased ventilation to the affected lung also leads to loss of tactile fremitus and hyporesonance.

III. Open sucking chest wound

A. Penetrating trauma to the chest wall and pleura can cause this condition.

B. If the diameter of the lesion approaches the diameter of the trachea, air will preferentially enter through the defect.

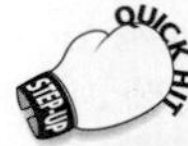

Flail chest is caused by multiple fractures of four or more consecutive ribs and leads to paradoxical movement of the injured area of the chest wall with respiration.

PULMONARY VASCULAR DISEASES

A variety of diseases primarily affect the vasculature of the lungs (Table 4-3).

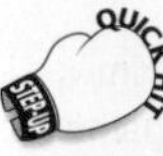
The clinical settings in which a pulmonary embolus can occur include cancer, multiple fractures, oral contraceptive use, prolonged bed rest, or CHF.

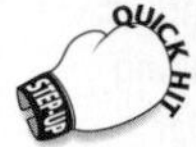
Fat emboli are often caused by crush injury with fracture of the long bones and orthopedic surgery.

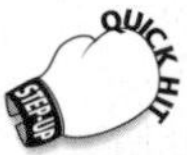
Pulmonary edema caused by heart failure is characterized histologically by hemosiderin-laden macrophages ("heart failure cells") and congested alveolar capillaries.

Chronic obstructive pulmonary disease (COPD) is characterized by airflow obstruction. This is in contrast to restrictive pulmonary diseases, which demonstrate defective lung expansion. Obstructive disorders have increased TLC, decreased FEV_1, and decreased FEV_1/FVC. Restrictive disorders show reduced lung volumes and normal or increased FEV_1/FVC. Normal FEV_1/FVC ratio is approximately 80%.

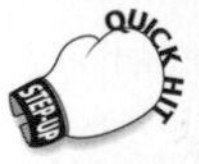
Reid Index: Ratio (normally < 0.4) between the thickness of the submucosal mucous secreting glands and the thickness between the epithelium and cartilage overlying the bronchus.

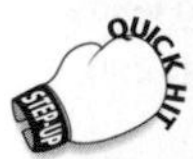
Two types of emphysema: Centriacinar primarily affects the respiratory bronchioles, is associated with smoking, and predominantly involves the upper lobes; panacinar is dilation of the entire alveolus, predominantly involves the lower segments, and involves α_1-antitrypsin deficiency.

TABLE 4-3 Pulmonary Vascular Diseases

Disease	Etiology	Features	Complications
Pulmonary hypertension	Primary—may be associated with proliferation of vascular smooth muscle	Loud S2	Leads to cor **pulmonale**
	Secondary—owing to COPD or increased pulmonary blood flow (as seen with a left-to-right shunt)	**Left parasternal heave due to right ventricular hypertrophy** Heart-failure cells	
Pulmonary embolism	Commonly from proximal **deep vein thrombosis** (usually lower limb such as femoral veins) as a result of **Virchow's triad:** blood stasis, endothelial damage (fat, infection, trauma), and hypercoagulable states	**Respiratory alkalosis, increased A–a gradient, hemorrhagic,** red, wedge-shaped infarct Acute-onset dyspnea, chest pain, tachycardia, hypotension *V/Q* ratio approaches infinity Saddle embolus—an embolus lodged at the pulmonary artery bifurcation, often fatal	Can lead to cardiovascular collapse and sudden death
Pulmonary edema	Obliteration of alveoli as a result of intra-alveolar accumulation of fluid	Heart failure or overload leads to **increased hydrostatic pressure** Inflammatory alveolar reactions (caused by drugs, pneumonia, sepsis, and uremia) leads to **increased capillary permeability**	Hypoxia
Wegener granulomatosis	Etiology is unknown but thought to be autoimmune in nature	Focal necrotizing **vasculitis** affecting small-size to medium-size vessels Acute necrotizing **granulomas of upper and lower respiratory tract** Bilateral nodular and cavitary infiltrates seen on chest radiograph Mucosal ulceration of nasopharynx seen on examination Associated with c-ANCA	Untreated disease is fatal within several years

c-ANCA, cytoplasmic antineutrophil cytoplasmic antibody; COPD, chronic obstructive pulmonary disease.

CHRONIC OBSTRUCTIVE PULMONARY DISEASE

I. Types of COPD (Table 4-4)

II. Therapeutic agents used in asthma and COPD (Table 4-5)

A. Inhaled agents
1. β_2-Agonists
a. β_2-Agonists are useful for treatment of an acute asthma attack characterized by SOB, chest tightness, wheezing, and cough as a result of bronchoconstriction.

TABLE 4-4 Types of COPD

Disease	Pathophysiology	Clinical Features and Management
Asthma	**Increased sensitivity** of bronchioles causes bronchoconstriction; muscle hypertrophy; **Curschmann spirals** (twisted, mucus casts of small airways); and **Charcot-Leyden crystals** (enzymes present within eosinophils)	**Wheezing;** SOB; dyspnea common treatment options include inhaled steroids and β_2-agonists
Chronic bronchitis	Caused by persistent irritants and infections; most common cause is smoking; hyperplasia of goblet cells and submucosal glands **(increased Reid index); excess mucus;** possible cor pulmonale	**Productive cough** for at least 3 consecutive months over 2 consecutive years; cyanosis due to decreased O_2 saturation, wheezing; "Blue bloater"; chronic respiratory acidosis as mucus plugs block the exhalation of CO_2; patients must quit **smoking**
Emphysema	Dilated alveoli; damaged alveolar walls; **damaged alveolar septae** leads to **enlarged alveolar airspaces;** destruction of structural support to lymphatic vessels leads to heavy pigment deposition; **decreased elastic recoil;** centrilobular (associated with smoking), panacinar (a_1-antitrypsin deficiency), paraseptal (associated with scarred tissue, may lead to spontaneous pneumothorax in young patients) and irregular forms	"Pink puffer"; paraseptal type may lead to pneumothorax; patients must quit **smoking;** anteroposterior diameter increased ("barrel chested"); hypertrophy of accessory respiratory muscles; episodes of nonproductive cough
Bronchiectasis	**Chronic infection leads to irreversible, bronchial dilation;** destruction of bronchial wall; commonly caused by bronchial **obstruction** (e.g., tumor)	Copius amounts of purulent sputum; hemoptysis; possible lung abscess; associated with CF and Kartagener syndrome

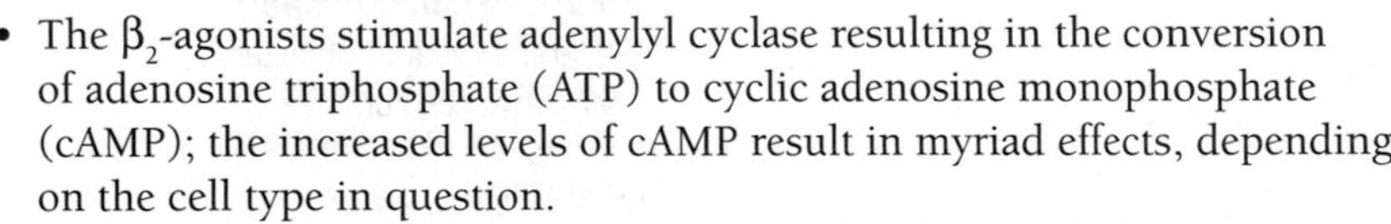

- The β_2-agonists stimulate adenylyl cyclase resulting in the conversion of adenosine triphosphate (ATP) to cyclic adenosine monophosphate (cAMP); the increased levels of cAMP result in myriad effects, depending on the cell type in question.
- β_2-Agonists are potent dilators of the bronchi. They act by relaxing smooth muscle in the airways.
- Systemic activation of β_2-specific receptors (which is minimal with inhaled β_2-agonists) may result in vasodilation, a slight decrease in peripheral resistance, bronchodilation, increased glycogenolysis in muscle and in the liver, increased release of glucagons, and relaxation of uterine smooth muscle.

b. Side effects include tachycardia, hyperglycemia, hypokalemia, and hypomagnesemia.

c. β_2-Agonists have no effect on the inflammation associated with asthma.

d. Selected β_2-agonists:
- **Albuterol** or **terbutaline** provides immediate relief of acute attacks without β_1-adrenoceptor stimulation.
- **Salmeterol** has a longer duration of action and a slower onset of action.

2. Corticosteroids

a. In cases of moderate asthma, corticosteroids (inhaled or systemic) can be used to decrease the associated inflammation.

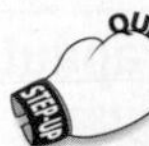

In emphysema, smoking attracts neutrophils which release elastase. α_1-antitrypsin normally inhibits elastase; however, free radicals caused by smoking inhibit α_1-antitrypsin, allowing elastase to damage the alveolar walls causing dilation.

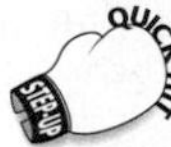

"Blue bloater": Blue refers to cyanosis; bloater refers to the peripheral edema in these patients from pulmonary hypertension and right ventricular overload.

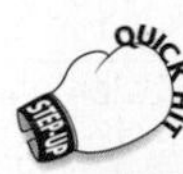

"Pink puffer": Pink refers to the lack of cyanosis from the nearly normal arterial oxygen pressures; puffer refers to the severe dyspnea seen in these patients.

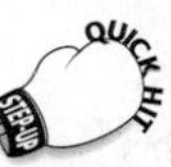

Status asthmaticus is a prolonged asthmatic attack that does not respond to therapy and can be fatal.

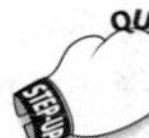

There are many types of asthma, including extrinsic (children), intrinsic (adults), exercise-induced, and cold-air induced.

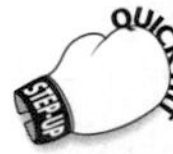

Emphysema and bronchitis often coexist in the same patient.

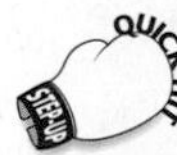

Order of β-agonist potency (most potent to least potent): isoproterenol, epinephrine, and norepinephrine. Order of α-agonist potency (most potent to least potent): epinephrine, norepinephrine, and isoproterenol.

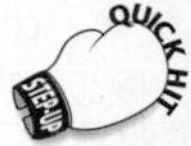

β_2-Selective agents such as terbutaline can be used in premature labor to prevent contractions.

TABLE 4-5 Therapeutic Agents for Asthma and COPD

Therapeutic Agent (common name, if relevant) [trade name, where appropriate]	Class—Pharmacology and Pharmacokinetics	Indications	Side or Adverse Effects	Contraindications or Precautions to Consider; Notes
Isoproterenol [Isuprel]	β-agonist (nonselective)—relaxes bronchial smooth muscle through β_2 receptor activity	Asthma	Tachycardia (β_1 receptor activity)	
Albuterol [Proventil, Ventolin]	**β_2 agonist—leads to relaxation of smooth muscle**	Asthma; COPD; bronchitis	**Tremor, tachycardia, arrhythmia,** headache, nausea, vomiting	
Salmeterol [Serevent]	**Long acting β_2 agonist—leads to relaxation of smooth muscle**	Asthma prophylaxis	**Hand tremor;** headache; nervousness; dizziness; cough; stuffed nose; runny nose; ear pain; muscle pain/cramps; sore throat	Not in acute asthmatic attack
Theophylline [Aerolate, Elixophyllin, Respbid, Slo-bid, Slo-Phyllin, Theo-24, Theo-Dur, Theolair, Uniphyl]	Methylxanthines—unknown mechanism; postulated to inhibit phosphodiesterase → decreases cAMP hydrolysis → promotes bronchodilation; stimulates CNS, cardiac muscle; relaxes smooth muscle; produces diuresis; increases cerebral vascular resistance	Asthma	Cardiotoxicity, neurotoxicity	Metabolized by cytochrome P450. Narrow therapeutic window
Ipratropium [Atrovent]	Muscarinic antagonist—competitively blocks muscarinic receptors → prevents bronchoconstriction	Asthma; COPD		
Cromolyn	Prevents release of mediators from mast cells → prevents bronchoconstriction and inflammation	Asthma prophylaxis		Not used during acute exacerbation
Beclomethasone, prednisone	Corticosteroids—inhibits leukotriene synthesis → reduces inflammation and leads to bronchodilation	Asthma; COPD	**Osteoporosis; Cushingoid reaction; psychosis; glucose intolerance; infection; hypertension; cataracts**	
Zileuton	Antileukotriene—**5-lipoxygenase inhibitor** → inhibits conversion of arachidonic acid to leukotriene → prevents bronchoconstriction and inflammatory cell infiltrate	Asthma		
Zafirlukast [Accolate], montelukast [Singulair]	Antileukotriene—**blocks leukotriene receptors (LTD_4)** → prevents bronchoconstriction and inflammatory cell infilate	Asthma (especially aspirin induced asthma)		
Nedocromil [Tilade]	Stabilizes membranes of mast cells and prevents mediator release	Asthma	Unpleasant taste	Not for acute asthmatic attacks

b. Inhaled corticosteroids such as beclomethasone, triamcinolone, and flunisolide decrease the effect that inflammatory cells (mast cells, eosinophils, macrophages) have on the airway.
c. In cases of severe asthma, intravenous methylprednisolone or oral prednisone may be necessary for a short period.
d. The side effects of inhaled steroids are minimal when compared with systemic steroid use. However, adverse reactions can occur and include oral candidiasis, and, with long-term use, osteoporosis.

B. Other asthma medications
1. **Cromolyn**, a prophylactic anti-inflammatory agent
2. **Ipratropium**, a derivative of atropine that blocks the vagal aspect of airway smooth muscle contraction and mucous secretion
3. **Theophylline**, a bronchodilator, which may result in seizures and arrhythmias
4. Newer agents
a. **Zileuton**, a 5-lipoxygenase inhibitor, blocks the conversion of arachidonic acid into leukotrienes, which are responsible for chemotaxis, increased secretion, and bronchospasm.
b. **Zafirlukast** prevents the chemotactic and bronchospastic effects of LTD_4 by blocking its receptor.

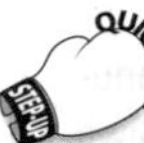
Agents useful in treating acute asthmatic exacerbation include albuterol, ipratropium, systemic corticosteroids, and magnesium. The use of leukotriene receptor antagonists may also be helpful in the acute setting, although this is controversial.

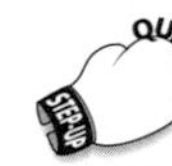
Agents useful in the treatment of an acute COPD exacerbation include albuterol, ipratropium, systemic corticosteroids, and doxycylcine. Even in the absence of a respiratory infection, doxycyline has anti-inflammatory properties that are useful in an acute exacerbation.

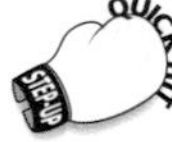
Agents useful in the long term management of chronic asthma include inhalcd β- agonsits (both short acting and long acting), inhaled corticosteroids, cromolyn, theophyline, and antileukotrienes.

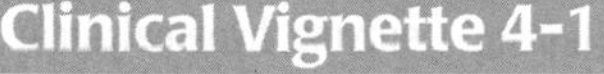

Clinical Vignette 4-1

Clinical Presentation: A 59-year-old female presents with a chief complaint of **SOB**. Patient states she has been experiencing worsening SOB with minimal physical exertion. She has been experiencing bouts of **productive cough** every morning for the past two years. She has smoked two packs of cigarettes a day for the past 35 years. Patient denies any fevers or bloody sputum. Physical exam reveals an **increased anteroposterior diameter of the chest wall** and **wheezes** and **rhonchi** on inspiration. T = 98.3 °F, BP = 142/92 mm Hg, HR = 93 bpm, RR = 23 breaths/min.

Differentials: COPD, asthma, CHF. Given the patient's presentation and long-standing history of smoking, this patient most likely has COPD.

Laboratory Studies: Proper follow-up management would include an **arterial blood gas** to provide information regarding the patients O_2 status as hypoxemia and hypercapnia may be present. **Spirometry** is the next best step in the evaluation process. **Flow volume loops** will assist in identifying restrictive from obstructive pulmonary disease. A FEV_1/FVC ratio in obstructive pulmonary diseases will be below the normal ratio of 0.8.

Management: Initial step in management is smoking cessation. **β-agonists and anticholinergic agents** provide bronchodilation via nebulizers. Administration of **oxygen** is necessary to correct hypoxemia. **Corticosteroids** can be used in acute exasperations along with **antibiotics** if there is suspicion of an underlying infection.

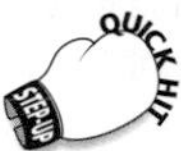
Interstitial lung disease (ILD) can be a side effect of bleomycin, methotrexate, and amiodarone.

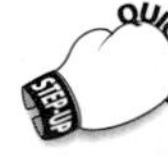
Interstitial lung diseases demonstrate alveolar wall fibrosis.

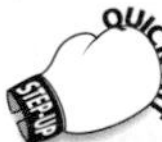
The three most common causes of hemoptysis are tuberculosis (TB), malignancy, and Goodpasture syndrome.

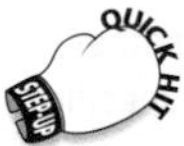
Bloody pleural effusions are most commonly from TB, malignancy, or trauma.

INTERSTITIAL LUNG DISEASE (Table 4-6)

ILD is a noninfectious, nonmalignant condition characterized by inflammation and pathologic changes of the alveolar wall. Differentiation and diagnosis often require histologic evaluation of the lung. It is characterized as having decreased lung volumes and a normal to increased FEV_1/FVC ratio.

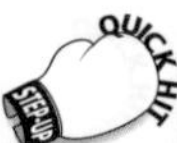

Rifampin decreases the half-lives of oral contraceptives as well as of warfarin, digitoxin, ketoconazole, propanolol, and prednisone. Consequently, higher doses of these medications may be required to achieve the same therapeutic effect.

Sudden infant death syndrome (SIDS) is the death of a child who is younger than 1 year of age from unexplained causes (even after autopsy). The infant is usually asleep in the prone position and has a history of an **upper respiratory infection.**

D. Etiology
1. Bacterial and *Mycoplasma* pneumonias (Table 4-8)
2. Viral pneumonia (Table 4-9)
3. Fungal pneumonia (Table 4-10)
4. Clinical diagnosis of pneumonia (Tables 4-11 and 4-12)

TABLE 4-8 Bacterial and Mycoplasma Pneumonia

Bacteria	Presentation	Population Most at Risk	Clinical Features
S. pneumoniae	Typical	**Adults**	Most common cause of community-acquired pneumonia
H. influenzae	Typical	Elderly	Complicates viral infection; chronic respiratory disease
S. aureus	Typical	Can cause typical community-acquired pneumonia but also infects immunocompromised and hospitalized patients	Abscesses; complicates viral infection
Streptococcus agalactiae	Typical	**Neonates**	Similar to *S. pneumoniae*
M. pneumoniae	Atypical	**Young adults**	Most common cause of atypical pneumonia; positive coldagglutinin test
Legionella pneumophila	Atypical	Immunocompromised patients	Found in drinking water and air conditioners
Klebsiella pneumoniae	Atypical	Patients with alcoholism	Aspiration of gastric contents
Chlamydia psittaci	Atypical	**Pet bird** owners	Bradycardia; splenomegaly
Chlamydia trachomatis (trachoma)	Atypical	**Neonates**	Most common cause of *trachoma,* preventable blindness
Chlamydia pneumoniae	Atypical	**Young adults**	Upper and lower pulmonary tract infection
Coxiella burnetii	Atypical	Dairy workers (via inhalation)	Fever
Francisella tularensis	Atypical	Hunters, veterinarians, livestock workers	Granulomatous nodules

TABLE 4-9 Viral Pneumonia

Virus	Pathophysiology	Clinical Features
Respiratory syncytial virus (types 1 and 2)	Atypical	Also causes bronchiolitis; more common in winter months; can cause serious respiratory distress in infants
Influenza	Atypical	**Often complicated by secondary bacterial infection**

TABLE 4-10 Fungal Pneumonia

Etiology	Pathophysiology	Clinical Features
Histoplasma capsulatum	Atypical	Most infections are subclinical; tiny yeast forms in macrophages; found in Ohio, Mississippi, and Missouri River Valleys; yeast with a thin cell wall but no true capsule
Coccidioides immitis	Atypical	Most infections are subclinical; spherules filled with endospores; "valley fever" found in southwestern deserts of United States; nonbudding spherule filled with endospores
P. carinii	Atypical	Often fatal common opportunistic infection in immunocompromised patients (such as HIV patients)
Paracoccidioides brasiliensis	Atypical	Budding yeast resemble spokes of a "pilot's wheel"; found in Central and South Americas; yeast with multiple budding
Sporotrichosis	Atypical	Skin lesions in rose gardeners
Aspergillus	Atypical	Fungal ball of hyphae (aspergilloma) in pre-existing lung cavities
Blastomyces dermatitidis	Atypical	Yeast forms in body; 5–25-mm yeast with thick refractile wall and broad-based budding; found in Mississippi–Ohio River basins and North America (especially mid-Atlantic states)
Candida albicans	Atypical	Yeast and hyphae
Cryptococcus	Atypical	Yeast with broad slimy capsule

TABLE 4-11 Clinical Diagnosis of Pneumonia

	Bacterial	Viral	Mycoplasma
Age	Any; often younger than 2 years old	Any	Young adults (teenagers)
Fever	>102.28 °F	<102.28 °F	<102.28 °F
Onset	Abrupt	Gradual	Gradual fever; gradual cough
Relatives	Healthy	Sick (concurrent)	Sick (2–3 weeks previous)
Cough	Productive	Dry	Paroxysmal
Pleuritic chest pain	Yes (splinting)	No	No
Physical examination	Tubular breath sounds; dull to percussion	Bilateral, diffuse rales	Rales in one or two segments
Radiographic findings	Consolidated "whited out" lobe	Diffuse; patchy; bilateral	Patchy; one or two lobes; no consolidation

THE RESPIRATORY SYSTEM

TABLE 4-14 Therapeutic Agents for Allergy, Cough, and Cold

Therapeutic Agent (common name, if relevant) [trade name, where appropriate]	Class—Pharmacology and Pharmacokinetics	Indications	Side or Adverse Effects	Contraindications or Precautions to Consider; Notes
Diphenhydramine, dimenhydrinate, chlorpheniramine	H_1 blocker (1st generation)	Allergy, motion sickness, insomnia	Sedation, antimuscarinic, anti-alpha adrenergic	
Loradatine, fexofenadine, desloratadine, cetirizine	H_1 blocker (2nd generation)	Allergy	Sedating	Less sedating than first generation H_1 blocker due to decreased CNS entry
Fluticasone [Flonase], beclomethasone, flunisolide [Nasarel], budesonide [Rhinocort], mometasone furoate	Intranasal glucocorticoids—decrease cytokine synthesis, down regulate inflammatory response in the nasal mucosa	Nasal congestion, allergic rhinitis	Local irritation of nasal mucosa, epistaxis	
Guaifenesin [Robutussin]	Expectorant—thins mucus and lubricates irritated respiratory tract	Cough associated with common cold and minor upper respiratory tract infections		Does not suppress cough reflex
N-acetylcysteine	Mucolytic—loosens mucus plugs	Cough (especially in CF patients), Acetaminophen overdose		
Glyceryl guaiacolate	Expectorant—increases bronchial secretions	Promotes cough		

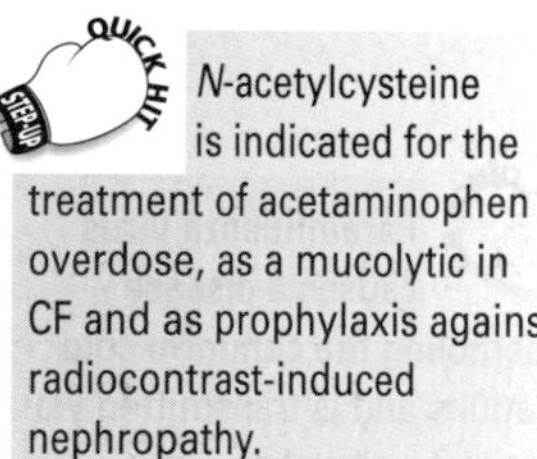

N-acetylcysteine is indicated for the treatment of acetaminophen overdose, as a mucolytic in CF and as prophylaxis against radiocontrast-induced nephropathy.

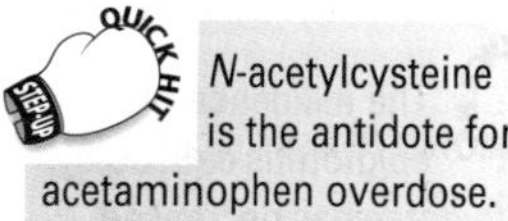

N-acetylcysteine is the antidote for acetaminophen overdose.

CYSTIC FIBROSIS

I. Cystic Fibrosis (CF) is the most common lethal genetic disease in Caucasians.

II. Autosomal recessive mutation occurs on chromosome 7, the CF transmembrane conductance regulator (CFTR) gene. This leads to

A. Deletion of phenylalanine at position 508 in 90% of CF patients in the United States.
B. Altered **chloride** and water transport in epithelial cells.
C. High sodium and chloride concentrations on sweat test.
D. Increased mucosal viscosity obstructs exocrine glands, which leads to organ failure.
E. An abnormally high rate of Na^+ absorption from luminal secretions and a decreased rate of Cl^- secretion into luminal secretions reduce the salt and water content of causing dehydrated secretions in bronchioles.

III. Chronic pulmonary disease

A. Most serious complication and **leading cause of death** in patients with CF.
B. *P. aeruginosa* infections are the most common followed by *S. aureus* and *H. influenzae*.
C. Increased RV and increased total lung capacity (TLC) are characteristics of chronic obstructive pulmonary disease.
D. Atelectasis.
E. Bronchiectasis.

IV. Pancreatic insufficiency

A. Nutritional deficiencies (especially of fat-soluble vitamins A, D, E, and K).
B. Steatorrhea.
C. β-Cells are initially spared but become functionally inactive with age leading to an increased need for insulin.

V. Meconium ileus

A. Usually presents in infant with abdominal distention, small bowel obstruction, and emesis

VI. Treatment of CF includes symptomatic treatment and gene therapy.

A. Mucolytics: *N*-acetylcysteine lyses the disulfide linkages between mucoproteins resulting in decreased mucus viscosity.
B. **Inhaled bronchodilators.**
C. Corticosteroids: prednisone has been shown to increase pulmonary function and body weight in CF patients.
D. **Antibiotics as needed to manage infections.**

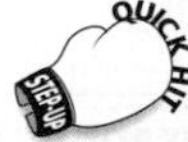

Superior sulcus tumors (**Pancoast tumors**) involve the apex of the lung and result in **Horner syndrome** (ptosis, miosis, anhydrosis). **Superior vena cava syndrome** occurs when the superior vena cava (SVC) is obstructed, resulting in facial cyanosis and swelling.

MNEMONIC

To remember the symptoms of Horner syndrome, think "PAM is Horny." P is ptosis, A is anhydrosis, M is miosis.

LUNG NEOPLASMS (Tables 4-15 to 4-17)

I. Lung neoplasms are the leading cause of cancer death for both men and women in the United States.

II. Lung is the second most common type of cancer (with the first being prostate cancer in men and breast cancer in women).

III. Lung cancer deaths among women are rising rapidly as a result of increased smoking in this population.

IV. Symptoms include cough, hemoptysis, airway obstruction, weight loss, and paraneoplastic syndromes.

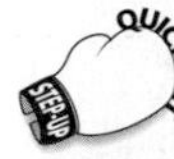

Nasopharyngeal carcinoma, common in Southeast Asia and East Africa, is caused by the Epstein-Barr virus.

MNEMONIC

To remember the location, risk factors, and hormone-producing properties for small cell and squamous cell carcinoma, think **s** with **c**entral, **s**moking, and **s**ecretions.

TABLE 4-15 Lung Neoplasms

Tumor	Location and Histology	Clinical Features
Adenocarcinoma	**Peripheral;** subpleural; usually on pre-existing parenchymal **scars;** glandular	**Most common type;** may be related to smoking; CEA-positive; K-*ras* oncogenes
Bronchioalveolar	**Peripheral;** subtype of adenocarcinoma; tumor cells line alveolar walls	**Less strongly associated with smoking;** autoantibodies to surfactant may exist
Carcinoid	Major bronchi; spread by direct extension	Increased secretion of **5-HT;** flushing; wheezing; recurrent diarrhea; heart disease; low malignancy
Large cell	**Peripheral;** undifferentiated; giant cells with pleomorphism	Poor prognosis; metastasis to the brain; smoking
Metastasis	**Cannonball** lesions	**Higher incidence than primary lung cancer**
Small cell (oat cell)	**Central;** undifferentiated; **most aggressive;** small, dark blue cells; arise from neuroendocrine (Kulchitsky) cells	Poor prognosis; strongly associated with smoking; ectopic ACTH, and ADH secretion
Squamous cell	**Central;** mass from bronchus; keratin pearls; cavitation	Strongly associated with smoking; secretion of **PTH-like peptide**

ACTH, adrenocorticotropic hormone; ADH, antidiuretic hormone; CEA, carcinoembryonic antigen; 5-HT, serotonin; PTH, parathyroid hormone.

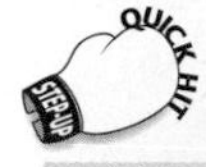

Paraneoplastic syndrome is a clinical and biochemical disturbance caused by a neoplasm that is not directly related to the primary tumor or metastases. Secretion of parathyroid hormone (PTH)-like hormone results in hypercalcemia. Ectopic antidiuretic hormone (ADH) production leads to syndrome of inappropriate antidiuretic hormone (SIADH) secretion with urinary retention and high urine osmolality. Adrenocorticotropic hormone (ACTH)-producing tumors lead to Cushing syndrome.

TABLE 4-16 Other Respiratory Carcinomas

Tumor	Histology	Risk Factors
Nasopharyngeal carcinoma	Lymphoepithelioma (rich in lymphocytes)	Epstein–Barr virus infection; common in Southeast Asia (adult) and East Africa (childhood)
Laryngeal carcinoma	Squamous cell carcinoma	Smoking

TABLE 4-17 Paraneoplastic Syndromes of Lung Cancer

Disorder	Causes and Clinical Presentation
Horner syndrome	Superior sulcus tumors (Pancoast tumors); Ptosis, miosis, anhydrosis
Superior vena cava syndrome	Insidious compression or obstruction of the SVC; facial cyanosis, facial swelling, headache, venous distension of the neck, upper chest, and arms
Ectopic Cushing syndrome	**ACTH** secretion; associated with small cell carcinoma; Fat deposition of the face (moon facies), upper back (buffalo hump), truncal obesity, muscle weakness, purple stria
Hypercalcemia	Secretion of **PTH**—related protein;
SIADH	Ectopic **antidiuretic hormone (ADH)** production; Hyponatremia (Na^+ below 120 mEq/L)
Eaton Lambert syndrome	Proximal muscle weakness with autonomic dysfunction; antibodies produced against presynaptic calcium channels of the neuromuscular junction, no improvement with administration of anticholinesterase agents

Clinical Vignette 4-2

Clinical Presentation: A 74-year-old male presents with **SOB**, a chronic **bloody cough, increased fatigue, and a weight loss of 20 lbs over a 3-month period**. Past medical history is significant for **hypertension, emphysema, coronary artery disease**, and a 26 pack-years of **smoking**. Physical examination reveals wheezing in the right upper lobe. *T* = 98.7°F, BP = 140/92 mm Hg, HR = 80 bpm, and RR = 25 breaths/min.

Differentials: Lung cancer, TB, pneumonia, left heart failure. Given the patient's presentation and long-standing history of smoking, this patient most likely has lung cancer. The two most common causes of hemoptysis in the United States are bronchitis and lung cancer.

Laboratory Studies: Proper follow-up for this patient would include imaging such as a chest **CT scan** or a **chest X-ray**. If imaging reveals a mass, **bronchoscopy** can be performed to obtain cells via brushings, bronchoalveolar lavage, or biopsy. **CT-guided fine needle biopsy** can also be performed to gather cells.

Management: Treatments include **surgical resection** and **chemotherapy** independently or in combination with **radiation**. Non-small cell lung cancer should be staged using the TNM (tumor, node, metastasis) system. Patients with stage I or II non-small cell lung cancers can be cured with surgical resection and radiotherapy. Small cell lung cancer often has metastasized at the time of diagnosis, making surgical resection futile and limiting radiotherapy and chemotherapy as the only treatment options.

DRUGS THAT CAUSE ADVERSE EFFECTS TO THE RESPIRATORY SYSTEM

I. **Pulmonary fibrosis:** bleomycin (antineoplastic), amiodarone (antiarrhythmic), busulfan (antineoplastic)

II. **Cough:** angiotensin-converting enzyme inhibitors (versus angiotensin II receptor blockers = no cough)

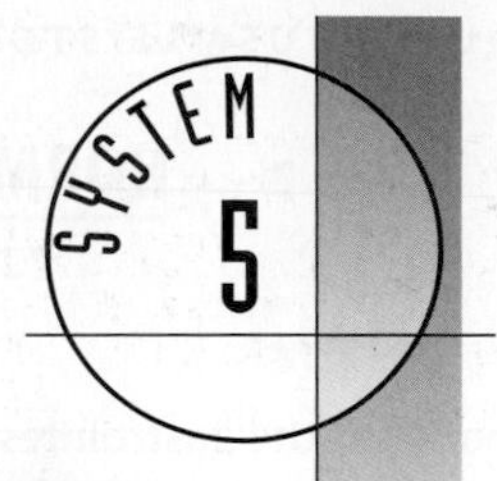

The Gastrointestinal System

INNERVATION AND BLOOD SUPPLY OF THE GASTROINTESTINAL TRACT (Figure 5-1)

FIGURE 5-1 **Innervation and blood supply of the gastrointestinal tract**

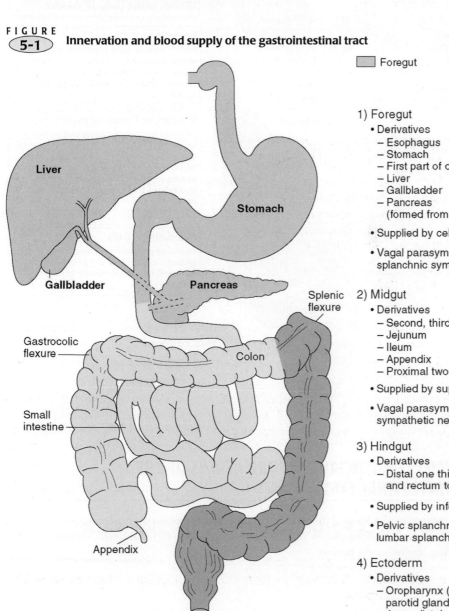

Foregut Midgut Hindgut

Liver
Stomach
Gallbladder
Pancreas
Splenic flexure
Gastrocolic flexure
Colon
Small intestine
Appendix
Rectum

1) Foregut
- Derivatives
  - Esophagus
  - Stomach
  - First part of duodenum
  - Liver
  - Gallbladder
  - Pancreas (formed from fusion of dorsal and ventral buds)
- Supplied by celiac trunk
- Vagal parasympathetic nerve, thoracic nerve, and splanchnic sympathetic nerve

2) Midgut
- Derivatives
  - Second, third, and fourth parts of duodenum
  - Jejunum
  - Ileum
  - Appendix
  - Proximal two thirds of colon (up to splenic flexure)
- Supplied by superior mesenteric artery
- Vagal parasympathetic nerve, thoracic splanchnic sympathetic nerve

3) Hindgut
- Derivatives
  - Distal one third of colon including sigmoid colon and rectum to pectinate line
- Supplied by inferior mesenteric artery
- Pelvic splanchnic (S2–S4) parasympathetic nerve and lumbar splanchnic sympathetic nerve

4) Ectoderm
- Derivatives
  - Oropharynx (anterior two thirds of tongue, lips, parotid glands, tooth enamel)
  - Anus, distal rectum (from pectinate line outward)

HORMONES OF THE GASTROINTESTINAL SYSTEM (Figure 5-2)

FIGURE 5-2 Hormones of the gastrointestinal system

Notilin
Secreted in upper GI tract to increase smooth muscle contraction in esophageal sphincter, stomach, and duodenum

Nitric oxide
Causes smooth muscle relaxation (e.g., lower esophageal sphincter [LES] relaxation)

Peptide YY
Secreted by endocrine cells of ileum and colon to inhibit gastric H^+ secretion

Glucagon
Secreted by cells of the pancreatic islets to promote glycogenolysis and gluconeogenesis

Gastrin
From antrum of stomach; secreted in response to gastric distention, vagal stimulation, and amino acid entering the stomach; causes gastric H^+ secretion

Cholecystokinin (CCK)
From cells in duodenum and jenunum and neurons of ileum and colon; Secreted in response to amino acids and fatty acids entering the duodenum; causes contraction of gallbladder and pancreatic secretion of enzymes and HCO_3^-

Secretin
From S cells of small intestines; secreted in response to H^+ and fatty acids entering the duodenum; causes pancreatic secretion of HCO_3^- and inhibits gastric H^+ secretion

Somatostatin
Produced by D cells of stomach and duodenum and δ cells of pancreatic islets to inhibit gastrin H^+ secretion, pancreatic secretion, and lower bile flow and to promote intestinal SMC contraction

Vasoactive intestinal peptide (VIP)
Secreted by smooth muscle and nerves of intestines; relaxes intestinal smooth muscle, causes pancreatice HCO_3^- secretion, and inhibits gastric H^+ secretion; enteric nervous system (ENS) peptide neurotransmitter, also relaxes lower esophageal sphincter, possibly as part of NO response

Parasympathetic (ACh)
Increases production of saliva; increased gastric H^+ secretion; increases pancreatic enzyme and HCO_3^- secretion; causes gallbadder contraction; allows for gastric receptive relaxation; stimulates enteric nervous system to create intestinal peristalsis; relaxes sphincters

Sympathetic (NE)
Increases production of saliva; decreases splanchnic blood flow in fight-or-flight response; decreases motility; constricts sphincters

Liver
Stomach
Gallbladder
Pancreas
Duodenum
Colon
Small intestine
Cecum
Appendix
Sigmoid
Rectum
1
2
3
4

Retroperitoneal
Partially peritonealized
Completely peritonealized

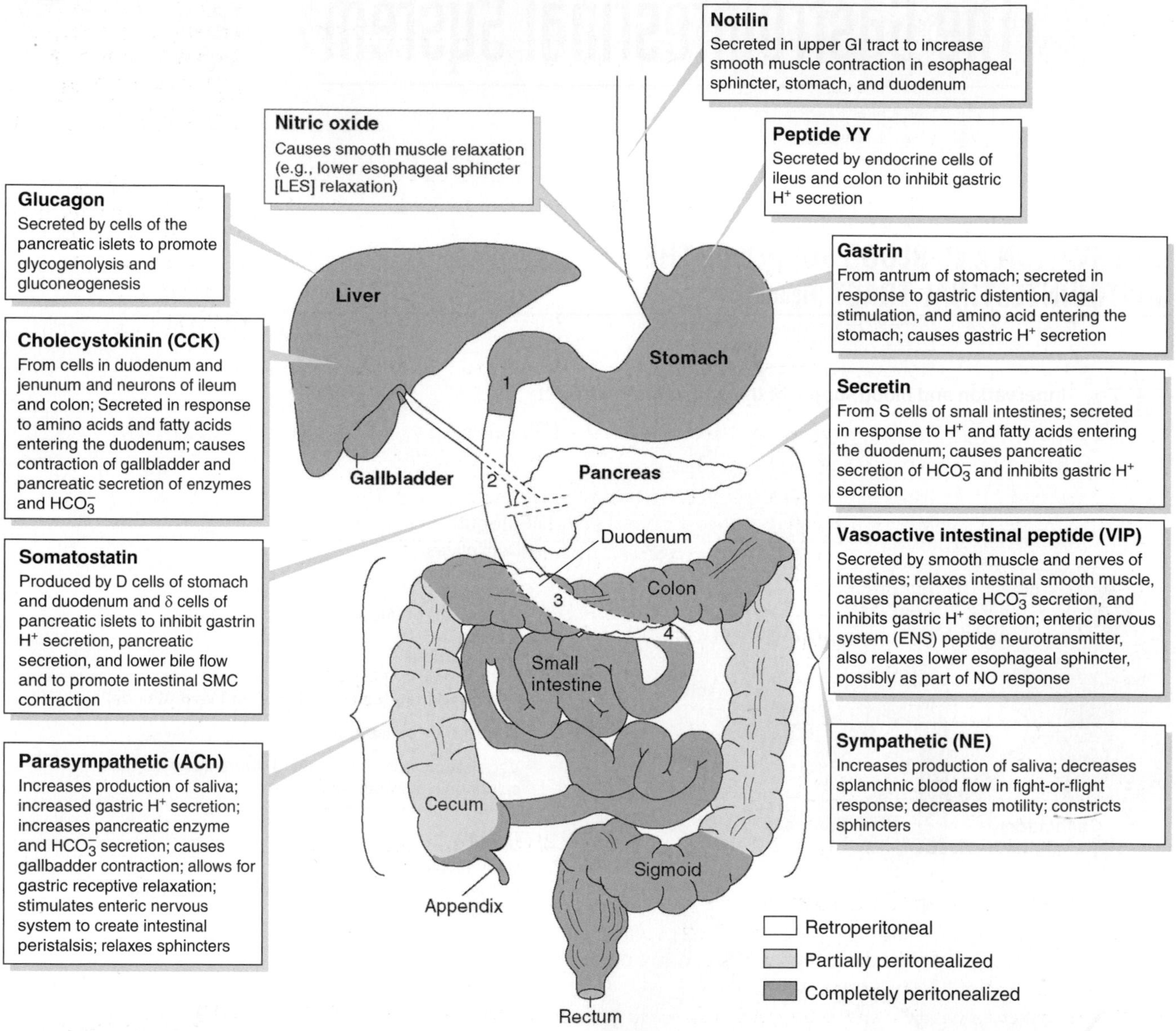

QUICK HIT: The boundaries of the epiploic foramen of Winslow (opening of the lesser sac) are the hepatoduodenal ligament (containing **the common bile duct (CBD), the proper hepatic artery, and the portal vein**) located anteriorly, the caudate lobe of the liver located superiorly, the duodenum located inferiorly, and the inferior vena cava located posteriorly.

IMPORTANT CONGENITAL MALFORMATIONS OF THE GASTROINTESTINAL SYSTEM (Table 5-1)

With the exception of a Meckel diverticulum, which can remain asymptomatic throughout the life, congenital malformations of the gastrointestinal (GI) tract will manifest themselves during the neonatal period.

TABLE 5-1 Important Congenital Malformations of the GI System

Malformation	Clinical Features
Hypertrophic pyloric stenosis	Thickening of the pylorus musculature **Projectile vomiting** Palpable knot "olive" in the pyloric region
Extrahepatic biliary atresia	Incomplete recanalization of the bile duct during development Presents shortly after birth Dark urine Clay-colored stool Jaundice
Annular pancreas	Abnormal fusion of ventral and dorsal pancreatic buds forming a constricting ring around the duodenum Duodenal obstruction (bilious vomiting) presents shortly after birth
Meckel diverticulum	Persistent remnant of the vitelline duct Forms an outpouching (true diverticulum) in the ileum Ulceration and bleeding 50% contain either gastric or pancreatic tissue when symptomatic
Malrotation of the midgut	Normal 270 degree rotation is not completed Cecum and appendix lie in upper abdomen Associated with **volvulus** (twisting of intestine) causing an obstruction
Intestinal stenosis or atresia	Results from failure of the normal recanalization of the lumen May produce failure to thrive
Hirschsprung disease (congenital or toxic megacolon)	Failure of **neural crest cells** to migrate to colon No peristalsis Constipation and abdominal distention in newborn **Bowel movement precipitated by digital rectal examination**
Anal agenesis	Lack of anal opening as a result of improper formation of the urorectal septum May cause rectovesical (anus to bladder), rectovaginal, or rectourethral fistula

MNEMONIC

Rule of 2s for Meckel diverticulum: 2 ft from ileocecal junction; 2 in long; 2% of the population affected; 2 times more common in men; and 2 types of ectopic tissue involved (gastric or pancreatic). Remember Meckel **di**verticulum as the disease associated with 2 as "**di-**" means "**2.**"

QUICK HIT

Duodenal atresia is associated with Down syndrome and demonstrates a characteristic **"double-bubble"** sign on radiograph and ultrasound.

THE OROPHARYNX, ESOPHAGUS, AND STOMACH

I. The digestion of food begins in the oral cavity with salivary enzymes.

II. The esophagus transports food to the stomach

A. The upper third of the esophagus is skeletal muscle.
B. The middle third is both skeletal and smooth muscle.
C. The lower third is smooth muscle.
D. The lower esophageal sphincter (LES) relaxes in preparation for the passage of food into the stomach.

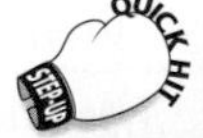

Many GI disorders present with abdominal pain—use the quality of pain to help you: **sharp, stabbing epigastric pain** that radiates to the back suggests pancreatitis; **burning epigastric pain** *suggests a gastric or duodenal* ulcer; and **pain that shifts** from the epigastrium to the right lower quadrant suggests appendicitis.

III. The stomach receives and stores food

A. **Receptive relaxation**—the stomach relaxes to accommodate the entering food (a vagovagal reflex).
B. Three phases of gastric secretion
   1. **Cephalic phase**—the sight, smell, taste, or thought of food stimulates secretion
   2. **Gastric phase**—secretion is caused by the entry of food into the stomach
   3. **Intestinal phase**—food entering the intestine causes a feedback stimulation of gastric secretion
C. Important gastric secretions
   1. **Hydrochloric acid (HCl)** is secreted by parietal cells of the fundus
      a. Stimulated by gastrin, histamine, and vagal stimulation
      b. Inhibited by **omeprazole** (proton pump inhibitor), **cimetidine** (H_2-blocker), chyme in small intestine via gastric inhibitory peptide (GIP), and secretin

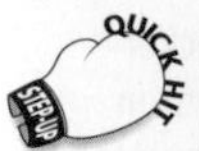

GERD, a common gastroesophageal disorder, is usually treated with H_2-blockers such as cimetidine or ranitidine or, in more severe cases, with proton pump inhibitors such as omeprazole or lansoprazole.

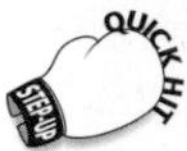

Cyclooxygenase-2 (COX-2) inhibitors such as celecoxib and rofecoxib not only reduce the adverse GI side effects and ulcers of normal nonsteroidal anti-inflammatory drugs (NSAIDs) but also do not inhibit platelet function.

2. **Intrinsic** factor is secreted by parietal cells of the fundus
   a. Binds to vitamin B_{12} (extrinsic factor)
   b. **Vitamin B_{12}-intrinsic factor complex absorbed in terminal ileum**
3. **Pepsinogen** is secreted by chief cells
   a. Pepsinogen is converted to pepsin by the low pH of the stomach.
   b. Pepsin begins the digestion of protein.
4. **Gastrin** secreted by the G cells of the antrum and pylorus stimulates the release of HCl from parietal cells.
5. **Somatostatin is secreted by a variety of cells throughout the GI tract and has a global inhibitory effect.**

D. The stomach grinds food into small particles and forces it into the duodenum.
   1. Grinding (trituration) takes place in peristaltic waves occurring at a rate of three to five waves per minute.
   2. **Migrating motor complexes (MMCs)**, stimulated by motilin, occur in the interdigestive period and serve to flush undigested food through the GI system.

IV. Nonneoplastic disorders of the oropharynx, esophagus, and stomach (Table 5-2)

TABLE 5-2 Nonneoplastic Disorders of the Oropharynx, Esophagus, and Stomach

Disorder	Etiology and Pathology	Clinical Features	Notes
Sialolithiasis	Blockage of salivary gland duct preventing release of saliva; follows chronic sialadenitis (inflammation of the salivary glands)	Acute pain; usually in submandibular gland or Stensen duct of the parotid gland	Passage of stone can be induced by stimulating the secretion of saliva (e.g., by sucking on a lemon)
Pleomorphic adenoma	Increased risk with radiation exposure	Benign, recurring, mixed cell tumor of the parotid; may lead to facial nerve injury	Most frequent salivary gland tumor; more common in women 20–40 years of age
Esophageal variceal bleeding	Bleeding from esophageal varices owing to portal HTN	Hematemesis; signs of portal HTN (i.e., caput medusae, ascites)	Usually treated with vasoconstrictors (vasopressin); endoscopy required for diagnosis (to rule out bleeding ulcers)
Boerhaave syndrome	Complete rupture of the esophagus (all layers); caused by severe retching	Often presents as left pneumothorax; surgical correction necessary	Esophageal reflux disease predisposes to this condition
Mallory-Weiss tear	Laceration of the gastroesophageal junction; usually caused by severe retching	Poststretching hematemesis	Alcoholics and bulimics are at an increased risk
Acute gastritis	NSAIDs; smoking; alcohol; aspirin; steroids; burn injury (Curling ulcer); brain injury (Cushing ulcer)	Erosive; acute inflammation; necrosis; hemorrhage; **"coffee-ground" vomitus**	Blood in the nasogastric tube
Chronic gastritis	Type A (fundal): autoimmune pernicious anemia, aging	Nonerosive; mucosal inflammation and atrophy of mucosa	Risk factor for gastric carcinoma
	Type B (antral): *Helicobacter pylori*		
Gastric ulcers	***H. pylori*** (70% of cases); bile-induced gastritis; increased permeability of gastric mucosa; associated with the use of aspirin and NSAIDs	Postprandial pain; bleeding; perforation; obstruction	Usually near the lesser curvature; not dependent on increased gastric acid secretion; not precancerous
Dumping syndrome	Postvagotomy; unimpeded passage of hypertonic food to the small intestine causing distention as a result of osmotic flow of water into the lumen	Nausea; diarrhea; palpitations; sweating; lightheadedness; reactive hypoglycemia	Can be prevented by eating only small meals and ingesting solids and liquids separately

NSAIDs, nonsteroidal anti-inflammatory drugs.

V. Neoplastic disorders of the oropharynx, esophagus, and stomach (Table 5-3 and Figure 5-3)

Nonneoplastic and neoplastic disorders originating proximal to the pyloric sphincter often present with hematemesis and dysphagia as a result of alcohol and tobacco abuse.

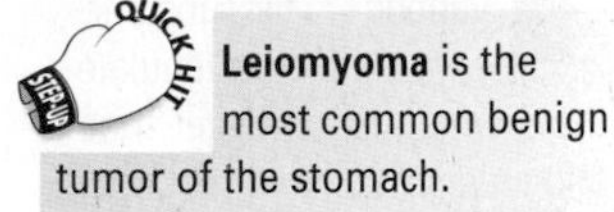

Leiomyoma is the most common benign tumor of the stomach.

TABLE 5-3 Neoplastic Disorders of the Oropharynx, Esophagus, and Stomach

Disorder	Etiology and Pathology	Clinical Features	Notes
Oral cancer	**Smoking;** chewing tobacco; alcohol	Squamous cell carcinoma; may involve tongue	Leukoplakia (white patch on the mucus membrane that cannot be wiped off) is a common precursor lesion
Esophageal adenocarcinoma	**Barrett esophagus;** complication of GERD	**Columnar metaplasia of esophageal squamous epithelium;** distal third of the esophagus	More common in Whites
Esophageal squamous cell carcinoma	Alcohol and tobacco use; esophagitis	Dysphagia; anorexia; pain	More common in Blacks
Gastric carcinoma	***H. pylori;*** gastritis; low-fiber diet, nitrosamines; blood group A; high-salt diet; increased incidence in Japan owing to greater consumption of smoked foods	Aggressive spread from antrum to nodes and liver; **Virchow node** (enlarged left-sided supraclavicular lymph node); **Krukenberg tumor** (metastatic disease to the ovaries from the stomach characterized by mucinous, signet ring cells)	More common in men older than 50 years of age; infiltration of stomach walls with tumor cells and subsequent fibrosis leads to linitis plastica (leather-bottle stomach)

FIGURE 5-3 Barium-swallow radiograph of achalasia

(Reproduced with permission from Humes DH, Dupont HL, Gardner LB, et al. Kelley's Textbook of Internal Medicine. 4th Ed. Philadelphia, PA: Lippincott Williams & Wilkins, 2000:821.)

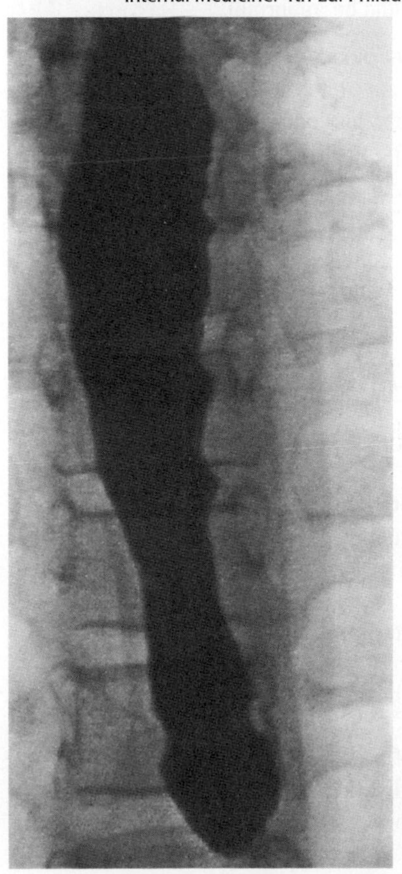

MNEMONIC

Various emetic substances in the blood stimulate the chemoreceptor trigger zone and area postrema to produce feelings of nausea and vomiting. Remember the extraintestinal causes of vomiting as part of your differential:

- **V**estibular disturbance/**V**agal
- **O**piates
- **M**igraine/**M**etabolic (diabetic ketoacidosis, gastroparesis, hypercalcemia)
- **I**nfections
- **T**oxicity
- **I**ncreased intracranial pressure (ICP)/**I**ngested alcohol
- **N**eurogenic, psychogenic
- **G**estation

MNEMONIC

To remember one cause and treatment of a**CHA**lasia, think **CHA**gas disease and calcium-**CHA**nnel blocker.

Clinical Vignette 5.1

Clinical Presentation: During a visit to her primary care physician, a 39-year -old female complains of **difficulty swallowing**. She also reports some heartburn and weight loss but denies pain on swallowing. She is an otherwise healthy female with no medical problems. Physical examination shows intact cranial nerves, swallowing mechanisms, and motor function of extremities. Vital signs are stable. Barium-swallow radiograph is shown previously.

Differentials: Mechanical obstruction—cancer, strictures, and rings; **oropharyngeal motility disorders**—multiple sclerosis, stroke, poliomyelitis, Parkinson disease, and myasthenia gravis; **esophageal motility disorders**—achalasia, scleroderma, and diffuse esophageal spasm. To remember the differentials for dysphagia, group them according to the phase of swallowing that has been disturbed and the type of pathology present (obstruction or motility disorder). To sort through the differentials, look for three symptoms specific to esophageal pathology: dysphagia (difficulty swallowing), odynophagia (pain on swallowing), and heartburn. Odynophagia would suggest diffuse esophageal spasm, whereas heartburn would suggest gastroesophageal reflux disease (GERD). Determine the type of dysphagia: difficulty with solids indicates mechanical obstruction; trouble with both solids and liquids suggests esophageal motility disorders; and problems in transferring food from the oral cavity suggest oropharyngeal disorders. For oropharyngeal disorders, look for details in the history and physical examination, such as aspiration pneumonia, nasal regurgitation, and cranial nerve pathology.

Laboratory Studies: In this case, the **barium-swallow chest radiograph** shows dilation of the esophagus with narrowing at the LES confirming a diagnosis of achalasia. Other significant findings on chest radiograph include pneumonia, thickened esophageal folds, ulcerations, and strictures. **Manometry** is also helpful in esophageal motility disorders, and in achalasia, it would classically show a lack of ordered peristalsis, increased LES pressures, and failure of LES relaxation after swallowing. **Esophagoscopy** is helpful in visualizing and qualifying obstruction and mucosal wall integrity and important to rule out cancer. **Esophageal pH monitoring** would also be done in this case to rule out GERD. If an oropharyngeal disorder is suspected, a **swallowing electromyography** is indicated and electromyelograms would be abnormal.

Management: Achalasia is treated by calcium-channel blockers and nitrates to decrease LED pressure. Patients refractory to medical treatment can undergo endoscopic injection of botulinum toxin at the LES to block the release of acetylcholine locally. Surgical management options include myotomy of the gastroesophageal junction to relieve LES pressure with partial fundoplication to prevent reflux.

THE SMALL INTESTINE, LARGE INTESTINE, AND RECTUM

I. Muscular layers of the GI tract is shown in Figure 5-4.

II. The small intestine digests and absorbs the food

A. Digestion is mediated by a variety of GI hormones including cholecystokinin (CCK), secretin, somatostatin, and others (Figure 5-2).

B. Carbohydrates

1. Pancreatic amylase hydrolyzes glycogen, starch, and most other complex carbohydrates to disaccharides.
2. Disaccharides are broken down to monosaccharides by intestinal brush border enzymes and absorbed.
3. Monosaccharides are absorbed by a variety of mechanisms:
   a. Glucose and galactose are absorbed by sodium (Na^+)-dependent transport.
   b. Fructose is absorbed by facilitated diffusion.

Lactose intolerance is caused by a genetic absence or decrease in lactase. Lactose cannot be broken down; it remains in the lumen of the gut and causes **osmotic** diarrhea.

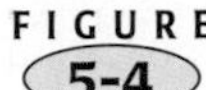
FIGURE 5-4 Picture of muscular layer of the GI tract

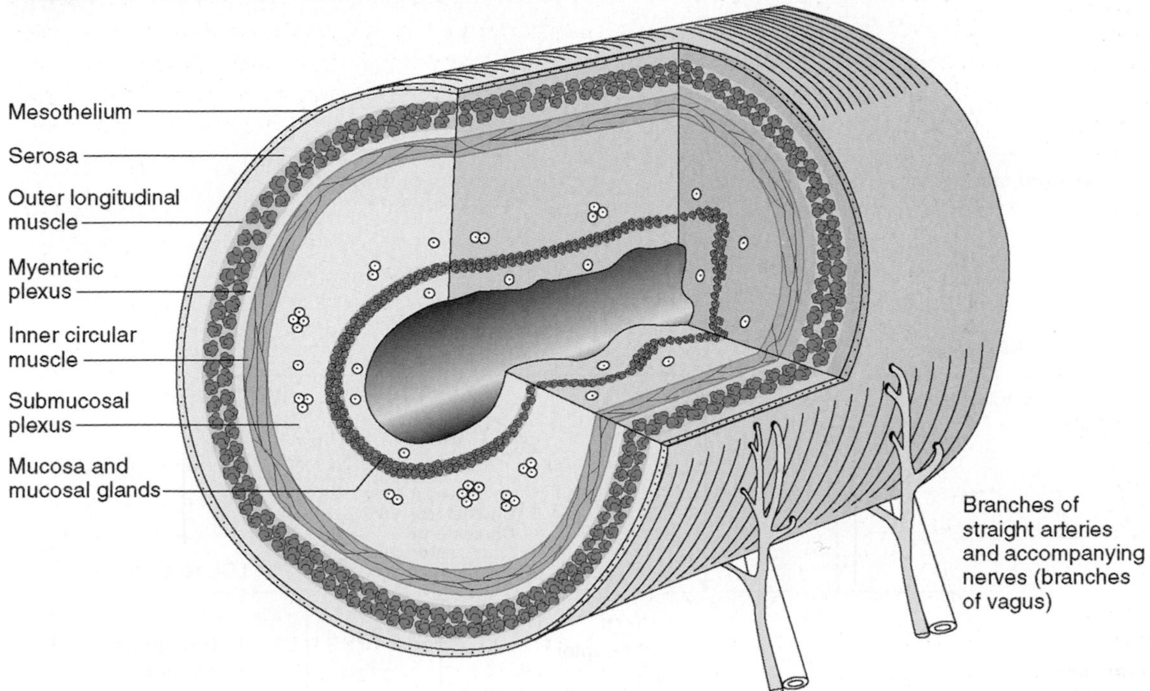

C. Protein
 1. It is degraded to amino acids, dipeptides, and tripeptides by proteases produced by the pancreas
  a. Activation of **trypsinogen to trypsin**
   - Autoactivated
   - Activated by intestinal brush border enterokinases
  b. Trypsin degrades the peptide bonds of arginine or lysine.
  c. Trypsin also **activates the other proteolytic pancreatic enzymes.**
 2. Proteins are absorbed by an Na^{+}-dependent transport.
  a. There are separate carriers for acidic, basic, and neutral amino acids.
  b. Dipeptides and tripeptides are absorbed faster than single amino acids.

D. Fats
 1. Lipids are broken into droplets by the mixing action of the stomach.
 2. **Pancreatic lipase** (and to a lesser extent salivary lipase) **hydrolyzes triacylglycerol to fatty acids and 2-monoacylglycerol. Chronic pancreatitis** decreases fat digestion and absorption due to decreased lipase release from the exocrine pancreas.
 3. Bile salts (amphipathic molecules) emulsify the hydrolyzed products and form micelles.
 4. **Micelles** allow for fat absorption (Figure 5-5).
 5. A variety of familial and acquired disorders may disrupt lipid metabolism, resulting in **hyperlipidemia**
  a. Hyperlipidemia, especially high levels of low-density lipoproteins (LDLs), is associated with coronary artery disease (CAD).
  b. Typically, treatment first involves dietary intervention and then drug therapy, regardless of the cause of the hyperlipidemia
   - **3-Hydroxy-3-methylglutaryl coenzyme A (HMG-CoA) reductase inhibitors**, also known as **"statins"** such as atorvastatin, lovastatin, and pravastatin, are an effective and widely used means of lowering LDL.

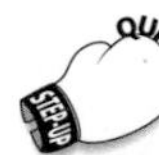

Often, the amino acid transporter found in the intestines is identical to the amino acid transporter found in the renal tubules. As such, diseases that affect these transporters have multiorgan system effects. One of these diseases is Hartnup disease, which is a defect in the intestinal and renal tubular absorption of neutral amino acids leading to excretion of tryptophan derivatives and causing pellagra-like symptoms.

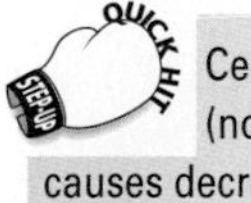

Celiac disease (nontropical sprue) causes decreased absorption of fat and fat soluble vitamins, leading to skeletal and hematological conditions due to decreased vitamin D and K.

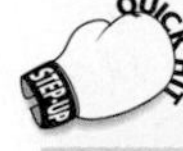

Although the statins work well as cholesterol-lowering agents, they can be **hepatotoxic**. Consequently, patients who take them should undergo routine liver function tests.

FIGURE 5-5 **Absorption and digestion of fats (lipid metabolism)**

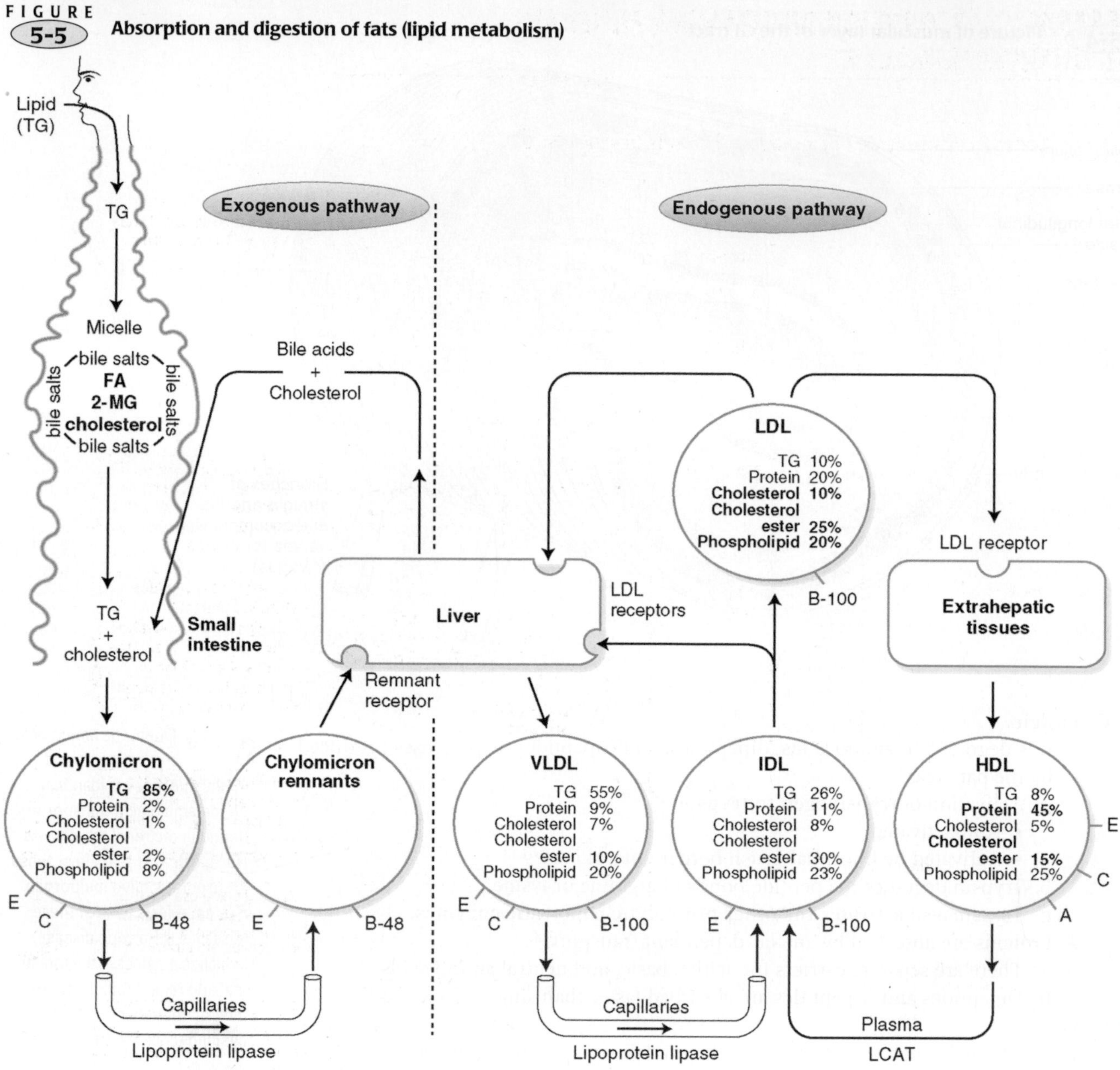

- **Bile acid-binding resins** such as cholestyramine and colestipol work by binding bile acids in the intestine and promoting their subsequent loss in the stool, which ultimately lowers LDL levels.
- **Nicotinic acid (niacin)** inhibits the release of lipoproteins from the liver, lowering very-low-density lipoproteins (VLDLs) and LDL.

III. The large intestine stores and excretes nondigestible material.

A. Absorbs 2 to 3 L per day of water

B. **Secretes potassium** (K^+)

C. Mediates defecation of undigested material through both voluntary and involuntary (rectosphincteric reflex) mechanisms

LOCATION OF ABSORPTION OF VITAMINS, MINERALS, AND NUTRIENTS (Figure 5-6)

FIGURE 5-6 Location of absorption of vitamins, minerals, and nutrients

COMMON CLINICAL DISORDERS OF THE SMALL INTESTINE, LARGE INTESTINE, AND RECTUM (Table 5-4)

Common clinical disorders of the GI tract, distal to the pyloric sphincter, will usually present as vague abdominal pain as a result of stimulation of the visceral afferent nerves. If the parietal peritoneum (the abdominal wall), innervated by the somatic afferent nerves, is irritated owing to the lesion, the pain will become more localized (as is seen in acute appendicitis).

Diarrhea, the passage of abnormal amounts of fluid or semisolid fecal matter, can be mediated by a number of mechanisms. Osmotic diarrhea results when unabsorbed solutes increase intraluminal oncotic pressure, causing an outpouring of water. Surgical resection can lead to an inadequate surface for absorption of nutrients, resulting in a form of **osmotic diarrhea**. Active ion secretion causing obligatory water loss is termed **secretory diarrhea**.

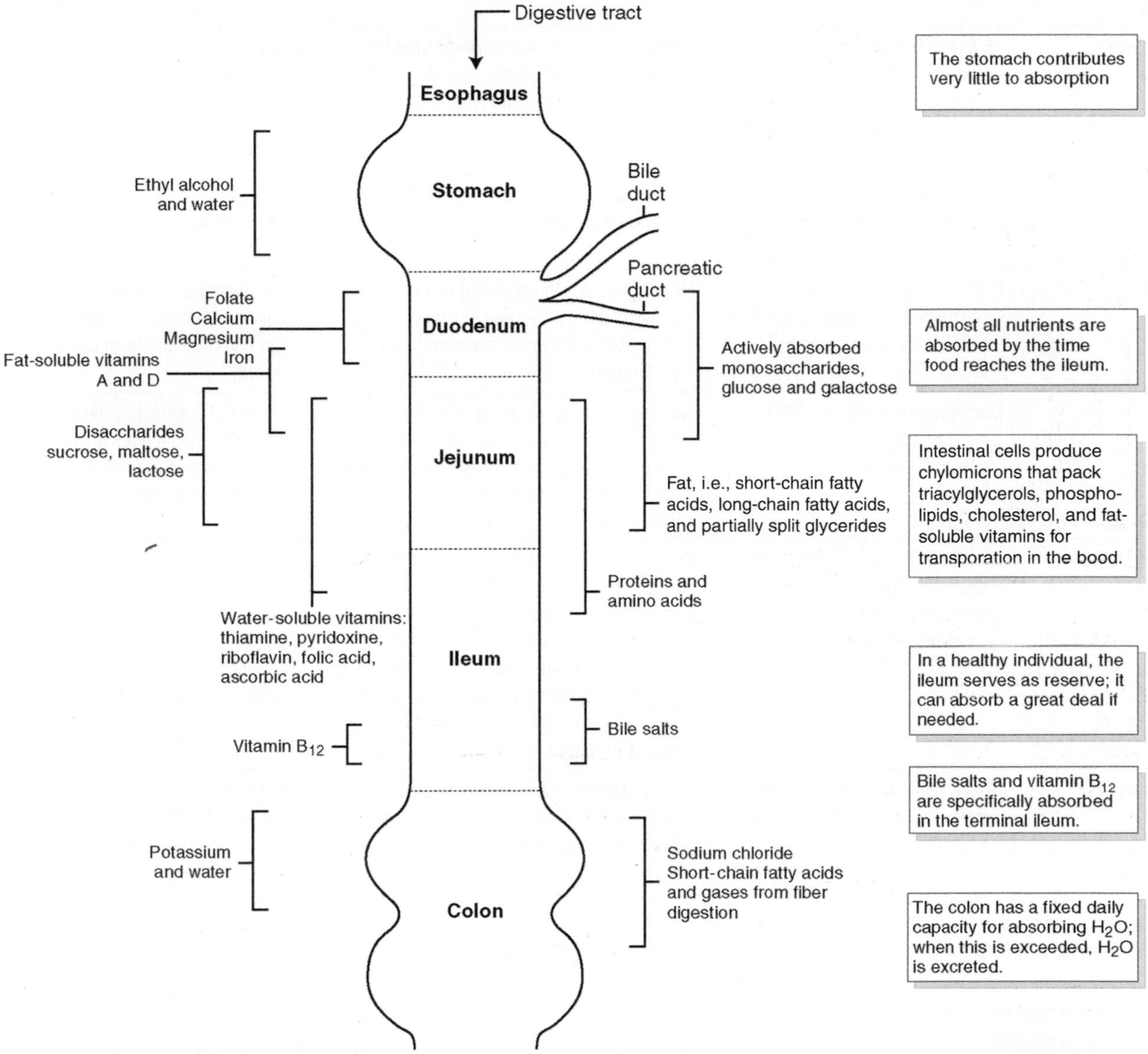

QUICK HIT: The sweetener sucralose, a chloride derivative of sucrose, is absorbed at a level only 11% to 27% of intake and most of it is excreted, unmetabolized, in feces.

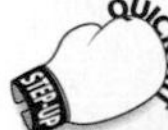

QUICK HIT: Posterior duodenal ulcers are associated with erosion of the gastroduodenal artery and subsequent hemorrhage.

TABLE 5-4 Common Clinical Disorders of the Small Intestine, Large Intestine, and Rectum

Disorder	Etiology and Pathology	Clinical Features	Notes
Hiatal hernia	Saclike herniation of stomach through diaphragm; smoking; obesity	Retrosternal pain (worse in supine position); can lead to **GERD**	Usually occurs in the sliding (versus rolling) form
Duodenal ulcers	***H. pylori*** (in 90% of cases); hypersecretion of acid; smokers; Zollinger–Ellison syndrome; blood group O; associated with NSAID use	Coffee-ground vomitus; **smooth border;** clean base; black stools; pain at night or 2 h postprandial; perforation may result in acute pancreatitis	Not precancerous
Ischemic bowel disease	Atherosclerosis of celiac artery or mesenteric artery	Abdominal pain; nausea; vomiting; stool positive for blood test	Usually affects water-shed areas (splenic flexure or rectosigmoid junction)
Diverticulitis	Outpouchings of the colon obstructed with fecalith leading to inflammation or infection; low-fiber diet	Usually involves the **sigmoid colon;** fever; leukocytosis; colicky pain; usually multiple in number and causes increased risk of perforation	False diverticula: pockets of mucosa and submucosa herniated through muscular layer (not all layers)
Appendicitis	Obstruction (usually fecalith or lymphoid hyperplasia); bacterial proliferation and mucosal invasion	Nausea; vomiting; anorexia; abdominal pain that migrates from epigastrium to right lower quadrant; pain at **McBurney point;** psoas sign or obturator sign; increased WBCs in blood	Differential diagnosis in females includes ectopic pregnancy, ovarian torsion, ruptured ovarian cyst, and pelvic inflammatory disease
Adenocarcinoma	Chronic IBD; low-fiber diet; older age; hereditary polyposis or adenomatous disorders	**Increased CEA** (not diagnostic, used to assess treatment); rectosigmoid tumors present in an **annular manner** producing early obstruction and constipation; **left-sided tumors present with blood in the stool, whereas right-sided tumors typically present with anemia as a result of occult blood loss**	Screen for occult blood in stool and flexible sigmoidoscopy; screening colonoscopy with a positive family history; third most common cause of cancer death (after lung and prostate/breast)
Carcinoid tumor	Arises from **neuroendocrine cells** (Kulchitsky cells); releases vasoactive peptides such as histamine, serotonin, and prostaglandins	**Increased 5-HIAA in urine;** diarrhea; **flushing;** right-sided heart valve lesions; hypotension; bronchospasm	Most common tumor of the appendix, but also found in the ileum, rectum, and bronchus

CEA, carcinoembryonic antigen; 5-HIAA, 5-hydroxyindoleacetic acid; NSAID, nonsteroidal anti-inflammatory drug; WBC, white blood cell.

QUICK HIT

Helicobacter pylori infection is pharmacologically treated with **"triple therapy."** The therapeutic regimen typically includes a proton pump inhibitor (omeprazole) and two of the following antibiotics: clarithromycin, amoxicillin, and metronidazole.

MNEMONIC

To quickly remember the pH changes associated with GI losses, think with vomiting, both the pH and food come up. With diarrhea, both the pH and food go down.

Altered intestinal motility, in which there is an alteration of the normally coordinated control of intestinal propulsion, may also result in diarrhea (often alternating with constipation). Finally, sloughing of colonic mucosa, caused by inflammation and necrosis, often as a result of infection, causes an **exudative form of diarrhea.**

- **Bacterial Causes of Diarrhea** (Table 5-5)
- **Viral Causes of Diarrhea** (Table 5-6)
- **Protozoal Causes of Diarrhea** (Table 5-7)
- **Inflammatory Bowel Conditions** (Table 5-8)

It is speculated that the pathogenesis of inflammatory bowel disease (IBD) is related to the activation of the immune system and the consequent release of cytokines and inflammatory mediators. The cause of IBD has yet to be discovered; however, there is some suggestion of a genetic component.

(text continues on page 148)

TABLE 5-5 Bacterial Causes of Diarrhea

Infectious Agent	Clinical Features	Treatment	Notes
Shigella	**Shiga-toxin** causes **bloody** diarrhea, mild to severe, 1–2 weeks in duration; fever for 3–4 days; lactose (–)	Bismuth, ampicillin, ciprofloxacin, or trimethoprim-sulfamethoxazole	Fecal leukocytes and stool culture necessary for diagnosis
Salmonella	**Bloody** diarrhea; fever; cramps; nausea; motile; lactose (–)	Supportive therapy only; no opiates; tetracycline may be used if needed, symptoms may be prolonged with antibiotics	Commonly acquired from **eggs, poultry, or turtles;** dia gnosis based on stool culture; increased susceptibility in immun ocompromised patients
Campylobacter jejuni	**Bloody** diarrhea; fever; crampy abdominal pain; self-limited, but may persist for 3–4 weeks	Supportive therapy or possibly erythromycin	**Leading cause of food-borne diarrhea** in United States, comma shaped, oxidase (+)
Vibrio cholerae	**Watery** diarrhea **(rice-water stools),** vomiting, and dehydration occur after 12–48 h of incubation	Supportive therapy only; no opiates	Caused by **toxin;** most often occurs in underdeveloped nations; commonly associated with consumption of raw oysters; comma shaped
Clostridium difficile	**Watery** diarrhea caused by antibiotic-induced suppression of normal colonic flora and *C. difficile* overgrowth; **pseudomembranes** on the colonic mucosa	Metronidazole, oral vancomycin	Exotoxin-mediated; termed pseudomembranous colitis because of the false membranes created on the colon by the bacterial infection
Enterotoxigenic *Escherichia coli* (traveler's diarrhea)	**Watery** diarrhea; 3–6 days' duration; occasional fever and vomiting	Bismuth, trimethoprim-sulfamethoxazole, doxycycline, and ciprofloxacin	Antibiotics reduce duration of infection to 1–2 days
Enterohemorrhagic *E. coli* (O157:H7)	**Shiga-like toxin** causes **bloody** diarrhea	Supportive therapy	Typically, food-borne transmission (e.g., **uncooked hamburger**); diagnosis made by stool culture
Yersinia enterocolitica	**Bloody** diarrhea; fever; cramps; nausea	Supportive therapy only; no opiates	Transmitted by food or contaminated domestic animal feces; clinically indistinguishable from *Salmonella* and *Shigella*

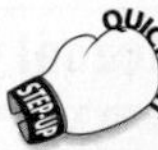

Duodenal versus gastric ulcer: In duodenal ulcers, pain *decreases after meals/antacids* whereas in gastric ulcers, *pain persists after meals/antacids.* Also, duodenal ulcers are associated with *increased acid production* whereas patients with gastric ulcers have *decreased to normal acid production.* Finally, although all gastric ulcers should be biopsied to rule out gastric *carcinoma,* duodenal ulcers require no such intervention.

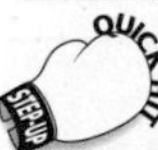

Small-bowel obstructions are usually caused by adhesions, whereas large-bowel obstructions are most commonly a result of neoplasms. Ileus, a common cause of temporary small-bowel paralysis, commonly occurs postoperatively.

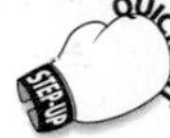

Diverticulosis, the most common cause of bleeding from the lower GI tract, can be differentiated from diverticulitis because diverticulitis typically does not cause bleeding but is painful, whereas diverticulosis does cause bleeding but is typically painless.

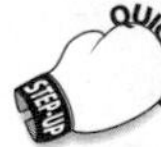

Salmonella requires at least 100,000 organisms to be infectious; *Shigella*, however, requires only 100.

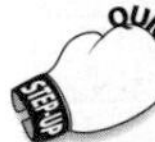

Norwalk virus, in contrast to most viruses transmitted via the fecal-oral route, is uncommon in children.

TABLE 5-6 Viral Causes of Diarrhea

Infectious Agent	Clinical Features	Treatment	Notes
Rotavirus	Severe, dehydrating diarrhea; vomiting; low-grade fever	Supportive therapy only	**Most common cause of diarrhea in infants;** usually occurs during **winter** months
Norwalk virus	Mild diarrhea and vomiting	Supportive therapy only	Epidemics in underdeveloped countries; **affects older children and adults**
Adenovirus (serotypes 40 and 41)	Diarrhea and moderate vomiting	Supportive therapy only	Second to rotavirus as the cause of gastroenteritis in children

TABLE 5-7 Protozoal Causes of Diarrhea

Infectious Agent	Clinical Features	Treatment	Notes
Entamoeba histolytica	**Bloody** diarrhea; lower abdominal pain; may lead to dysentery with 10–12 bloody and mucous stools per day	Metronidazole	Caused by ingestion of viable cysts via fecal-oral route
Giardia lamblia	**Watery,** foul-smelling diarrhea; nausea; anorexia; cramps lasting weeks to months	Metronidazole	Fecal-oral transmission; often contracted while **camping**
Cryptosporidium	**Watery** diarrhea with large fluid loss; symptoms persist in immunocompromised patients; self-limited in healthy individuals	Supportive therapy	Immunocompromised patients (especially **AIDS patients**); fecal-oral transmission of oocysts

TABLE 5-8 Comparison of Inflammatory Bowel Conditions

	Crohn Disease	Ulcerative Colitis
Typical patient	• Young person of Jewish descent • Bimodal age distribution: 25–40 years of age and 50–65 years of age • Female > male	• Person of Jewish descent • Recently quit smoking • Bimodal age distribution: 20–35 years of age and 65+ years of age • Male > female
Clinical findings	• Diarrhea • Abdominal pain • Fever • Malabsorption • Obstruction	• Bloody, mucous diarrhea • Abdominal pain • Fever • Weight loss • Toxic megacolon
Location	• Small intestine • Colon • "Mouth to anus"	• Colon • Rectum
Histologic findings	• Full-thickness inflammation • **Granulomas**	• Mucosal inflammation • **Crypt abscesses**
Gross findings	• **Cobblestone appearance** • Wall thickening with narrowed lumen • **Skipped areas** • **Fistulas**	• Pseudopolyps • Widened lumen • Toxic megacolon
Diagnostic evaluation	• Colonoscopy • Barium enema • Upper GI series with small-bowel follow-through	• Colonoscopy • Barium enema • Upper GI series with small-bowel follow-through
Risk of malignancy	• Small increase	• Large increase
Associated systemic manifestations	• Arthritis • Eye lesions • Erythema nodosum • Pyoderma gangrenosum • Aphthous ulcers (chancre sores)	• Arthritis • Eye lesions • Erythema nodosum • Pyoderma gangrenosum • Sclerosing cholangitis
Medical treatment	• Sulfasalazine • Steroids • Metronidazole	• Sulfasalazine • Steroids • Metronidazole
Indications for surgery	• Obstruction • Massive bleeding • Perforation • Refractory to medical treatment • Cancer • Toxic megacolon	• Toxic megacolon • Cancer • Massive bleeding • Failure to mature • Refractory to medical treatment

Clinical Vignette 5-2

Clinical Presentation: A 21-year-old female presents to the emergency department with **right lower quadrant pain** of several hours' duration. She reports that the **pain began in the epigastrium** and has since moved to the right lower quadrant. Since the onset of the pain, she reports **no appetite and nausea.** She is otherwise a healthy young female. Physical examination reveals **tenderness at McBurney point.** No peritoneal signs, psoas sign, or obturator sign. Rectal examination gives a negative result. T = 100.3 °F; BP = 120/80 mm Hg; HR = 95 bpm; and RR = 20 breaths/min.

Differentials: Appendicitis, mittelschmerz, ovarian cyst rupture, pelvic inflammatory disease, ectopic pregnancy, kidney stones, and Meckel diverticulum. The shift in pain described above is classic for appendicitis. Also, anorexia, nausea, and vomiting beginning after the onset of pain are typical for appendicitis. Further, gynecologic history is needed on this patient to determine if midcycle pain associated with ovulation (mittelschmerz) was occurring. Also, a pelvic examination is indicated in this patient to further determine the pelvic pathology.

Laboratory Studies: If this were a young male, the history and physical examination would be sufficient to indicate surgery for appendicitis. In a young female, however, there is a longer differential list and a **computerized tomography (CT) scan** would be helpful in determining the cause of the pain. A **complete blood count (CBC)** often shows a mildly elevated white blood cell (WBC) count, but this is not a consistent finding. A **human chorionic gonadotropin (hCG) pregnancy test** and **pelvic ultrasound** should also be performed on this patient to rule out pelvic pathology.

Management: Laparoscopic or open appendectomy should be performed emergently because of the risk of rupture.

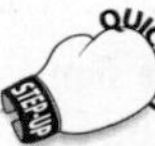

Vibrio cholerae produces an exotoxin that activates adenylate cyclase in the crypt cells. The increase in cyclic adenosine monophosphate (cAMP) activates Cl^- secretory channels. Consequently, sodium and water accompany Cl^- into the lumen, which results in an osmotic diarrhea.

MNEMONIC

Remember the causes of constipation by the three Cs: **C**ancer/**C**rohn/ulcerative **C**olitis. Also, recall **DOPED:**

- **D**iverticulosis
- **O**piates
- **P**ain
- **E**ndocrine (hypothyroid)
- **D**epression

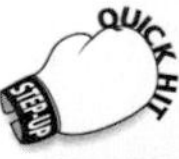

The *Giardia trophozoite* has a very characteristic appearance. It is pear shaped with four pairs of flagella and two nuclei that resemble eyes.

MNEMONIC

Left-sided valvular lesions are not observed in carcinoid syndrome because the lung metabolizes serotonin (5-HT). Remember the symptoms of **CARC**inoid syndrome as **C**utaneous flushing, **A**sthmatic wheezing, **R**ight-sided valvular lesions, and **C**ramping diarrhea.

Clinical Vignette 5-3

Clinical Presentation: A 54-year-old female presents to the emergency department with **severe abdominal pain** of 36 h-duration. Her past medical history is significant for **CAD, hypertension (HTN), and diabetes.** Physical examination reveals a **soft, nondistended, nontender abdomen** with **normal bowel sounds** and no palpable masses. T = 98.9 °F; BP = 140/90 mm Hg; HR = 99 bpm; and RR = 21 breaths/min.

Differentials: Acute mesenteric ischemia, appendicitis, diverticulitis, colon adenocarcinoma, IBD, and pseudomembranous colitis. Pain disproportionate to the physical findings is strongly suggestive of mesenteric ischemia. As the ischemia progresses, peritonitis, sepsis, and shock may occur.

Laboratory Studies: Mesenteric angiogram is the definitive diagnostic test for mesenteric ischemia. **Plain abdominal radiographs** are obtained to rule out other causes of acute abdominal pain. **Abdominal radiographs with barium enema** often show "thumbprinting" as a result of thickened edematous mucosal folds.

Management: Supportive therapy with intravenous (IV) fluids and broad-spectrum antibiotics should be started. Further treatment depends on the cause of the ischemia. Given the history of CAD in this patient, this is most likely **thrombotic** in nature and direct **intra-arterial injection of papaverine** (a vasodilator) into the superior mesenteric system during arteriography will relieve the occlusion and vasospasm. An **embolic** occlusion indicates direct **intra-arterial infusion of thrombolytics or embolectomy.** If it is a **venous thrombosis, heparin anticoagulation** should be started. If signs of peritonitis develop, the **nonviable bowel should be resected.**

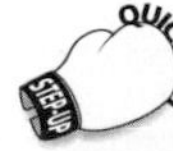

The shift of pain that is observed classically in appendicitis occurs because the visceral peritoneum is irritated first, which produces diffuse sensation of pain. As the appendicitis progresses, the parietal peritoneum becomes inflamed, resulting in a more localized sensation of pain in the right lower quadrant.

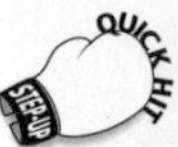

A **positive psoas sign** elicited by pain on extension of the leg indicates retroperitoneal inflammation and suggests the appendix is located behind the cecum retroperitoneally. A **positive obturator sign** elicited by pain on abduction/adduction at the hip joint of a leg flexed at the knee suggests the appendix is located in the pelvic region; a pelvic appendix can also be palpated on rectal examination.

Clinical Vignette 5-4

Clinical Presentation: A 6-year-old boy presents to the emergency department with multiple episodes of **nausea and vomiting** of 2 days' duration, and today his **"stomach hurts."** The worried mother reports finding the Tylenol bottle half empty this morning. On physical examination, the patient is **jaundiced** and diaphoretic, with **right upper quadrant (RUQ) tenderness.** *T* = 98.6 °F; BP = 110/70 mm Hg; HR = 103 bpm; and RR = 22 breaths/min.

Differentials: Acetaminophen-induced liver toxicity and gastroenteritis. The chemical structure of acetaminophen is *N*-acetyl-*p*-aminophenol (APAP). APAP itself is nontoxic but it is metabolized primarily in the liver by cytochrome P450 to a toxic metabolite, *N*-acetyl-*p*-benzoquinoneimine (NAPQI). Glutathione can bind NAPQI and lead to the excretion of nontoxic mercapturate conjugates in the urine. As the glutathione stores are diminished, NAPQI accumulates and covalently binds to the hepatocyte lipid bilayer, causing centrilobular necrosis. Inducers of cytochrome P450, such as ethanol, isoniazid, rifampin, phenytoin, barbiturates, and carbamazepine, can lead to an increased production of NAPQI.

Laboratory Studies: Elevated **serum APAP levels** and **transaminase levels** greater than 1,000 U/L support the diagnosis of APAP hepatotoxicity. **Coagulation studies** should also be obtained to monitor the liver function.

Management: Glutathione stores can be replaced orally or intravenously by sulfhydryl-containing compounds like ***N*-acetylcysteine.** *N*-acetylcysteine also directly detoxifies NAPQI to nontoxic metabolites by acting as a substrate for sulfation. In addition to *N*-acetylcysteine, if the patient presents within hours of the incident, **gastric lavage** and **oral charcoal** could also be performed.

MALABSORPTION SYNDROMES OF THE SMALL INTESTINE (Table 5-9)

Malabsorption may produce a variety of symptoms ranging from diarrhea to steatorrhea to specific nutrient deficiencies. For example, iron, vitamin B_{12}, fat-soluble vitamins (A, D, E, and K), or protein may be poorly absorbed and lead to systemic manifestations.

TABLE 5-9 Malabsorption Syndromes of the Small Intestine

Syndrome	Pathology	Clinical Features	Notes
Abetalipoproteinemia	Lack of apoprotein B; defective chylomicron assembly; enterocytes congested with lipid	Acanthocytes ("burr" cells) in blood; **no chylomicrons, VLDL, or LDL in blood**	Autosomal recessive
Celiac disease (nontropical sprue)	Gluten sensitivity	Foul-smelling, pale stool; **villi of small intestine blunted;** stunted growth; symptoms disappear when gluten is removed from diet	Associated with HLA-B8 and DQW2; predisposes to T-cell lymphoma and GI and breast cancer; if unmanaged, causes vitamin deficiency resulting in skeletal, hematological, and neurological symptoms

(continued)

TABLE 5-9 Malabsorption Syndromes of the Small Intestine *(Continued)*

Syndrome	Pathology	Clinical Features	Notes
Disaccharidase deficiency	Enzyme deficiency; bacterial digestion of unabsorbed disaccharide	Diarrhea; bloating	Most commonly lactase deficiency
Tropical sprue	Etiology unclear	Affects small intestine; may cause vitamin deficiencies and megaloblastic anemia	Possible infectious cause, does not improve with gluten removal
Whipple disease	Systemic disease caused by *Tropheryma whippelii*	Diarrhea; weight loss; lymphadenopathy; hyperpigmentation; **macrophages laden with *T. whippelii***	Older white males
Bacterial overgrowth	Bacterial overpopulation of small intestine owing to stasis, raised pH, impaired immunity, or **clindamycin** or **ampicillin** therapy	Inflammatory infiltrate in bowel wall	Treat with antibiotics, metroidazole or vancomycin

GI, gastrointestinal; HLA-B8, human leukocyte antigen-B8; LDL, low-density lipoprotein; VLDL, very-low-density lipoprotein.

NEOPLASTIC POLYPS (Table 5-10)

GI polyps can be very diverse in their presentation. Individuals can be asymptomatic, as is usually the case with tubular adenomas, or can present with serious systemic manifestations such as anemia secondary to invasive cancer.

- **Comparison of Polyposis Conditions** (Table 5-11)

TABLE 5-10 Neoplastic Polyps

Tubular Adenoma	Tubulovillous Adenoma	Villous Adenoma
• Usually **benign**	• Greater potential of malignancy than tubular adenoma	• Highly **malignant**
• Multiple	• Morphologically, shares features of both tubular and villous adenomas	• **Sessile** tumors • Fingerlike projections
• **Pedunculated** tumors • Greater chance of malignancy if genetically predisposed • Most common polyp		

TABLE 5-11 Comparison of Polyposis Conditions

Disease	Inheritance	Clinical Features
Familial adenomatous polyposis	Autosomal dominant	Colon lined with hundreds of polyps; potential for malignancy approaches 100%
Turcot syndrome	Autosomal dominant	Colonic polyps and **central nervous system (CNS) tumors;** potential for malignancy approaches 100%
Gardner syndrome	Autosomal dominant	Colonic polyps; soft-tissue and **bone tumors;** potential for malignancy approaches 100%
Peutz–Jeghers syndrome	Autosomal dominant	Benign hamartomatous polyps of the gastrointestinal tract (especially the small intestine); **hyperpigmented mouth, hands, and genitalia;** increased incidence of tumors of the uterus, breast, ovaries, lung, stomach, and pancreas; no malignant potential
Familial nonpolyposis syndrome	Autosomal dominant	**Defect in DNA repair** causing large number of colonic lesions (especially proximal); potential for malignancy approaches 50%

MNEMONIC

Remember the drugs that cause hepatic necrosis by the phrase "**V**ery **A**ngry **H**epatocytes": **V**alproic acid, **A**cetaminophen, and **H**alothane.

THE HEPATOBILIARY SYSTEM

I. Microscopic organization of the liver (Figure 5-7)

FIGURE 5-7 Microscopic organization of the liver

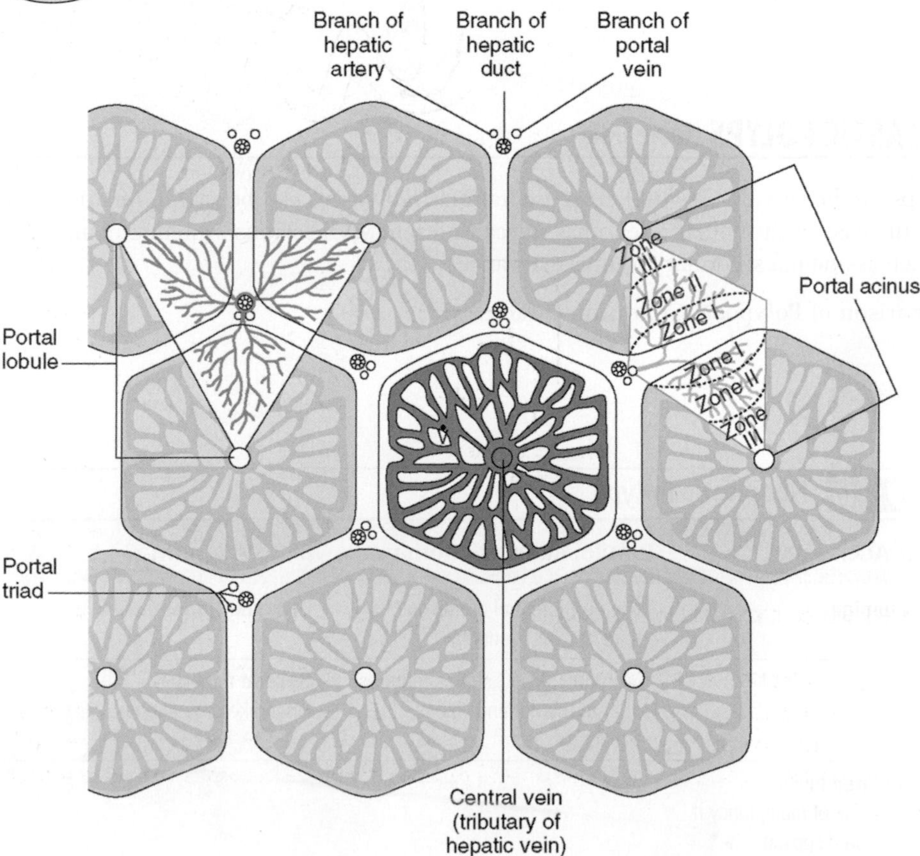

II. Enterohepatic cycling and the excretion of bilirubin (Figure 5-8)

FIGURE 5-8 Enterohepatic cycling and the excretion of bilirubin

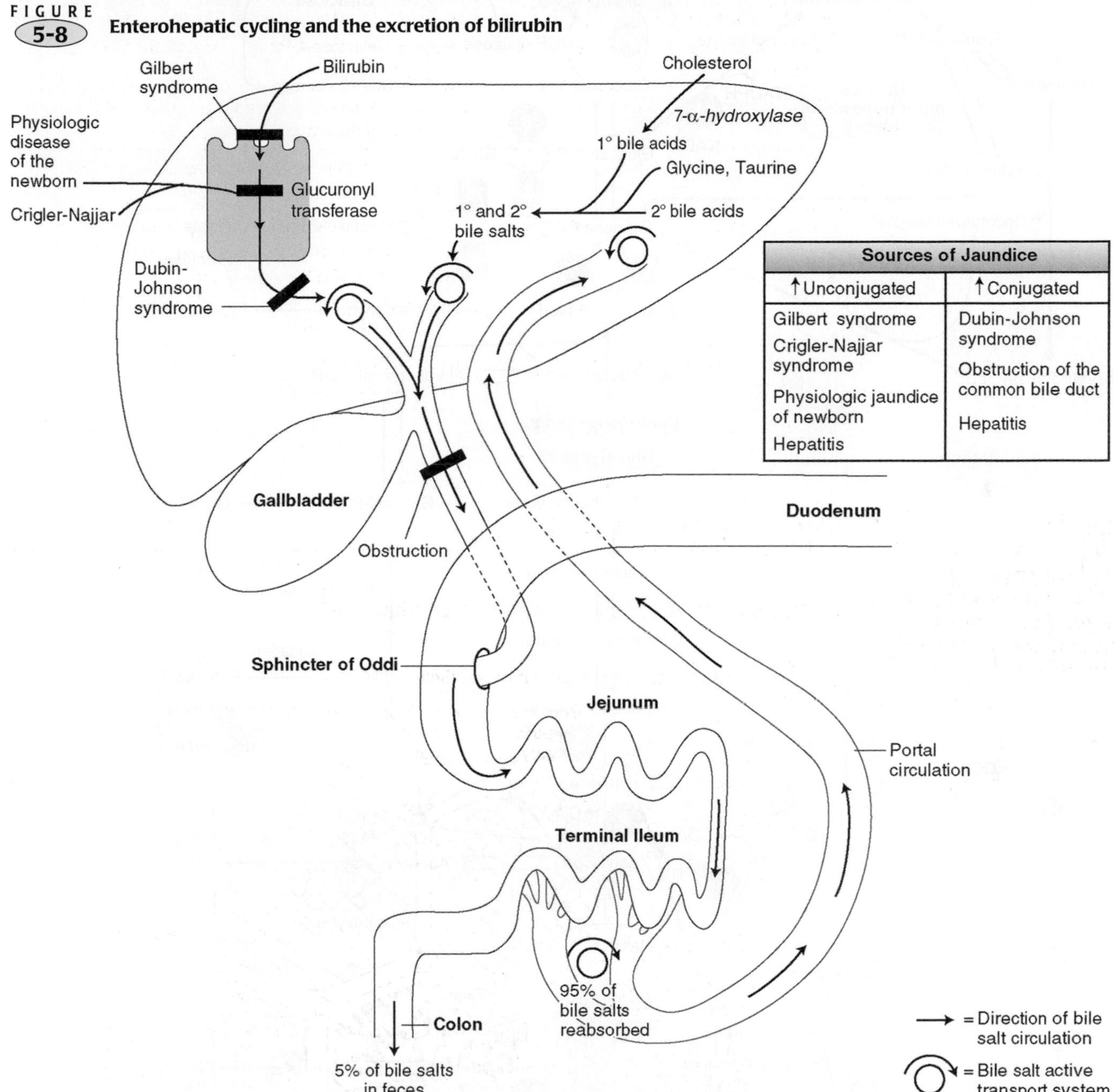

Sources of Jaundice	
↑Unconjugated	↑Conjugated
Gilbert syndrome	Dubin-Johnson syndrome
Crigler-Najjar syndrome	Obstruction of the common bile duct
Physiologic jaundice of newborn	Hepatitis
Hepatitis	

III. Important biochemical pathways of the liver and digestion (Figure 5-9)

IV. Glycolysis versus gluconeogenesis versus glycogenolysis (Table 5-12)

As food is absorbed, the **glycolysis** pathway is activated and energy is stored as glycogen in the liver. **Glycogenolysis** provides food for the periods between regular meals. After 30 h of fasting, glycogen is completely depleted and **gluconeogenesis** becomes the only source of blood glucose.

FIGURE 5-9 **Important biochemical pathways of the liver and digestion**

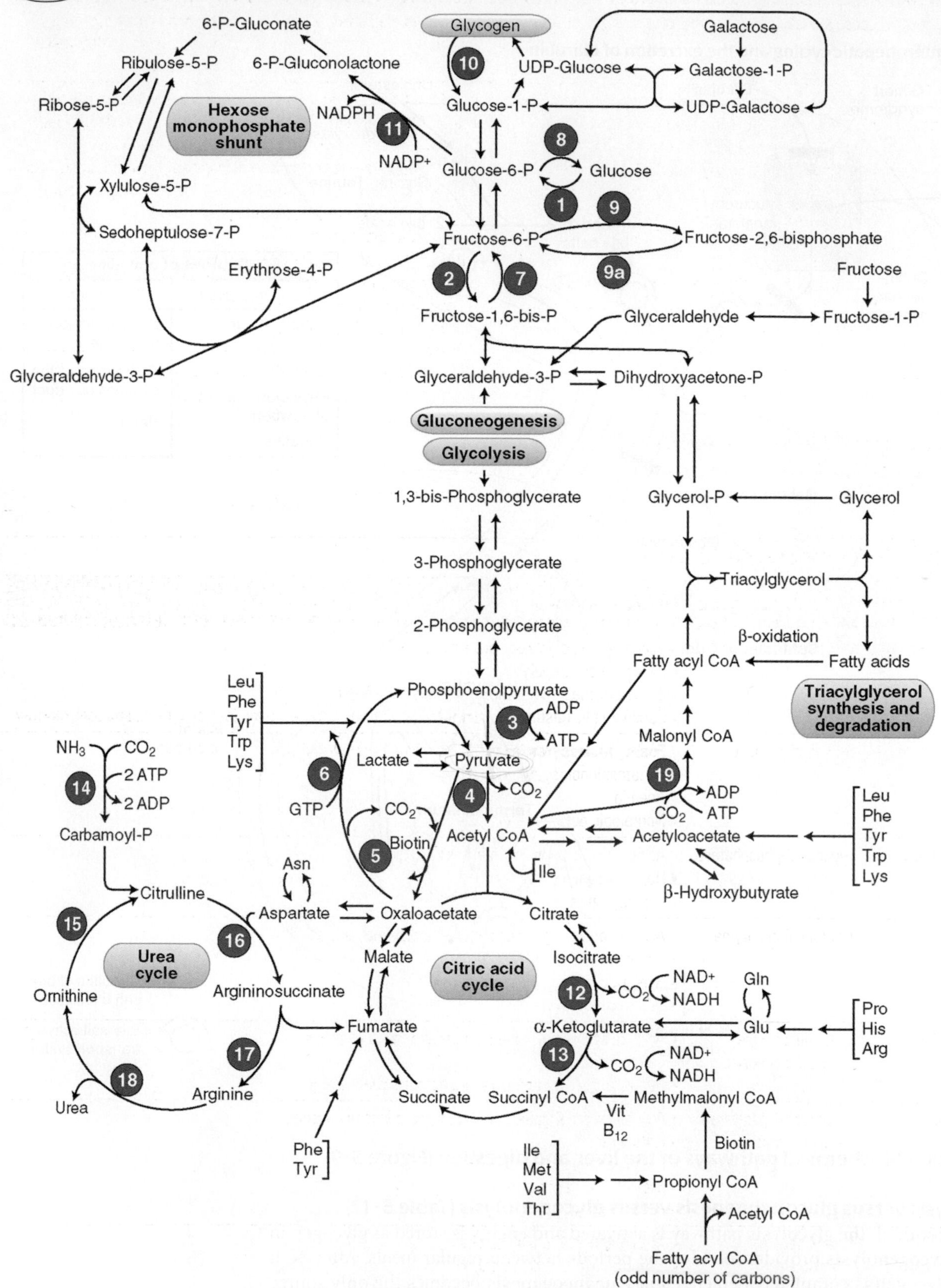

THE GASTROINTESTINAL SYSTEM

TABLE 5-12 Glycolysis versus Gluconeogenesis versus Glycogenolysis

	Glycolysis	Gluconeogenesis	Glycogenolysis
Description of the process	Glucose is broken down to form pyruvate and energy is released	Glucose is formed after 4–6 h of fasting	**Glucose** is produced from glycogen stores after **2–3 h of fasting**
Key enzymes and their regulation	Glucokinase (in liver), hexokinase (all tissues); requires ATP; (–) glucose-6-P; see enzyme 1, Figure 5-9 Phosphofructokinase-1 (PFK-1); requires ATP; **rate-limiting step in glycolysis;** (+) AMP, fructose-2-6-bis-P; (–) ATP, citrate; see enzyme 2, Figure 5-9 Pyruvate kinase; produces ATP; (+) fructose-1-6-bis-P; (–) alanine, phosphorylation, ATP; see enzyme 3, Figure 5-9 Pyruvate dehydrogenase; (+) pyruvate, insulin, ADP; (–) NADH, acetyl CoA, phosphorylation; see enzyme 4, Figure 5-9	Pyruvate carboxylase; requires **biotin, CO_2, and ATP;** (+) acetyl CoA; see enzyme 5, Figure 5-9 Phosphoenolpyruvate carboxykinase (PEPCK); requires GTP; (+) cortisol, glucagon; see enzyme 6, Figure 5-9 Fructose-1-6-bisphosphatase; (+) glucagon; (–) AMP, fructose-2-6-bis-P; see enzyme 7, Figure 5-9 Glucose-6-phosphatase; (+) glucagon; see enzyme 8, Figure 5-9	Glycogen phosphorylase; (+) AMP, phosphorylation; see enzyme 10, Figure 5-9 Phosphoglucomutase converts glucose-1-P to glucose-6-P

ADP, adenosine triphosphate; AMP, adenosine monophosphate; ATP, adenosine triphosphate; CoA, coenzyme A; CO_2, carbon dioxide; GTP, guanosine triphosphate; NADH, reduced nicotinamide adenine dinucleotide; P, phosphate.

V. Defective enzyme diseases (Table 5-13)

With a few exceptions, most defective enzyme diseases are autosomal recessive. Since the liver contains a high proportion of metabolic enzymes, it is often affected by these diseases.

TABLE 5-13 Defective Enzyme Diseases

Disease	Defective Enzyme	Clinical Features
Gaucher disease	Glucocerebrosidase	• Accumulation of **glucocerebroside** • Hepatosplenomegaly • Erosion of the head of the long bones (e.g., femur) • Gaucher cells (distinctive, **wrinkled paper** appearance) found in liver, spleen, and bone marrow
Niemann–Pick disease	Sphingomyelinase	• **Foamy histiocytes** in liver, spleen, lymph nodes, and skin • Hepatosplenomegaly • Anemia • Neurologic deterioration
von Gierke disease	Glucose-6-phosphatase	• Accumulation of glycogen in liver and kidney • Hepatomegaly • Hypoglycemia
Cori disease	Debranching enzyme	• Accumulation of glycogen in liver and striated muscle • Hepatomegaly • Hypoglycemia • Failure to grow
Pompe disease	α_1,4-Glucosidase (lysosomal enzyme)	• Accumulation of glycogen in liver and striated muscle • Cardiomegaly • Death caused by cardiac failure before 3 years of age
Galactosemia	Galactose-1-phosphate uridylyl transferase	• Accumulation of galactose-1-phosphate in many tissues • **Cataracts** • Cirrhosis • Mental retardation • Failure to thrive
Phenylketonuria	Phenylalanine hydroxylase	• Accumulation of phenylalanine • Cerebral myelin degeneration • **Mental retardation**
Maple syrup urine disease	Branched-chain α-ketoacid dehydrogenase	• Inability to metabolize leucine, isoleucine, and valine • Neurologic symptoms • High mortality

QUICK HIT

McArdle disease is a glycogen-storage disease similar to von Gierke, Pompe, and Cori diseases but has no GI manifestations. It is a deficiency of muscle glycogen phosphorylase with consequent accumulation of glycogen in skeletal muscle.

MNEMONIC

To remember that hepatitis A and E are transmitted by the fecal-oral route, think of the phrase **"vowels are bowels."**

VI. Viral hepatitis (Table 5-14 and Figure 5-10)

Viral hepatitis can lead to **direct hyperbilirubinemia**, elevated serum transaminases, icterus, or hepatomegaly but not ascites. Morphologically, changes range from multifocal hepatocellular necrosis (hepatitis A and hepatitis B) to ballooning degeneration (hepatitis B and hepatitis C) to piecemeal necrosis (hepatitis C).

TABLE 5-14 Viral Hepatitis

	Hepatitis A	Hepatitis B	Hepatitis C	Hepatitis D	Hepatitis E
Virus family	Picornavirus	Hepadnavirus	Flavivirus	Delta agent	Calicivirus
Viral morphology	Single-stranded RNA	Circular, double-stranded DNA	Single-stranded RNA	Incomplete genome of single-stranded RNA	Single-stranded RNA
Mode of transmission	Fecal-oral	Sexual and parenteral, transplacental	Parenteral; limited sexual; transplacental	Sexual and parenteral, transplacental	Fecal-oral
Diagnostic test	IgM anti-HAV	HBsAg; anti-HBsAg; HBeAg; HBV DNA; IgM anti-HBcAg	Anti-HCV	Anti-Δag	None
Severity	Mild	Moderate	Mild	Severe	Mild
Chronic infection	No	10% of adults, 80%–90% of infants, and immunocompromised patients	80%–90%	No increase over hepatitis B alone	No
Carrier state	No	Yes	Yes	Yes	No
Hepatocellular carcinoma	No	Yes	Yes	No	No
Prophylaxis and treatment	Immune globulin; vaccine	Hepatitis B immune globulin; vaccine Interferon and nucleoside analog inhibitors of viral DNA synthesis	Interferon and ribavirin	Hepatitis B immune globulin; vaccine	None
Notes	Incubation period of 14–15 days	**Dane particle:** viral DNA genome, DNA polymerase, HBcAg, HBeAg, HBsAg; HAS **reverse transcriptase;** incubation period 60–90 days	**Most frequent cause of transfusion-mediated hepatitis**	Defective in replication; **requires coinfection with hepatitis B**	Hepatitis infection in Third World nations; mortality in pregnant females

Ag, antigen; HAV, hepatitis A virus; HBcAg, hepatitis B core antigen; HBeAg, hepatitis B envelope antigen; HBsAg, hepatitis B surface antigen; HBV, hepatitis B virus; HCV, hepatitis C virus.

FIGURE 5-10 **Hepatitis B serology and interpretation of hepatitis B panel**

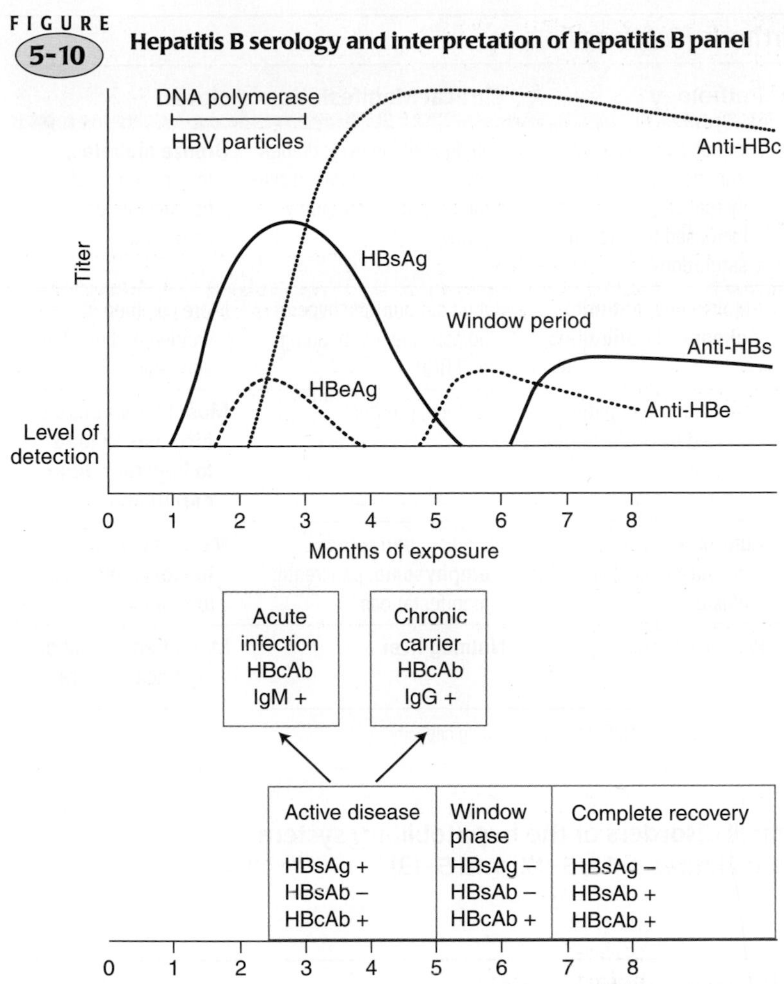

QUICK HIT: Hepatitis B viral DNA, hepatitis B surface antigen (HBsAg), and hepatitis B envelope antigen (HBeAg) are indicators of virus replication. Antibody to hepatitis B surface antigen (HBsAb) is indicative of recovery and immunity. HBsAb is also positive following vaccination. Antibody to hepatitis B core antigen (HBcAb) is positive in early infection; in addition, HBcAb acts as a marker for hepatitis infection during the "window" period, which is the period during acute infection when HBsAg is undetectable and HBsAb has not yet appeared. During the window period, equivalent amounts of surface antigen and antibody neutralize each other and, thus, are not detectable by testing.

VII. Cirrhosis (Table 5-15)

Cirrhosis is a disease of the liver characterized by fibrosis and disorganization of the lobular and vascular structure owing to the destruction and regeneration of hepatocytes.

TABLE 5-15 Cirrhosis

Etiology	Pathology	Clinical Manifestation	Notes
Chronic alcohol abuse	**Micronodular** fatty liver; decreased metabolism of estrogen; decreased synthesis of coagulation factors	**Jaundice;** bleeding; gynecomastia; testicular atrophy; edema; **asterixis;** portal HTN (**esophageal varices,** spider angiomata, and splenomegaly); encephalopathy	**Most common cause of cirrhosis in the United States**
Wilson disease	**Decreased ceruloplasmin**	Copper deposits in liver, basal ganglia (causing extrapyramidal signs), and Descemet membrane of cornea **(Kayser–Fleischer ring)**	Autosomal recessive

(continued)

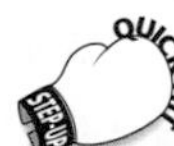

QUICK HIT: Cirrhosis often leads to **portal hypertension.** There are three major collateral circulation pathways that allow blood to return to the heart: (a) left gastric to esophageal plexus to azygous to the superior vena cava (SVC) **(esophageal varices);** (b) inferior mesenteric to superior rectal to inferior rectal to inferior vena cava (IVC) **(hemorrhoids);** and (c) ligamentum teres to superficial abdominals to SVC or IVC **(caput medusae).**

TABLE 5-15 Cirrhosis *(Continued)*

Etiology	Pathology	Clinical Manifestation	Notes
Hemochromatosis	Familial; increased total iron; decreased TIBC; increased ferritin; increased transferrin saturation	Iron deposits in liver; diabetes mellitus; increased skin pigmentation; cardiomyopathy	**Bronze diabetes;** increased risk of hepatocellular carcinoma
Primary biliary cirrhosis	Autoimmune; **antimitochondrial antibodies**	Jaundice; pruritus; hypercholesterolemia, beading on ERCP	More common in women and middle-age people
Posthepatitic cirrhosis	Chronic active hepatitis caused by HBV and HCV infection	Jaundice; pruritus	**Most likely cause of cirrhosis to lead to hepatocellular carcinoma**
α_1-Antitrypsin deficiency	Autosomal recessive; decreased inactivation of elastase	Jaundice; **panacinar emphysema;** pancreatic manifestations	**More severe in homozygous form** (piZZ alleles)
Congestive heart failure	Passive congestion	**Nutmeg liver**	Most often a result of right-heart failure

HBV, hepatitis B virus; HCV, hepatitis C virus; TIBC, total iron-binding capacity.

QUICK HIT: Hepatobiliary diseases vary in their presentation and etiology. Cholelithiasis is very common and curable with surgery whereas hepatocellular carcinoma is much less common but usually fatal.

QUICK HIT: Metastatic disease is the most common source of malignancy in the liver.

QUICK HIT: Renal cell carcinoma also typically spreads via the **hematogenous route.**

VIII. Common clinical disorders of the hepatobiliary system (Table 5-16 and Figures 5-11, 5-12, and 5-13)

TABLE 5-16 Common Clinical Disorders of the Hepatobiliary System

Disorder	Etiology and Pathology	Clinical Features	Notes
Cholelithiasis (gallstones)	Very common disease; women older than 40 years of age; obesity; multiparity	Steatorrhea; nausea; vomiting; bile duct obstruction; jaundice; may lead to cholangitis or cholecystitis; malignancy; positive Murphy sign	Cholesterol stones (large); pigment stones (seen in hemolytic anemia or excess bilirubin production); mixed stones (majority)
Primary biliary cirrhosis	**Autoimmune** disease leading to the destruction of intrahepatic bile ducts; middle-age women	**Pruritus, jaundice, hypercholesterolemia;** RUQ discomfort; portal HTN	Positive **antimitochondrial antibodies;** associated with other autoimmune diseases
Primary sclerosing cholangitis	Fibrosis and stenosis of intrahepatic or extrahepatic bile ducts	Jaundice; pruritus; weight loss	Strong association with **ulcerative colitis**; increased incidence of cholangiocarcinoma
Hepatocellular adenoma (hepatoma)	Benign tumor; women 20–30 years of age taking **oral contraceptives**	Usually found incidentally; may cause pain or hemorrhage	10% may become malignant; oral contraceptive use should be stopped, lesion regresses with the cessation of contraceptive
Adenocarcinoma of the gallbladder	Gallstones	Obstructive jaundice; enlarged gallbladder	**Courvoisier law:** obstruction of CBD enlarges the gallbladder whereas obstructing stones do not; caused by scarring of the gallbladder
Hepatocellular carcinoma	Cirrhosis; **hepatitis B; hepatitis C;** aflatoxin B (carcinogen in contaminated peanuts)	Increased α-fetoprotein; jaundice; abdominal distention; ascites	**Hematogenous spread**

FIGURE 5-11 **Approach to liver studies**

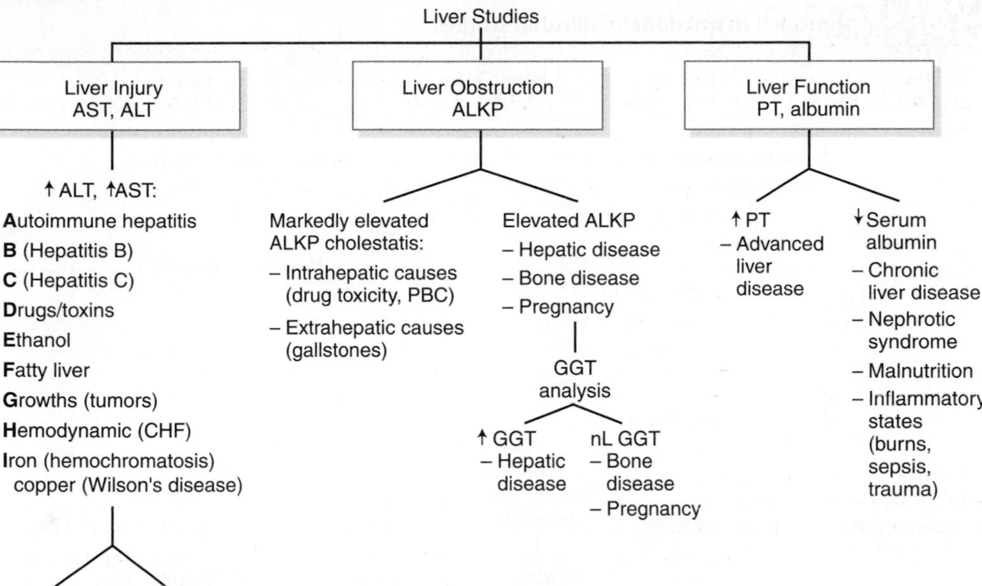

*AST and ALT are produced by hepatocytes; liver necrosis or inflammation leads to release of these enzymes into the circulation.

*AlKP and GGT are produced by cells of the biliary tract; obstruction of the biliary tree results in release of these enzymes into the circulation.

*Liver synthesizes albumin and coagulation factors I, II, V, VII, IX, X, XII, XIII; destruction of 90% liver results in decreased synthetic capacity.

QUICK HIT: Pigment gallstones occurring in children or young adults with no history of pregnancy may be a result of a congenital hemoglobinopathy (e.g., sickle cell disease or thalassemia).

FIGURE 5-12 **Diseases of the gallbladder and biliary tract**

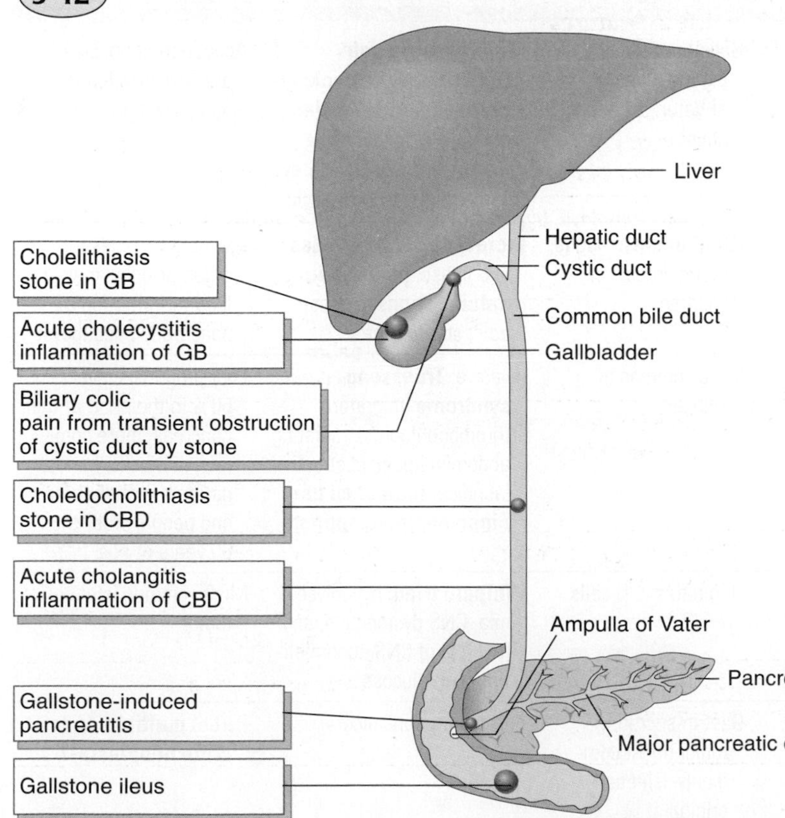

FIGURE 5-13 Approach to fractionate bilirubin studies

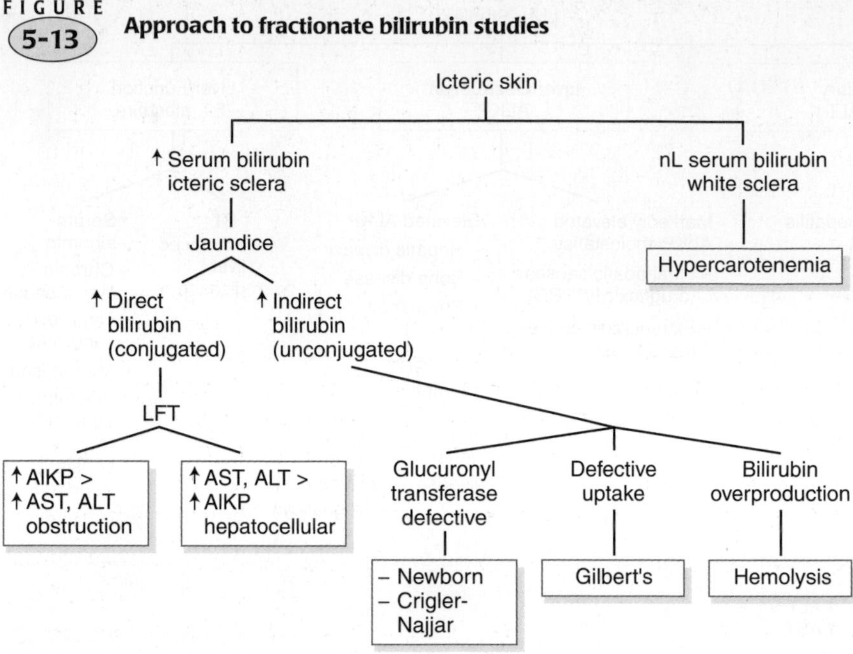

THE PANCREAS

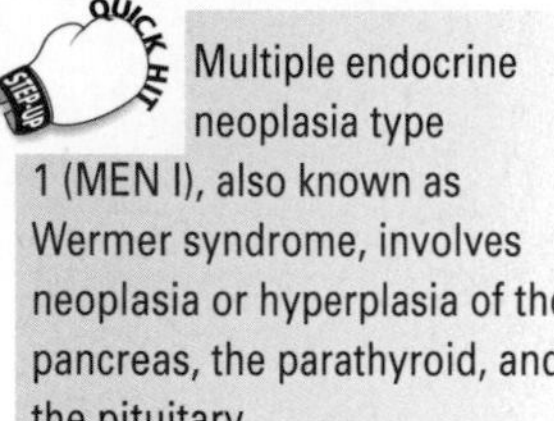

QUICK HIT: The presence of **C-peptide** in the blood distinguishes endogenous insulin secretions (as in an insulinoma) from exogenous insulin administration (as seen in Münchhausen syndrome).

QUICK HIT: Multiple endocrine neoplasia type 1 (MEN I), also known as Wermer syndrome, involves neoplasia or hyperplasia of the pancreas, the parathyroid, and the pituitary.

- Common Clinical Disorders of the Pancreas (Table 5-17)

In the United States, alcohol is the most common cause of pancreatic pathology.

TABLE 5-17 Common Clinical Disorders of the Pancreas

Disorder	Etiology and Pathology	Clinical Features	Notes
Acute pancreatitis	Gallstones (obstructing the ampulla of Vater); alcohol abuse	**Midepigastric pain radiating to the back; increased serum amylase** and lipase; hemorrhage may lead to Cullen or Grey Turner sign; hypocalcemia	Activation of pancreatic enzymes leads to autodigestion
Chronic pancreatitis	**Alcoholism** in adults; cystic fibrosis in children	**Increased serum amylase** and lipase; **pancreatic calcifications;** epigastric pain; steatorrhea	Irreversible; leads to organ atrophy; may lead to formation of pancreatic pseudocyst
Adenocarcinoma of the exocrine pancreas	More common in smokers	Invasive; **Trousseau syndrome** (migratory thrombophlebitis); radiating abdominal pain; obstructive jaundice; **increased carcinoembryonic antigen**	Poor prognosis; over 50% in the head of the pancreas; more common in Blacks, males, patients with diabetes, and people older than 60 years of age
Insulinoma (endocrine pancreas)	Originates in β cells	**Whipple triad:** hypoglycemia, CNS dysfunction, and reversal of CNS abnormalities with glucose	Most common islet cell tumor
Gastrinoma (Zollinger–Ellison syndrome)	Gastrin-secreting tumor (most commonly, islet cell origin)	Recurrent peptic ulcers	Part of **multiple endocrine neoplasia-1**

Clinical Vignette 5-5

Clinical Presentation: During a visit to her primary care physician, a 42-year-old female complains of intermittent **RUQ pain** of several months' duration, which is worse after **large and fatty meals.** Pain is **steady** and **lasts 1 to 4 h** and is sometimes associated with nausea and vomiting. Physical exam reveals a soft, nondistended abdomen with mild tenderness in the RUQ, normal bowel sounds, and no palpable masses. No cough tenderness, rebound tenderness, or tenderness to percussion. $T = 98.7\,°F$; BP = 130/80 mm Hg; HR = 85 bpm; and RR = 20 breaths/min.

Differentials: Biliary colic/cholelithiasis, acute cholecystitis, choledocholithiasis, and acute cholangitis. When differentiating between the various causes of RUQ pain, use these findings to guide your approach: (a) when **obstructive symptoms (jaundice, pruritus, light-colored stools, tea-colored urine, etc.)** are present, consider a stone in the CBD (i.e., choledocholithiasis or acute cholangitis); (b) **inflammation of the parietal peritoneum** elicited by **cough tenderness, rebound tenderness, tenderness to percussion, and still posture** indicates an inflammatory condition (i.e., acute cholecystitis or acute cholangitis; and (c) look for specific signs: **Murphy sign** (acute cholecystitis), **Charcot triad** (acute cholangitis), and **Reynold pentad** (acute suppurative cholangitis).

Laboratory Studies: Ultrasound is the most effective imaging study for diagnosing cholelithiasis and is superior to CT and radiography. Relevant findings include stones, a thickened gallbladder wall, and pericholecystic fluid. Dilation of the CBD suggests obstruction. To sort through the differentials, look for an obstructive pattern on **fractionate bilirubin** and **liver enzyme studies** to support choledocholithiasis and acute cholangitis: elevated direct bilirubin and marked increases in alkaline phosphatase in comparison to mild increases in aspartate aminotransferase (AST) and alanine aminotransferase (ALT). **CBC studies** showing an increase in WBC with a left shift would support an inflammatory condition (acute cholecystitis or cholangitis).

Management: Uncomplicated cholelithiasis and acute cholecystis are treated surgically with a cholecystectomy. Choledocholithiasis and acute cholangitis are treated by endoscopic retrograde cholangiopancreatography (ERCP); if this fails, surgical exploration of the CBD is attempted. In acute cholecystitis and cholangitis, antibiotics are also given to resolve the underlying infection.

Murphy sign: Cessation of inspiration as a result of deep palpation of RUQ by examiner during inspiration; **Charcot triad:** Fever, RUQ pain, and jaundice; **Reynold pentad:** Charcot triad plus hypotension and mental status changes.

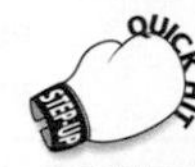

Use patient **history** to determine whether the cause of pancreatitis is gallstones or alcohol abuse. The **amylase/lipase levels** are markedly elevated in gallstone pancreatitis (thousands) in comparison to the increase seen in alcoholic pancreatitis (hundreds); chronic alcohol consumption may lead to less functioning pancreatic tissue.

BUGS OF THE GASTROINTESTINAL TRACT

I. Bacterial

Enterobacteriaceae	*Vibrio cholerae*	*Clostridium botulinum*
Salmonella	*Staphylococcus aureus*	*Clostridium difficile*
Shigella	*Campylobacter jejuni*	*Bacillus fragilis*
Escherichia coli	*Helicobacter pylori*	

II. Parasitic

Entamoeba histolytica	*Cryptosporidium*	*Ascaris lumbricoides*
Giardia lamblia	*Trichuris trichiura*	*Strongyloides stercoralis*

III. Viral

Adenovirus	Echovirus	Norwalk agent
Coronavirus	Rotavirus	Reovirus

THERAPEUTIC AGENTS FOR THE GASTROINTESTINAL SYSTEM

Various therapeutic agents have been designed to treat GI diseases such as heartburn (Table 5-18), diarrhea (Table 5-19), constipation (Table 5-20), and nausea (Table 5-21).

TABLE 5-18 Therapeutic Agents for Heartburn

Therapeutic Agent (common name, if relevant) [trade name, where appropriate]	Class—Pharmacology and Pharmacokinetics	Indications	Side or Adverse Effects	Contraindications or Precautions to Consider; Notes
Cimetidine, ranitidine [Zantac]	**H_2 blocker—blocks histamine H_2 receptors reversibly → decreases proton secretion by parietal cells**	**Peptic ulcer disease, gastritis, esophageal reflux**	**Gynecomastia; impotence;** decreased libido in males; **confusion, dizziness, and headaches**	**Crosses placenta decreases renal excretion of creatinine; P450 inhibitor**
Famotidine [Pepcid], nizatidine	**H_2 blocker—reversibly blocks histamine H_2 receptors → reduces gastric acid secretion**	**Peptic ulcer disease, gastritis, esophageal reflux**	**Gynecomastia;** rare; confusion, dizziness, and headaches	**Crosses placenta; milder side effect profile** than cimetidine and ranitidine
Omeprazole [Prilosec], lansoprazole	**Proton pump inhibitor—irreversibly inhibits H^+/K^+-ATPase in gastric parietal cells → decreases proton secretion by parietal cells**	Peptic ulcer disease, gastritis, esophageal reflux, and **Zollinger–Ellison syndrome**		**Inhibits cytochrome P450**; given with clarithromycin and **amoxicillin** for ***H. pylori***
Bismuth [Pepto-Bismol], sucralfate	**Cytoprotectant—binds to ulcer base → protection, allows bicarbonate ion secretion to re-establish pH gradient in the mucous layer**	**Traveler's diarrhea**, peptic ulcer disease		
Misoprostol	**Cytoprotectant—PGE_1 analog → increased production and secretion of gastric mucosa barrier, decreased acid production**	**Prevents NSAID induced peptic ulcers;** maintains patent ductus arteriosus	**Diarrhea**	**Abortion inducing drug**, contraindicated in women of childbearing age
Pirenzipine, propantheline	**Muscarinic antagonist—blocks M_1 receptors on ECL cells → decreases histamine secretion; blocks M_3 receptors on parietal cells → decreases acid secretion**	Peptic ulcer	**Tachycardia, dry mouth, blurry vision** (difficulty accommodating)	
Aluminum hydroxide	**Antacid**—buffers gastric acid by raising pH	Peptic ulcer, gastritis, esophageal reflux, and diarrhea	**Constipation**, hypophosphatemia, muscle weakness, **osteodystrophy**, seizures, and **hypokalemia**	Can affect the **absorption, bioavailability,** or **urinary excretion** of drugs by changing the **gastric pH, urinary pH,** or **gastric emptying**

(continued)

TABLE 5-18 Therapeutic Agents for Heartburn *(Continued)*

Therapeutic Agent (common name, if relevant) [trade name, where appropriate]	Class–Pharmacology and Pharmacokinetics	Indications	Side or Adverse Effects	Contraindications or Precautions to Consider; Notes
Magnesium hydroxide [Milk of Magnesia]	**Antacid**—buffers gastric acid by raising pH	Peptic ulcer, gastritis, esophageal reflux, and constipation	**Diarrhea, hyporeflexia, hypotension, cardiac arrest, hypokalemia**	**Can affect the absorption, bioavailability, or urinary excretion of drugs by changing the gastric pH, urinary pH, or gastric emptying.**
Calcium carbonate [TUMS, Caltrate]	**Antacid**—buffers gastric acid by raising pH	Peptic ulcer, gastritis, esophageal reflux, and calcium deficiency	**Hypercalcemia, rebound acid increase, and hypokalemia**	**Can affect the absorption, bioavailability, or urinary excretion of drugs by changing the gastric pH, urinary pH, or gastric emptying.**

TABLE 5-19 Therapeutic Agents for Diarrhea, Ulcerative Colitis, and Crohn Disease

Therapeutic Agent (common name, if relevant) [trade name, where appropriate]	Class–Pharmacology and Pharmacokinetics	Indications	Side or Adverse Effects	Contraindications or Precautions to Consider; Notes
Loperamide [Imodium]	**Antidiarrheal—similar to opioid agonist**	**Oral antidiarrheal**		
Aluminum hydroxide	**Antidiarrheal—delays gastric emptying**	Peptic ulcer, gastritis, esophageal reflux, and diarrhea	**Constipation**, hypophosphatemia, muscle weakness, **osteodystrophy**, seizures, and **hypokalemia**	Can **affect the absorption, bioavailability, or urinary excretion of drugs** by changing the **gastric pH, urinary pH**, or **gastric emptying**.
Sulfasalazine	**Anti-inflammatory—Sulfapyridine (antibacterial)** and **mesalamine (anti-inflammatory)**	Ulcerative colitis, Crohn disease	Malaise, nausea, **sulfonamide toxicity**, reversible **oligospermia**	**Activated by colonic bacteria**
Infliximab	**Anti-inflammatory—monoclonal antibody** that binds TNF → **inhibits proinflammatory effects** of TNF	**Crohn disease**, rheumatoid arthritis	Respiratory infection, fever, and hypotension	

TABLE 5-20 Therapeutic Agents for Constipation

Therapeutic Agent (common name, if relevant) [trade name, where appropriate]	Class—Pharmacology and Pharmacokinetics	Indications	Side or Adverse Effects	Contraindications or Precautions to Consider; Notes
Methylcellulose [Citrucel]	**Bulk-forming laxative**—dietary fiber	Constipation	Impaction above strictures, fluid overload, gas, and bloating	
Psyllium [Per diem Fiber]	**Bulk-forming laxative**—dietary fiber	Constipation	Impaction above strictures, fluid overload, gas, and bloating	
Lactulose [Chronulac]	**Osmotic laxative**	Decreases ammonia in hepatic encephalopathy; constipation	Abdominal bloating and flatulence	
Magnesium hydroxide [Milk of Magnesia]	**Osmotic laxative**	Constipation; peptic ulcer, gastritis, and esophageal reflux	Diarrhea	
Magnesium sulfate, Magnesium citrate	**Osmotic laxative**		Magnesium toxicity (in renal insufficiency)	
Docusate	**Stool softener;** by emulsifying stool, it makes the passage of stool easier	Constipation	Skin rash	
Bisacodyl [Dulcolax]	**Stimulant laxative;** increases peristalsis	Constipation	Electrolyte imbalances (chronic use); gastric irritation	
Senna [Senokot]	**Stimulant laxative;** increases peristalsis	Constipation	Electrolyte imbalances (chronic use); melanosis coli	
Phenolphthalein [Ex-Lax]	**Stimulant laxative**—reduces the absorption of electrolytes and water from the gut	Constipation	Tumorigenic	
Anthraquinones	**Stimulant laxative**—reduces the absorption of electrolytes and water from the gut	Constipation		
Castor oil	**Stimulant laxative**—reduces the absorption of electrolytes and water from the gut; active component is ricinoleic acid	Constipation, labor induction		
Mineral oil [Fleet Mineral Oil Enema]	**Hyperosmolar agent**—draws water into the gut lumen → gut distension → promotes peristalsis and evacuation of bowel	**Preoperative patients;** short term treatment of constipation		May interfere with the absorption of fat-soluble vitamins

(continued)

TABLE 5-20 Therapeutic Agents for Constipation *(Continued)*

Therapeutic Agent (common name, if relevant) [trade name, where appropriate]	Class–Pharmacology and Pharmacokinetics	Indications	Side or Adverse Effects	Contraindications or Precautions to Consider; Notes
Cisapride	**Prokinetic agent—increases acetylcholine release at myenteric plexus** → increases esophageal tone and gastric/duodenal contractility (improves colon transit time)	Constipation	**Torsades des pointes**	Rarely used; interacts with **erythromycin, ketoconazole, nefazodone, and fluconazole** to produce **Torsades des pointes**
Metoclopramide [Reglan]	**Prokinetic agent—D_2 receptor antagonist**; increases resting tone, contractility, LES tone, and motility (does not affect colon transit time)	**Diabetic** and **postoperative gastroparesis**	Sleepiness; fatigue; headache; insomnia; dizziness; nausea; akathisia, **dystonia**, and tardive dyskinesia	Interacts with **digoxin** and **diabetic agents; contraindicated in small bowel obstruction**

TABLE 5-21 Therapeutic Agents for Nausea

Therapeutic Agent (common name, if relevant) [trade name, where appropriate]	Class–Pharmacology and Pharmacokinetics	Indications	Side or Adverse Effects	Contraindications or Precautions to Consider; Notes
Scopolamine	**Anticholinergic**—M_1-muscarinic receptor antagonist	**Motion sickness;** prophylaxis	**Dry mouth,** drowsiness, and **vision disturbances**	**Delivered transdermally**
Promethazine [Phenergan]	**Antihistamine**—D_2-receptor antagonist; H_1-blocker	Counteracts nausea of **migraine**; allergies; **motion sickness**	Sedation; CNS depression; atropine-like effects; allergic dermatitis; blood dyscrasias; **teratogenicity;** acute antihistamine poisoning	
Prochlorperazine [Compazine]	**Dopamine antagonist**—D_2-receptor antagonist	**Nausea**; counteracts nausea of **migraine**	Teratogenic	
Metoclopramide [Reglan]	**Dopamine antagonist—central and peripheral D_2 antagonism at low doses and** weak 5-HT_3 antagonism at high doses; enhances acetylcholine release, prokinetic	**Nausea;** counteracts nausea of **migraine;** increases stomach motility	Sleepiness; fatigue; headache; insomnia; dizziness; nausea; akathisia, **dystonia,** and tardive dyskinesia	
Ondansetron [Zofran]	**Serotonin antagonist—5-HT_3 blocker**	**Nausea** (caused by **cancer therapy** or **postoperative state**)	Headache, constipation, and dizziness	

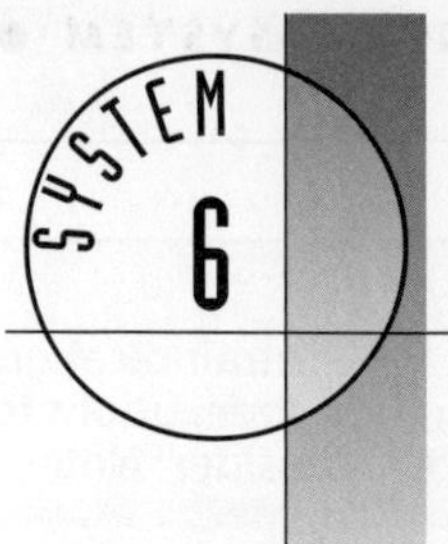

The Renal System

DEVELOPMENT

I. Intermediate mesoderm

A. This forms the **urogenital ridges** on each side of the aorta.

B. The **nephrogenic cord** arises from the urogenital ridge and gives rise, wholly or in part, to the pronephros, the mesonephros, and the metanephros.

II. Pronephros

A. Forms in the fourth week

B. Quickly regresses by the fifth week

C. Nonfunctional

III. Mesonephros

A. Forms late in the fourth week and is functional until the permanent kidney is able to develop.

B. The **mesonephric duct** forms from the mesonephros:

1. Forms the ductus deferens, epididymis, ejaculatory duct, and seminal vesicle in the male.
2. Forms the **ureteric bud** from which the **ureter, renal pelvis, calyces**, and **collecting tubules** in both the male and female are derived.
3. No important genital or reproductive derivatives of the mesonephric duct specific to females are formed.

QUICK HIT: In the adult male, the ureter passes posterior to the ductus deferens; in the adult female, the ureter passes posterior to the uterine artery.

MNEMONIC

To remember the relationship of the arteries to the ureter, think "water under the bridge"; the ureters (which carry water) are posterior to the ovarian/testicular artery and uterine artery.

IV. Metanephros

A. Develops into the **adult kidney**.

B. Formed during the fifth week from the **ureteric bud** and the metanephric mass (which is induced to form by contact with the ureteric bud) and begins to function in the ninth week.

C. Metanephric mesoderm forms the nephrons.

D. "Ascends" from sacral levels to low thoracic levels during its development because of longitudinal growth of the fetus.

E. Urogenital sinus forms the **bladder**, which is continuous with allantois. Allantois is equivalent to the median umbilical ligament in the adult.

F. Urethra

1. Formed from endoderm and urogenital sinus
2. Distal portion formed from ectoderm

QUICK HIT: The entire collecting system arises from the **ureteric bud**. The remainder of the renal system arises from the metanephric mesoderm.

V. Congenital anomalies of the renal system (Table 6-1)

QUICK HIT: Fanconi syndrome is a **hereditary** or **acquired** dysfunction of the proximal renal tubules. As a result of impaired glucose, amino acid, phosphate, and bicarbonate reabsorption, it manifests clinically as glycosuria, hyperphosphaturia, aminoaciduria, and acidosis.

GROSS DESCRIPTION OF THE KIDNEY

I. Paired adult kidneys weigh approximately 150 g each.

II. They are located posterior to the peritoneum and at approximately the level of the first lumbar vertebra.

TABLE 6-1 Congenital Anomalies

Anomaly	Characteristics
Bilateral renal agenesis (Potter syndrome)	• Occurs when the ureteric bud does not form • **Oligohydramnios** • Limb deformities • Facial deformities • **Pulmonary hypoplasia** • Bilateral agenesis is not compatible with life
Accessory renal arteries	• Arise from the aorta • Feed a particular section of the kidney • Are end arteries • **Cutting will produce ischemic** infarct in the area they supply
Congenital polycystic kidney disease	• Multiple small and large cysts causing renal insufficiency • Cysts are "closed"—not continuous with collecting system • Enlarged kidneys palpable on newborn examination • Death within days to weeks
Horseshoe kidney	• Inferior poles of the kidneys are fused • Ascent is arrested at the level of the inferior mesenteric artery • Increases probability of Wilms tumor

III. The right kidney is slightly lower than the left owing to downward displacement by the liver.

IV. The left renal vein lies posterior to the superior mesenteric artery and anterior to the abdominal aorta.

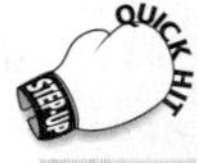

The left gonadal (testicular or ovarian) vein drains into the left renal vein; the right gonadal vein drains directly into the inferior vena cava.

V. The kidney is highly vascularized; it filters more than 1,700 L of blood per day to produce about 1 L of urine.

VI. Kidney and urinary tract (Figure 6-1).

VII. Distribution of body water (Figure 6-2).

NORMAL KIDNEY FUNCTION

I. Renal blood flow (RBF)

A. 25% of cardiac output.

B. RBF = **renal plasma flow** (RPF)/[1 – **hematocrit** (Hct)].

C. Renal vasculature **autoregulates** RBF, keeping it constant even when arterial pressure varies from 100 to 200 mm Hg.

II. Renal plasma flow

A. Effective RPF is measured by clearance of para-aminohippuric acid (PAH), which is filtered and secreted.

B. This measurement underestimates by 10%.

III. Glomerular filtration rate (GFR)

A. Normal GFR is 90 to 125 mL/min based on creatinine.

B. It is measured by **inulin** clearance. Inulin is an ideal marker for the measurement of GFR because it is a substance that is **filtered** by the kidney but **not reabsorbed or secreted**. Therefore, urine levels of inulin vary directly with GFR. However, inulin clearance is not practical for clinical use.

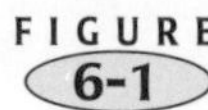

FIGURE 6-1 **The kidney and urinary tract**
(Adapted with permission from Damjanov I. A Color Atlas and Textbook of Histopathology. Baltimore, MD: Williams & Wilkins, 1996:258–259.)

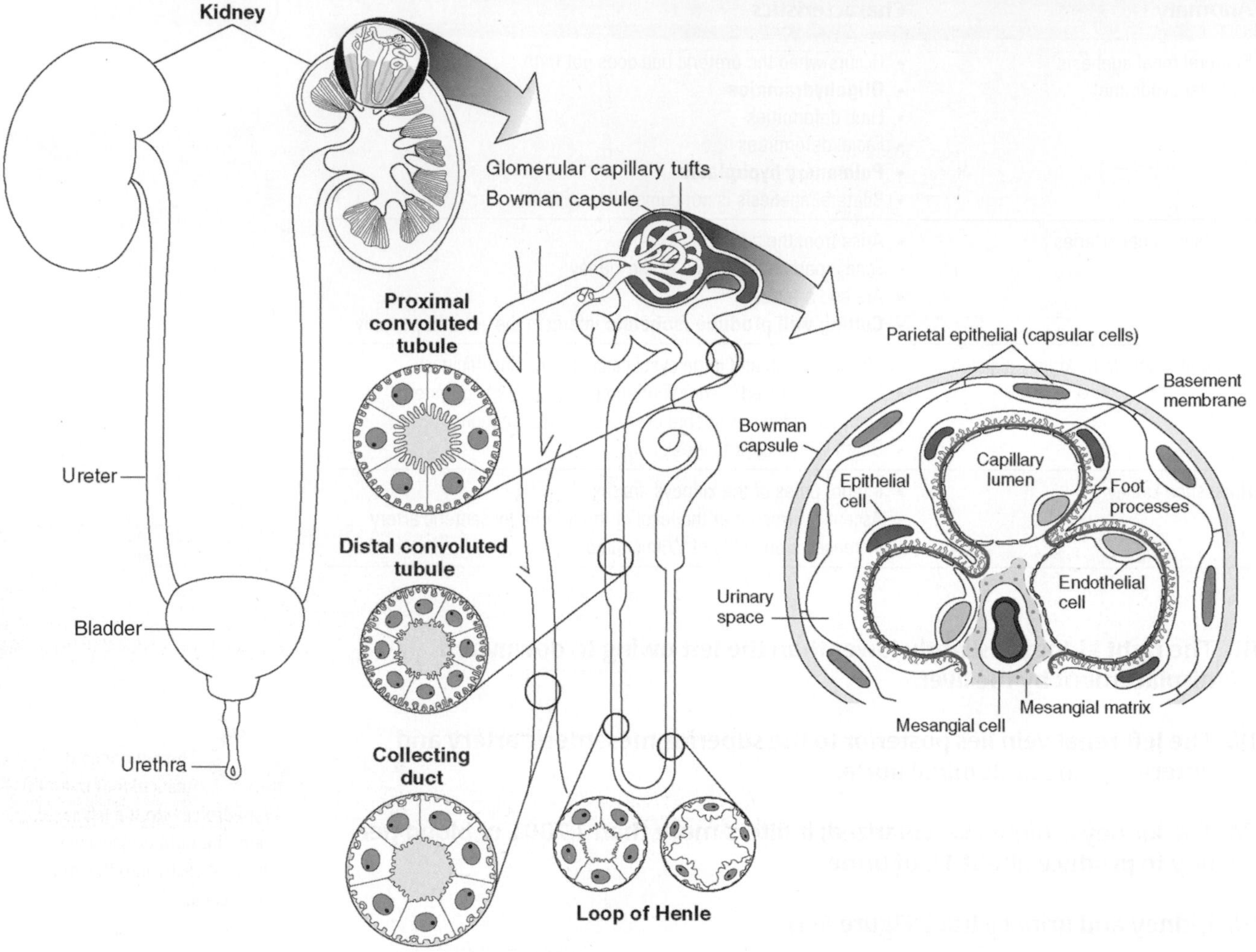

C. GFR is clinically measured with **creatinine** clearance. Endogenous creatine is the most common clinical marker because it is **filtered**, **minimally secreted**, and **not reabsorbed** by the kidneys. While creatinine excretion is generally 10% to 20% greater than filtration, this discrepancy is cancelled by the overestimation of plasma creatinine. Therefore, creatinine is relatively accurate for GFR calculation
   1. Decreases in GFR cause a rise in blood urea nitrogen (BUN) and creatinine levels.
   2. GFR decreases with age.

D. GFR is driven by Starling forces (filtration is always favored) (Figure 6-3).

E. Renal clearance
   1. Removal of a substance from the blood by renal excretion
   2. Determined by the following equation:

$$\text{Clearance} = [U \times V]/P \text{ (in mL/min)}$$

where U = concentration of substance in urine in mg/mL
V = urine volume (urine flow rate) in mL/min
P = plasma concentration of substance in mg/mL

Note: One common pitfall to using creatinine is **muscle mass**. Plasma creatinine varies directly with muscle mass, so individuals with lower muscle mass (e.g., emaciated, elderly) may have an artificially higher GFR and individuals with high muscle mass (e.g., bodybuilders) may have an artificially lower GFR. Similarly, with age and loss of muscle mass, GFR may remain stable when in fact there is a decline in glomerular function and a decrease in GFR.

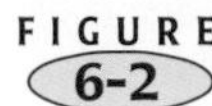

Distribution of body water

Cl, chloride; D_2O, heavy water; HCO_3^-, bicarbonate; H_2O, water; K^+, potassium; Mg_2^+, magnesium; Na^+, sodium.

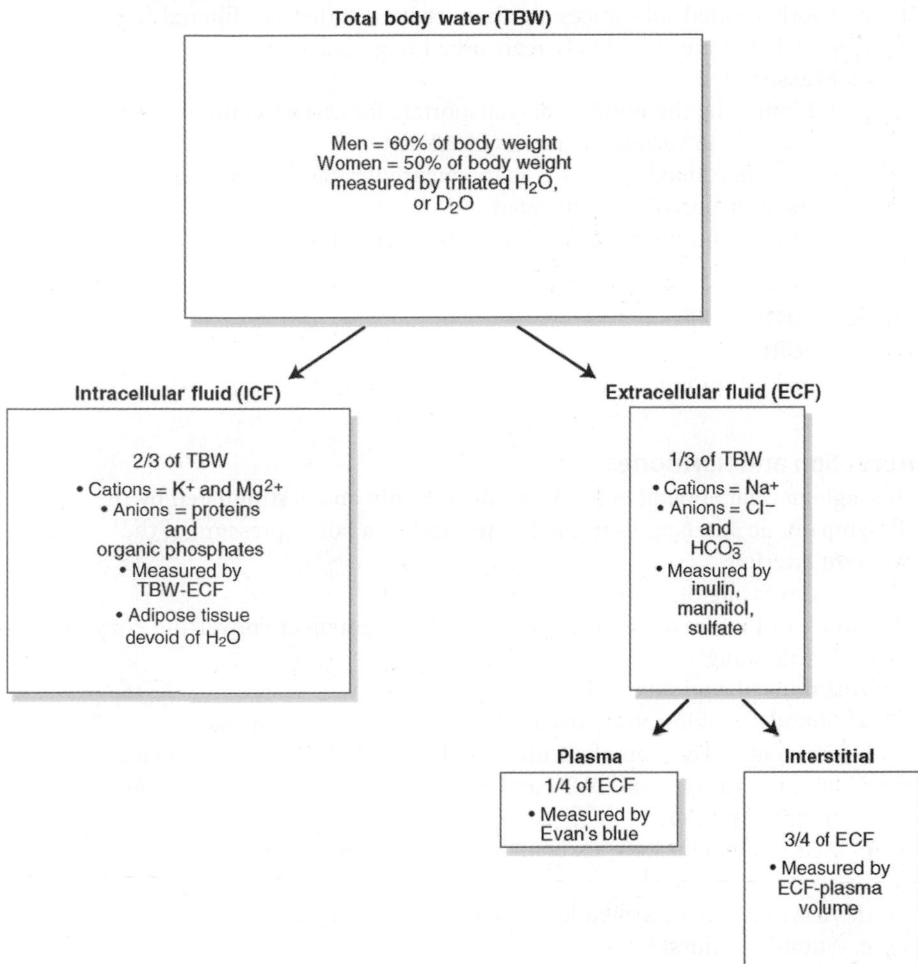

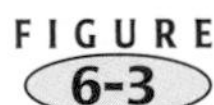

Starling forces on the glomerular capillary

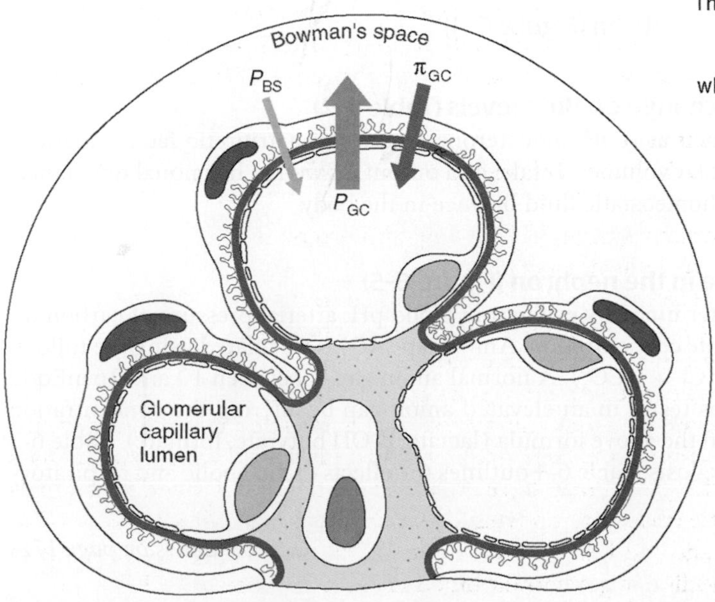

The Starling forces influence the Glomerular filtration rate (GFR)

$$GFR = K_F\,[(P_{GC}-P_{BS}) - (\pi_{GC}-\pi_{BS})]$$

where K_F: The filtration coefficient of the glomerular capillaries

P_{GC}: The hydrostatic pressure exerted by the fluid in the glomerular capillary. A dilated afferent arteriole increases P_{GC}, as does a constricted efferent arteriole.

P_{BS}: The hydrostatic pressure exerted by the fluid in Bowman's space. Blockage or constriction of the ureters increases P_{BS}.

π_{GC}: The oncotic pressure of the glomerular capillary. The value of π_{GC} increases along the length of the capillary because the protein concentration in the capillary increases as water is forced into Bowman's space.

π_{BS}: The oncotic pressure in Bowman's space. This value is usually zero.

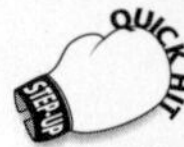

The T_m for glucose is reached at approximately 350 mg/dL. Greater concentrations result in an osmotic diuresis, such as that seen in diabetics with hyperglycemia.

3. Factors that determine clearance
   a. Highly cleared substances (e.g., PAH) are those that are filtered and secreted and not reabsorbed.
   b. Poorly cleared substances are those that are either not filtered (e.g., protein) or are completely reabsorbed (e.g., glucose).
   c. Reabsorption
      - Limited by the number of transporters for certain compounds (e.g., glucose) in various segments of tubule.
      - Transport maximum (T_m) is the maximum rate of reabsorption at which the transporters are saturated.
      - At concentrations above T_m, excess is excreted.

IV. Filtration fraction (FF)

A. FF = GFR/RPF.

B. The normal filtration fraction is 20%.

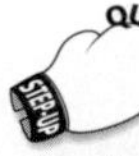

ACE inhibitors, **captopril** and **enalapril**, reduce hypertension by inhibiting the conversion of angiotensin I to angiotensin II, thereby decreasing the release of aldosterone. The angiotensin II receptor blocker, **losartan,** prevents angiotensin II from interacting with its receptor. This prevents angiotensin II from causing constriction of efferent arterioles.

V. Innervation and hormones

A. Juxtaglomerular apparatus (JGA) produces renin and is stimulated by the β-sympathetic adrenergics in the kidney and by a fall in pressure of the afferent arteriole.

B. **Renin** cleaves angiotensinogen to **angiotensin I**.

C. Angiotensin I is cleaved to **angiotensin II** by angiotensin-converting enzyme (ACE) in the lung

1. Functions of angiotensin II
   a. Stimulates aldosterone release from the zona glomerulosa
   b. Stimulates secretion of antidiuretic hormone (ADH, also known as arginine vasopressin, AVP) and adrenocorticotropic hormone (ACTH) from the pituitary
   c. Acts as a potent local vasoconstrictor of the renal arterioles at low plasma levels
   d. Acts as a general systemic vasoconstrictor at high plasma levels
   e. Stimulates thirst
   f. Stimulates epinephrine and norepinephrine release from adrenal medulla
2. Angiotensin II is inactivated to angiotensin III, a potent stimulator of aldosterone secretion but not an effective vasoconstrictor.

VI. Hormones and the nephron (Figure 6-4)

VII. Effects of volume change on fluid levels (Table 6-2)

A variety of hormones, such as ADH, aldosterone, and atrial natriuretic factor, regulate extracellular and intracellular volumes. Intake and output, as well as hormonal imbalance, can significantly alter the homeostatic fluid balance in the body.

VIII. Electrolyte balance in the nephron (Figure 6-5)

Acidosis or alkalosis is determined by evaluating blood pH, arterial pressure of carbon dioxide PCO_2, and bicarbonate concentration. Anion gap (AG) is calculated using the following equation: $AG = Na^+ - (Cl^- + HCO_3^-)$. A normal anion gap is between 10 and 16 mEq/L. Certain acidotic conditions result in an elevated anion gap by altering the concentration of anions not considered in the above formula (lactate, β-OH butyrate, formate). Table 6-3 compares acidosis with alkalosis. Table 6-4 outlines the effects of metabolic and respiratory acid–base disturbances.

(text continues on page 172)

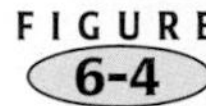

Hormones and the nephron

ACE, angiotensin-converting enzyme; AT I, angiotensin I; Ca_2^+, calcium; cAMP, cyclic adenosine monophosphate; cGMP, cyclic guanosine monophosphate; DCT, distal convoluted tubule; GFR, glomerular filtration rate; H^+, hydrogen ion; HCO_3^-, bicarbonate; H_2O, water; JGA, juxtaglomerular apparatus; K^+, potassium; Na^+, sodium; PCT, proximal convoluted tubule; PO_4^{3-}, phosphate; V2, vasopressin receptor, type 2.

Atrial natriuretic factor (ANF)
• released by cardiac muscle in response to ↑plasma volume, vasodilation, ↓renal blood flow
↑cGMP → ↑GFR → ↑Na^+ excretion
Aldosterone:
• released by adrenal cortex
⊕ New protein synthesis
Principal cell
• ↑Na^+ reabsorption
• ↑K^+ secretion
Intercalated cell
• ↑H^+ secretion
Angiotensin II (AT II)
↑Na^+-H^+ exchange and ↑HCO_3^- reabsorption
JGA
Renin
DCT
Angio-tensinogen
AT I
ACE (Lung)
AT II
Liver
Collecting duct
Parathyroid hormone
PCT
↑cAMP → ↓PO_4^{3-} reabsorption (PCT)
→ ↑Ca^{2+} reabsorption (DCT)
→ ⊕ 1α *hydroxylase* (PCT)
25 hydroxycholecalciferol
1,25 dihydroxycholecalciferol
↑Ca^{2+} and PO_4^{2-} reabsorption (DCT)
Antidiuretic hormone (ADH), aka arginine vasopressin (AVP), vasopressin
V_2 receptor (principal cells)
↑cAMP
↑Aquaporin II channels
↑H_2O reabsorption
ADH is released from the posterior pituitary in response to increased osmolarity in the hypothalamus.
Note: ADH changes water secretion. Aldosterone changes the solutes
Loop of Henle
⊕ Stimulates

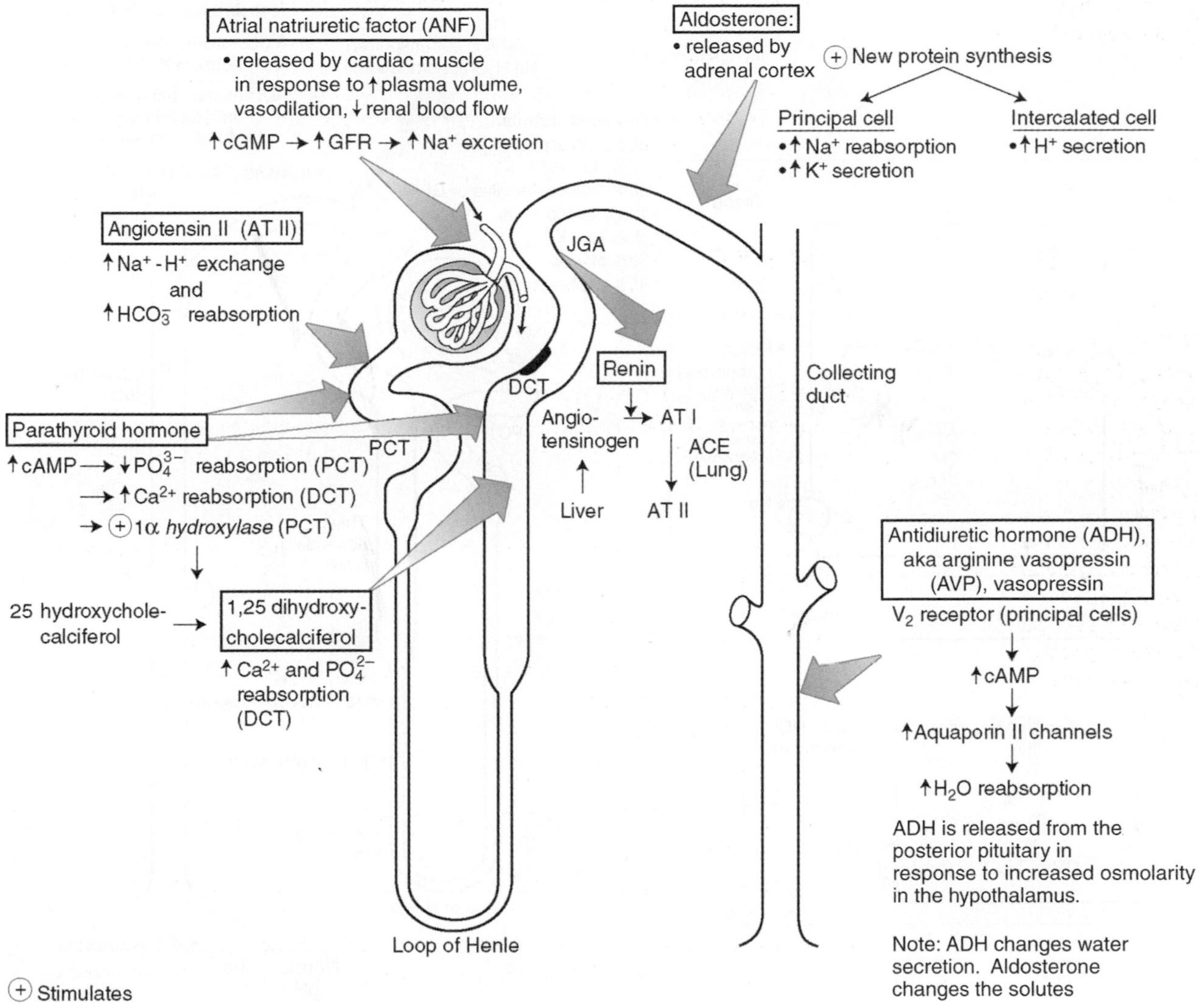

TABLE 6-2 Effects of Volume Change on Fluid Levels

Type	Key Examples	ECF Volume	ICF Volume	ECF Osmolarity	Hct and Serum [Na+]
Isosmotic volume expansion	Isotonic fluid infusion (e.g., normal saline or lactated Ringer solution)	↑	No change	No change	↓Hct [Na+]
Isosmotic volume contraction	Diarrhea	↓	No change	No change	↑ Hct – [Na+]
Hyperosmotic volume expansion	High NaCl intake	↑	↓	↑	↓ Hct ↑ [Na+]
Hyperosmotic volume contraction	Sweating, fever, diabetes insipidus	↓	↓	↑	– Hct ≠ [Na+]
Hyposmotic volume expansion	SIADH	↑	↑	↓	– Hct ↓ [Na+]
Hyposmotic volume contraction	Adrenal insufficiency	↓	↑	↓	↑ Hct ↓ [Na+]

–, no change; ECF, extracellular fluid; Hct, hematocrit; ICF, intracellular fluid; SIADH, syndrome of inappropriate secretion of antidiuretic hormone. (Reproduced with permission from Costanzo LS. BRS Physiology. 2nd Ed. Baltimore, MD: Williams & Wilkins, 1998:139.)

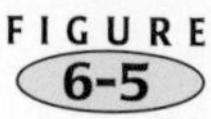

FIGURE 6-5 Electrolyte balance in the nephron

ADH, antidiuretic hormone; CA, carbonic anhydrase; Cl^-, chloride; CO_2, carbon dioxide; DCT, distal convoluted tubule; H^+, hydrogen ion; HCO_3^-, bicarbonate; H_2CO_3, carbonic acid; H_2O, water; HPO_4^{2-}, $H_2PO_4^-$, two forms of phosphate ions; JGA, juxtaglomerular apparatus; K^+, potassium; Mg^{2+}, magnesium; Na^+, sodium; NH_3, ammonia; NH_4^+, ammonium; PCT, proximal convoluted tubule.

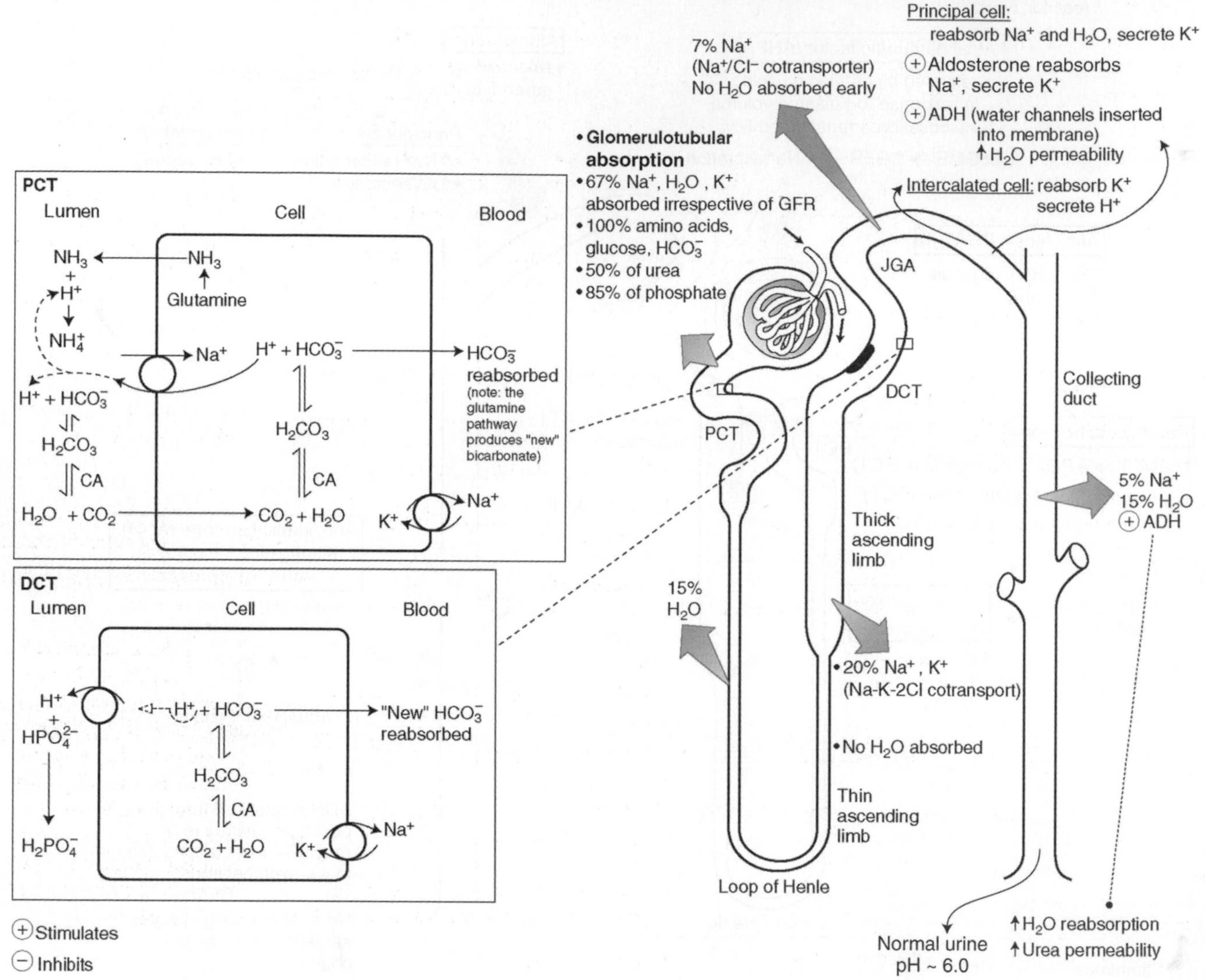

PCT
Lumen | Cell | Blood
NH_3 ← NH_3 ↑ Glutamine
$+ H^+$ → NH_4^+
Na^+
$H^+ + HCO_3^-$ → HCO_3^- reabsorbed (note: the glutamine pathway produces "new" bicarbonate)
$H^+ + HCO_3^-$ ⇌ H_2CO_3 ⇌ CA
H_2CO_3 ⇌ CA
$H_2O + CO_2$ → $CO_2 + H_2O$
K^+ Na^+

DCT
Lumen | Cell | Blood
H^+ + HPO_4^{2-} → $H_2PO_4^-$
$H^+ + HCO_3^-$ → "New" HCO_3^- reabsorbed
H_2CO_3
CA
$CO_2 + H_2O$
K^+ Na^+

(+) Stimulates
(−) Inhibits

• Glomerulotubular absorption
• 67% Na^+, H_2O, K^+ absorbed irrespective of GFR
• 100% amino acids, glucose, HCO_3^-
• 50% of urea
• 85% of phosphate

7% Na^+ (Na^+/Cl^- cotransporter) No H_2O absorbed early

Principal cell: reabsorb Na^+ and H_2O, secrete K^+
(+) Aldosterone reabsorbs Na^+, secrete K^+
(+) ADH (water channels inserted into membrane) ↑ H_2O permeability
Intercalated cell: reabsorb K^+ secrete H^+

JGA
DCT
PCT
Collecting duct
5% Na^+
15% H_2O
(+) ADH
Thick ascending limb
15% H_2O
• 20% Na^+, K^+ (Na-K-2Cl cotransport)
• No H_2O absorbed
Thin ascending limb
Loop of Henle
Normal urine pH ~ 6.0
↑ H_2O reabsorption
↑ Urea permeability

Clinical Vignette 6-1

Clinical Presentation: A 24-year-old male medical student is brought to the emergency department after being found **unconscious** in his apartment by his roommate. It is unknown whether he suffered any trauma, but the roommate tells you that they just finished exam week at the medical school. There are no signs of injury on examination. The roommate tells you that the patient has no other medical problems. The patient cannot be aroused in the emergency department but does respond to pain. Vital signs: T = 100.8°F; **RR = 35 breaths/min;** BP = 150/90 mm Hg; HR = 104 bpm. Pupils are round and reactive to light bilaterally. Laboratory tests reveal the following: WBC = 8.4; Hgb = 14.2; Hct = 30.9; Na = 140; K = 3.8; Cl = 102; **HCO_2 = 13;** BUN = 16; Cr = 0.8; Gluc = 110. Arterial blood gasses are obtained and reveal the following: **pH = 7.19; P_aCO_2 = 26; P_aO_2 = 95.**

Differential: This patient has metabolic acidosis. In approaching a patient with metabolic acidosis, the **first step is the calculation of the anion gap:** anion gap = [Na] − ([Cl] + [HCO_3]). This patient has an increased anion gap metabolic acidosis (AG >15) for which differentials are diabetic ketoacidosis (DKA), alcoholic ketoacidosis, lactic acidosis, starvation, renal failure, and overdose of salicylate, methanol, or ethylene glycol. Given that the patient is not diabetic

(continued)

Clinical Vignette 6-1 *(Continued)*

and has a glucose of 114, DKA is unlikely. Also, renal function is not impaired. As the cause is unclear, further testing is necessary.

Laboratory Studies: To determine the cause of the anion gap metabolic acidosis in this patient, **serum ketone, salicylate, lactate, blood alcohol, methanol, and ethylene glycol levels** should be obtained. Next, determine whether this is a primary acid–base disorder or mixed disorder. Using **Winter's formula** [1.5 (measured HCO_2) + 8 ± 2], the expected P_aCO_2 level in this patient is 25.5 to 29.5. With a P_aCO_2 of 26, this patient has an appropriate respiratory compensation response (RR of 35 breaths/min). If actual P_aCO_2 is higher than expected, there is an additional acidotic process occurring. If actual P_aCO_2 is lower than expected, then there is an additional alkalotic process occurring.

Management: Management depends on the cause of metabolic acidosis. **Sodium bicarbonate** may be needed in cases of severe acidemia and **mechanical ventilation** may be required if patient is fatigued from hyperventilation.

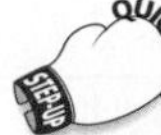

Kussmaul respiration is an increase in both the rate and the volume of respirations. It is classically described as occurring in diabetic ketoacidosis. The Kussmaul sign is a loss of the normal 5- to 10-mm Hg drop in blood pressure that accompanies inspiration. This is seen in pericarditis, restrictive cardiomyopathy, and after massive pulmonary embolism.

TABLE 6-3 Acidosis and Alkalosis

Metabolic Disturbance	Presentation	Causes
Metabolic acidosis	• Fatigue • Shortness of breath • Abdominal pain • Vomiting • **Kussmaul respirations** • Hypotension • Tachycardia	• Chronic renal failure • Lactic acidosis • Uremia • **Ketoacidosis** • Intoxication (aspirin, methanol, ethylene glycol) • **Diarrhea**[a] • **Renal tubular acidosis**[a] • Acetazolamide[a]
Respiratory acidosis	• **Hypercapnia** • Confusion • Blunted sensation and pain • **Asterixis** • Papilledema	• Respiratory depression by drugs • Cerebral disease • Cardiopulmonary arrest response • Neuromuscular disease (e.g., myasthenia gravis) • Poor ventilation secondary to disease (e.g., asthma, pneumonia, bronchitis, emphysema)
Metabolic alkalosis	• No specific signs or symptoms • Can cause apathy, stupor, and confusion • If coupled with low calcium, can cause tetany	• Diuretics (loop and thiazide) • Vomiting • Milk alkali syndrome • Large intake of alkaline substance • **Cushing syndrome** • Primary aldosteronism
Respiratory alkalosis	• **Hyperventilation** • Numbness • Tingling • Paresthesia • Tetany, if severe	• Asthma • Pneumonia • Pulmonary edema • Heart disease with cyanosis • Pulmonary fibrosis • Aspirin intoxication • **Gram-negative sepsis** • Fever • Anxiety • Pregnancy • Drugs • Conditions that stimulate the medullary respiratory center (e.g., altitude) • Aspirin intoxication (via stimulation of respiratory center)

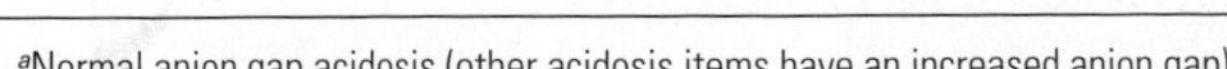

[a]Normal anion gap acidosis (other acidosis items have an increased anion gap).

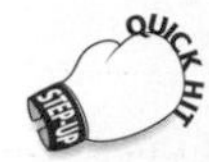

Emphysema and bronchitis often cause chronic respiratory acidosis.

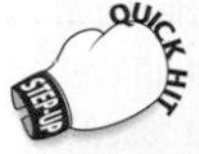

Renal tubular acidosis (RTA) is characterized by a normal anion gap. Type 1 (distal) RTA is caused by a failure to excrete titratable acid and NH_4^+. Type 2 RTA is caused by renal loss of HCO_3^-. Type 4 RTA is caused by hypoaldosteronism, which leads to poor excretion of NH_4^+ and hyperkalemia.

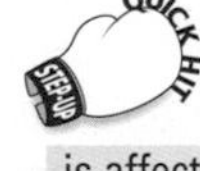

A patient's respiratory status affects and is affected by his or her acid–base status. This is because of the reversible conversion of CO_2 to H^+ in the following way: $H_2O + CO_2 \leftrightarrow H_2CO_3 \leftrightarrow HCO_3^- + H^+$.

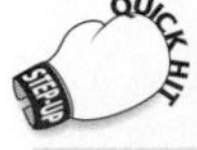

The first reaction is catalyzed by the enzyme carbonic anhydrase.

MNEMONIC

To remember the causes of increased anion gap metabolic acidosis, think **KUSMAL: K**etoacids, **U**remia, **S**alicylate, **M**ethanol/ethylene glycol, **A**lcohol, **L**actate.

TABLE 6-4 Effects of Metabolic and Respiratory Acid–Base Disturbances

Primary Disorder	pH	[H+]	[HCO_3^-]	PCO_2	Respiratory Compensation	Renal Compensation
Metabolic acidosis	↓	↑	↓* (lost by buffering)	↓	Hyperventilation	↑ H+ excretion (NH_3) ↑ "New" HCO_3^- reabsorption
Metabolic alkalosis	↑	↓	↑*	↑	Hypoventilation	↑ HCO_3^- excretion
Acute respiratory acidosis	↓	↑	↑	↑*	None	Not yet
Chronic respiratory acidosis	↓ (more normal)	↑	↑↑	↑*	None	↑ H+ excretion (NH_4^+) ↑ "New" HCO_3^- reabsorption
Acute respiratory alkalosis	↑	↓	↓	↓*		Not yet
Chronic respiratory alkalosis	↑ (more normal)	↓	↓↓	↓*		↓ H+ excretion ↓ HCO_3^- reabsorption

*, primary disorder; ↑, increased; ↓, decreased.

GLOMERULAR DISEASES

MNEMONIC

To remember the hallmark findings of nephrotic syndrome, think **Protein LEAC: Protein**uria, **L**ipid increased, **E**dema, **A**lbumin decreased, **C**holesterol increased.

I. Nephrotic syndrome

A. Features
1. **Proteinuria** of more than 3.5 to 4.0 g of protein per day
2. Hypoalbuminemia
3. Edema
4. Hyperlipidemia

B. Etiology
1. Idiopathic—75%
2. Systemic disease—25%

C. Common types (Table 6-5)

TABLE 6-5 Nephrotic Glomerular Diseases

Glomerular Disease	Etiology	Clinical Features	Notes
Minimal change disease (lipoid nephrosis)	Fusion of foot processes on the basement membrane leads to loss of negative charge and changes in the protein selectivity; altered appearance of villi on epithelial cells	Electron microscopy shows **fusion of podocyte foot processes** (Figure 6-6), and lipid-laden renal cortices	**Common in young children** (usually younger than 5 years of age); responds well to steroids; albumin usually selectively secreted
Membranous glomerulonephritis	Idiopathic; secondarily caused by SLE, hepatitis B, syphilis, gold, penicillamine, malignancy	Basement membrane thickening; **"spike and dome"** with **subepithelial IgG and C3 deposits**	Common in young adults
Diabetic nephropathy	Microangiopathy leading to thickening of basement membrane	Basement membrane thickening	Two types: diffuse and nodular glomerulosclerosis; nodular glomerulosclerosis has **Kimmelstiel–Wilson nodules** (Figure 6-7); usually leads to renal failure
Renal amyloidosis	Subendothelial or mesangial amyloid deposits; associated with multiple myeloma	Stains: periodic acid–Schiff (PAS) (–); **Congo Red (+)**	Increasing severity leads to renal failure
Focal and segmental glomerulosclerosis	Has four possible etiologies: idiopathic; superimposed on preexisting pathology; associated with loss of renal mass; secondary to other disorders (e.g., heroin abuse or HIV)	Sclerosis of some glomeruli; only capillary tuft is involved in affected glomeruli	Clinically similar to minimal change disease, but affects older population

C3, third component of complement; SLE, systemic lupus erythematosus.

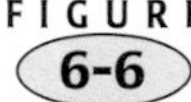

FIGURE 6-6 **Minimal change disease. Electron micrograph showing effacement of the podocyte foot processes**

EC, endothelial cell; US, urinary space; V, vacuole; BM, basement membrane.

(Reproduced with permission from Rubin E, Farber JL. Pathology. 3rd Ed. Philadelphia, PA: Lippincott Williams & Wilkins, 1999.)

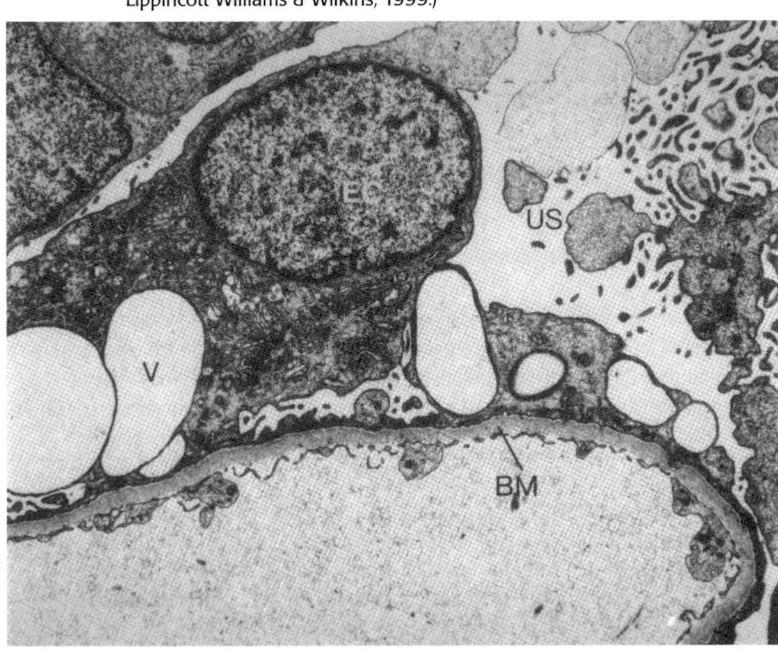

FIGURE 6-7 **Diabetic nodular glomerulosclerosis. A periodic acid–Schiff stain demonstrates nodular Kimmelstiel–Wilson lesions at the periphery of the glomerulus which are pathognomonic of diabetic glomerulosclerosis**

(Reproduced with permission from Rubin E, Farber JL. Pathology. 3rd Ed. Philadelphia, PA: Lippincott Williams & Wilkins, 1999.)

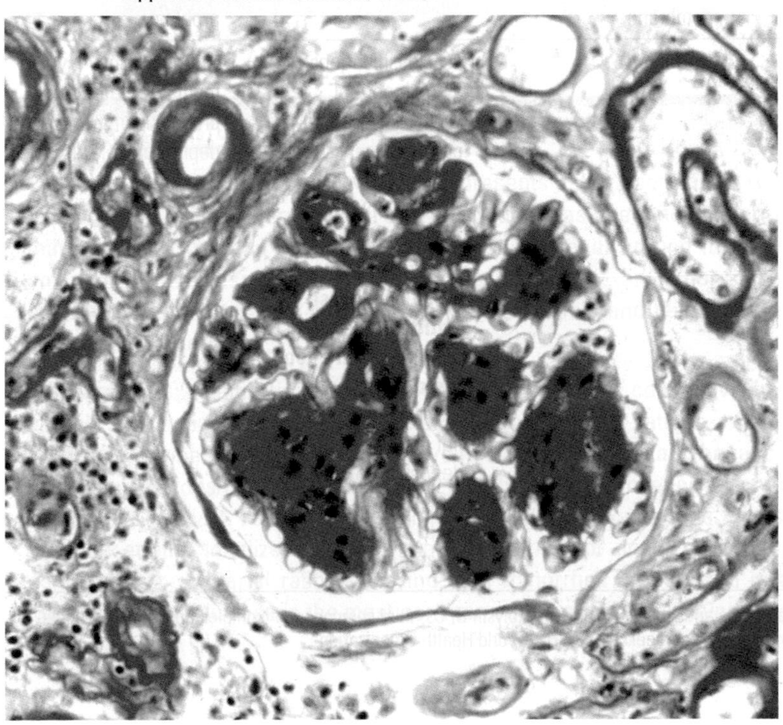

Clinical Vignette 6-2 *(Continued)*

Laboratory Studies: **Urinalysis** shows **proteinuria** in both nephrotic and nephritic syndromes but is more severe in nephrotic syndrome. **Hematuria** is seen in nephritic syndrome. **Blood studies** would reveal **hypoalbuminemia** and **hyperlipidemia** in nephrotic syndrome and **azotemia** in nephritic syndrome.

Management: Nephrotic syndrome is best treated by **albumin infusion** followed by **diuretics** and **corticosteroids.** Many children grow out of minimal change disease.

III. Nonnephritic, nonnephrotic glomerular diseases (Table 6-7)

IV. Glomerular deposits in disease (Figure 6-9)

TABLE 6-7 Nonnephritic, Nonnephrotic Glomerular Diseases

Disease	Etiology	Clinical Features	Notes
IgA nephropathy (Berger disease)	IgA deposits in mesangium; hematuria usually follows infection	Mesangial cell proliferation on electron microscopy	Minimal clinical significance; common
Membranoproliferative glomerulonephritis	Type 2 has IgG autoantibody; C3 is reduced in both types	Basement membrane thickens and appears as two layers; **"train-track"** appearance on electron microscopy	Two types: type 1 and type 2 (dense deposit disease); may lead to either nephrotic or nephritic syndromes

C3, third component of complement.

FIGURE 6-9 Glomerular deposits in disease
BM, basement membrane; C3, third component of complement; Ig, immunoglobulin; SLE, systemic lupus erythematosus.

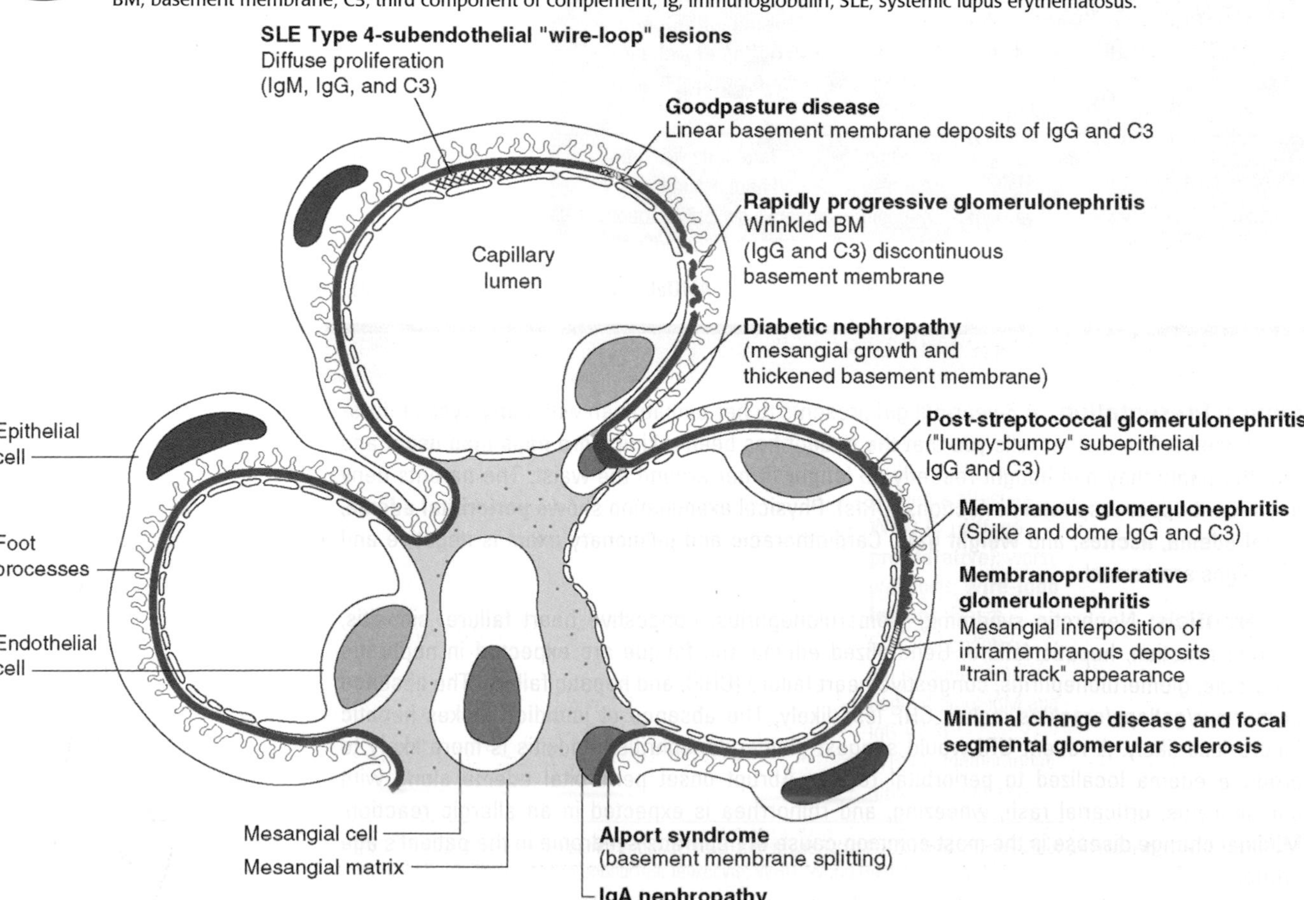

URINARY TRACT INFECTIONS

I. Cystitis

A. Characteristic clinical features
  1. **Dysuria**
  2. **Frequency**
  3. **Urgency**
  4. Suprapubic pain

B. Etiology and pathogenesis
  1. Bacteria gain access to the urinary tract via the urethra.
  2. Cystitis most frequently involves normal colonic flora.
     a. ***Escherichia coli*** is the most common cause (approximately 80%).
     b. *Proteus*, *Klebsiella*, and *Enterobacter* are also implicated.
     c. *Staphylococcus saprophyticus* causes 10% to 15% of infections in young women.
  3. **Women** have a higher incidence of infection because they have shorter urethras.
  4. Other risk factors include sexual activity, pregnancy, urinary obstruction, neurogenic bladder, and vesicoureteral reflux.

C. Diagnostic findings
  1. Characteristic clinical features are present.
  2. **Pyuria** (more than 8 leukocytes/high-power field).
  3. Bacterial culture yields **greater than 10^5 organisms/mL**.

D. Treatment
  1. Cystitis is treated with antibiotics.
  2. Recurrent cystitis may require prophylactic antibiotics.

MNEMONIC

To remember the most common pathogens of UTIs, think **KEEPS: *Klebsiella***, *Enterobacter*, ***E.*** *coli*, ***P****roteus*, ***S.*** *saprophyticus*.

II. Acute pyelonephritis

A. **Characteristic clinical features**
  1. **Flank pain** or **costovertebral angle tenderness**
  2. **Dysuria**
  3. **Fever**
  4. Chills
  5. Nausea and vomiting
  6. Diarrhea

B. Etiology and pathogenesis
  1. Bacteria **ascend** from an infected urinary bladder to the kidney via the **vesicoureteral** reflux.
  2. Infection may also spread **hematogenously** to the kidney (may not necessarily be preceded by acute cystitis).
  3. Causative organism is usually *E. coli*.

C. **Diagnostic findings**
  1. Characteristic clinical features are present.
  2. Bacteriuria, pyuria, and **white blood cell casts** are seen on urine microscopy.
  3. Urine and blood cultures are performed to determine infection.

D. Treatment
  1. Treatment is with **antibiotics**, often **intravenously**.
  2. Recurrent infection can lead to chronic pyelonephritis. This condition has several complications:
     a. **Scarring and deformity of the renal pelvis and calyces**
     b. Interstitial fibrosis and tubular atrophy
     c. Ischemia of the tubules leading to microscopic "**thyroidization**" of the kidney

MAJOR CAUSES OF ACUTE RENAL FAILURE (Figure 6-10)

I. Prerenal failure is defined as oliguria and an increase in BUN and creatinine with inherently normal renal function.

QUICK HIT: COX is inhibited by aspirin and other nonsteroidal anti-inflammatory drugs (NSAIDs), but not by acetaminophen (APAP).

QUICK HIT: Acute renal failure and acute tubular necrosis are often used synonymously. However, acute renal failure can occur without acute tubular necrosis.

QUICK HIT: Fractional excretion of Na^+ is calculated using the formula:

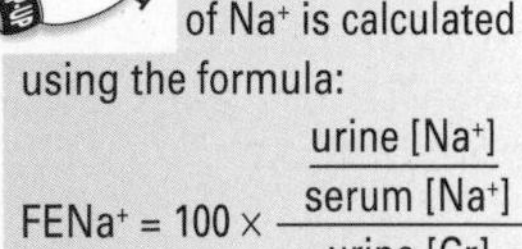

$$FENa^+ = 100 \times \frac{\dfrac{\text{urine }[Na^+]}{\text{serum }[Na^+]}}{\dfrac{\text{urine }[Cr]}{\text{serum }[Cr]}}$$

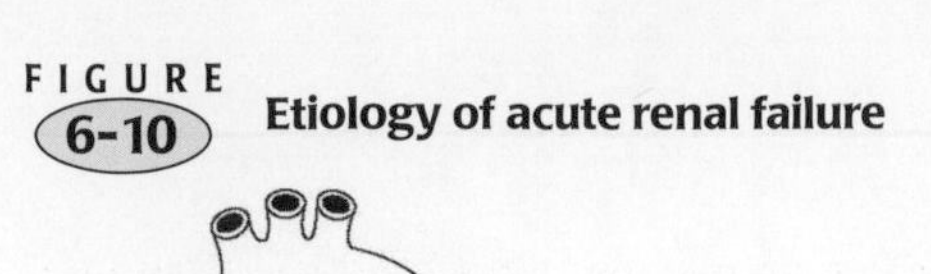

FIGURE 6-10 Etiology of acute renal failure

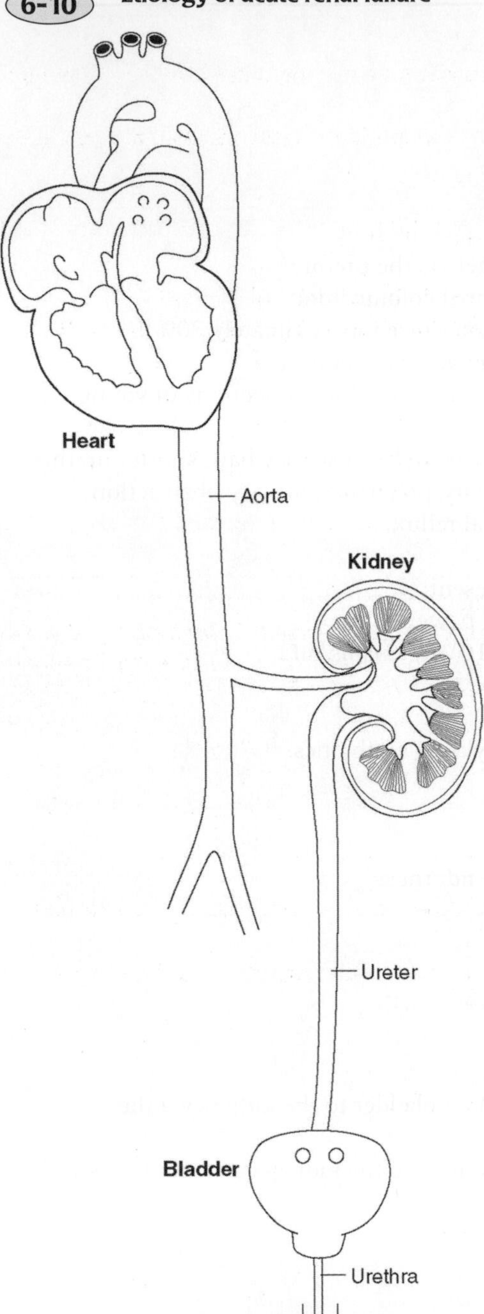

A. Hypovolemic states
   1. Hemorrhage
   2. Burns
   3. Dehydration
   4. Vomiting
   5. Diarrhea
   6. Diuretics
   7. Pancreatitis
B. Low cardiac output states
   1. Arrhythmias
   2. Pulmonary embolus

3. Myocardial or valvular disease
4. Cardiac tamponade
5. Pulmonary hypertension

C. **Renal vasoconstrictive states** resulting in ischemia may be caused by the following:
1. Cirrhosis with ascites
2. Vasoconstrictive drugs: epinephrine, norepinephrine, cyclosporine, amphotericin B

D. Intrinsic decrease of renal perfusion
1. Cyclo-oxygenase (COX) inhibitors
2. Angiotensin-converting enzyme (ACE) inhibitors

II. Acute intrinsic renal failure is the inherent malfunction of the renal tissue. It may be glomerular, tubular, or interstitial. Table 6-8 compares prerenal failure with intrinsic renal failure.

A. Acute tubular necrosis (ATN)
1. Drugs that may lead to ATN are exogenous toxins (contrast, cyclosporine, aminoglycosides, ethylene glycol, acetaminophen, heavy metals) or endogenous toxins (myoglobin, uric acid, oxalate).
2. Ischemia can result in ATN via causes related to prerenal failure.

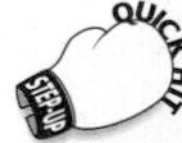

Sheehan syndrome (pituitary necrosis) is also caused by postpartum hemorrhage and leads to the loss of gonadotropins, thyroid-stimulating hormone (TSH), and ACTH, which clinically manifests as fatigue, weight loss, and amenorrhea.

TABLE 6-8 Prerenal Versus Intrinsic Renal Failure

	Prerenal Renal Failure	Intrinsic Renal Failure
Fractional excretion of Na^+	<1	>1
Urine sodium concentration	<10 mg/dL	>20 mg/dL
Urine creatinine to plasma creatinine	>40	>20
Urine casts	Hyaline	Muddy brown and granular
Plasma blood-urea-nitrogen-to-creatinine ratio	>20	<10–15

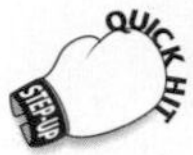

HUS and TTP cause a "flea-bitten" kidney.

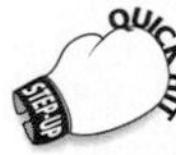

The most **common** cause of acute renal failure (ARF) is therapeutic drugs.

B. Obstruction of renal vasculature from atherosclerosis, vasculitis, or other factors may also cause acute intrinsic renal failure.

C. Diseases that affect the glomeruli or microvasculature include the following:
1. Disseminated intravascular coagulopathy (DIC)
2. Glomerulonephritis
3. Hemolytic uremic syndrome (HUS)
4. Thrombotic thrombocytopenic purpura (TTP)
5. Pregnancy
6. Scleroderma
7. Systemic lupus erythematosus (SLE)

D. **Interstitial nephritis** can have many causes
1. β-Lactams
2. Sulfonamides
3. Trimethoprim (TMP)
4. Rifampin
5. COX inhibitors
6. Diuretics
7. Captopril
8. Infection
9. Idiopathic

E. Acute renal transplant rejection is a cause of ATN.

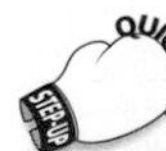

Renal transplant rejection rates can be decreased by administration of cyclosporine and muromonab-CD3 (OKT3).

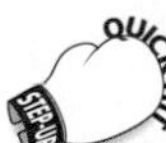

Finasteride, a 5α-reductase inhibitor, is used to treat benign prostatic hyperplasia (BPH). Cold medicines and α-agonists exacerbate BPH.

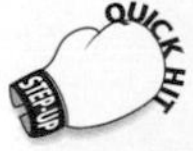

Uremia causes burr cells. Burr cells are misshapen red blood cells (RBCs) with irregular fingerlike projections from their surface.

III. Postrenal failure is bilateral obstruction of the ureters or obstruction of the urethra. It accounts for less than 5% of acute renal failure (ARF) and has a variety of causes.

A. Urolithiasis (see section on stone formation)
B. Prostatic hyperplasia
C. Tumor obstructing the bladder or the ureters bilaterally
D. Neurogenic bladder

CHRONIC RENAL FAILURE AND UREMIA (Figure 6-11)

I. Major causes of chronic renal failure (CRF)

A. Hypertension

B. Diabetes mellitus

II. Profound loss of renal function leads to uremia

A. GFR is reduced to 50% to 65% of normal.

B. Byproducts of amino acid and protein metabolism (especially urea) cause a variety of signs and symptoms

1. **Endocrine and electrolyte findings**
   a. Hyperkalemia
   b. Hypertriglyceridemia
   c. Hyperuricemia
   d. Hypocalcemia and osteomalacia as a result of decreased 1,25-dihydroxycholecalciferol levels
   e. Impaired growth and development
   f. Infertility and sexual dysfunction
   g. Metabolic acidosis
2. **Gastrointestinal findings**
   a. Anorexia
   b. Nausea
   c. Peptic ulcer
   d. Vomiting

FIGURE 6-11 **Manifestations of chronic renal failure and uremia**
BUN, blood urea nitrogen.

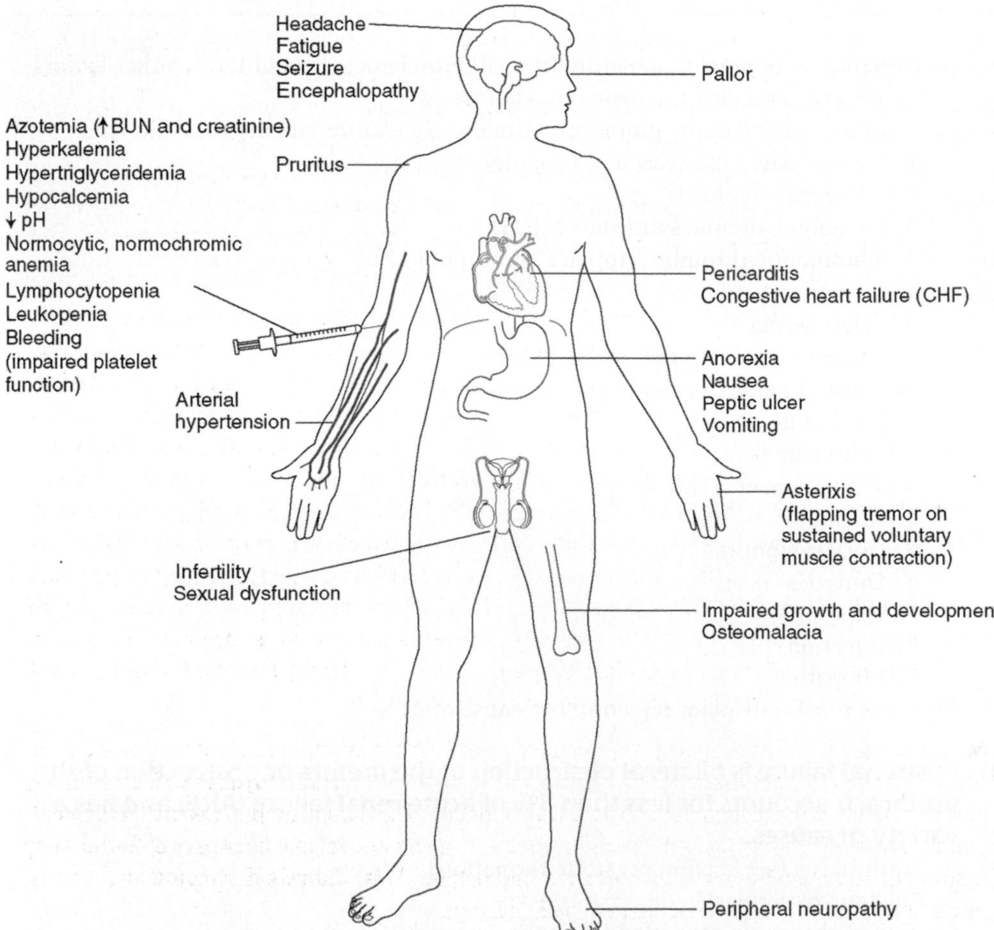

3. **Renal findings:** azotemia
4. **Cardiovascular and pulmonary findings**
   a. Arterial hypertension
   b. Congestive heart failure
   c. Pericarditis
5. **Dermatologic findings**
   a. Pallor
   b. Pruritus
6. **Neuromuscular findings**
   a. Asterixis
   b. Headache and fatigue
   c. Peripheral neuropathy
7. **Hematologic findings**
   a. Increased susceptibility to infection
   b. Lymphocytopenia and leukopenia
   c. Normocytic, normochromic anemia

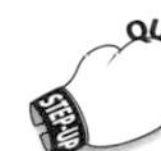

Exogenous toxins causing acute tubular necrosis include contrast, cyclosporine, ethylene glycol, and acetaminophen. Endogenous toxins include myoglobin, uric acid, and oxalate.

Clinical Vignette 6-3

Clinical Presentation: A 55-year-old female presents to her primary care physician with the chief complaint of **nausea, vomiting,** and **feeling "out of it"** over the past 2 days. She also reports **urinating less frequently** and **weight gain,** although she does not have much of an appetite. Her past medical history is significant for **CHF.** Physical examination reveals generalized edema and a 10-lb weight gain since her last visit 1 month ago.

Differentials: Acute renal failure, chronic renal failure, acute tubular necrosis. Acute renal failure is defined as rapid, progressive decrease in renal function characterized by elevation in blood urea nitrogen/creatinine (BUN/Cr) and possibly oliguria. Renal failure can be prerenal, intrinsic renal, or postrenal. Prerenal failure is caused by insufficient renal perfusion as in CHF, whereas postrenal failure is caused by obstructed renal outflow. Intrinsic renal failure is caused by parenchymal damage to the glomerulus, tubules, interstitium, or vasculature. There are a number of causes for each type of renal failure (Figure 6-10). In this patient, hypovolemia from CHF is the cause of insufficient renal perfusion. Acute tubular necrosis causes 85% of intrinsic renal failure, but we would expect some history of renal ischemia or toxin exposure (see Quick Hit). Chronic renal failure has lab findings in common with acute renal failure, but we would expect clinical manifestations of uremia and multiple instances of abnormal BUN, Cr, and urinalysis.

Laboratory Studies: A urinalysis would be obtained looking for the presence of casts. Presence of muddy brown casts (seen in acute tubular necrosis), red blood cell (RBC) casts (glomerular disease), or white blood cell (WBC) casts (pyelonephritis, acute interstitial nephritis) would not be expected in acute renal failure. **Urine chemistry** consisting of BUN/Cr, fractional excretion of sodium (FE_{Na}), and urine osmolality would also be obtained. In prerenal and postrenal failure, the **BUN:Cr ratio** is typically greater than 20:1 because of increased urea absorption as compared to intrinsic renal failure. In prerenal failure, the **FE_{Na}** is less than 1% because the decreased glomerular filtration rate causes massive reabsorption of sodium and water, whereas in intrinsic renal failure, the FE_{Na} is greater than 2% to 3% because Na is poorly reabsorbed. Similarly, we expect increased **urine osmolality** in prerenal failure because the kidney is able to reabsorb water, whereas we see decreased urine osmolality in intrinsic renal failure because renal water reabsorption is impaired. Also, **renal ultrasound** would be obtained to rule out obstruction. Renal ultrasound showing small, echogenic kidneys are pathognomic of chronic renal failure (CRF).

Management: The most important part of therapy is to follow urinary output: acute renal failure (ARF) patients first experience an **oliguric phase** followed by a **diuretic phase.** Approximately 40% of patients go on to a **recovery phase** with normalization of urine output. **Correct fluid imbalance**—some ARF patients are dehydrated whereas others are volume overloaded. Correct any **electrolyte abnormalities** and **optimize cardiac output.** Order **dialysis** if symptomatic uremia, acidemia, hyperkalemia, or volume overload develops.

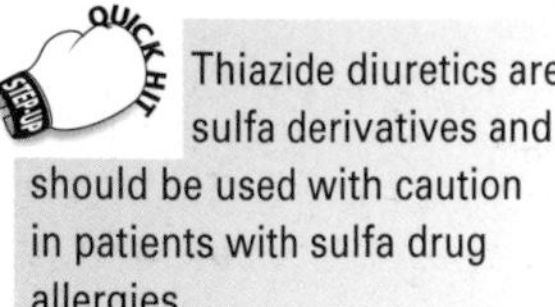
Thiazide diuretics are sulfa derivatives and should be used with caution in patients with sulfa drug allergies.

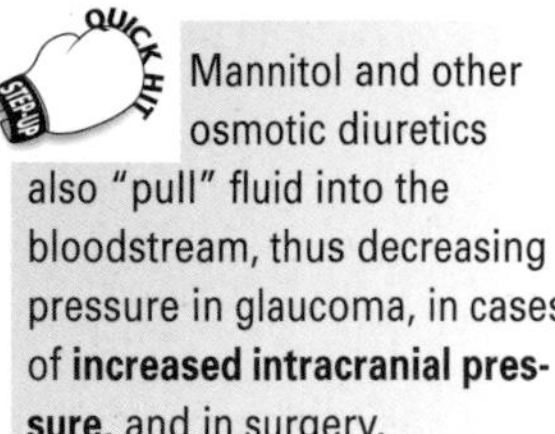
Mannitol and other osmotic diuretics also "pull" fluid into the bloodstream, thus decreasing pressure in glaucoma, in cases of **increased intracranial pressure**, and in surgery.

THERAPEUTIC AGENTS

I. Effects of diuretics on the nephron (Figure 6-14)

A. The **diuretics** in Figure 6-14 can be grouped into five main categories, each with a different mechanism of action (Table 6-10). The side effects of each type of diuretic are also different, which means that certain diuretics are better suited for certain patients.

B. **ADH** causes an increase in the expression of **water channels** in the collecting tubule, which results in an increase in the reabsorption of water. Urine output drops, and concentration increases.

1. In the syndrome of inappropriate secretion of antidiuretic hormone (SIADH), **lithium** or **demeclocycline**, which blocks the effects of ADH, can be administered to prevent excessive water retention.
2. In central diabetes insipidus, either **desmopressin**, an ADH analog, or ADH can be given to prevent the excessive loss of dilute urine. These drugs are not useful in the nephrogenic (also known as the peripheral) form of diabetes insipidus in which the kidneys do not respond to ADH.

FIGURE 6-14 **Effects of diuretics on the nephron**
Cl^-, chloride; DCT, distal convoluted tubule; HCO_3^-, bicarbonate; JGA, juxtaglomerular apparatus; K^+, potassium; Na^+, sodium; PCT, proximal convoluted tubule.

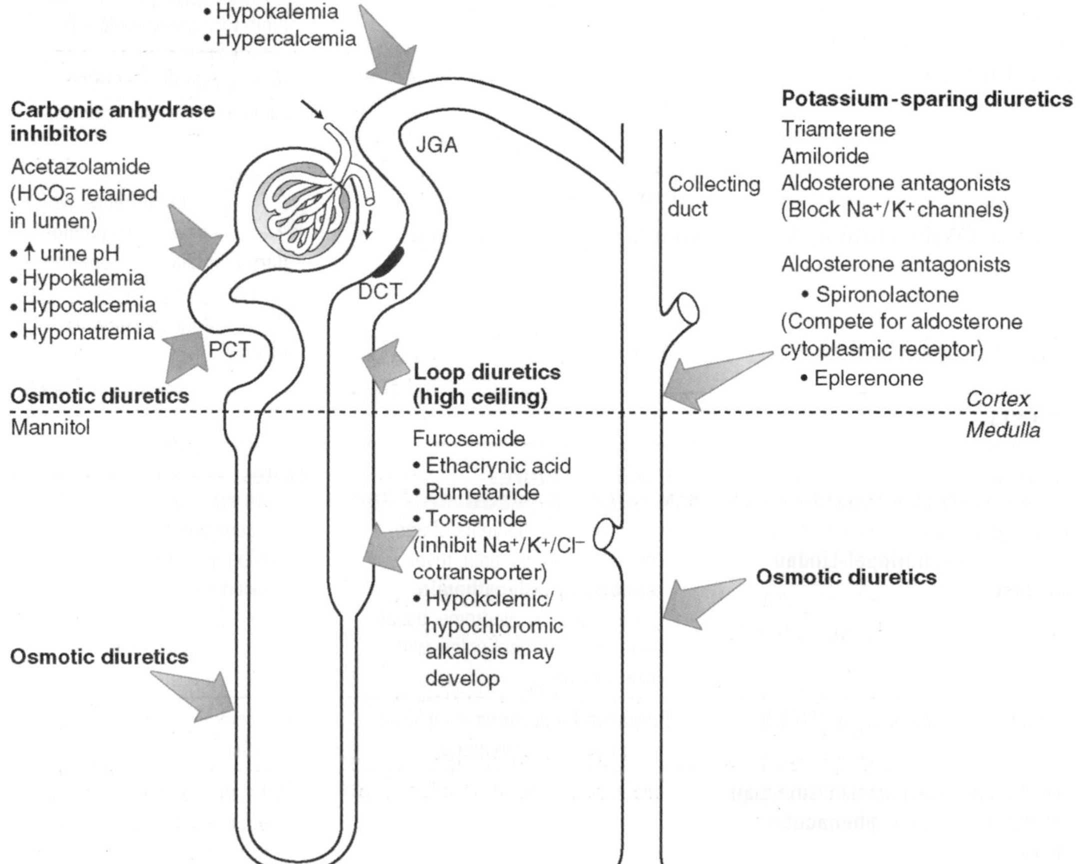

TABLE 6-10 Diuretics

Therapeutic Agent	Mechanism of Action	Electrolytes Lost in Urine	Indications	Side Effects	Notes
Acetazolamide	Carbonic anhydrase inhibitors—Inhibit carbonic anhydrase in **PCT,** which prevents HCO_3^- reabsorption	Na^+, HCO_3^-, K^+	Glaucoma, urinary alkalinization, metabolic alkalosis, altitude sickness	**Hyperchloremic metabolic acidosis**, **sulfa drug allergy**, neuropathy, ammonium toxicity	Causes decreased secretion of HCO_3^- in aqueous humor
Furosemide	Loop diuretic—Prevents cotransport of Na^+, K^+, and Cl^- in **thick ascending limb**	Na^+, Cl^-, Ca^{2+}, K^+	**Congestive heart failure**, Cirrhosis, Nephrotic syndrome, pulmonary edema, hypertension, hypercalcemia	**Ototoxicity**, **hypokalemic metabolic alkalosis**, dehydration, **sulfa drug allergy**, nephritis, gout	Has rapid onset and short duration of action, which is ideal for relieving acute edema
Mannitol	Osmotic diuretic—Prevents isosmotic reabsorption of filtrate in **PCT, loop of Henle,** and **collecting tubule**	Na^+ and all other filtered solutes	Shock, drug overdose, decrease intracranial or intraocular pressure; maintenance of urine flow in rhabdomyolysis	Pulmonary edema, dehydration; contraindicated in anuria and congestive heart failure	Results in increased urine volume; readily filtered and not reabsorbed
Spironolactone, Triamterene, Amiloride, Eplerenone	Potassium sparing diuretics—Bind to intracellular aldosterone steroid receptors in **collecting tubules**; blocks induction of Na^+ channels and Na^+/ATPase synthesis or block Na^+ channels directly (amiloride, tramterene)	Na^+, Cl^-	Hyperaldosteronism, potassium depletion, congestive heart failure	**Hyperkalemic metabolic acidosis**, **gynecomastia** (spironolactone), antiandrogen effects	Results in decreased secretion of K^+ and H^+, which can lead to **hyperkalemic metabolic acidosis;** often given in combination with a thiazide
Hydrochlorothiazide	Thiazides—Inhibit transport of Na^+ and Cl^- into cells of **DCT**	Na^+, Cl^-, K^+	Hypertension, congestive heart failure, idiopathic hypercalciuria, nephrogenic diabetes insipidus	**Hypokalemic metabolic alkalosis**, hyponatremia, **hyperglycemia**, **hyperlipidemia**, hyperuricemia, hypercalcemia, **sulfa drug allergy**	Causes decreased Ca^{2+} excretion, can lead to K^+ wasting with chronic therapy
Ethacrynic acid	Phenoxyacetic acid derivative— Prevents cotransport of Na^+, K^+, and Cl^- in **thick ascending limb**	Na^+, Cl^-, Ca^{2+}, K^+	**Diuresis in patients with sulfa drug allergy**	**Ototoxicity**, **hypokalemic metabolic alkalosis**, dehydration	**Can be given to patients with sulfa drug allergy**, hyperuricemia, acute gout

ATPase, adenosine triphosphatase; Ca^{2+}, calcium; Cl^-, chloride; DCT, distal convoluted tubule; PCT, proximal convoluted tubule.

II. Gout is a condition in which uric acid crystals in joints trigger intermittent inflammatory reactions. The etiologic process can be blocked at different stages (Table 6-11).

A. Inhibition of the production of uric acid from the breakdown of DNA **purines**
B. Increased excretion of uric acid in the urine
C. Blunting the body's **inflammatory response** to the gout crystals (the body's reaction to gout crystals actually causes the pain and damage associated with gout)

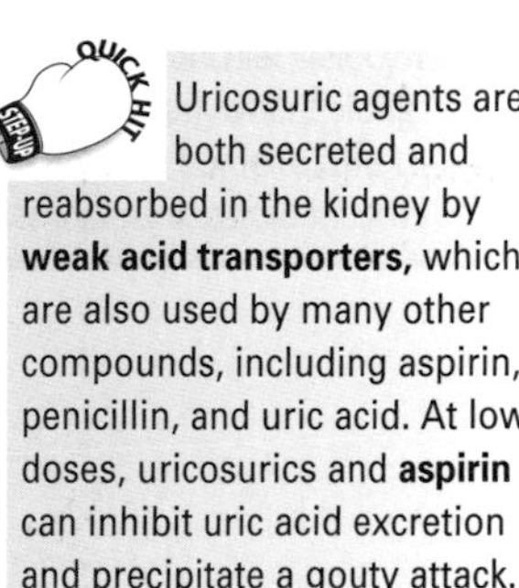

Uricosuric agents are both secreted and reabsorbed in the kidney by **weak acid transporters,** which are also used by many other compounds, including aspirin, penicillin, and uric acid. At low doses, uricosurics and **aspirin** can inhibit uric acid excretion and precipitate a gouty attack.

FIGURE 7-2 Hormones of the adrenal gland

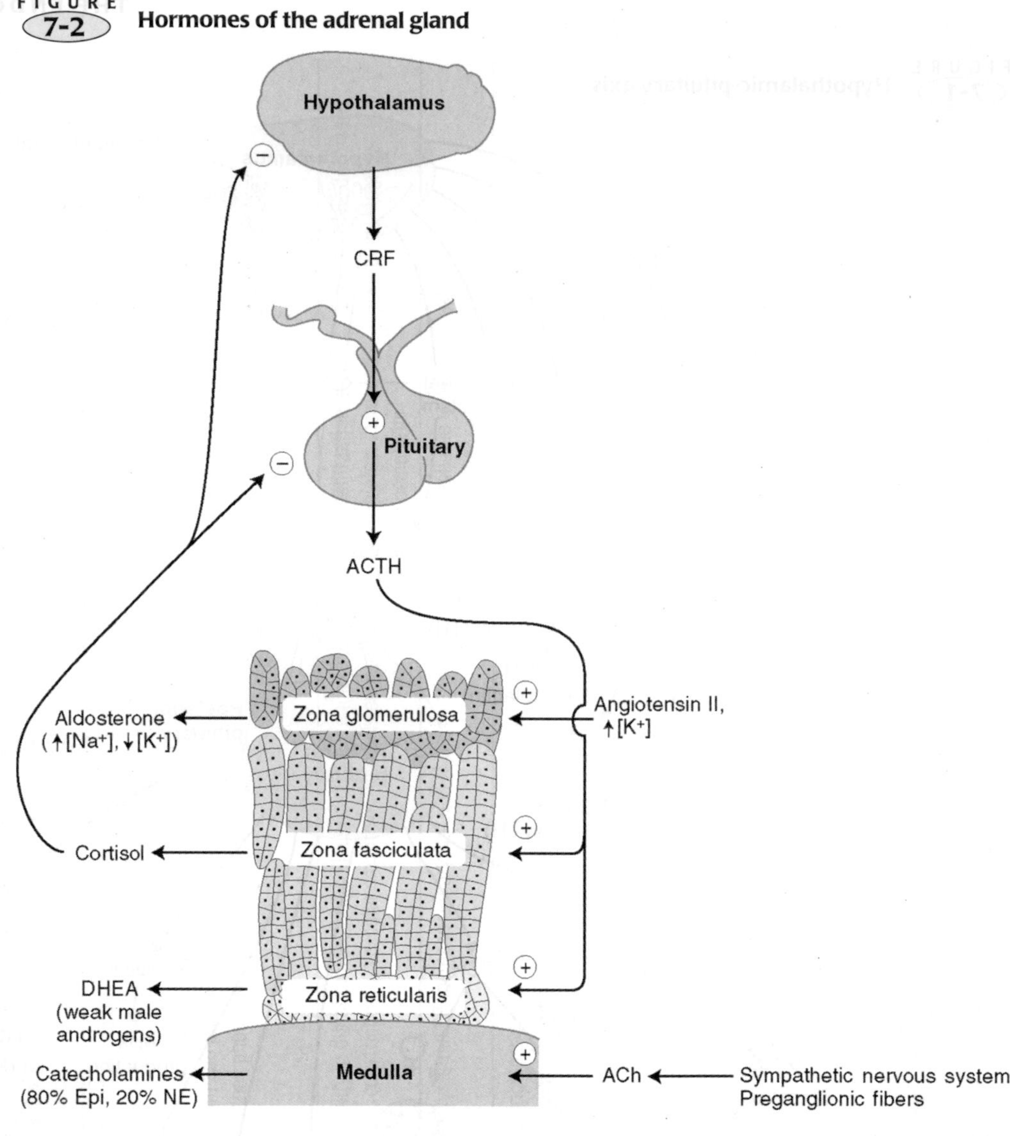

TABLE 7-3 **Hormone Second Messenger Systems**

cAMP	cGMP	IP3	Steroid	Tyrosine Kinase
β_1-agonists	ANF	α_1-agonists	Aldosterone	Insulin
β_2-agonists	EDRF	GnRH	Estrogen	IGF-1
LH		TRH	Glucocorticoids	Prolactin
FSH		GHRH	Testosterone	GH
TSH		Angiotensin II	Progesterone	
ADH (V2)		ADH (V1)	Thyroid	
hCG		Oxytocin	Vitamin D	
CRH				
PTH				
Calcitonin				
Glucagon				

ADH, antidiuretic hormone; ANF, atrial natriuretic factor (also known as ANP, atrial natriuretic peptide); cAMP, cyclic adenosine monophosphate; cGMP, cyclic guanine monophosphate; CRH, corticotropin-releasing hormone; EDRF, endothelium-derived relaxing factor; FSH, follicle stimulating hormone; GH, growth hormone; GHRH, growth hormone-releasing factor; GnRH, gonadotropin-releasing hormone; hCG, human chorionic gonadotropin; IGF, insulin-like growth factor; IP3, inositol-1,4,5-triphosphate; LH, luteinizing hormone; PTH, parathyroid hormone; TRH, thyrotropin-releasing hormone; TSH, thyroid-stimulating hormone.

FIGURE 7-3 **Hormone second-messenger systems**

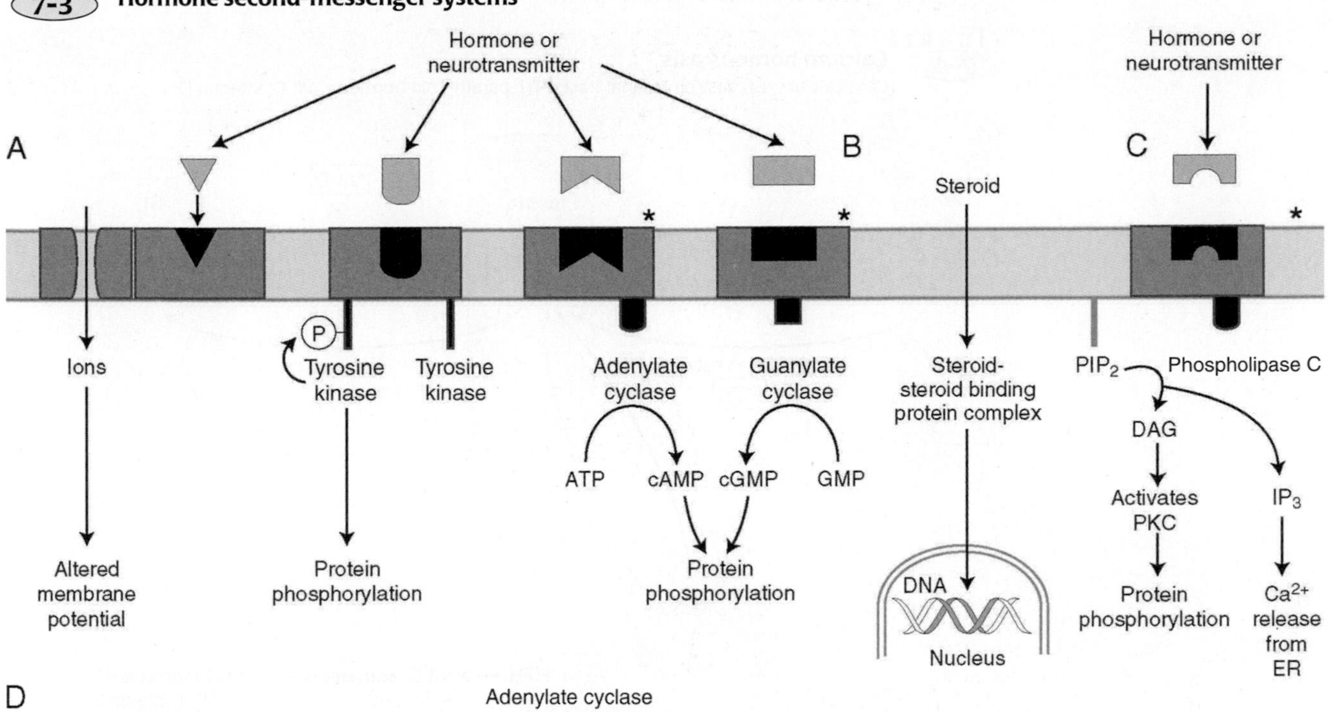

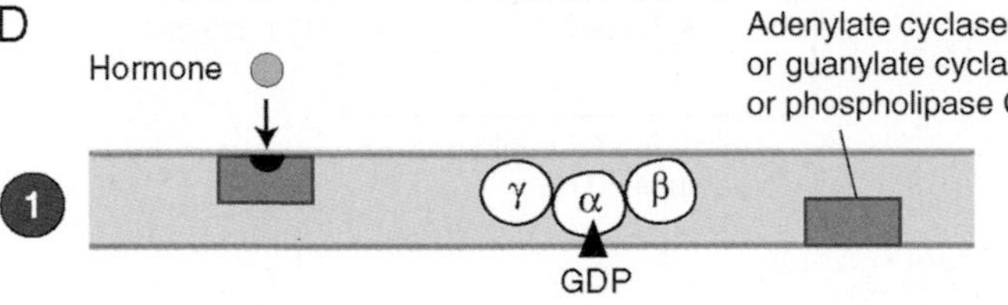

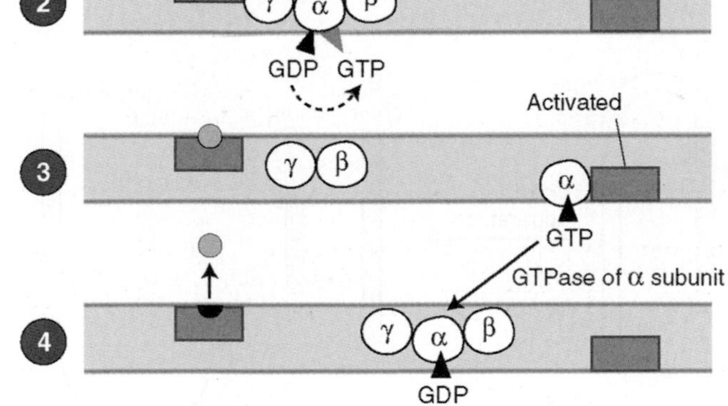

A. Peptide mechanism. Peptide binds to hormone receptor site and influences various second messenger systems. These hormones are typically short-acting and do not involve gene regulation, in contrast to steroid hormones, which have a slower onset of action.

B. Steroid mechanism. Lipid-soluble steroid penetrates cell membrane and binds to steroid binding protein. This complex enters the nucleus and influences DNA synthesis.

C. Phospholipase C mechanism.

D. G-protein mechanism.
1. Messenger system before hormone binding.
2. After hormone binding, GTP replaces GDP on G-protein.
3. GTP, attached to α subunit, dissociates from the β–γ complex and converts ATP to cAMP.
4. Hormone is released from binding site and complex returns to inactive state when GTPase cleaves GTP to GDP.

*Mechanism utilizing a G-protein, as shown in D

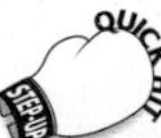

Glucose enters cells through facilitated transporters designated GLUT-1 through GLUT-5. These transporters have the following locations:
GLUT 1: Erythrocytes, blood–brain barrier
GLUT 2: Liver, kidney, pancreatic β cell, intestinal mucosa
GLUT 3: Neurons
GLUT 4*: Adipose tissue, skeletal and cardiac muscle
GLUT 5: Intestinal epithelium
*insulin-responsive transport to membrane

tissue and stimulates glucose absorption and triacylglycerol synthesis. In the liver, insulin inhibits gluconeogenesis and glycogen breakdown.

Insulin is formed from two polypeptides linked by disulfide bridges (Figure 7-5). The insulin receptor is **tyrosine kinase** linked; binding of insulin to the α subunit causes phosphorylation of the tyrosine kinase connected to the β subunit. This stimulates recruitment of glucose transporters (GLUTs) to the cell membrane (GLUT-4 in skeletal muscle) and increases the uptake of glucose (Figure 7-6). Glucagon counteracts the actions of insulin. It is a single polypeptide secreted by the β cells of the islets of Langerhans. Glucagon is secreted in response to low blood glucose increased amino acids in the blood and epinephrine and leads to a rise in blood glucose concentration via **gluconeogenesis** and **glycogenolysis.** Release of glucagon is inhibited by insulin. Glucagon is also responsible for the formation of ketone bodies and increased uptake of amino acids by the liver muscle is not responsive to glucagon.

- **Blood Levels of Insulin and Glucagon after a High Carbohydrate Meal** (Figure 7-7)

FIGURE 7-4 **Calcium homeostasis**
Ca^{2+}, calcium; GI, gastrointestinal tract; PTH, parathyroid hormone; Vit D, vitamin D.

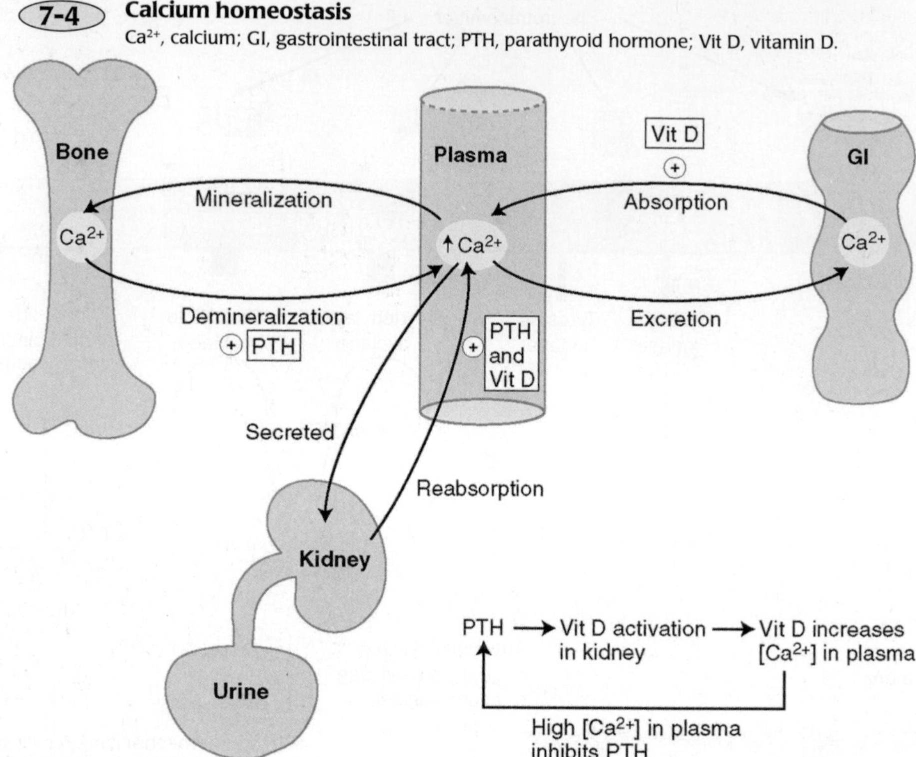

FIGURE 7-5 **Formation of insulin**

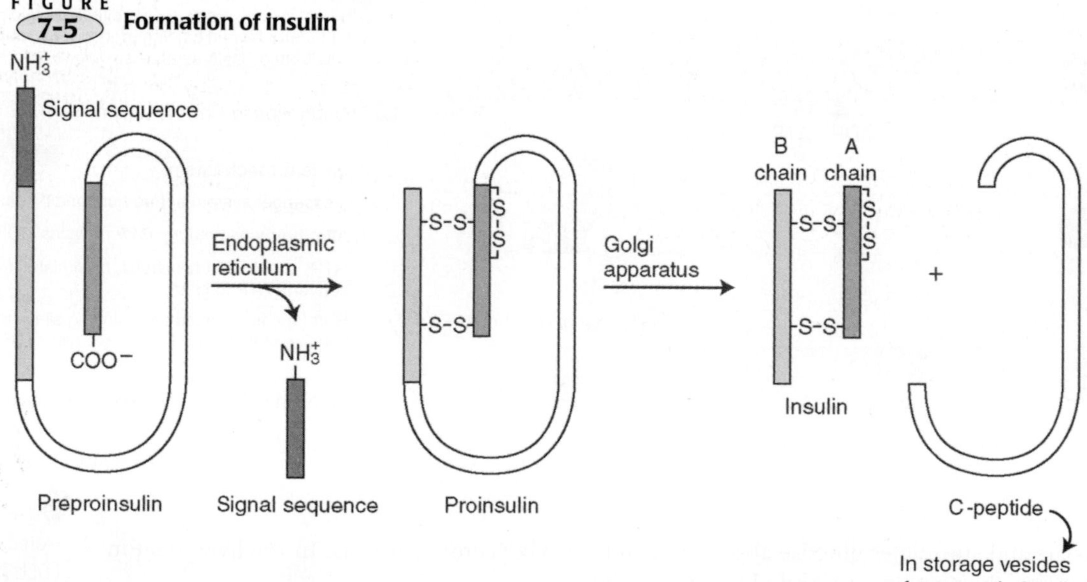

BLOOD GLUCOSE LEVELS

I. Hypoglycemia

A. Causes
   1. Excess insulin administration (in a diabetic patient)
   2. Sulfonylurea administration
   3. Alcohol ingestion
   4. Insulinoma
   5. Factitious hyperinsulinism

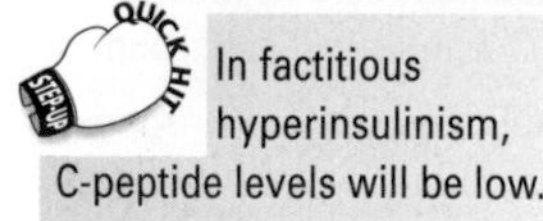

In factitious hyperinsulinism, C-peptide levels will be low.

FIGURE 7-6 Insulin recruitment of glucose transporters

(Adapted with permission from Champe PC, Harvey RA. Lippincott's Illustrated Reviews: Biochemistry. 2nd Ed. Philadelphia, PA: Lippincott-Raven, 1994:274.)

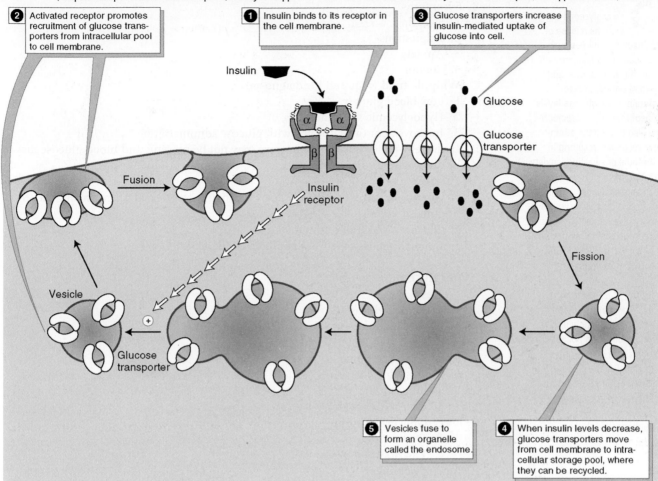

❷ Activated receptor promotes recruitment of glucose transporters from intracellular pool to cell membrane.

❶ Insulin binds to its receptor in the cell membrane.

❸ Glucose transporters increase insulin-mediated uptake of glucose into cell.

Insulin

α α

S-S

β β

Glucose

Glucose transporter

Fusion

Insulin receptor

Fission

Vesicle

Glucose transporter

❺ Vesicles fuse to form an organelle called the endosome.

❹ When insulin levels decrease, glucose transporters move from cell membrane to intracellular storage pool, where they can be recycled.

FIGURE 7-7 Blood levels of glucose, insulin, and glucagon after a high-carbohydrate meal

(Adapted with permission from Champe PC, Harvey RA. Lippincott's Illustrated Reviews: Biochemistry. 2nd Ed. Philadelphia, PA: Lippincott-Raven, 1994:272.)

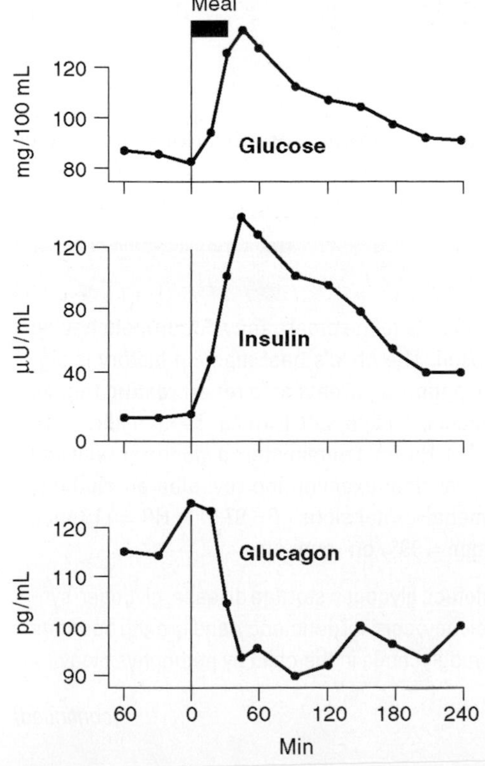

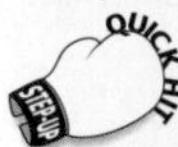

Hypoglycemia triggers the release of anti-insulin hormones such as glucagon, cortisol, growth hormone, epinephrine, and norepinephrine, to help maintain blood glucose levels. Epinephrine and norepinephrine also turn on the adrenergic response, resulting in symptoms of sweating, anxiety, palpitations, and tremor. Decreased availability of glucose to the central nervous system (CNS) eventually results in neuroglycopenic symptoms of lethargy, confusion, slurred speech, coma, and death.

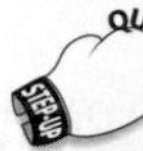

Hyperinsulinemic state results in low ketone production because insulin shuts down lipolysis at the level of the adipose cell, decreasing the amount of fatty acids released into the blood stream, which decreases the substrate for ketone production.

B. **Symptoms**
  1. Sweating
  2. Palpitations
  3. Anxiety
  4. Tremor

C. **Whipple triad** (required for diagnosis)
  1. Low blood glucose
  2. Hypoglycemic symptoms
  3. Improvement of symptoms with glucose administration

D. In diabetic patients, these symptoms may not be present, and blood glucose may be allowed to drop to dangerous levels; coma or death may result.

E. Therapy
  1. Glucose or intravenous (IV) dextrose should be given after measuring blood glucose levels.
  2. Glucagon should be administered.
  3. Epinephrine is sometimes appropriate therapy.

II. Hyperglycemia

A. Causes
  1. Diabetes mellitus
  2. Chronic pancreatitis
  3. Acromegaly
  4. Cushing syndrome
  5. Adverse drug reactions
     a. Furosemide
     b. Glucocorticoids
     c. Growth hormone
     d. Oral contraceptives
     e. Thiazides

B. Acute symptoms
  1. Ketoacidosis or hyperosmolar nonketotic coma
  2. Polyuria
  3. Polydipsia
  4. Polyphagia
  5. Weight loss
  6. Encephalopathy
     a. Tremulousness
     b. Convulsions
     c. Coma

The chronic symptoms of hyperglycemia mimic the chronic complications of diabetes (Table 7-7).

Clinical Vignette 7-1

Clinical Presentation: A 4-year-old male child presents to the emergency department having woken up this morning feeling **lethargic** and **confused.** The child's past medical history is significant for two prior episodes of hypoglycemia. The patient's parents also report **resting tremor.** Mother denies **seizure activity, loss of consciousness,** and recent trauma. Mother did urine dipstick, which showed glucose level of 42 mg/dL (low). Parents administered glucose orally and brought the patient to the emergency department. Physical examination revealed an **anxious, diaphoretic** child with **slurred speech.** No hepatomegaly. Vital signs: T = 97.5 °F; HR = 119 bpm; RR = 30 breaths/min; BP = 109/55 mm Hg; O_2 saturation = 99% on room air.

Differentials: Hyperinsulinism, fatty acid oxidation defect, glycogen storage disease, glycogen synthesis defect, gluconeogenesis defect, glucagon deficiency, cortisol deficiency, and growth hormone deficiency. Figure 7-8 groups the various causes of hypoglycemia in the child by pathophysiology.

(continued)

Clinical Vignette 7-1 *(Continued)*

Laboratory Studies: Urine ketones should be assessed via urinalysis. If urine ketones are low, it indicates the presence of a hyperinsulinemic state or a defect in fatty acid oxidation (resulting in an inability to produce ketones). These are best differentiated by obtaining an **insulin level.** If urine ketones are high, further workup is necessary to differentiate liver metabolism from endocrine defects. Consequently, **serum lactate, pyruvate, liver function tests,** and **uric acid** levels should be obtained to help rule out possibilities such as maple syrup urine disease, glycogenolysis defect, glycogen storage disease, and gluconeogenesis defect. Also, **serum cortisol** levels should be obtained to rule out cortisol deficiency. Eventually, the patient should be screened for **growth hormone** and **pituitary hormones.**

Management: Key point is to **treat first** and evaluate lab studies later. After blood samples are drawn, a quick bedside glucose reading should be done. If hypoglycemia is mild and the patient is able to tolerate oral dosing, treat with **oral glucose.** If severe hypoglycemia occurs and/or if the patient is unable to tolerate oral dosing, provide dextrose bolus followed by appropriate **maintenance infusion.**

FIGURE 7-8 **Causes of hypoglycemia**

1. Decreased intake
   - Fasting
   - Malnutrition

2. Decreased absorption
   - Acute diarrhea

Intake → Blood glucose

Absorption → Blood glucose

3. Decreased glycogen reserves
   - Defect in enzymes of glycogen synthesis pathway

4. Inability to mobilize glycogen
   - Glucagon deficiency

5. Ineffective glycogenolysis
   - Defect in enzyme of glucogenolytic pathway

Glycogen stores → Glycogenolysis → Blood glucose

6. Decreased or absent fat stores

7. Ineffective gluconeogenesis
   - Enzymatic defect in gluconeogenic pathway
   - Enzymatic defect in fatty acid oxidation

Alternative fuels (fatty acids, amino acids) → Gluconeogenesis → Blood glucose

Blood glucose → Utilization by peripheral tissues

8. Hyperinsulinism
   - Islet cell adenoma
   - Oral hypoglycemic agents
   - Insulin therapy

9. Anti-insulin deficiency
   - Cortisol deficiency
   - Growth hormone deficiency
   - Hypopituitarism

10. Increased catabolic states
    - Large tumors
    - Illness

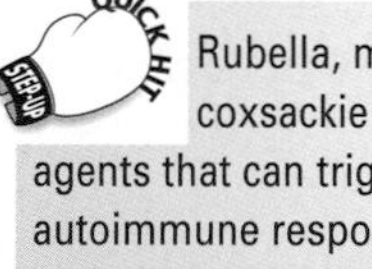

Rubella, mumps, and coxsackie are viral agents that can trigger the autoimmune response of the body to pancreatic β cells and cause type 1 diabetes (also called juvenile-onset diabetes).

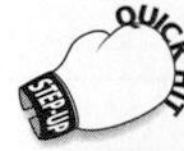

The ketone bodies **(acetoacetate, β-hydroxybutyrate)** are produced by the liver from acetyl coenzyme A (CoA) in the fasting state. The body (including the brain after 4 to 5 days) uses the ketone bodies for energy instead of glucose and amino acids. Red blood cells (RBCs), however, can only use glucose.

DIABETES MELLITUS

Diabetes mellitus (or, simply, diabetes) refers to a group of disorders that are characterized by hyperglycemia and affect 1% to 2% of the US population. Although the pathogenesis of these disorders is varied, individuals with diabetes lack the ability to produce sufficient insulin or respond to secreted insulin in order to meet their metabolic needs. Furthermore, all diabetic patients are vulnerable to complications such as nephropathy, neuropathy, and retinopathy. Monitoring and control of blood sugar, insulin replacement, proper diet, and exercise can significantly reduce the morbidity and mortality of this disease.

I. Diagnosis of diabetes mellitus (Table 7-4)

TABLE 7-4 Diagnosis of Diabetes Mellitus

	Normal	Impaired Glucose Tolerance	Diabetes Mellitus
Fasting blood glucose level	<115 mg/dL	<140 mg/dL	126 mg/dL
		or	or
Blood glucose level after oral glucose tolerance test (OGTT)	<140 mg/dL	140–199 mg/dL	200 mg/dL

II. Table 7-5 compares type 1 with type 2 diabetes mellitus

III. DKA and NKH states (Table 7-6)

IV. Chronic symptoms of diabetes (Table 7-7)

V. Treatment of diabetes mellitus (Table 7-8 and Table 7-9)

The goal of treatment of both type 1 and type 2 diabetes mellitus is steady control of blood glucose levels. However, because the pathogenesis underlying these two disease processes is different, the therapy is also different.

QUICK HIT: IDDM can be distinguished from NIDDM by low C-peptide levels, which also indicates the need for treatment with insulin.

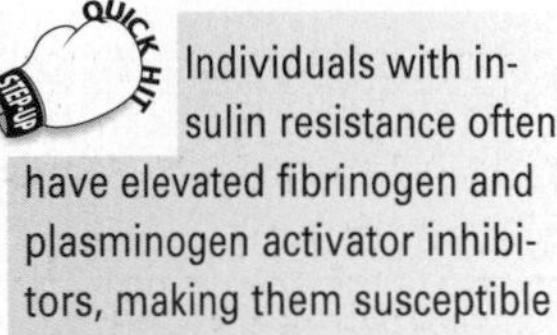

QUICK HIT: Individuals with insulin resistance often have elevated fibrinogen and plasminogen activator inhibitors, making them susceptible to thrombosis.

Type 1 diabetes mellitus, which can be viewed simply as a total deficiency of insulin, may be treated with careful administration of exogenous **insulin**. This agent has been the only treatment option for type 1 diabetes mellitus for many years and remains so today. However, advances have been made in both the type of insulin and the method of delivery. To maintain steady glucose levels, different preparations of human insulin have been designed, each with a characteristic rate of onset and duration of action (Table 7-8). Insulin, a peptide hormone, cannot be given orally. It is typically administered subcutaneously and, in emergencies, intravenously.

TABLE 7-5 Type 1 versus Type 2 Diabetes Mellitus

	Type 1 Diabetes (IDDM) 15%	Type 2 Diabetes (NIDDM) 85%
Cause	Possible **autoimmunity** to β cells triggered by viral cause	Increased **insulin resistance,** decreased receptors, or decreased conversion of proinsulin to insulin
Chromosomal association	6 (HLA-DQ)	Unknown
Family history	Weak predictor	Strong predictor
Age of onset	Younger than 25 years of age	Older than 40 years of age
Body habitus	Normal to thin	Obese
Plasma insulin	Low	Normal to high
Plasma glucagon	High but suppressible	High and resistant to suppression
Pancreas morphology	Atrophy and fibrosis; β-cell depletion	Atrophy and amyloid deposits; variable β-cell population
Acute complication (Table 7-6)	Ketoacidosis	Hyperosmolar nonketotic coma
Common symptoms	**Polydipsia, polyuria, polyphagia (symptoms of hyperglycemia)**	Variable: from asymptomatic to polydipsia, polyuria, and polyphagia
Response to insulin therapy	Responsive	Variable
Response to sulfonylurea therapy	Unresponsive	Responsive

IDDM, insulin-dependent diabetes mellitus; NIDDM, noninsulin-dependent diabetes mellitus.

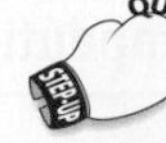

Diabetic ketoacidosis (DKA) and nonketotic hyperosmolar state (NKH) are not mutually exclusive. Patients may present with features of both.

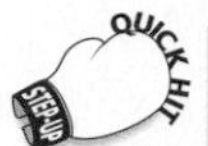

Kussmaul respirations are rapid and deep.

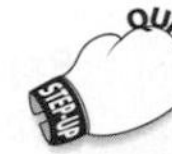

There tends to be minimal ketosis in NKH, because a small amount of insulin is released in these patients to counteract anti-insulin hormones (like glucagon). However, in DKA, there is no release of insulin and nothing to counteract the anti-insulin hormones. This hormonal profile encourages the lipolysis at the adipose cell, churning out fatty acids taken up by the liver for ketone production.

TABLE 7-6 DKA and NKH State

	DKA	NKH
Pathology	Increased serum **ketone bodies** (>2 mmol/L); anion gap metabolic acidosis (pH <7.2); **hyperglycemia** (glucose >300 mg/dL because of increased production and decreased uptake)	**Hyperglycemia** (250–600 mg/dL); **hyperosmolarity** (>320 mg/dL); pH >7.3
Patient	Type 1 (IDDM)	An elderly type 2 (NIDDM) patient
Precipitating event	**50% infection** (look for fever); 25% insufficient insulin	**Decreased ability to sense thirst or obtain enough water;** infection; vascular event (CVA, MI)
Fluid loss	5–7 L	9 L
Clinical presentation	Nausea and vomiting; **Kussmaul respiration;** osmotic diuresis; shock; coma	Usually **coma** if serum osmolarity >350 mg/dL
Mortality	10%	17%
Treatment	Insulin; saline; K^+ replacement	Saline (essential); insulin
Complications	**Cerebral edema;** hyperchloremic (nongap) metabolic acidosis	Dehydration is more severe (older patients have lower body water stores)

CVA, cerebrovascular accident; IDDM, insulin-dependent diabetes mellitus; MI, myocardial infarction; NIDDM, noninsulin-dependent diabetes mellitus.

TABLE 7-7 Chronic Symptoms of Diabetes Mellitus

Anatomic Location	Clinical Features
Red blood cells	**Glycosylation (HbA1c);** measure of long-term control of diabetes (reflects past 3 months)
Blood vessels/Cardiovascular system	**Atherosclerosis;** dyslipidemia; coronary artery disease; gangrene; peripheral vascular disease
Eyes	**Retinopathy;** hemorrhage; hard exudates; cotton-wool spots; cataracts; glaucoma
GI tract	Constipation; **gastroparesis**
Kidneys	Nephropathy; **nodular sclerosis; Kimmelstiel-Wilson nodules;** chronic renal failure; azotemia
Penis	**Impotence** as a result of autonomic neuropathy
Extremities	**Stocking-glove peripheral neuropathy;** nonhealing ulcers

TABLE 7-8 Commonly Used Insulin Preparations

Insulin Preparation	Onset of Activity	Time of Peak Activity	Duration of Action
Lispro insulin	12–30 min	1.5–2.5 h	3–4 h
Aspart insulin	12–30 min	1–3 h	3–5 h
Regular insulin	30 min	2–4 h	6–8 h
NPH (neutral protamine Hagedorn) insulin	1–2 h	6–12 h	18–24 h
Lente insulin	1–3 h	6–12 h	18–24 h
Ultralente insulin	3–4 h	No peak	24 h or longer
Glargine	3–4 h	No peak	24 h or longer

TABLE 7-9 Therapeutic Agents for Diabetes

Therapeutic Agent (common name, if relevant) [trade name, where appropriate]	Class–Pharmacology and Pharmacokinetics	Indications	Side or Adverse Effects	Contraindications or Precautions to Consider; Notes
Insulin				
Lispro [Humalog]	**Rapid acting insulin**—*see mechanism for regular insulin*	**Diabetes mellitus** (typically **Type 1**), **hyperkalemia, stress induced hyperglycemia**	**Hypoglycemia** (diaphoresis, vertigo, tachycardia); insulin allergy; insulin antibodies; lipodystrophy	
Aspart [Novolog]	**Rapid acting insulin**—*see mechanism for regular insulin*	**Diabetes mellitus** (typically **Type 1**), **hyperkalemia, stress induced hyperglycemia**	**Hypoglycemia** (diaphoresis, vertigo, tachycardia); insulin allergy; insulin antibodies; lipodystrophy	
Regular insulin [Humulin R, Novolin R]	**Short acting insulin—Liver:** Promotes glucose storage as glycogen, increases trigylceride synthesis **Muscle:** facilitates protein and glycogen synthesis **Adipose tissue:** improves trigycleride storage by activating plasma lipoprotein lipase; reduces circulating free fatty acids	**Diabetes mellitus** (typically **Type 1**), **hyperkalemia, stress induced hyperglycemia**	**Hypoglycemia** (diaphoresis, vertigo, tachycardia); insulin allergy; insulin antibodies; lipodystrophy	
NPH [Humulin N, Novolin N]	**Intermediate acting insulin**—*see mechanism for insulin*	**Diabetes mellitus** (typically **Type 1**)	**Hypoglycemia** (diaphoresis, vertigo, tachycardia); insulin allergy; insulin antibodies; lipodystrophy	
Lente [Humulin L, Novolin L]	**Intermediate acting insulin**—*see mechanism for regular insulin*	**Diabetes mellitus** (typically **Type 1**)	**Hypoglycemia** (diaphoresis, vertigo, tachycardia); insulin allergy; insulin antibodies; lipodystrophy	
Ultralente [Humulin U, Novolin U]	**Long acting insulin**—*see mechanism for regular insulin*	**Diabetes mellitus** (typically **Type 1**)	**Hypoglycemia** (diaphoresis, vertigo, tachycardia); insulin allergy; insulin antibodies; lipodystrophy	
Glargine [Lantus]	**Long-acting insulin**—*see mechanism for regular insulin*	**Diabetes mellitus** (typically **Type 1**)	**Hypoglycemia** (diaphoresis, vertigo, tachycardia); insulin allergy; insulin antibodies; lipodystrophy	
Sulfonylureas				
Tolubutamide, Chlorpropamide	**First generation sulfonylureas**—closes potassium channel in β-cell membrane → reduces K^+ efflux, increases Ca^{2+} influx → increases secretion of insulin	Oral treatment for **NIDDM (type 2 diabetes)**	**Hypoglycemia;** GI disturbances; muscle weakness; mental confusion	
Glyburide [DiaBeta, Micronase], **glimepiride** [Diabinese], **glipizide** [Glucotrol]	**Second generation sulfonylureas**—closes potassium channel in pancreatic β-islet cell membrane → reduces K^+ efflux, increases Ca^{2+} influx → increases secretion of insulin	Oral treatment for **NIDDM (type 2 diabetes)**	**Hypoglycemia;** GI disturbances; muscle weakness; mental confusion; weight gain	Not useful in Type 1 DM because it requires some islet function.

(continued)

TABLE 7-9 Therapeutic Agents for Diabetes *(Continued)*

Therapeutic Agent (common name, if relevant) [trade name, where appropriate]	Class–Pharmacology and Pharmacokinetics	Indications	Side or Adverse Effects	Contraindications or Precautions to Consider; Notes
Biguanides				
Metformin [Glucophage]	**Biguanide**—unknown mechanism, postulated to decrease gluconeogenesis, increase glycolysis → decreases serum glucose levels	Oral treatment for **NIDDM (type 2 diabetes)**	**Lactic acidosis,** GI upset (diarrhea, nausea, abdominal pain), metallic taste	Stop use in patients undergoing studies or procedures involving **contrast.** Can be used in patients without islet function.
Thiazolidinedione				
Pioglitazone [Actos], **rosiglitazone** [Avandia]	Glitazone—improves target cell response to insulin	Oral treatment for **NIDDM (type 2 diabetes)**	**Weight gain,** edema, hepatotoxicity, increases LDL, triglycerides	
α-Glucosidase inhibitors				
Acarbose [Precose]	**α-Glucosidase inhibitor**—inihibit intestinal brush border enzyme α-glucosidase → delays sugar hydrolysis and glucose absorption from gut → decreases **posprandial hyperglycemia**	Oral treatment for **NIDDM (type 2 diabetes)** postprandially	**Flatulence,** cramps, diarrhea; may reduce absorption of iron	Does not cause reactive hypoglycemia; decreases HbA1c
Miglitol	**α-Glucosidase inhibitor**—inhibit intestinal brush border enzyme α-glucosidase → delays sugar hydrolysis and glucose absorption → decreases **posprandial hyperglycemia**	Oral treatment for **NIDDM (type 2 diabetes)** postprandially	**Flatulence,** cramps, diarrhea; may reduce absorption of iron	Does not cause reactive hypoglycemia; decreases HbA1c

Some combination of these types of insulin usually can be found that provides adequate glucose control during both the fed and fasting states. Treatment of type 1 diabetes mellitus is essentially a balancing act—too much insulin causes hypoglycemia, and too little leads to hyperglycemia, which, over time, leads to the long-term complications of diabetes mellitus.

Type 2 diabetes mellitus, which is more complex than type 1 disease, is characterized primarily by insulin resistance. In some cases, a strict regimen of diet and exercise completely reverses the course of the disease. In many cases, however, drugs are required to control blood sugar levels. The most commonly used drugs in type 2 diabetes mellitus are metformin and the insulin sensitizers. **Metformin**, in the biguanide class of agents, is considered by many to be the first-line drug of choice in type 2 diabetes mellitus and acts primarily by decreasing hepatic glucose production. Advantages include the very low risk of hypoglycemia as well as the weight loss and improvement in lipid profiles in many patients. The one feared adverse reaction is lactic acidosis, a rare but serious complication. Also, nausea and diarrhea are side effects of this medication.

Pioglitazone and **rosiglitazone**, of the class thiazolidinedones, are the two most common insulin sensitizers. Their mechanism of action is poorly understood. Like metformin, these agents can be used alone or as part of a multidrug regimen for diabetic blood sugar control. Both drugs have a low risk of hypoglycemia. However, they have been known to exacerbate congestive heart failure and frequent monitoring of liver function is required.

Sulfonylureas were once the mainstay of treatment for type 2 diabetes, but they are used infrequently today. These drugs, which include agents such as glipizide and glyburide, act by increasing the release of insulin from the pancreas. To a lesser extent, these agents also decrease glucagon levels and increase insulin binding at target sites in the periphery. The primary side effect of these drugs is hypoglycemia.

MNEMONIC

To remember the duration of action for the various insulin types, think: **Lis is a pro at sports** (lispro and aspart, rapid-acting). **Ultralente** is **ultralong** (long). **Glargine** remains for a **large** amount of time (long). Remember **regular** is **short acting**, and **everything else (NPH, lente) is intermediate acting.**

MNEMONIC

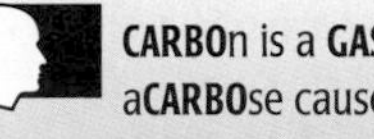

CARBOn is a **GAS**, and a**CARBO**se causes **GAS.**

Clinical Vignette 7-2

Clinical Presentation: An 8-year-old female child presents to the emergency department with complaints of several days of **vomiting** and **thirst.** The mother also reports that the patient has **not been acting like herself** lately and has been **urinating** more than usual. The patient recently recovered from an **upper respiratory infection** with high fevers. On examination, the patient is breathing rapidly and deeply **(Kussmaul respirations),** and a **sweet smell** is noticed on her breath. Her **skin and oral mucosa are dry.**

Differentials: DKA, nonketotic hyperglycemia hyperosmolar (NKH) coma, gastroenteritis, hypoglycemic coma, metabolic acidosis (from causes other than DKA).

Laboratory Studies: An **urinalysis** should be obtained with interest in glucose and ketone levels—high glucose and ketone levels suggest DKA. **In NKH, the glucose levels are elevated but there is no ketosis.** NKH is more often seen more in type 2 diabetics, and DKA is more often seen in type 1 diabetics. A **blood chemistry** would also be key in differentiating causes; in DKA, it would show high glucose, high ketones, and an acidotic profile with low pH, low bicarbonate, and elevated anion gap from the ketones (organic acids). Also in DKA, serum K is high because the acidosis causes a shift of serum hydrogen ions into cells in exchange for intracellular potassium ions. Serum sodium appears decreased because hyperglycemia increases serum osmolality shifting water out of cells. Blood glucose and serum osmolality are significantly higher in NKH than in DKA, and ketones are not found because there are sufficient levels of insulin to prevent lipolysis, thereby preventing ketogenesis. NKH usually presents with a nonacidotic profile. Metabolic acidosis can also cause vomiting, Kussmaul respirations, a low blood pH, and bicarbonate. Causes of metabolic acidosis with a normal anion gap include: diarrhea, renal tubular acidosis, or acetazolamide overdose. Causes of metabolic acidosis with an elevated anion gap include chronic renal failure, lactic acidosis, DKA, uremia, salicylate overdose, methanol ingestion, and ethylene glycol ingestion. To determine the cause of the metabolic acidosis in this patient, **salicylate, lactate, blood alcohol, methanol, and ethylene glycol levels** should be obtained. Finally, in gastroenteritis, a metabolic alkalosis from the vomiting is expected. In hypoglycemic coma, the glucose levels are low.

Management: Three-tiered approach: (1) **Rehydration**—a fluid bolus is indicated because the patient is severely dehydrated. Monitor rehydration status by noting resolution of mental status changes. The most common complication of this treatment is **cerebral edema** from too rapid a change in serum osmolality. (2) **Insulin**—to facilitate peripheral uptake of glucose, decrease ketone body formation. (3) **Potassium replacement**—although blood studies show high serum K^+ levels, that is misleading because the acidosis caused the potassium to shift out of cells and the body is actually potassium starved.

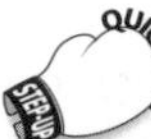

Sheehan syndrome is panhypopituitarism caused by postpartum pituitary necrosis resulting from blood loss and ischemia during childbirth.

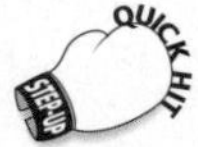

Surprisingly, diabetes insipidus can be treated with hydrochlorothiazide (a diuretic).

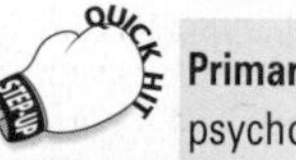

Primary polydipsia, a psychological condition of drinking excess water, causes a decrease in plasma osmolality, and thus can be differentiated from diabetes insipidus, which causes an increase in plasma osmolality. Patients who present with primary polydipsia are generally young or middle-age women with a history of neurosis.

MNEMONIC

Both nephrogenic and central diabetes insipidus present with dilute urine after dehydration. In diagnosing these subtypes of diabetes insipidus, think after administering antidiuretic hormone: **C**oncentrated urine = **Central**, **N**o effect = **N**ephrogenic.

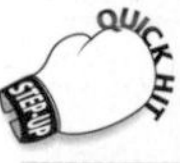

Diabetes insipidus may be transiently induced during pregnancy due to greater metabolism of vasopressin (ADH).

OBESITY

Obesity is a multifactorial disease with a variable genetic component and is associated with diet, lifestyle, drugs, and endocrine disorders. Multiple therapeutic strategies including diet, exercise, bariatric surgery, and drugs can be attempted. Table 7-10 summarizes pharmacological agents available in treating obesity.

PITUITARY DISORDERS (Table 7-11)

The pituitary gland sits in the sella turcica. The anterior portion is regulated by the hypothalamus. The posterior portion contains extensions of hypothalamic neurons. Excess prolactin can result from estrogen therapy or drugs, such as antipsychotics, that interfere with dopamine (prolactin-inhibiting hormone).

DIABETES INSIPIDUS (Table 7-12)

Diabetes insipidus is a disease characterized by excessive low-osmolality urine output. There are two forms: central and nephrogenic.

TABLE 7-10 Therapeutic Agents for Obesity

Therapeutic Agent (common name, if relevant) [trade name, where appropriate]	Class–Pharmacology and Pharmacokinetics	Indications	Side or Adverse Effects	Contraindications or Precautions to Consider; Notes
Orlistat	**Inhibits pancreatic lipases** → alters fat metabolism	**Obesity** (long term)	**Steatorrhea,** GI irritation, reduced absorption of fat soluble vitamins, and headache	**Used in conjunction with modified diet.**
Sibutramine	**Sympathomimetic serotonin and norepinephrine reuptake inhibitor**	Obesity (short term and long term)	Hypertension, tachycardia	

TABLE 7-11 Pituitary Disorders

Disorder	Etiology	Clinical Features	Laboratory Diagnosis	Treatment
Prolactinoma	Lactotrophic (chromophobic) anterior pituitary tumor; **most common** pituitary tumor	Decreased libido; amenorrhea; gynecomastia; galactorrhea; virilization	Minimal or no increase in serum prolactin after TRH given	Bromocriptine or surgery
Acromegaly (adults)/gigantism (children)	Somatotrophic (acidophilic) anterior pituitary adenoma	Prominent forehead, jaw; **large hands, feet; enlargement of viscera;** hyperglycemia; renal failure; hypertension; mental disturbances	Excess growth hormones and somatomedins (IGF-1)	Transsphenoidal surgery, bromocriptine, radiation, or octreotide
Cushing disease	Hypersecretion of ACTH from basophilic adenoma of pituitary	(Table 7-11)	Suppression of ACTH secretion during high-dose dexamethasone test	Surgery or pituitary irradiation
Panhypopituitarism (Simmonds disease, Sheehan syndrome)	Pituitary tumors, ischemia, trauma; DIC; sickle cell anemia	Marked wasting; **panhypopituitarism;** headache; vomiting	Decreased levels of FSH, LH, ACTH, TSH	Hormone replacement
SIADH	Pituitary hypersecretion; ectopic production of ADH **(small cell lung cancer)**	Decreased urinary output; fatigue; mental disturbances	Hyponatremia; high urine osmolality	Fluid restriction
Diabetes insipidus	**Neurogenic** (central): ADH insufficiency **Nephrogenic:** lack of end-organ (kidney) response	Dehydration; thirst; polyuria; recent trauma to the head or anoxia	(Table 7-10); hypernatremia	Neurogenic: desmopressin (DDAVP) acts as ADH Nephrogenic: fluid restriction and thiazide response diuretics (works by a paradoxical effect)

ACTH, adrenocorticotropic hormone; ADH, antidiuretic hormone (vasopressin); DDAVP, 1-deamino-8-D-arginine vasopressin; DIC, disseminated intravascular coagulation; FSH, follicle stimulating hormone; IGF, insulin-like growth factor; LH, luteinizing hormone; SIADH, syndrome of inappropriate secretion of antidiuretic hormone; TRH, thyrotropin-releasing hormone; TSH, thyroid-stimulating hormone.

TABLE 7-12 Diabetes Insipidus

	Urine Osmolarity Greater than 280 mOsm/kg with Dehydration	Response to Antidiuretic Hormone after Dehydration
Normal	+	–
Central diabetes insipidus	–	+
Partial diabetes insipidus	+	+
Nephrogenic diabetes insipidus	–	–
Primary polydipsia	+	+

THE ADRENAL GLANDS

21-Hydroxylase deficiency is the **most common** adrenal enzyme deficiency.

I. Congenital adrenal hyperplasia (Figure 7-9)

The adrenal glands are anatomically divided into a medulla and a cortex. The cortex itself is divided into three anatomic layers. The four anatomic layers of the adrenal glands are responsible for various metabolic functions in the body.

II. Adrenal cortex pathology (Table 7-13)

III. Adrenal medulla pathology (Table 7-14)

FIGURE 7-9 Congenital adrenal hyperplasia (CAH)

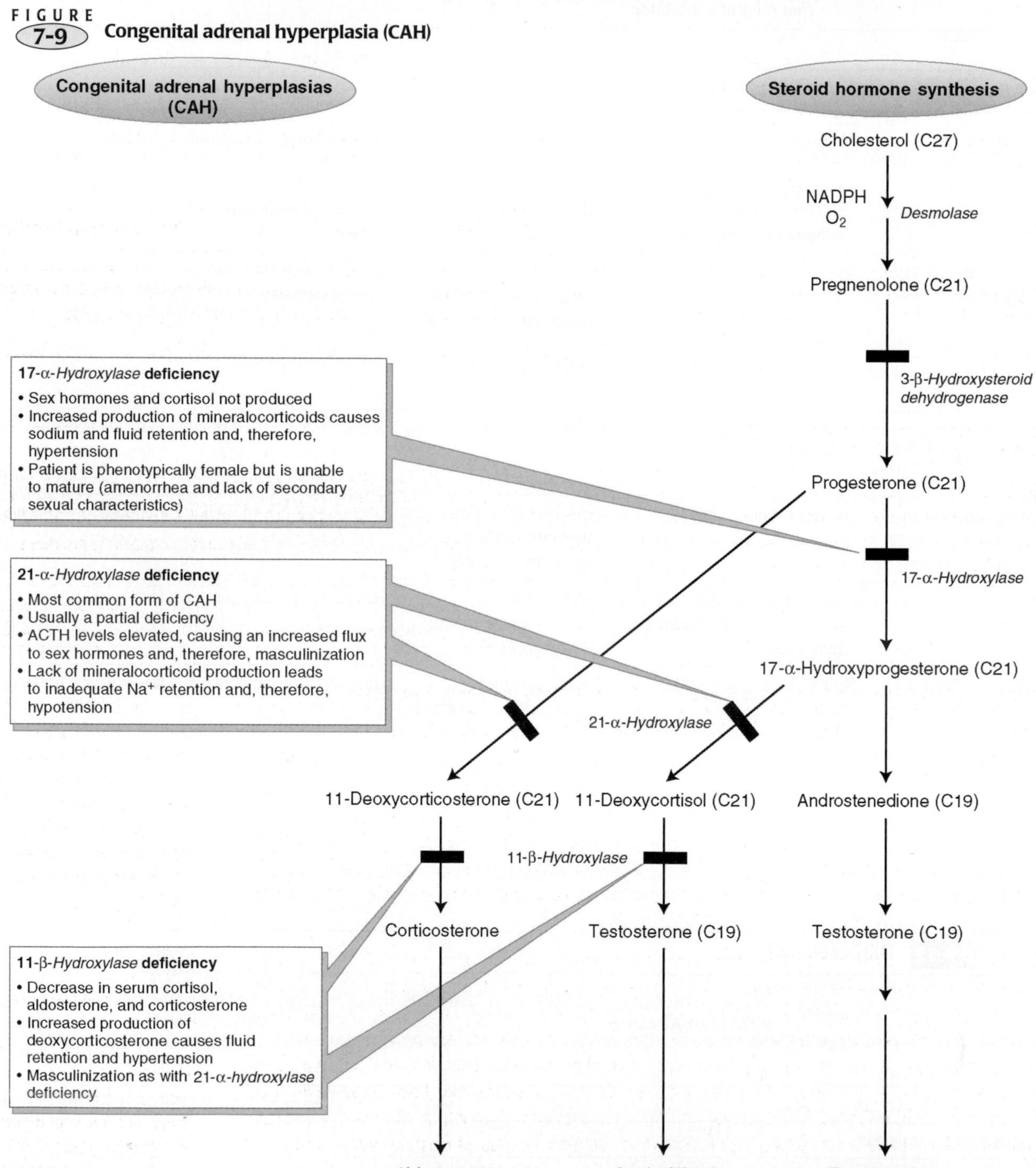

Congenital adrenal hyperplasias (CAH)
Steroid hormone synthesis
Cholesterol (C27)
NADPH
O_2
Desmolase
Pregnenolone (C21)
3-β-*Hydroxysteroid dehydrogenase*
Progesterone (C21)
17-α-*Hydroxylase*
17-α-Hydroxyprogesterone (C21)
21-α-*Hydroxylase*
11-Deoxycorticosterone (C21)
11-Deoxycortisol (C21)
Androstenedione (C19)
11-β-*Hydroxylase*
Corticosterone
Testosterone (C19)
Testosterone (C19)
Aldosterone
Cortisol(C21)
Estradiol (C18)
17-α-*Hydroxylase* **deficiency**
• Sex hormones and cortisol not produced
• Increased production of mineralocorticoids causes sodium and fluid retention and, therefore, hypertension
• Patient is phenotypically female but is unable to mature (amenorrhea and lack of secondary sexual characteristics)
21-α-*Hydroxylase* **deficiency**
• Most common form of CAH
• Usually a partial deficiency
• ACTH levels elevated, causing an increased flux to sex hormones and, therefore, masculinization
• Lack of mineralocorticoid production leads to inadequate Na^+ retention and, therefore, hypotension
11-β-*Hydroxylase* **deficiency**
• Decrease in serum cortisol, aldosterone, and corticosterone
• Increased production of deoxycorticosterone causes fluid retention and hypertension
• Masculinization as with 21-α-*hydroxylase* deficiency

(text continues on page 207)

TABLE 7-13 Adrenal Cortex Pathology

Disease	Etiology	Clinical Features
Cushing syndrome	Excess cortisol as a result of **iatrogenic corticosteroid therapy (most common cause),** adrenal adenoma (more common than carcinoma); ectopic ACTH from neoplasm (especially **small cell lung carcinoma**)	Peripheral muscle wasting and weakness; **central obesity** with rounds facies and increased fat deposition at upper back, easy bruising with abdominal striae; bone demineralization, osteoporosis, psychosis, acne; hirsutism; hyperglycemia; hypertension
Cushing disease	Excess cortisol as a result of **pituitary hypersecretion of ACTH;** bilateral hyperplasia of adrenal cortex; **second most common** cause of Cushing syndrome	Identical to Cushing syndrome
Conn syndrome (primary hyperaldosteronism)	Adrenal cortex **adenoma** (more common than hyperplasia, which is more common than carcinoma); sodium retention; **low plasma renin**	**Hypertension;** hypokalemic alkalosis
Secondary hyperaldosteronism	Renal tumors; renal ischemia; edematous conditions (cirrhosis, nephrotic syndromes, congestive heart failure); **increased plasma renin**	**Hypertension;** hypokalemic alkalosis
Addison disease	Most commonly **idiopathic** cortisol deficiency; possibly autoimmune; may be caused by tumor, infections (i.e., tuberculosis)	**Hypotension;** low serum sodium; **hyperpigmentation;** increased serum potassium
Waterhouse-Friderichsen syndrome	***Neisseria meningitis*** infection leads to disseminated intravascular coagulation (**DIC**); hemorrhagic adrenal **necrosis** and circulation collapse	Acute hypotension and salt wasting; **shock;** more common in children; death within hours if not treated

ACTH, adrenocorticotropic hormone.

TABLE 7-14 Adrenal Medulla Tumors

Tumor	Pathology	Clinical Manifestation
Neuroblastoma	**Malignant;** excess catecholamine secretion; N-*myc* (oncogene) amplification	**Children;** degree of N-*myc* amplification related to prognosis
Pheochromocytoma	**Benign** (10% malignant); tumor of chromaffin cells; seen in MEN IIa and IIb	**Adults;** hypertension (usually paroxysmal); palpitations, sweating, and headache; increased urinary vanillylmandelic acid **(VMA)**

Clinical Vignette 7-3

Clinical Presentation: A 37-year-old female presents to her primary care physician with a chief complaint of **weight gain, fatigue, acne,** and **hirsutism.** After further questions, the patient reports that she has not had her period for 3 months. Her past medical history is significant for a bone marrow transplantation for which the patient is currently on medication. Patient denies a family history of diabetes or hypertension. Physical examination reveals **central obesity, abdominal striae, bruising** on thighs and buttocks, and **muscle weakness.** Vital signs: T = 97.5 °F; HR = 80 bpm; RR = 20 breaths/min; **BP = 140/90 mm Hg.**

Differential: Iatrogenic Cushing syndrome, adrenocorticotropic hormone (ACTH) producing pituitary adenoma (Cushing **disease**), adrenal adenoma, ectopic ACTH production, and obesity. This patient is exhibiting signs and symptoms of high cortisol, termed Cushing syndrome. Some findings (i.e., **obesity, hypertension, osteoporosis, diabetes mellitus**) are nonspecific and less helpful in diagnosis of Cushing syndrome. **Easy bruising, striae, virilization,** and **myopathy** are more helpful in the diagnosis. Also, patients with **Cushing disease** can have **hyperpigmentation** as a result of elevated ACTH levels, whereas patients with **Cushing syndrome** due to other causes will not have hyperpigmentation. The most common cause of Cushing syndrome is an unfavorable response to prescribed steroids; patient's recent transplantation history suggests the possibility that she received immunosuppressive steroids.

(continued)

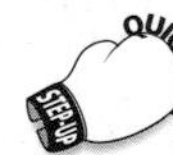

Hyperpigmentation in Addison disease is caused by increased production of proopiomelanocortin (POMC) by the pituitary. POMC is enzymatically split to yield adrenocorticotropin (ACTH) and melanocyte-stimulating hormone (**MSH**).

MNEMONIC

To remember the anatomic layers of the adrenal cortex, think **GFR: G**lomerulosa, **F**asciculata, and **R**eticularis. To remember the hormones produced by each layer, think the **deeper you go, the sweeter it gets:** aldosterone (**salt** hormone), glucocorticoid (**sugar** hormone), and androgens (**sex** hormone).

Clinical Vignette 7-3 *(Continued)*

Laboratory Studies: Figure 7-10 outlines the approach. The first step is to determine whether cortisol levels are elevated in this patient, which can be done via a **urine 24-h free cortisol level** or an **overnight dexamethasone suppression test.** In this latter test, dexamethasone is given at night, and serum cortisol levels are measured in the morning. In normal individuals, dexamethasone should suppress the pituitary–adrenal axis, resulting in decreased cortisol in the morning. In Cushing syndrome, the serum cortisol remains elevated. The next step is to determine the cause of the cortisol elevation, which could be from (a) **increased ACTH production** at the level of the pituitary or ectopically, (b) **increased cortisol production** at the level of the adrenal gland, or (c) **exogenous cortisol** in the form of prednisone. To determine the cause, measure **ACTH levels,** which would be low in the case of exogenous cortisol and adrenal adenoma, because cortisol feedback inhibits the pituitary from secreting ACTH. Knowing which medications the patient is using helps in differentiating these causes. ACTH levels are high in patients with obesity, ectopic ACTH, or pituitary ACTH adenoma. The key differentiating factor is that **low-dose dexamethasone** will suppress ACTH production in obese individuals, **high-dose dexamethasone** will suppress ACTH production in pituitary adenoma cases, and nothing will suppress ACTH levels in the ectopic ACTH patients.

Management: This patient most likely has iatrogenic Cushing syndrome, which is remedied by **tapering of the glucocorticoid.** Pituitary or adrenal adenoma requires **surgical removal of the neoplasm.**

MNEMONIC

To remember the side effects of steroids, think:
CUSHINGOID:
Cataract
Ulcers
Skin: striae, thinning, bruising
Hypertension/**H**irsutism/
Hyperglycemia
Infections
Necrosis (avascular necrosis of the femoral head)
Glycosuria
Osteoporosis/Obesity
Immunosuppression
Diabetes

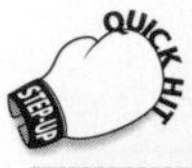

Small cell lung carcinoma is a potential source for ectopic ACTH production resulting in paraneoplastic syndrome.

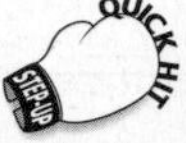

Extra-adrenal chromaffin cell tumors are called paragangliomas (e.g., tumors originating in the organ of Zuckerkandl).

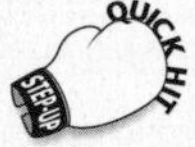

The pheochromocytoma rule of 10s: 10% are malignant, 10% multiple, 10% bilateral, 10% familial, and 10% extra-adrenal, 10% children.

FIGURE 7-10 **Approach to Cushing syndrome**
ACTH, adrenocorticotropin; CT, computed tomography; MRI, magnetic resonance imaging.

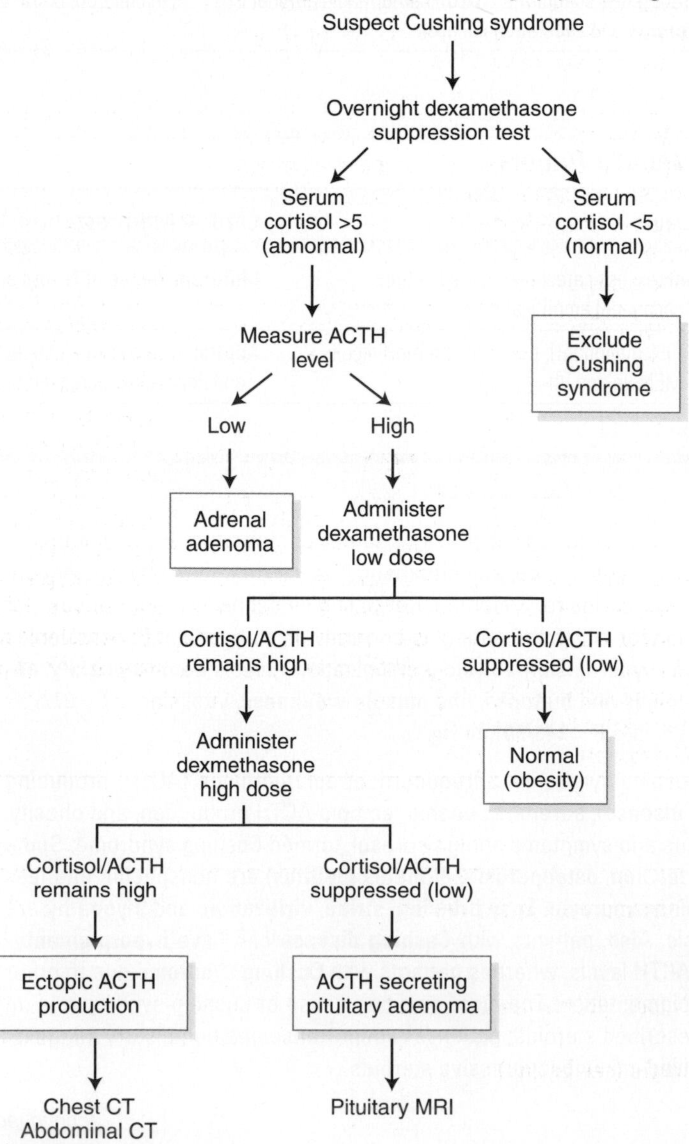

THERAPEUTIC AGENTS FOR THE HYPOTHALAMUS, PITUITARY, AND ADRENAL GLANDS (Table 7-15)

TABLE 7-15 Therapeutic Agents for Hypothalmic, Pituitary, and Adrenal Conditions

Therapeutic Agent (common name, if relevant) [trade name, where appropriate]	Class–Pharmacology and Pharmacokinetics	Indications	Side or Adverse Effects	Contraindications or Precautions to Consider; Notes
Growth hormone (somatotropin) [Somatrem]	**Synthetic analog of growth hormone—causes liver to produce insulin-like growth factors (somatomedins)**	Replacement therapy in children with **growth hormone deficiency, Turner syndrome; burn victims**		
Growth hormone-releasing hormone (GH-RH)	**Synthetic analog of GHRH—stimulates release of GH**	**Dwarfism**	**Pain at injection**	
Octreotide [Sandostatin]	**Synthetic analog of somatostatin**—decreases release of GH, gastrin, secretin, VIP, CCK, glucagon, insulin	**Acromegaly; glucagonoma; insulinoma; carcinoid syndrome**	Nausea; cramps; gallstones	
Oxytocin [Pitocin, Syntocinon]	**Synthetic analog of oxytocin—stimulates uterine contraction and contraction of breast myoepithelial cells; milk letdown reflex**	**Induces labor; control uterine hemorrhage**		
Desmopressin (DDAVP)	**Synthetic analog of ADH**—recruits water channels to luminal membrane in collecting duct	Antidiuresis; central (pituitary) diabetes insipidus	Overhydration; allergic reaction; larger doses result in pallor, diarrhea, hypertension; coronary constriction; chronic rhinopharyngitis	**Synthetic analog to vasopressin; intranasal administration**
Prednisone, hydrocortisone, triamcinolone, dexamethasone, beclomethasone	**Glucocorticoid**—inhibits protein synthesis; reduces lymph node and spleen size; inhibits cell cycle activity of lymphoid cells; lyses T cells; suppresses antibody, prostaglandin, and leukotriene synthesis; blocks monocyte production of IL-1	Addison disease; rheumatic arthritis; autoimmune disorders; allergic reaction; asthma; organ transplantation (especially during rejection crisis)	**Osteoporosis; Cushingoid reaction; psychosis; glucose intolerance; infection; hypertension; cataracts; peptic ulcers**	

THYROID

I. Formation of thyroid hormone (Figure 7-11)

II. Myxedema

A. Can be described as hypothyroidism of the **adult**

B. Causes

1. **Hashimoto thyroiditis** (see below)
2. Idiopathic causes

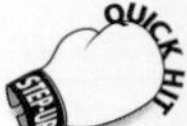

Thyroxine (T_4) is converted to triiodothyronine (T_3) in the periphery, with T_3 being 35 times more potent than T_4. T_4 has a half-life of 5 to 7 days, whereas T_3 has a half-life of 1 day.

FIGURE 7-11 Formation of thyroid hormone

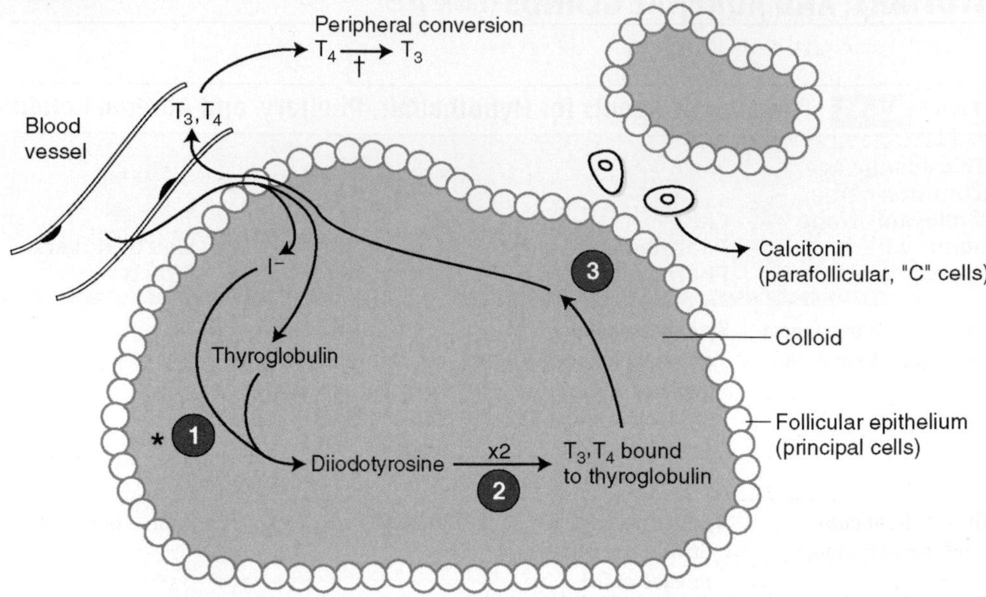

1 Oxidation of I^- by peroxidase followed by iodination of thyroglobulin
2 Condensation
3 Proteolytic release of hormone from follicle
* Inhibited by propylthiouracil and methimazole
† Inhibited by propylthiouracil

3. Iodine deficiency
   a. A problem in geographic areas with poor nutrition.
   b. Deficiency in pregnant women can lead to cretinism in the child (see below).
4. Paradoxically, high doses of iodine lead to a decrease in thyroid hormone production.
5. **Overirradiation** of the thyroid using iodine-131 for treatment of hyperthyroidism

C. Clinical features of the hypothyroid state
   1. Cold intolerance
   2. Weight gain
   3. Constipation
   4. Lowering of voice
   5. Menorrhagia
   6. Slowed mental and physical function
   7. Dry skin with coarse and brittle hair
   8. Reflexes showing slow return phase ("hung reflex")

D. Treatment is usually with levothyroxine (T_4).

III. Cretinism

A. Can be describe as **hypothyroidism** of the **fetus or child**
B. Causes
   1. **Iodine-deficient diet** in the mother or during the early life of the child
   2. Thyroid-related enzyme deficiency
   3. Thyroid developmental defect
   4. Failure of thyroid descent during development
   5. Transfer of antithyroid antibodies from the mother with an autoimmune disease to the fetus

Because of the devastating effects that hypothyroidism can have on children (**cretinism**), thyroid hormone levels (along with galactosemia and phenylketonuria) are routinely evaluated at birth in the United States.

C. Clinical features
  1. Impaired physical growth
  2. Mental retardation
  3. Enlarged tongue
  4. Enlarged, distended abdomen

IV. Hashimoto thyroiditis

A. An **autoimmune** disorder causing **hypothyroidism** and a **painless goiter**
  1. Dense infiltrate of lymphocytes into the thyroid gland
  2. Antithyroglobulin and antithyroid peroxidase (formerly antimicrosomal) antibodies
  3. **5:1 female predominance**
  4. Incidence increases with age
  5. Associated with human leukocyte antigen DR5 (**HLA-DR5**) and **HLA-B5**

B. Is the **most common form of hypothyroidism in those with adequate iodine** intake

C. Clinical features
  1. Slowly progressing course with stages of euthyroid state, hyperthyroid state, and hypothyroid state.
  2. May lead to a scarred and shrunken gland in hypothyroid state.
  3. Microscopically, thyroid resembles lymph node.

D. Associated with other autoimmune disorders
  1. Diabetes mellitus
  2. Pernicious anemia
  3. Sjögren syndrome

V. Subacute (de Quervain) thyroiditis

A. Transient hyperthyroidism with **painful** goiter
  1. Focal destruction of thyroid
  2. Granulomatous inflammation
  3. 3:1 female predominance
  4. Associated with HLA-B35

B. Causes—possibly as a result of recent viral infection with coxsackie virus, echovirus, adenovirus, measles, or mumps

C. Clinical features
  1. Acute febrile state
  2. Rapid, painful enlargement of the thyroid
  3. Transient hyperthyroidism owing to gland destruction

D. Self-limited disease

VI. Graves disease

A. **Autoimmune** disorder causing **hyperthyroidism** and a **goiter**
  1. Thyroid-stimulating immunoglobulin (**TSI**) is an immunoglobulin G (IgG) antibody to the thyroid-stimulating hormone (TSH) receptor.
  2. Binding of TSI to the TSH receptor stimulates thyroid hormone production and hyperplasia of the thyroid gland.
  3. It is associated with **HLA-DR3 and HLA-B8.**
  4. It has a **4:1 female** predominance.

B. Clinical features of Graves disease
  1. Hyperthyroidism and goiter caused by autoimmune immunoglobulins
     a. Increased total thyroxine (T_4)
     b. Increased triiodothyronine (T_3)
     c. Decreased TSH level
     d. Increased resin radioactive T_3 uptake
     e. Increased radioactive iodine
  2. Exophthalmos, proptosis
  3. Warm, moist, and flushed skin
  4. Thin, fine hair

5. Cardiovascular system
   a. Increased heart rate and cardiac output
   b. **Palpitations** and **fibrillations**
6. Muscle atrophy
   a. Weakening of skeletal muscles occurs
   b. Vital capacity of lungs decreases owing to weakened respiratory muscles
7. **Weight loss** occurs despite an increased appetite
8. Diarrhea is common
9. Menstrual flow may decrease or stop

C. Treatment (Table 7-16)
1. Antithyroid drugs (i.e., propylthiouracil or methimazole)
2. A **β-blocker** to reduce the cardiac effects
3. Radioactive iodine (iodine-131)
4. Surgery

QUICK HIT: Because of its long half-life, T_4 is ideal as a hormone replacement in patients with hypothyroidism. Even with once-a-day dosing, steady serum levels of T_4 and T_3 can be achieved.

TABLE 7-16 Therapeutic Agents for Thyroid Disorders

Therapeutic Agent (common name, if relevant) [trade name, where appropriate]	Class–Pharmacology and Pharmacokinetics	Indications	Side or Adverse Effects	Contraindications or Precautions to Consider; Notes
Propylthiouracil [Propyl-Thyracil]	Antithyroid agent—inhibits peroxidase enzyme in thyroid → decreases synthesis of thyroid hormone	**Hyperthyroidism**	**Agranulocytosis**	**Crosses the placenta and can cause fetal goiter and hypothyroidism;** Preferred to methimazole in treating pregnant females with moderate to severe hyperthyroidism.
Methimazole [Tapazole]	Antithyroid agent—inhibits peroxidase enzyme in thyroid → decreases synthesis of thyroid hormone	**Hyperthyroidism**	**Agranulocytosis**	**Crosses the placenta;** Can cause fetal goiter, hypothyroidism, and aplasia cutis (fetal scalp defect).
Levothyroxine (T_4) [Levothroid]	Synthetic analog of thyroxine T_4	**Hypothyroidism**	Tachycardia, heat intolerance, tremors, arrhythmia	
Triiodothyronine (T_3) [Triostat]	Synthetic analog of thyroid hormone T_3	**Hypothyroidism**	Tachycardia, heat intolerance, tremors, arrhythmia	

Clinical Vignette 7-4

Clinical Presentation: A 40-year-old female presents to your office with a 20-pound **weight loss** over the past 2 months despite **eating more.** She also reports **irregular menses, diarrhea,** and **difficulty sleeping and concentrating.** She denies chest pain and palpitations. Physical examination reveals **warm, moist skin** and **resting hand tremor.** Neck examination shows a **diffusely enlarged, nontender thyroid gland.** Vital signs: *T* = 99.0 °F; RR = 20 breaths/min; **HR = 99 bpm; BP = 140/90 mm Hg.**

Differential: Hyperthyroidism [Graves disease, factitious hyperthyroidism, subacute thyroiditis, multinodular goiter, thyroid adenoma], Hashimoto thyroiditis, menopause, panic disorder, and pheochromocytoma. The patient's symptoms are indicative of thyrotoxicosis. Of all the causes of thyrotoxicosis listed above, **exophthalmos** and **thyroid bruit** occur only in Graves disease. Also,

(continued)

Clinical Vignette 7-4 *(Continued)*

although Hashimoto thyroiditis eventually results in hypothyroidism, early findings in the disease are consistent with hyperthyroidism.

Laboratory Studies: Figure 7-12 outlines the approach to determining a cause of hyperthyroidism in a patient. **Serum TSH and T_3/T_4 levels** should be obtained. These tests would show elevated T_3/T_4 and suppressed TSH in hyperthyroidism and would be normal in menopause, panic disorder, and pheochromocytoma. A **thyroid scan with radioactive iodide uptake** is useful for distinguishing between the various causes of hyperthyroidism listed above. A negative scan would be expected for subacute thyroiditis and factitious hyperthyroidism. These can be further differentiated by a thorough history and physical examination. The patient with subacute thyroiditis has a tender thyroid, systemic flulike symptoms, and possible history of recent viral infection. Factitious hyperthyroidism is more often seen in healthcare workers with access to T_3/T_4 who are abusing it for weight-loss purposes. A positive scan of different types would be observed in Graves disease, multinodular goiter, and thyroid adenoma. In Graves disease, a diffuse hot scan would be seen, whereas in multinodular goiter, several nodules—both hot and cold—would be visualized. In thyroid adenoma, only one such hot nodule would be seen. Graves disease can be further supported by presence of **thyroid-stimulating IgG** that binds to thyrotropin receptors on the thyroid gland. These lab studies would be normal in menopause and panic disorder. Normal **urine metanephrines** and **vanillylmandelic acid** would rule out pheochromocytoma.

FIGURE 7-12 **Approach to thyrotoxicosis**

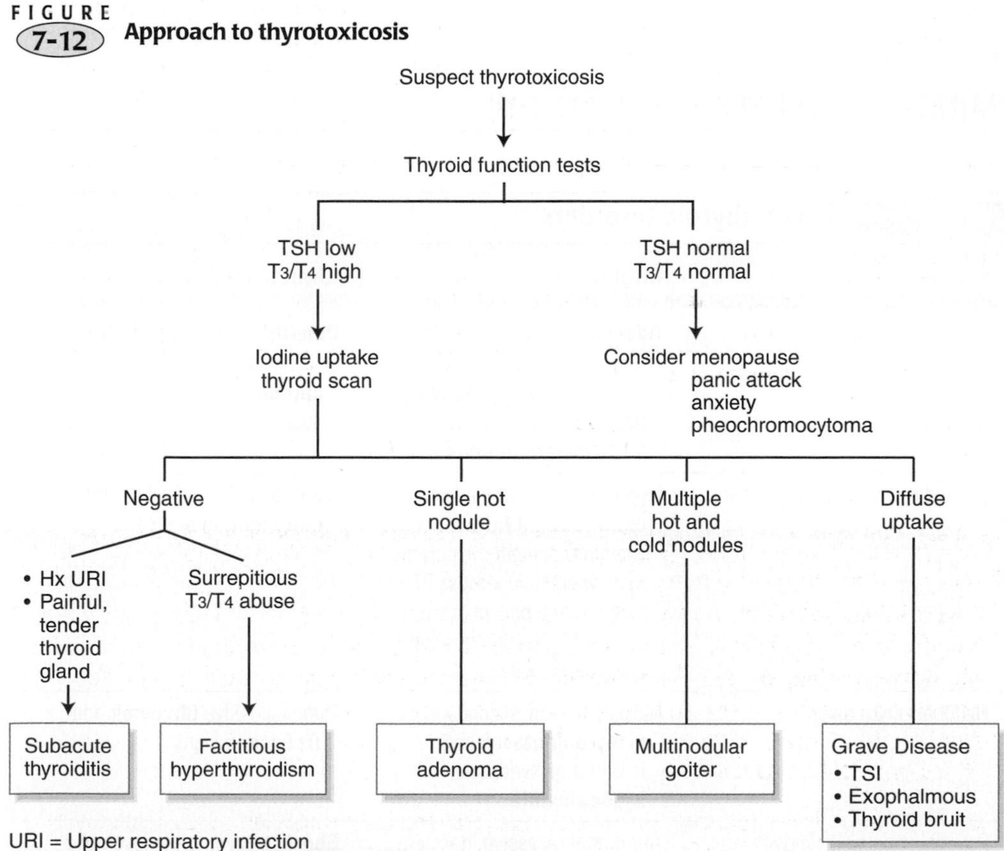

QUICK HIT: Thyrotoxicosis factitia is a factitious disorder in which the patient intentionally self-administers excess thyroid hormone (levothyroxine) to simulate the symptoms of hyperthyroidism.

VII. Thyroid neoplasms (Table 7-17)

TABLE 7-17 Thyroid Carcinomas

Tumor	Description
Papillary tumor	• **Most common** thyroid cancer • **Best prognosis** of the thyroid cancers • **3:1 female predominance** • Usually occurs in third to fifth decade of life • "Ground glass" nuclei of neoplastic cells, also called "Orphan Annie eyes" • **Psammoma bodies** may be present • Forms papillary projections covered with cuboidal epithelium within glandular spaces
Follicular tumor	• Worse prognosis than papillary • **3:1 female predominance** • Uniform cuboidal cells lining follicles • Lacks the distinctive nuclear features of papillary carcinoma
Medullary tumor	• Parafollicular cell neoplasm • **Secretes calcitonin** • Associated with MEN IIa and MEN IIb
Anaplastic thyroid carcinoma	• Anaplastic, undifferentiated neoplasm • More common in older patients • Rapidly fatal

QUICK HIT: Care must be taken when performing thyroid or parathyroid surgery as the **recurrent laryngeal nerves** run directly posterior to these glands. Cutting the recurrent nerve leads to paralysis of the muscles used for speech **(except the cricothyroid)** and hoarseness on the affected side.

QUICK HIT: If a patient presents with hypocalcemic symptoms status post thyroidectomy, think of accidental removal of the parathyroid glands.

QUICK HIT: Pancreatitis leads to fat necrosis because of release of pancreatic enzymes. The excess lipid binds calcium in a process called saponification and produces hypocalcemia.

MNEMONIC

To remember the symptoms of hypercalcemia, think:
Bones: pain in bones
Stones: renal stones
Groans: abdominal pain
Psychic moans/overtones: confused state

PARATHYROID PATHOLOGY (Table 7-18)

TABLE 7-18 Parathyroid Disorders

Condition	Etiology	Clinical Features
Primary hyperparathyroidism	**Adenoma** (most common); hyperplasia more common than carcinoma; seen in **MEN I** and **IIa**; excess parathyroid hormone (PTH); **hypercalcemia**	**Osteitis fibrosa cystica** (cystic "brown tumors" of bone); **renal calculi** and nephrocalcinosis; duodenal ulcers
Secondary hyperparathyroidism	**Hypocalcemia** caused by **chronic renal failure** (loss of vitamin D activation); parathyroid hyperplasia; excess PTH; high alkaline phosphatase; ectopic PTH (squamous cell lung carcinoma)	Cystic bone lesions; metastatic **calcification** of organs
Hypoparathyroidism	Most commonly secondary to **thyroidectomy;** seen in DiGeorge syndrome; **hypocalcemia**	Tetany; positive **Chvostek** and **Trousseau** signs
Pseudohypoparathyroidism	Autosomal recessive; deficient organ response to PTH	**Short stature;** underdeveloped fourth and fifth digits

MULTIPLE ENDOCRINE NEOPLASIA (MEN) SYNDROMES (Table 7-19)

TABLE 7-19 Multiple Endocrine Neoplasia Syndromes

Type I (Wermer)	Type IIa (Sipple)	Type IIb (or type III)
Hyperplasia or tumors of the thyroid, adrenal cortex, parathyroid, pancreas, or pituitary	Pheochromocytoma, medullary carcinoma of the thyroid, hyperparathyroidism	Pheochromocytoma, medullary carcinoma of the thyroid, multiple mucocutaneous neuromas (particularly of the GI tract)

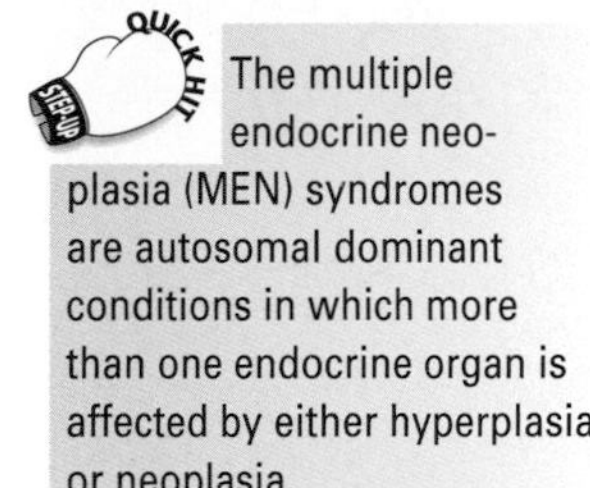

The multiple endocrine neoplasia (MEN) syndromes are autosomal dominant conditions in which more than one endocrine organ is affected by either hyperplasia or neoplasia.

MNEMONIC

MEN I is a disease of **3 Ps: P**ituitary, **P**arathyroid, and **P**ancreas.

MNEMONIC

MEN II is a disease of **2 Ms: M**edullary thyroid carcinoma and **M**edulla of adrenal (pheochromocytoma). Remember medullas with **MEN II.**

MNEMONIC

Men III is a disease of **3 Ms: M**edullary thyroid carcinoma, **M**edulla of adrenal (pheochromocytoma), and **M**ucocutaneous neuromas.

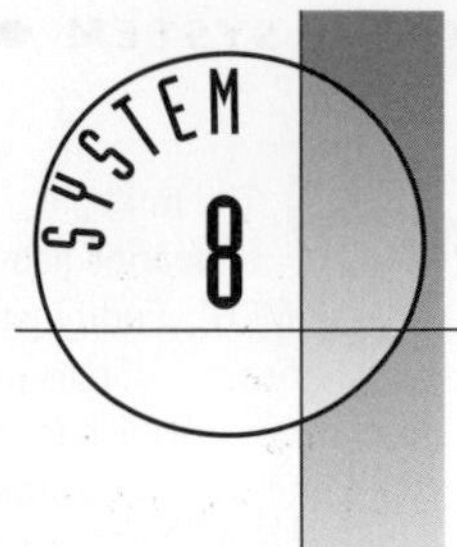

The Reproductive System

DETERMINATION OF SEX

Before the seventh week of gestation, the fetal gonads are not differentiated into either the male or female genotype. Primordial germ cells migrate into the genital ridge mesoderm to form testes and ovaries. The presence or absence of the Y chromosome and the sex-determining region of the Y chromosome (SRY) determine gonadal differentiation. Gender determination, which occurs after the seventh week, depends on the type of gonads present.

FEMALE REPRODUCTIVE SYSTEM DEVELOPMENT

I. Ovaries and other female reproductive structures

A. Primordial follicles contain **primary oocytes (XX genotype)** and follicular (granulosa) cells that form the ovaries.

B. As the upper abdomen grows, the ovaries "descend" toward the perineum.

C. The gubernaculum assists in this descent and then becomes the ovarian ligament and the round ligament of the uterus.

D. The **paramesonephric ducts** develop into the uterine tubes and eventually into the uterus.

II. Vagina and uterus (Figure 8-1)

III. Breasts

A. Only the main lactiferous ducts develop during the fetal life.

B. Glands enlarge during puberty owing to the increased levels of estrogens, progestins, prolactin, and growth hormone.

MALE REPRODUCTIVE SYSTEM DEVELOPMENT

I. Testes and other male reproductive organs

A. Primary sex cords contain primordial germ cells of **XY genotype**. The Y chromosome codes for the testes-determining factor that allows for male gonadal differentiation (i.e., formation of medullary cords and seminiferous tubules).

B. Müllerian-inhibiting factor **(MIF)** is secreted by **Sertoli cells.** MIF causes regression of the müllerian (paramesonephric) ducts and their associated female genital structures (uterine tubes and uterus).

C. The mesonephric ducts, under the influence of testosterone, become the ductus deferens, the seminal vesicles, and the ejaculatory ducts in the adult male.

MNEMONIC

To remember the path of the sperm through the male reproductive system, think of the phrase "SEVEN UP": **S**eminiferous tubules, **E**pididymis, **V**as deferens, **E**jaculatory duct, **N**othing, **U**rethra, **P**enis.

FIGURE 8-1 **Development of the female genital tract**
(Adapted with permission from Moore KL, Persaud TVN. The Developing Human: Clinically Oriented Embryology. 6th Ed. Philadelphia, PA: WB Saunders, 1998.)

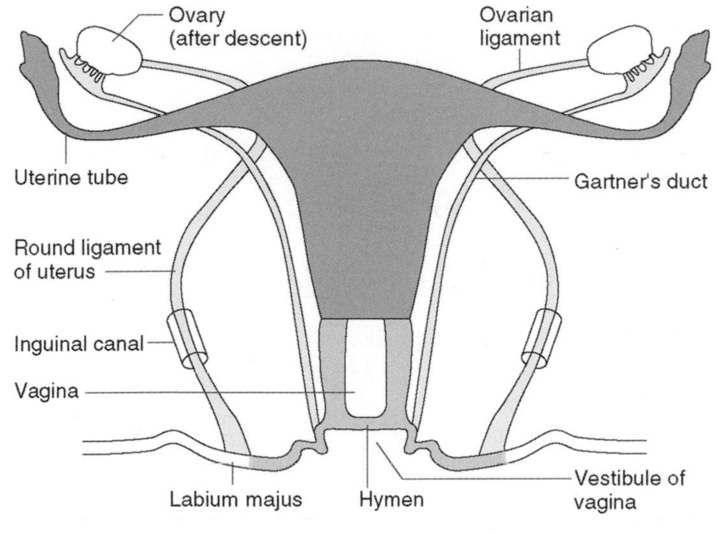

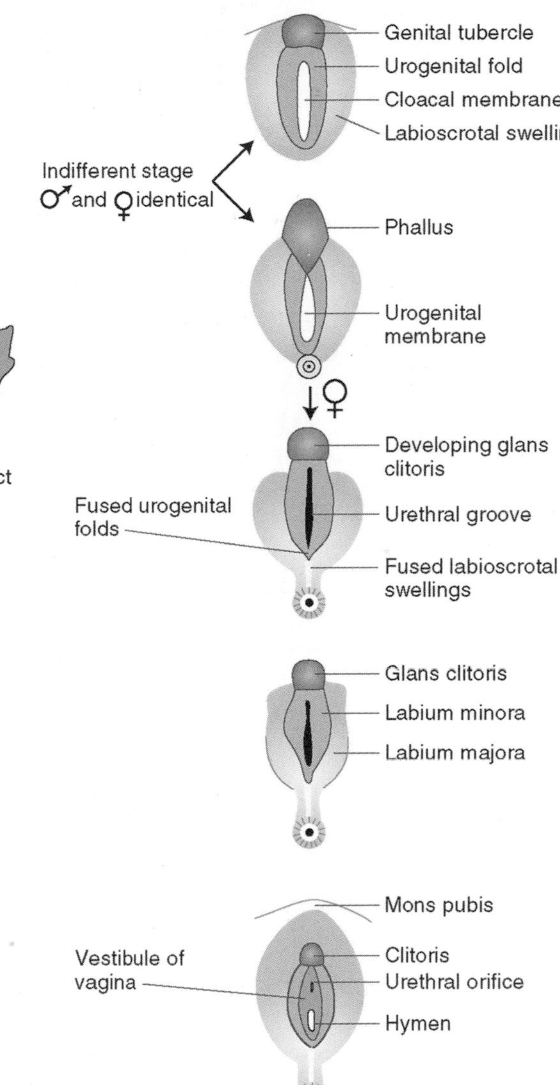

II. The prostate gland forms from the urogenital sinus (Figure 8-2)

III. External genitalia

A. Dihydrotestosterone (DHT) is responsible for the masculinization of genitalia.
B. The genital tubercle enlarges to become the glans penis.
C. The urogenital fold becomes the shaft of the penis.
D. The labioscrotal swellings fuse in the midline and become the scrotum.

- **Spermatogenesis Versus Oogenesis** (Figure 8-3)
- **Important Anatomic Features of the Perineum** (Figure 8-4)

CONGENITAL MALFORMATIONS

Congenital malformations are most often caused by exposure to teratogens during the third to eighth weeks of pregnancy, which is the period of organogenesis (Table 8-1).

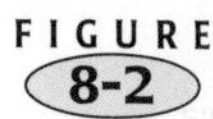

FIGURE 8-2 **Development of the male genital tract**
(Adapted with permission from Moore KL, Persaud TVN. The Developing Human: Clinically Oriented Embryology. 6th Ed. Philadelphia, PA: WB Saunders, 1998.)

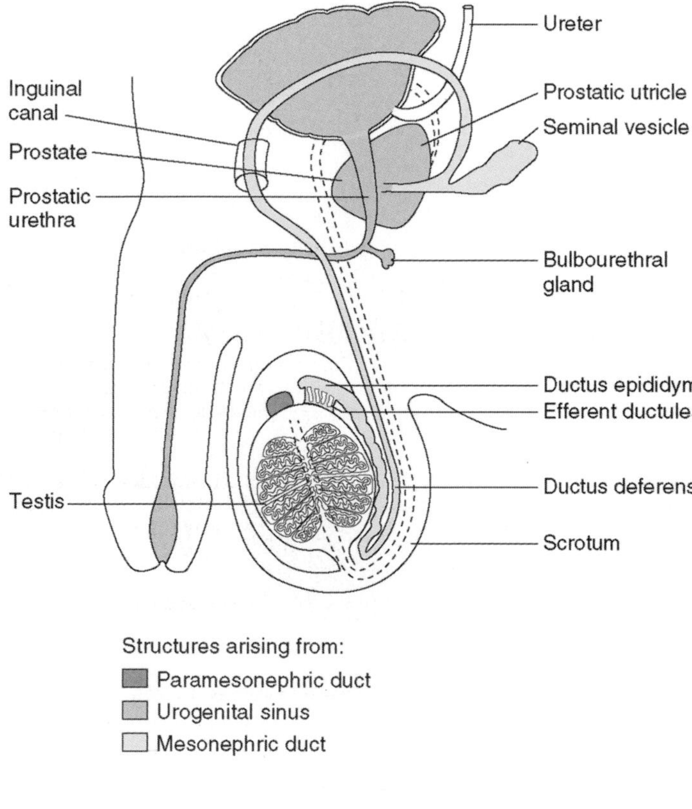

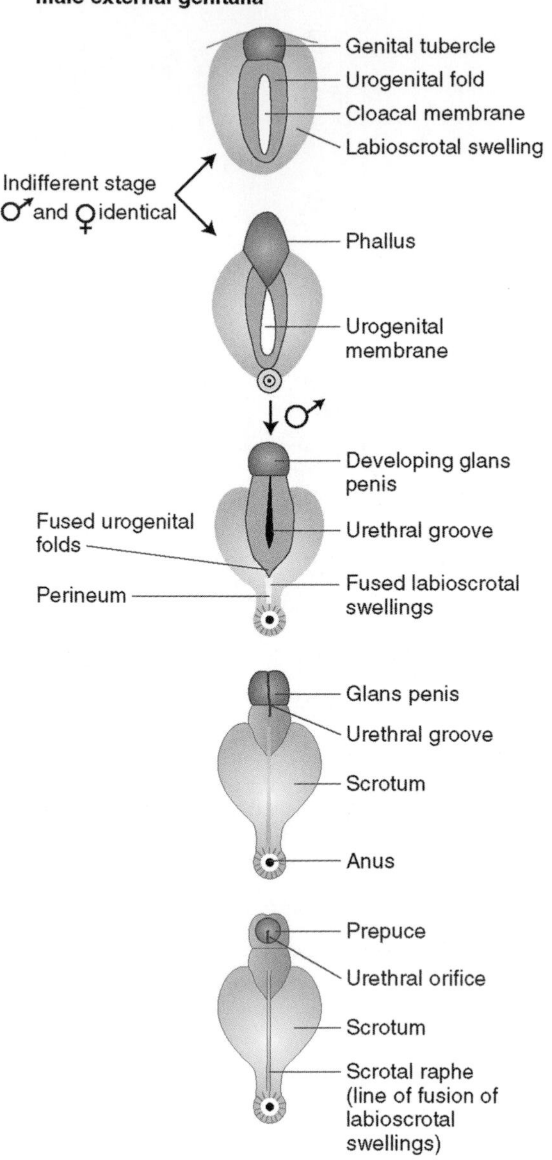

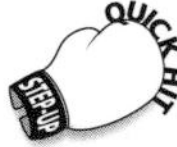

There is an increased incidence of trisomy 21 in women older than 35 years of age. The incidence of the robertsonian translocation type of Down syndrome is familial and does not increase with the age of the mother.

Breast surgery should not be performed in girls with precocious puberty because the excision of a "lump" in premature thelarche leads to the loss of an entire breast.

GENETIC ABNORMALITIES

The incidence of genetic abnormalities as a result of aberrant chromosomes significantly increases when the mother is older than 35 years of age. In these patients, additional consideration should be given to genetic testing.

- **Genetic Abnormalities Caused by Abnormal Somatic Chromosomes** (Table 8-2)
- **Genetic Abnormalities Caused by Abnormal Sex Chromosomes** (Table 8-3)

MENARCHE, MENSTRUATION, AND MENOPAUSE (Figure 8-5)

I. Menarche

A. First menstruation; usually occurs **between 11 and 14 years of age**
B. Follows thelarche (development of breast buds) by 2 years

FIGURE 8-3 **Spermatogenesis versus oogenesis**
(Adapted with permission from Moore KL, Persaud TVN. The Developing Human: Clinically Oriented Embryology. 6th Ed. Philadelphia, PA: WB Saunders, 1998.)

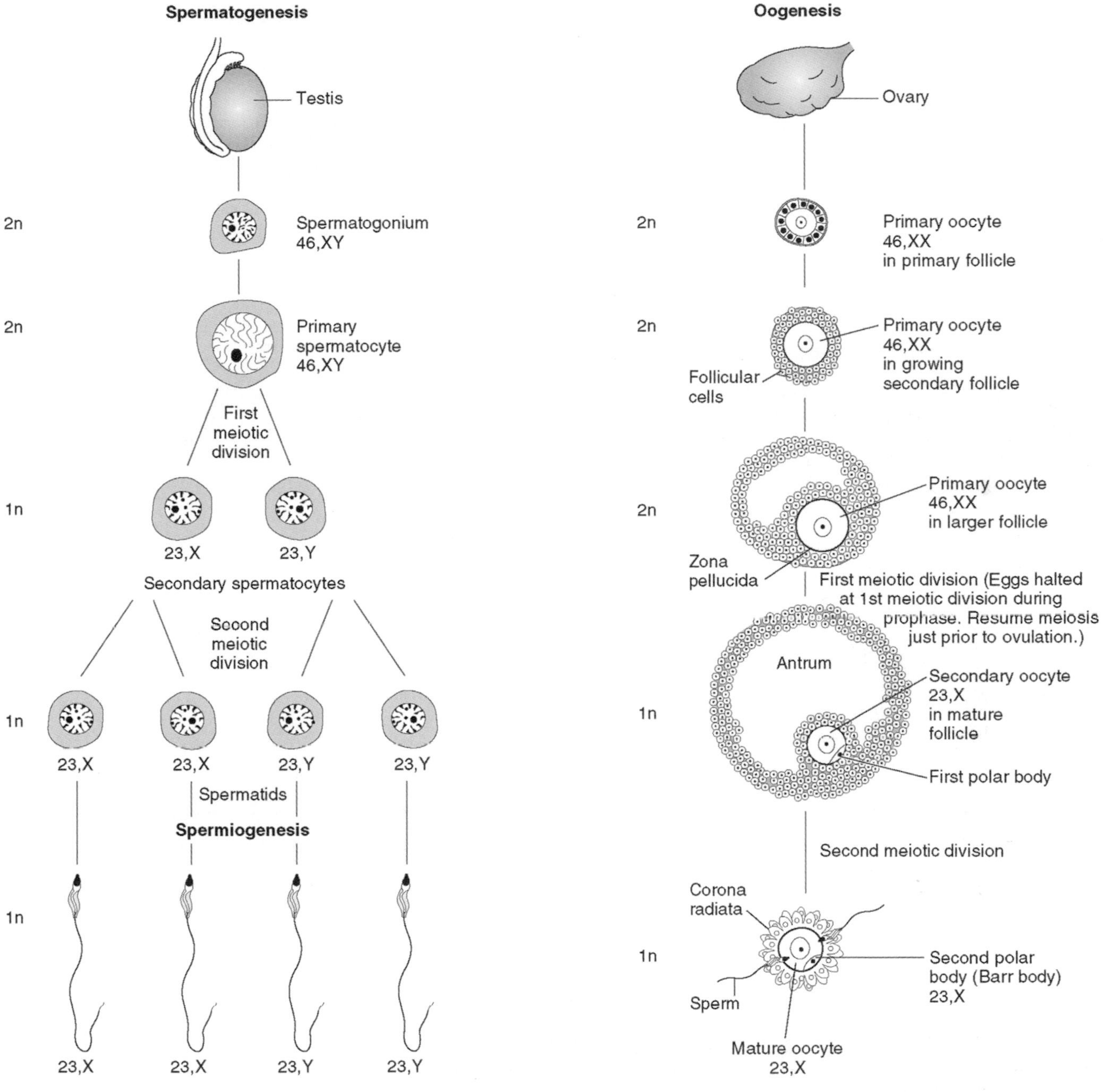

C. Precocious puberty
   1. Pubertal changes before 9 years of age in boys and 8 years of age in girls.
   2. True precocious puberty
      a. Early, but normal pubertal development
      b. **Usually idiopathic**
      c. May cause emotional and social adjustment problems
   3. Incomplete precocious puberty
      a. Premature development of a single pubertal characteristic
      b. Types
         - Premature thelarche: breast budding before 8 years of age
         - Premature adrenarche: growth of axillary hair
         - Premature pubarche: growth of pubic hair
      c. Generally self-limiting

(text continues on page 220)

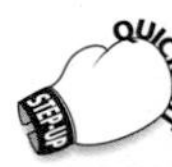

Puberty in males, usually occurring at age 15, is marked by an increased testosterone, leading to a greater hair distribution, growth of genitalia, nocturnal emissions, deepening of the voice, and increased muscle mass. Precocious puberty in males has a similar pathology to that in females, with the exception that it has a later age of onset.

MNEMONIC

To remember the layers of the scrotum, consider the phrase "Some Darn Englishman Called It The Testis"; from superficial to deep: **S**kin, **D**artos, **E**xternal spermatic fascia, **C**remaster, **I**nternal spermatic fascia, **T**unica vaginalis, and **T**estis.

MNEMONIC

Remember the function of luteinizing hormone (**LH**) and follicle-stimulating hormone (**FSH**) in the male; **LH** stimulates **L**eydig cells to produce testosterone and **FSH** stimulates **S**permatogenesis.

FIGURE 8-4 **Important anatomic features of the perineum**

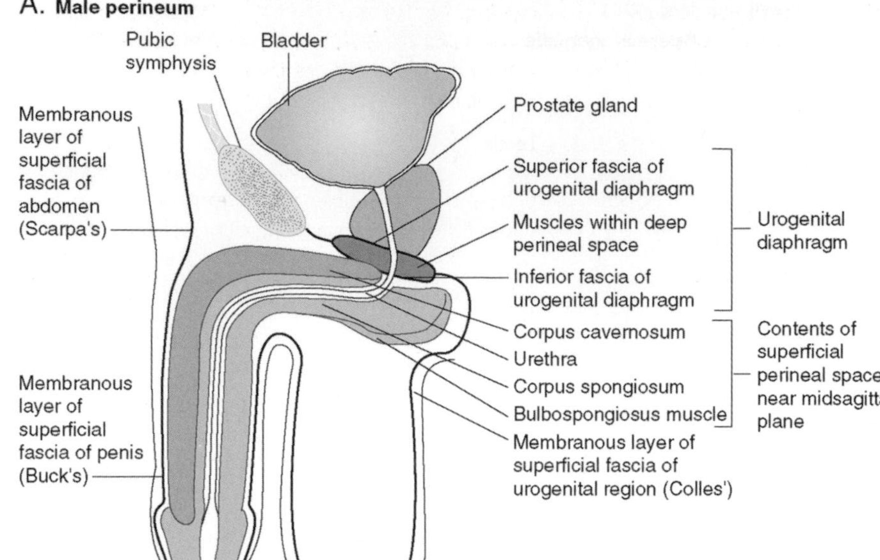

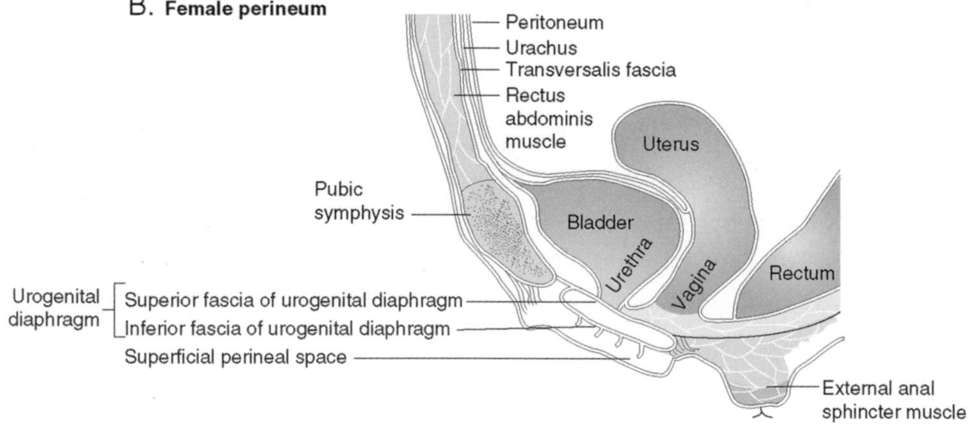

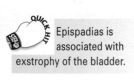

QUICK HIT: Epispadias is associated with exstrophy of the bladder.

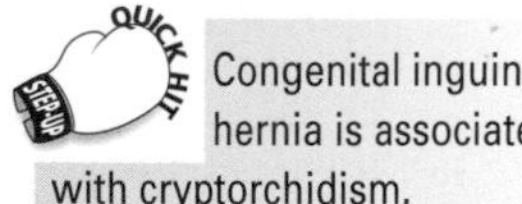

QUICK HIT: Congenital inguinal hernia is associated with cryptorchidism.

TABLE 8-1 **Congenital Malformations**

Malformation	Clinical Features
Hypospadias	• Urethra opens on the **ventral** side of the penis • Spongy urethra does not form properly or the **urogenital folds** do not fuse • Paucity of hormone receptors or too little hormone produced from the testes may play a role • More common than epispadias
Epispadias	• Urethra opens on the **dorsum** of the penis
Undescended testis (cryptorchidism)	• Most are of unknown cause • May be unilateral or bilateral • Most testes descend before 1 year of life • If testes remain undescended, **sterility or testicular cancer** can result
Congenital inguinal hernia (indirect hernia)	• A communication is formed between the **tunica vaginalis** (adjacent to the testis) and the peritoneal cavity • A loop of intestine may herniate into the opening and become entrapped, resulting in obstruction

(continued)

TABLE 8-1 Congenital Malformations *(Continued)*

Malformation	Clinical Features
True hermaphroditism	• **Both testicular** and **ovarian tissue** are present • External genitalia are ambiguous • Usually 46,XX
Female pseudohermaphroditism	• XX genotype with **virilization** of the external genitalia is present • The cause is **excess androgen exposure** • This malformation is most often caused by congenital adrenal hyperplasia, a **21-hydroxylase deficiency** (autosomal recessive disease with low cortisol and high ACTH)
Male pseudohermaphroditism	• XY genotype with varying ambiguities of the external genitalia • The cause is a **lack of MIF and testosterone**
Androgen insensitivity syndrome (testicular feminization)	• **XY** genotype with female phenotype • Caused by a **defective androgen receptor** • Vagina ends blindly (no uterus) • Normal female pubertal development occurs but pubic hair is scant and there are no menses
Double uterus completely	• The cause is failure of the **paramesonephric ducts** to fuse • The condition may appear in two forms: uterus divided internally by a thin septum or a division of only the superior part of the uterus (bicornuate uterus)
Kallmann syndrome	• A deficiency of GnRH results in decreased FSH and LH • No secondary sexual characteristics are present • Associated with hypoplasia of the olfactory bulbs **(anosmia)**

ACTH, adrenocorticotropic hormone; FSH, follicle-stimulating hormone; GnRH, gonadotropin-releasing hormone; LH, luteinizing hormone; MIF, müllerian inhibiting factor.

TABLE 8-2 Genetic Abnormalities Caused by Abnormal Somatic Chromosomes

Syndrome	Genotype	Description
Down syndrome	Trisomy 21 (95%) or robertsonian translocation of 14 and 21	• **Mental retardation** • Epicanthal folds • Large tongue • Brushfield spots on iris • Simian crease in hands • Increased incidence of congenital heart disease, acute leukemia, and dementia of the Alzheimer type later in life
Edward syndrome	Trisomy 18	• Duodenal atresia • Mental retardation • Micrognathia • **Rocker bottom feet** • Second digit overlaps third and fourth • Increased incidence of congenital heart disease
Patau syndrome	Trisomy 13	• Mental retardation • Microphthalmia • Polydactyly • Cleft lip and palate
Cri-du-chat syndrome	Deletion of 5p (5p–)	• Catlike cry • Mental retardation • Microcephaly • Hypertelorism

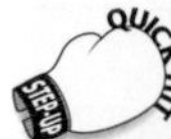

Fragile X is the second most common cause of mental retardation in males; Down syndrome is the most common cause.

MNEMONIC

To remember that Fragile X is due to a trinucleotide repeat **CGG**, think: "**See Giant Gonads.**"

TABLE 8-3 Genetic Abnormalities Caused by Abnormal Sex Chromosomes

Syndrome	Genotype	Description
Turner syndrome	45,XO	• **Monosomy** of the X chromosome • Absence of Barr body • Short stature • Webbed neck • Widely spaced nipples • Wide "shieldlike" chest • Wide carrying angle of arms • Lack of sexual maturity • Amenorrhea • Coarctation of the aorta
Klinefelter syndrome	47,XXY	• Tall with long limbs • Often presents with gynecomastia • Hyalinization of seminiferous tubules • Lack of spermatogenesis leading to sterility • One Barr body
XYY syndrome	47,XYY	• Normal-appearing male, often tall • Often associated with **aggressive behavior** • May be overrepresented in the population of incarcerated males
XXX syndrome	47,XXX	• Usually asymptomatic • Rarely associated with **menstrual irregularities** and mild mental retardation • Two Barr bodies
Fragile X syndrome	46,XY	• The end of the X chromosome appears delicate • **Macro-orchidism** • Common cause of **mental retardation** • Long face • Low-set, large ears
Prader–Willi syndrome	–15q12 (no paternal contribution, imprinting disorder)	• Obesity • **Hyperphagia** • **Hypogonadism** • Short stature • Mental retardation
Angelman syndrome	–15q12 (no maternal contribution, imprinting disorder)	• Ataxia • Mental retardation • **Inappropriate laughter** • Patient appears to act like a **"happy puppet"**

4. Etiology
   a. Central—increased FSH and LH
   b. Peripheral—caused by increased sex steroids

II. Menstruation and fertilization

A. Hormone formation and function (Figure 8-6)
   1. Ovarian **steroids** are synthesized from **cholesterol.**
   2. LH from the pituitary regulates the conversion of cholesterol to pregnenolone (the first step in estrogen synthesis) in the theca cells.
   3. FSH from the pituitary regulates the final step in estrogen synthesis in the granulosa cells.
   4. Estrogen
      a. Secreted by the follicular cells of the **ovary**
      b. Induces development of the secondary sex characteristics
         - Binds to the estrogen receptor
         - Activated estrogen-receptor complex interacts with nuclear chromatin
         - Initiates hormone-specific RNA synthesis
         - Results in protein synthesis

MNEMONIC

Associate **4** with the female reproductive system: **4** is the normal pH of the vagina; **40** weeks is the normal gestation period; **400** oocytes are released between menarche and menopause; **400,000** oocytes are present at puberty.

FIGURE 8-5 **Hormone regulation from infancy to menopause**

FSH, follicle-stimulating hormone; LH, luteinizing hormone. (Adapted with permission from Harrison TR, Fauci AS. Harrison's Principles of Internal Medicine. 14th Ed. New York: McGraw-Hill, 1997.)

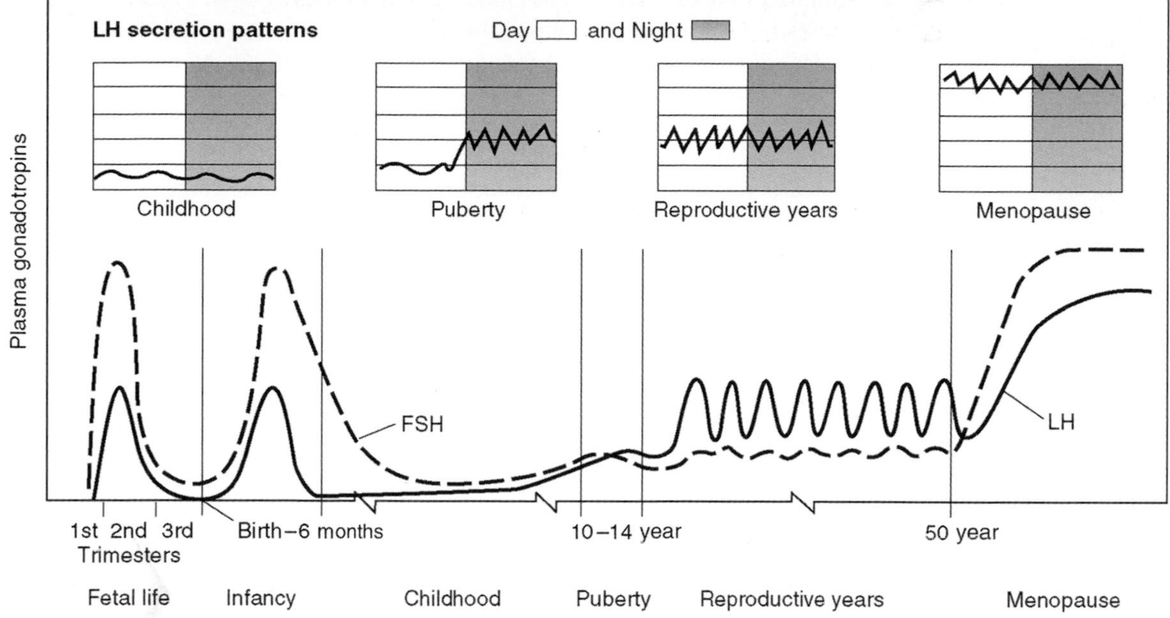

FIGURE 8-6 **Hormone function within the menstrual cycle**

FSH, follicle-stimulating hormone; LH, luteinizing hormone.

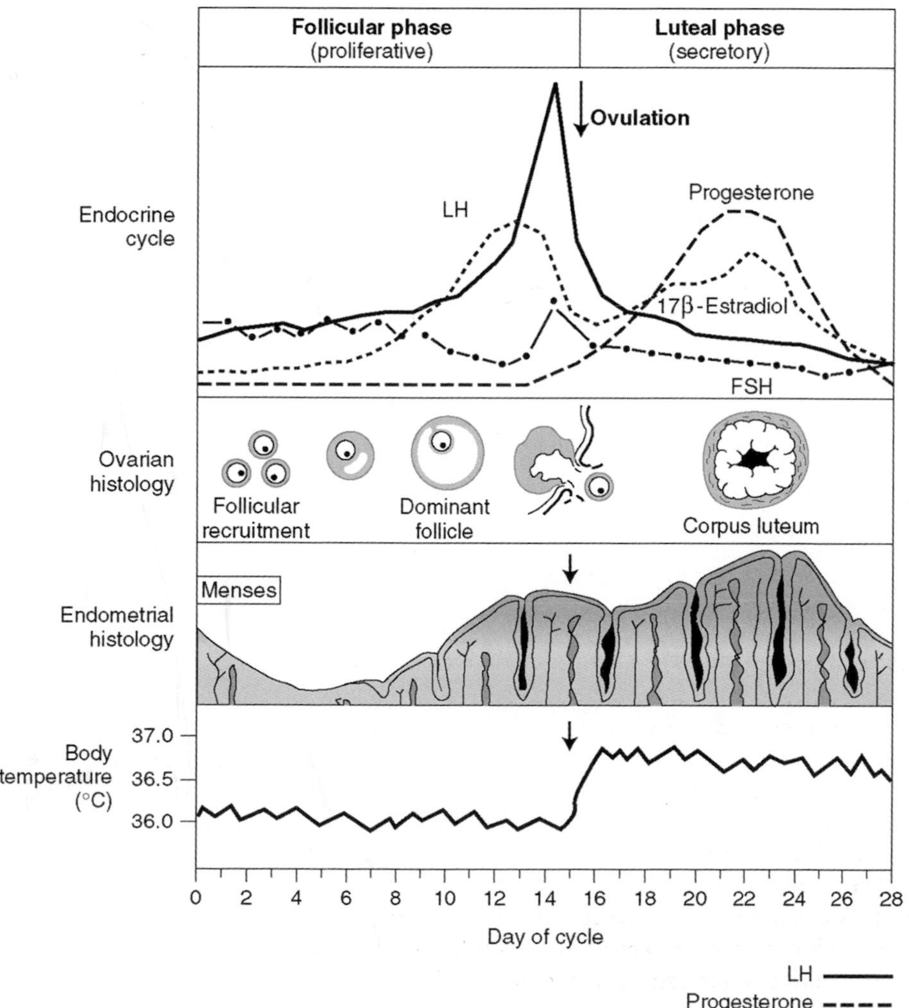

THE REPRODUCTIVE SYSTEM

c. Stimulates uterine growth and development
d. Stimulates the growth of endometrial spiral arteries
e. Causes thickening of the vaginal mucosa
f. Induces development of the breast ductal system
g. Causes bone growth (increased osteoblastic activity)

5. Progesterone
   a. Secreted by the **corpus luteum** produced in response to LH
   b. Converts proliferative endometrium to secretory endometrium
   c. Induces proliferation of endometrium
   d. Inhibits uterine contractions
   e. Increases the viscosity of cervical mucus
   f. Increases the basal body temperature
   g. Induces the development of breast glandular system

B. Menstrual cycle (Figure 8-7)
   1. One cycle is defined as the time from the onset of one menses to the next, an average of **28 days**.

FIGURE 8-7 **The menstrual cycle**
FSH, follicle-stimulating hormone; hCG, human chorionic gonadotropin; LH, luteinizing hormone.

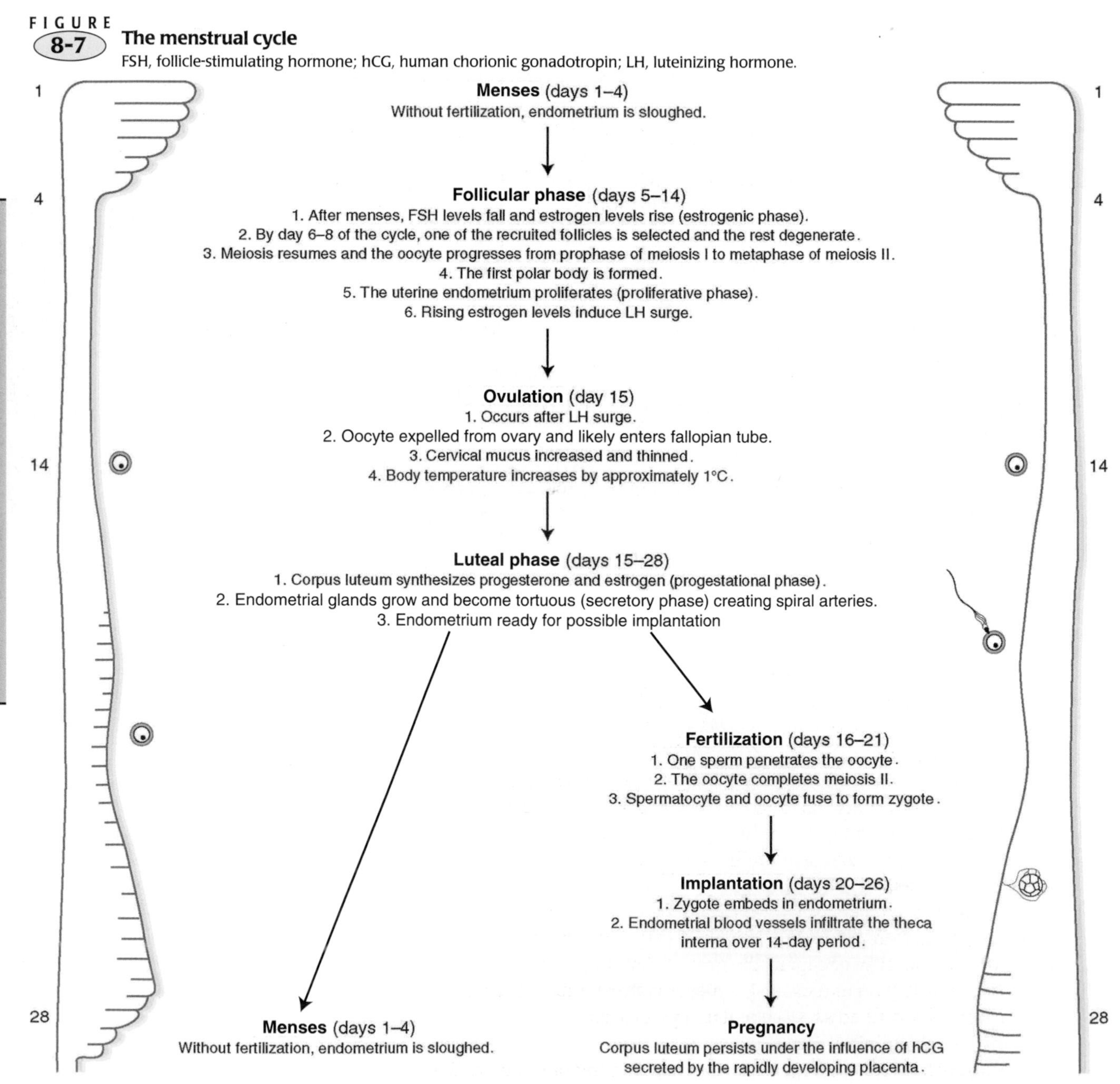

1
4
14
28
Menses (days 1–4)
Without fertilization, endometrium is sloughed.
Follicular phase (days 5–14)
1. After menses, FSH levels fall and estrogen levels rise (estrogenic phase).
2. By day 6–8 of the cycle, one of the recruited follicles is selected and the rest degenerate.
3. Meiosis resumes and the oocyte progresses from prophase of meiosis I to metaphase of meiosis II.
4. The first polar body is formed.
5. The uterine endometrium proliferates (proliferative phase).
6. Rising estrogen levels induce LH surge.
Ovulation (day 15)
1. Occurs after LH surge.
2. Oocyte expelled from ovary and likely enters fallopian tube.
3. Cervical mucus increased and thinned.
4. Body temperature increases by approximately 1°C.
Luteal phase (days 15–28)
1. Corpus luteum synthesizes progesterone and estrogen (progestational phase).
2. Endometrial glands grow and become tortuous (secretory phase) creating spiral arteries.
3. Endometrium ready for possible implantation
Fertilization (days 16–21)
1. One sperm penetrates the oocyte.
2. The oocyte completes meiosis II.
3. Spermatocyte and oocyte fuse to form zygote.
Implantation (days 20–26)
1. Zygote embeds in endometrium.
2. Endometrial blood vessels infiltrate the theca interna over 14-day period.
Menses (days 1–4)
Without fertilization, endometrium is sloughed.
Pregnancy
Corpus luteum persists under the influence of hCG secreted by the rapidly developing placenta.

FIGURE 8-8 Developmental changes in the ovary

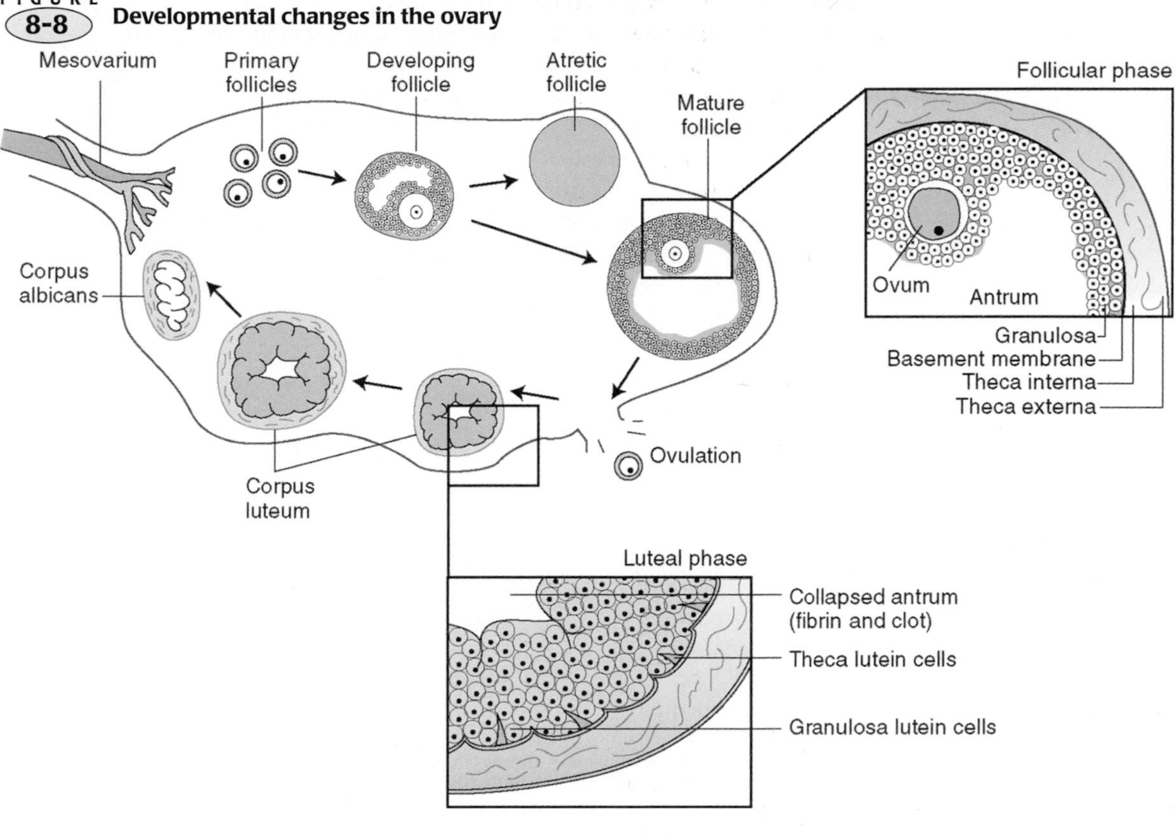

2. Some oocytes within the ovaries undergo developmental changes during the cycle (Figure 8-8).

C. **Disorders**

1. **Dysfunctional uterine bleeding (DUB)**
    a. A functional menstrual disorder with excessive bleeding during or between menstrual periods
    b. Most common gynecologic problem during reproductive years
    c. Caused by
        - Leiomyoma (fibroids)
        - Anovulatory cycle
        - Organic lesions (tumors, polyps)
        - Complications of pregnancy (ectopic pregnancy, cesarean section, abortion, etc.)
        - Endometrial hyperplasia
        - Corpus luteum cysts
        - Polycystic ovary syndrome
        - Endometriosis
2. **Polycystic ovary syndrome (Stein–Leventhal syndrome)**
    a. Triad of **secondary amenorrhea**, **obesity**, and **hirsutism**
    b. Increased LH and testosterone
    c. Stromal fibrosis and small follicular cysts in the ovary
3. **Endometriosis**
    a. Non-neoplastic endometrial tissue located outside the uterus
    b. Responds to hormonal variations of menstrual cycle
    c. Most commonly occurs in the ovary (bilateral)
    d. Presents as pain and excessive bleeding during menstruation
    e. Large, blood-filled sacs (**chocolate cysts**) seen
    f. May result in infertility
    g. **Danazol**, a mild androgen, can be used as a treatment modality

4. **Amenorrhea** (Figures 8-9 and 8-10)
   a. **Primary amenorrhea**: absence of menarche in a woman by age 16
      - Turner syndrome
      - Imperforate hymen
      - Androgen insensitivity syndrome
      - Müllerian duct agenesis
      - Delayed puberty
   b. **Secondary amenorrhea**: cessation of menstruation for >3 months in a woman of reproductive age with cyclic periods or >6 months in a woman with irregular periods
      - Pregnancy
      - Ovarian failure
      - Polycystic ovary syndrome
      - Hypothyroidism
      - Athleticism
      - Anorexia
      - Stress

QUICK HIT: In understanding müllerian duct agenesis and androgen insensitivity syndrome, it is important to remember that the ovaries and the lower vagina are not derived from the müllerian system. The ovaries are derived from germ cells that migrate from the primitive yolk sac into the mesenchyme of the peritoneal cavity and subsequently develop into ova and supporting cells. The lower one third of the vagina arises from the sinovaginal bulb which fuses with the müllerian-derived upper two thirds to form the complete vagina.

QUICK HIT: There are four causes of primary amenorrhea in the female: Turner syndrome (XO), müllerian duct agenesis (XX), imperforate hymen (XX), and androgen insensitivity syndrome (XY).

FIGURE 8-9 **Causes of amenorrhea**

In approaching the various causes of amenorrhea, it is easiest to conceptualize them within the hypothalamic-pituitary-ovarian-uterine framework. It is postulated that stress, exercise, and anorexia act at the level of the hypothalamus to stop the menstrual cycle. Prolactin tumors at the pituitary level disrupt the neuroendocrine regulation of GnRH, resulting in an abnormal menstrual function. At the ovarian level, ovarian failure, polycystic ovarian syndrome, and streak gonads of Turner syndrome result in menstrual dysfunction. Müllerian duct agenesis, imperforate hymen, and androgen insensitivity syndrome are abnormalities at the uterine and vaginal level. PCOS, polycystic ovarian syndrome.

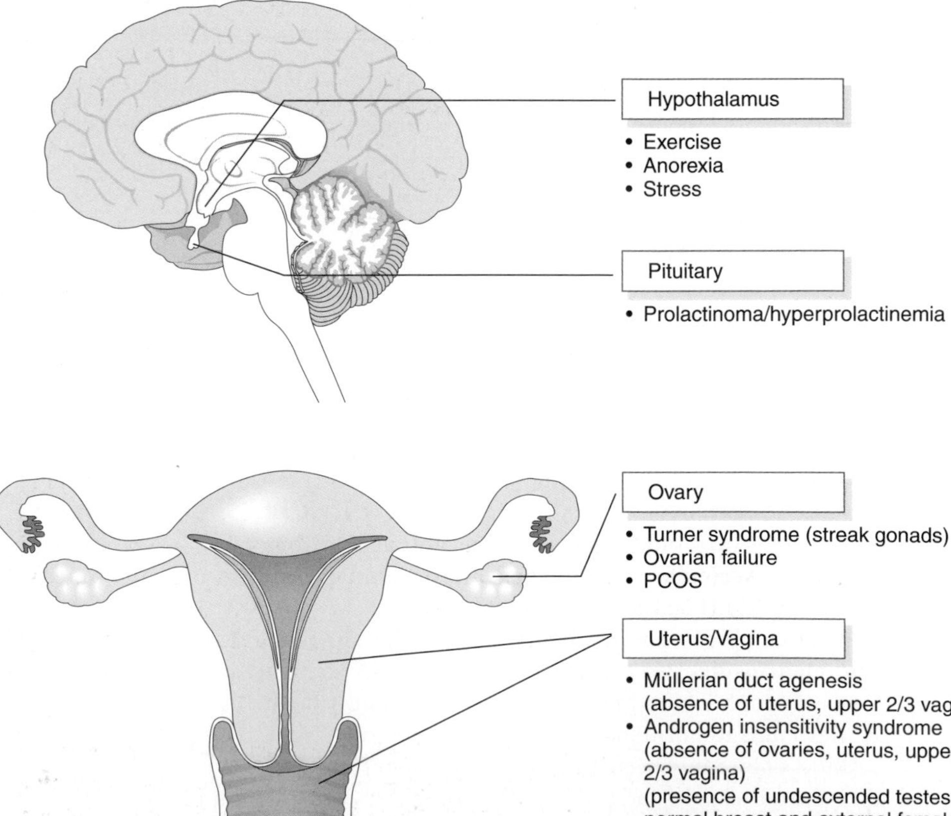

FIGURE 8-10 **Approach to amenorrhea**
DHEAS, dehydroepiandrosterone sulfate; PCOS, polycystic ovarian syndrome.

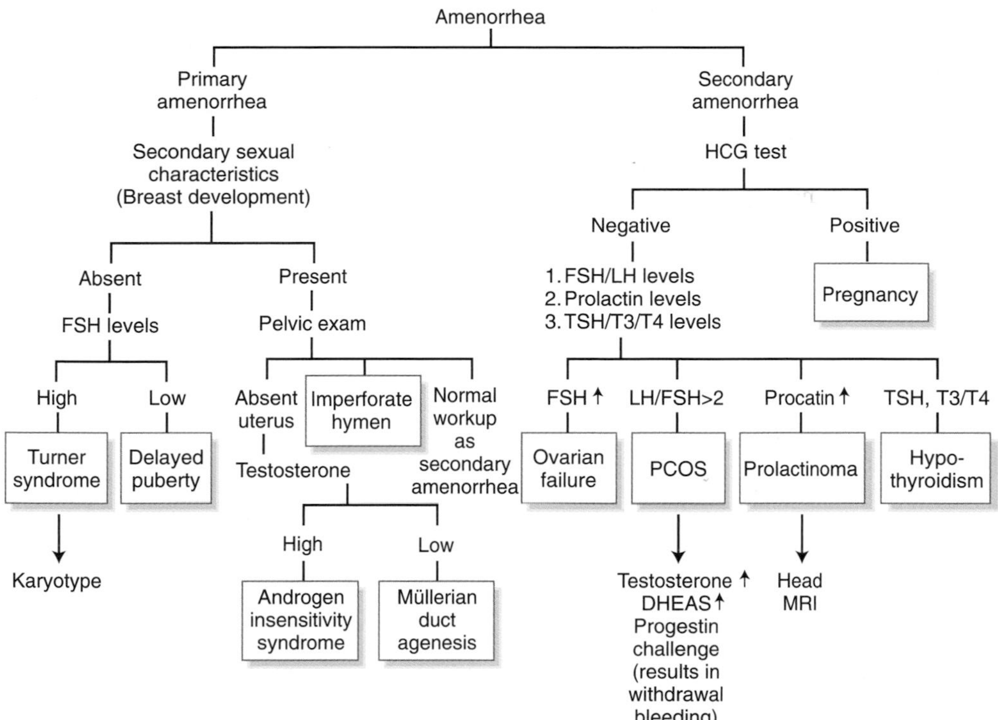

Clinical Vignette 8-1

Clinical Presentation: A 17-year-old girl presents to her primary care physician with the chief complaint that she has not **had her period for several months.** She previously had fairly regular menses, with menarche at age 13. She is the daughter of a **middle class family,** an **excellent student,** and **active in track** outside of class. Physical examination shows a well-developed female with **normal external female genitalia.** Pelvic examination is deferred.

Differentials: Pregnancy, anorexia nervosa, exercise, pituitary prolactinoma, polycystic ovary syndrome, ovarian failure, Turner syndrome, and hypothyroidism. **Any female who reports missing her period should be evaluated for pregnancy.** The first step in approaching amenorrhea is to determine whether the patient has had periods in the past (secondary amenorrhea) or has never experienced menstruation (primary amenorrhea). There are four diagnoses unique to primary amenorrhea: Turner syndrome, müllerian duct agenesis, imperforate hymen, and androgen insensitivity syndrome. These disorders can be ruled out in this case because the patient has a history of periods. (*Note:* Mosaic Turner syndrome can have some menstrual bleeding prior to the cessation of periods.) Figure 8-9 shows the various causes of amenorrhea. On the USMLEs, look for certain symptoms that suggest some disorders over others: hirsutism (polycystic ovary syndrome [PCOS]), obesity (PCOS), galactorrhea (prolactinoma), webbed neck (Turner), widely spaced nipples (Turner), presence of abdominal masses (testes gen insensitivity syndrome), and renal anomalies (müllerian duct agenesis). Pelvic examination would be helpful in assessing imperforate hymen, androgen insensitivity syndrome (blind ending short vaginal canal and absence of uterus and ovaries), and müllerian duct agenesis (blind ending short vaginal canal and absence of uterus).

Laboratory Studies: In approaching secondary amenorrhea (Figure 8-10), first obtain a **pregnancy test.** If negative, a battery of tests would be performed including **follicle-stimulating hormone (FSH), leuteinizing hormone (LH), thyroid-stimulating hormone (TSH)/ triiodothyronine (T_3)/ levothyroxine (T_4), and prolactin levels** to rule out hypothyroidism and prolactinoma,

(continued)

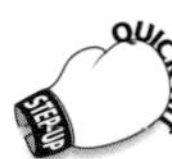

In androgen insensitivity syndrome (AIS), affected individuals have normal testes with normal production of testosterone and normal conversion to DHT, which differentiates this condition from 5α-reductase deficiency. Because the testes produce normal amounts of MIF, affected individuals do not have fallopian tubes, a uterus, or a proximal (upper) vagina. In AIS, the external female genitalia and breasts develop by default because of the **lack of responsiveness of androgen receptors to DHT** during development. In 5α-reductase deficiency, **lack of DHT** results in a female genotype. At puberty in these individuals, a testosterone surge results in adequate levels of DHT, resulting in growth of male genitalia and "penis at 12" syndrome.

Clinical Vignette 8-1 *(Continued)*

respectively. FSH and LH levels are expected to be high in cases of ovarian defects (Turner syndrome, ovarian failure, and PCOS) and low to normal in defects at the hypothalamic/pituitary level (pituitary tumors, anorexia, and athleticism). To further differentiate among these, if LH/FSH >2, it suggests PCOS and **testosterone and** dehydroepiandrosterone sulfate **(DHEAS) levels** should be measured (will likely be elevated). Also, progestin challenge should induce withdrawal from menstrual bleeding. Turner syndrome and ovarian failure can be distinguished by karyotype. In cases of suspected anatomical abnormalities, a pelvic ultrasound should be performed.

Management: Most treatments of secondary amenorrhea are directed to correct the underlying disease process via surgery or restore ovulatory cycle via estrogen–progestin therapy. PCOS is treated based on the reproductive desire of the female—**spironolactone** with **clomiphene citrate** is used if the patient is interested in conceiving; otherwise, **oral contraception** may be used.

III. Menopause

A. Last physiologic menstrual cycle usually occurs in the **mid-40s or early 50s.**
B. Estrogen levels fall (because of the reduced ovarian function) and FSH levels increase.
C. Early signs
   1. Anxiety
   2. Mood swings
   3. Irritability
   4. Depression
   5. **Hot flashes:** bouts of flushing and sweating
D. Late signs
   1. Vaginal dryness
   2. Painful intercourse
   3. Urinary tract infections
   4. Atrophy of breast tissue because of lack of estrogen stimulation
   5. **Osteoporosis**
   6. **Decreased high-density lipoproteins** (HDL), leading to an increased risk of **coronary artery disease**
   7. Does not result in a decreased libido
E. Management of patients who are menopausal or postmenopausal may involve estrogen replacement therapy.
   1. Effects
      a. Decreases sleep disturbances
      b. Increases HDL and decreases low-density lipoprotein (LDL)
      c. Decreases postmenopausal vaginal atrophy
      d. Decreases bone resorption and osteoporosis
      e. Decreases frequency of "hot flashes" by reestablishing hypothalamic control of norepinephrine secretion
   2. Risks and contraindications
      a. History of estrogen-dependent cancer
      b. Increased risk of breast and endometrial cancer
      c. In women with an intact uterus, estrogen increases the risk of developing endometrial carcinoma. Therefore, estrogen is combined with progestin to decrease the effects of unopposed estrogen.
      d. Women's Health Initiative showed that estrogen increased the absolute risk of stroke by 0.13% when compared to placebo.

IV. Oral contraceptives

A. Agents that interfere with ovulation to prevent pregnancy
B. Combination pills contain progestin and estrogen
   1. The estrogen component suppresses ovulation.
   2. The progestin component prevents implantation in the endometrium.

C. Other agents
   1. Progestin only
      a. Available as pills and progestin implants
      b. Higher failure rate
      c. Increased rate of menstrual irregularities
   2. Mifepristone (RU 486), a progestin antagonist
      a. Results in fetal abortion when given early in pregnancy (within first 6 weeks)
      b. Interferes with progesterone and decreases human chorionic gonadotropin (hCG)
D. Side effects
   1. Cardiovascular disease
      a. Women older than 35 years of age who smoke are at greatest risk from thromboembolism.
      b. Progestin-predominant preparations can lead to an increase in the LDL:HDL ratio.
   2. Benign liver hepatomas and hemangiomas
   3. Emotional changes

PREGNANCY AND ITS ASSOCIATED COMPLICATIONS

I. Normal pregnancy

A. For clinical purposes, assume that a **woman of childbearing age is pregnant** unless proven otherwise.
B. Normal gestation is **40 weeks.**
C. Clinical signs include missed periods, swollen breasts, fatigue, nausea, and **elevated** β-human chorionic gonadotropin (β-hCG) (serum).
D. Hormonal regulation
   1. During fertilization, **β-hCG** produced by the placenta **prevents corpus luteum regression.**
   2. During the first trimester, the **corpus luteum** produces estrogen and progesterone.
   3. Second and third trimester
      a. Progesterone is produced by the **placenta.**
      b. Estrogen production is regulated by the interplay among the fetal adrenal gland, fetal liver, and placenta.
   4. The initiating event in parturition is unknown, but delivery can be induced by oxytocin.
   5. Lactation
      a. Estrogen and progesterone block the effect of prolactin on the breast.
      b. Prolactin levels rise throughout pregnancy and suppress ovulation.
      c. Estrogen/progesterone levels fall after delivery.
E. Prenatal diagnostic procedures
   1. **Amniocentesis** is an aspiration of fluid from the amniotic sac at 10 to 14 weeks after fertilization.
      a. α-Fetoprotein (**AFP**) assay for neural tube defects
      b. **Spectrophotometry** to determine hemolytic disease of the newborn (see System 10)
      c. Sex chromatin studies for X-linked disease
      d. **Cell culture** studies for chromosomal abnormalities
      e. Enzyme and DNA analysis
   2. Maternal serum AFP
      a. Elevated in neural tube defects
      b. Reduced in Down syndrome
   3. Chorionic villus sampling
      a. It can be performed at 10 weeks of pregnancy.
      b. Cells are aspirated from the chorionic villi.
      c. Cells are evaluated for genetic abnormalities.

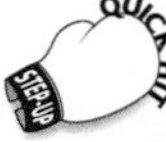

Clomiphene interferes with the negative feedback provided by estrogen and causes an increase in gonadotropin-releasing hormone (GnRH). This leads to stimulation of ovulation and can be used to treat infertility associated with anovulatory cycles.

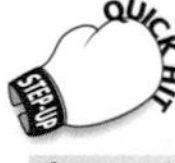

A pudendal nerve block can be performed to alleviate the pain of childbirth. One hand is inserted into the vagina to locate the ischial spine, which is used as a landmark, while the other hand inserts a needle, which contains anesthetic for the skin lateral to the vaginal opening.

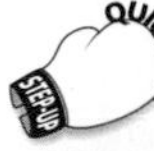

The narrowest diameter that the fetus must transverse during birth is the pelvic outlet, from ischial spine to ischial spine (interspinous distance).

MNEMONIC

Remember the causes of **I**ncreased **M**aternal **S**erum **A**lpha **F**eto **P**rotein: **I**ntestinal obstruction; **M**ultiple gestation/**M**yeloschisis; **S**pina bifida cystica; **A**nencephaly/**A**bdominal wall defects; **F**etal deaths; and **P**lacental abruption.

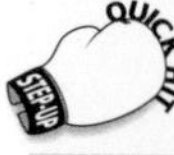

Some nonsexually transmitted infections of the genitourinary tract include *Candida albicans,* which causes vulvovaginitis, *Staphylococcus aureus,* which can result in toxic shock syndrome, and *Escherichia coli* and *Staphylococcus saprophyticus,* both of which can cause urinary tract infections (UTIs).

Salpingitis, often associated with PID, can lead to infertility if left untreated.

4. **Ultrasound**
   a. Can be performed at 12 weeks of pregnancy
   b. Measures the fetal size, determines the sex, and diagnoses the fetal malformations

F. Apgar score
1. It is used for physical assessment of child 1 min and 5 min after birth.
2. Five categories are scored 0, 1, or 2, with 2 being indicative of better performance.
   a. Color (blue = 0, trunk pink = 1, all pink = 2)
   b. Heart rate (0 = 0, <100 = 1, 100+ = 2)
   c. Reflexes (none = 0, grimace = 1, grimace and irritable = 2)
   d. Muscle tone (none = 0, some = 1, active = 2)
   e. Respiration (none = 0, irregular = 1, regular = 2)

II. Abnormal placental attachment

A. **Abruptio placentae**
1. Placenta separates from the uterine wall before parturition.
2. It usually leads to fetal **death.**
3. It may result in disseminated intravascular coagulation (**DIC**) in mother.

B. **Placenta accreta**
1. Direct connection of the uterus wall to placenta
2. Caused by prior surgery or trauma during pregnancy
3. Improper separation results in massive **hemorrhage**

C. **Placenta previa**
1. Placenta attaches to the lower uterus and blocks the cervical os.
2. It is associated with **bleeding.**

III. Ectopic pregnancy

A. Risk factors
1. **Pelvic inflammatory disease (PID)** (e.g., chronic salpingitis)
2. Previous surgery
3. Endometriosis
4. Previous ectopic pregnancy

B. Clinical features
1. Amenorrhea
2. Pelvic pain and cervical tenderness
3. Tissue mass (usually in the fallopian tubes)
4. Abnormally elevated β-hCG levels

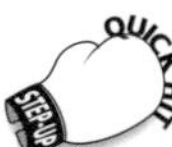

Treatment for pre-eclampsia includes magnesium sulfate or terbutaline. However, the treatment of choice to deliver a complete cure is the delivery of the fetus, if feasible.

IV. Pre-eclampsia

A. Triad of **hypertension, proteinuria,** and **edema**

B. Most common in the last trimester of first pregnancy

C. May result in eclampsia if untreated
1. Eclampsia has manifestations similar to pre-eclampsia, but it also includes seizures and possibly DIC.
2. Eclampsia can be characterized by **H**ypertension, **E**levated **L**iver enzymes, and **L**ow **P**latelets (**HELLP** syndrome).

Hydatidiform moles usually precede gestational choriocarcinoma (a malignant neoplasm of trophoblastic cells).

V. Hydatidiform mole

A. Placental villi that enlarge abnormally early in pregnancy

B. "**Cluster of grapes**" with a marked increase in β-hCG

C. Manifests as vaginal bleeding and an increase in uterine size

D. "Snowstorm" pattern seen on ultrasound

E. Two types
1. **Complete mole**
   a. Diploid XX karyotype
   b. No embryo present
   c. Completely paternal in origin

2. **Partial mole**
   a. Triploid (XXX or XXY) karyotype
   b. Embryo present

VI. Gestational diabetes

A. Insulin resistance occurs in normal pregnancy.
B. Mother may be unable to meet the increased metabolic demands of pregnancy.
C. Two or more of the following venous glucose values must be reached after a 100-g oral glucose load
   1. Fasting >105 mg/dL
   2. 1 h >190 mg/dL
   3. 2 h >165 mg/dL
   4. 3 h >145 mg/dL
D. High blood glucose leads to hypoglycemia in the infant, macrosomia (enlarged body), increased risk of trauma, and increased likelihood of cesarean section because of the large size of fetus.

VII. Infections causing birth defects (TORCHES)

A. The **TORCHES** are **T**oxoplasmosis, **O**ther infections, **R**ubella, **C**ytomegalovirus infection, **HE**rpes simplex, and **S**yphilis.
B. This group of infectious organisms can cause birth defects if the mother is infected during pregnancy, especially in the first trimester
   1. Infection with herpes simplex more commonly occurs during the passage through the birth canal.
C. Important agents in the "other" category are human immunodeficiency virus (HIV) and hepatitis B.

GYNECOLOGIC DIAGNOSTIC TESTS

I. Wet mount

A. Vaginal epithelial scrapings placed on a glass slide with a drop of saline
B. Microbes detected
   1. Trichomonas appears as a pear-shaped organism with sporadic movement.
   2. Bacterial vaginosis appears as vaginal epithelium with roughened edges (**clue cells**).

II. Potassium hydroxide (KOH) preparation

A. KOH is added to a microscope slide prepared with vaginal epithelial scrapings.
B. Epithelium is dissolved with KOH.
C. Microbes detected
   1. *Candida*, which is resistant to KOH, remains on the slide and is identified by its **budding cells with short hyphae.**
   2. KOH reacts with bacterial amines producing a "fishy odor" characteristic of bacterial vaginosis (whiff test).

III. Papanicolaou (Pap) smear

A. Cells from the cervix are scraped and fixed onto a glass slide.
B. Microbes detected
   1. Human papilloma virus (HPV) is characterized by **koilocytes** (large epithelial cells with perinuclear clearing).
   2. Cytomegalovirus (CMV) appears as intranuclear inclusions with a halo around them (**owl's eye** cells).
   3. Herpes simplex virus appears as intranuclear inclusions and multinucleated giant cells.
C. Precancerous lesions detected: cervical intraepithelial neoplasia (CIN) 1, 2, and 3
D. Cancers detected
   1. Invasive **squamous cell carcinoma** (most common)
   2. Endometrial adenocarcinoma

SEXUALLY TRANSMITTED DISEASES

Between 20% and 50% of those patients with one STD will have a coexisting infection with another. The sexual partners of those diagnosed with an STD should be treated. Physicians should encourage their patients to make partners aware of potential STD risk and urge them to seek diagnosis and treatment (Table 8-4).

> QUICK HIT: **Chlamydia is the most common sexually transmitted disease (STD) in the world** in part because of the fact that it goes undetected when the patient is coinfected with *Neisseria gonorrhoeae.* Treatment for gonorrhea should be supplemented with chlamydia therapy for both the patient and his/her partner.

TABLE 8-4 Sexually Transmitted Diseases

Microbe	Disease
Calymmatobacterium granulomatis	Granuloma inguinale; biopsy shows **Donovan bodies**
Chlamydia trachomatis	Urethritis; **acute pelvic inflammatory disease;** ulcerative lesions of the genitalia (L1, L2, and L3 serotypes)
Gardnerella vaginalis	Vulvovaginitis
Haemophilus ducreyi	Chancroid; **painful** ulcerative lesions of the genitalia
Herpes simplex virus-2	Genital herpes; urethritis; **painful** ulcerative lesions of the genitalia
HIV types 1 and 2	**AIDS**
Human papilloma virus (especially serotypes 6 and 11)	**Condyloma acuminatum** of vulva
Human papilloma virus (especially serotypes 16, 18, 31, and 45)	Genital or anal **warts; squamous cell carcinoma** of cervix, vagina, anus, or penis; CIN
Neisseria gonorrhoeae	Urethritis; **acute pelvic inflammatory disease;** pharyngitis; monoarticular **arthritis**
Treponema pallidum	Syphilis; **painless** ulcerative lesions of the genitalia Primary syphilis—hard chancres Secondary syphilis—gray wartlike lesions on the genitalia (condyloma lata) Tertiary syphilis—neurologic manifestations such as tabes dorsalis and ascending aortic aneurysm
Trichomonas vaginalis	Vulvovaginitis; male urethritis

> MNEMONIC: To remember the painful ulcers of the genitalia, think in *Haemophilus ducreyi* "you do cry" and HSV2 is painful **too.** Syphillus is pain**less**.

> QUICK HIT: PID can be diagnosed via bimanual pelvic examination eliciting **"the chandelier sign"** (exquisite cervical motion tenderness).

> MNEMONIC: Remember the features of *Trichomonas* with the four Fs: Flagella, Frothy discharge, Fishy odor, and Flagyl (treatment).

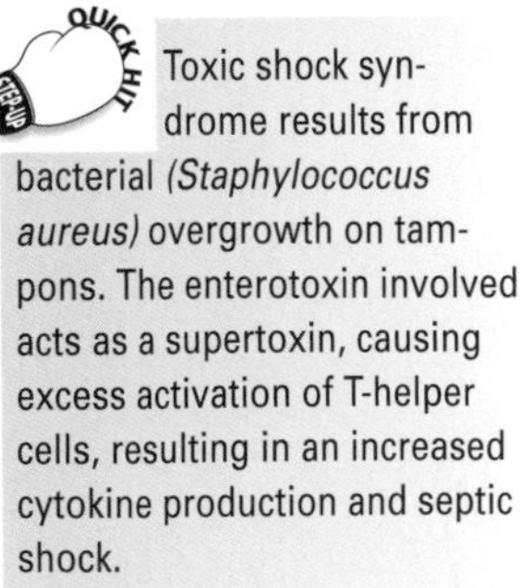

Toxic shock syndrome results from bacterial *(Staphylococcus aureus)* overgrowth on tampons. The enterotoxin involved acts as a supertoxin, causing excess activation of T-helper cells, resulting in an increased cytokine production and septic shock.

FEMALE GYNECOLOGIC NEOPLASMS

Tumors of the gynecologic organs may manifest themselves as DUB and, as such, a heightened level of suspicion must be maintained with this presentation. Many of these neoplasms can be detected, and even prevented (as is the case with cervical cancer), by routine gynecologic examinations.

I. Ovarian neoplasms of epithelial origin (Table 8-5)

II. Ovarian neoplasms of germ cell origin (Table 8-6)

III. Tumors of the uterus (cervix and body) (Table 8-7)

IV. Tumors of the vulva and vagina (Table 8-8)

BREAST PATHOLOGY

Risk factors for breast cancer include being older than 45 years of age, nulliparity, early menarche, late menopause, high-fat diet, *HER-2*/neu oncogene activation, first-degree relative with positive history, and a history of breast cancer in the contralateral breast (Table 8-9).

(text continues on page 233)

TABLE 8-5 Ovarian Neoplasms of Epithelial Cell Origin

Neoplasm	Morphology	Clinical Presentation
Serous cystadenoma	Cystic	Benign; frequently bilateral
Serous cystadenocarcinoma	Cystic	Malignant; frequently bilateral; most common (50% of ovarian neoplasms)
Mucinous cystadenoma	Mucin-filled cysts	Benign
Mucinous cystadenocarcinoma	Mucin-filled cysts	Malignant; **pseudomyxoma peritonei** (diffuse peritoneal metastasis secreting mucin)
Endometrioid adenocarcinoma	Resembles endometrium	Malignant
Brenner tumor	Resembles **transitional epithelium**	Benign; rare tumor
Clear cell cancer	Abundant **clear cytoplasm**	Usually unilateral; rare

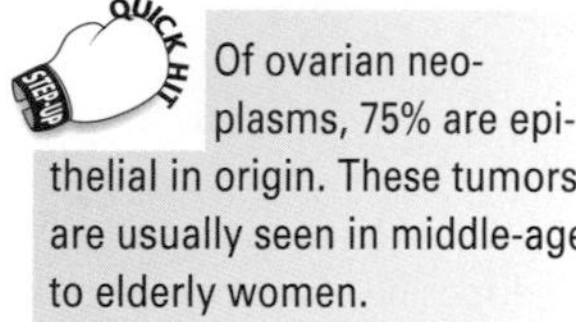

Of ovarian neoplasms, 75% are epithelial in origin. These tumors are usually seen in middle-age to elderly women.

TABLE 8-6 Ovarian Neoplasms of Germ Cell Origin

Neoplasm	Morphology	Clinical Features
Dysgerminoma	Large cells with clear cytoplasm	Malignant; **equivalent of seminoma;** occurs in children
Endodermal sinus (yolk sac)	Resembles yolk sac	Malignant; produces **AFP**
Immature teratoma	Elements from multiple embryonic layers; poorly differentiated; resembles fetal or embryonic tissue	Malignant
Mature teratoma (dermoid cyst)	Elements from multiple embryonic layers, including hair, bone, tooth, and nervous tissue; duplication of maternal genetics; resembles adult tissue	**Most common germ cell neoplasm** (90%); **benign** (vs. malignant in males)
Monodermal teratoma	Elements from multiple embryonic layers; one tissue type develops, most commonly thyroid tissue **(struma ovarii)**	Benign; hyperthyroidism
Choriocarcinoma	Usually seen in combination with other germ cell tumors	Malignant; produces **(β-hCG)**
Granulosa-theca tumor	Lipid-laden cells; fibroblast proliferation; cuboidal cells in cords; eosinophilic follicles **(Call–Exner bodies)**	Benign; may secrete estrogen, leading to precocious puberty or endometrial hyperplasia or carcinoma
Thecoma fibroma	Fibroblast proliferation	Benign; rare; in combination with ascites and hydrothorax, referred to as **Meigs syndrome**
Sertoli–Leydig cell tumor	Tubules containing Sertoli and Leydig cells	Produces testosterone; virilization
Metastasis	Most commonly from gastrointestinal tract, breast, or ovary; **Krukenberg tumor,** primary in stomach with signet-ring cells bilaterally	Only 5% of ovarian neoplasms

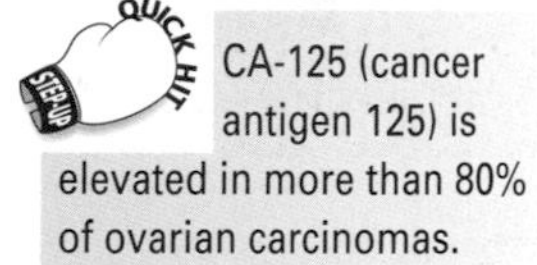

CA-125 (cancer antigen 125) is elevated in more than 80% of ovarian carcinomas.

Germ cell tumors account for only 25% of ovarian neoplasms but are the most common ovarian tumors found in women younger than 20 years of age.

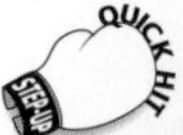

Estrogens can be synthesized by adipose tissue. This may be partially responsible for predisposing obese women to endometrial carcinoma.

TABLE 8-7 Tumors of the Uterus (Cervix and Body)

Neoplasm	Clinical Features
CIN	• May be classified as CIN I, CIN II, or CIN III • Neoplastic changes in the endometrium beginning at the **squamocolumnar junction** • CIN I: mild dysplasia extending less than one-third the thickness of the epithelium • CIN II: cells appear more malignant with increased mitotic figures and variation in nuclear size; approximately two-thirds of the epithelium involved • CIN III: also called carcinoma in situ; involves the full thickness of the cervical epithelium • Associated with HPV 16, 18, 31, 33, and 45 infection
Squamous cell carcinoma of the cervix	• Evolves from a progression of CIN • Increased incidence is associated with **early sexual activity** and **multiple sex partners**
Leiomyoma	• Benign tumor of the uterine body • The **most common tumor of women** (the most common malignancy in women is breast cancer) • Often multiple • Size increases with pregnancy and decreases with menopause
Leiomyosarcoma	• Uncommon • Does not arise from a preexisting dysplastic or neoplastic condition
Endometrial carcinoma	• The **most common malignancy** of the female genital tract • Associated with nulliparity • More often found in older women • Exogenous **estrogen** administration or estrogen-producing tumors may be the predisposing factors • Other risk factors are diabetes, tamoxifen, hypertension, and obesity • Usually presents as vaginal bleeding

TABLE 8-8 Tumors of the Vulva and Vagina

Tumor	Description
Papillary hidradenoma	• **Most common** benign tumor of the vulva • Often presents as an ulcerated and bleeding nodule • Originates from apocrine sweat glands • Can easily be surgically removed
Squamous cell carcinoma of the vulva	• Similar to squamous cell carcinoma of the cervix • Highest occurrence in **older women** • Vulvar dystrophy precedes carcinoma • Associated with the infections of HPV 16, 18, 31, 33, and 45
Paget disease of the vulva	• Histologically, similar to Paget disease of the breast • Not always associated with underlying adenocarcinoma (vs. Paget disease of the breast)
Malignant melanoma	• Similar to malignant melanoma of the skin • 10% of malignant tumors of the vulva
Squamous cell carcinoma of the vagina	• The vagina is rarely a primary site of cancer formation • Usually an extension of squamous cell carcinoma of the cervix
Clear cell adenocarcinoma	• A rare malignant tumor • Occurs in the daughters of women given **diethylstilbestrol (DES)** during pregnancy
Sarcoma botryoides	• A type of rhabdomyosarcoma • Usually occurs in **girls younger than 5** years of age • **"Bunch of grapes"** that protrude from the vagina

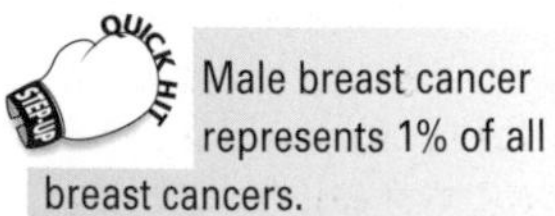

Male breast cancer represents 1% of all breast cancers.

TABLE 8-9 Breast Pathology

Condition	Pathology	Clinical Features
Acute mastitis	Entry of ***Staphylococcus aureus*** through nipple; abscess	Most often occurs during **nursing;** may be caused by eczema
Fibrocystic changes	Breast mass; tender during menstruation; usually **bilateral; "blue-domed"** cysts	**Most common breast disorder;** non-neoplastic; predisposition to cancer only with evidence of cellular atypia
Fibroadenoma	Painless; rubbery mass	Benign; **most common tumor in patients younger than 25 years of age**
Intraductal papilloma	Tumor of the lactiferous ducts	Benign; may present as serous or bloody discharge
Phyllodes tumor	Large mass; cysts; ulceration of the skin	Malignant potential; may recur
Invasive ductal carcinoma	Firm mass; cells form glands; fibrous stroma	Malignant; **most common** carcinoma of the breast
Lobular carcinoma	Cancer cells fill ducts; **bloody discharge;** may be bilateral; cells line up **"Indian file"**	Malignant; may be progression of lobular carcinoma in situ
Paget disease	Superficial lesion of nipple or areola; **Paget cells** in epidermis (large cell with marginal clearing seen)	Malignant; indicative of **underlying ductal carcinoma**
Medullary carcinoma	Soft, fleshy tumor; characterized by lymphocytic infiltrate	Malignant

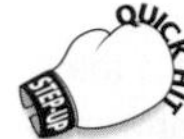

Breast cancer is the **most common cancer** of women, but the second leading cause of cancer death after lung cancer. The most common location is the upper outer quadrant.

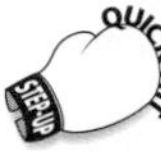

The presence of estrogen or progesterone receptors on breast cancer reflects a good prognosis because of the ability to use hormonal (antiestrogen) therapy.

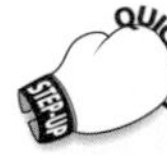

Gynecomastia (enlargement of the breast tissue in males) can be caused by alcoholism, cimetidine, ketoconazole, spironolactone, and digitalis.

Benign prostatic hyperplasia (BPH) develops in the transition zone of the prostate surrounding (and potentially obstructing) the urethra.

THE PROSTATE (Figure 8-11)

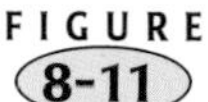

FIGURE 8-11 The prostate
DRE, digital rectal examination; PSA, prostate-specific antigen; UTI, urinary tract infection.

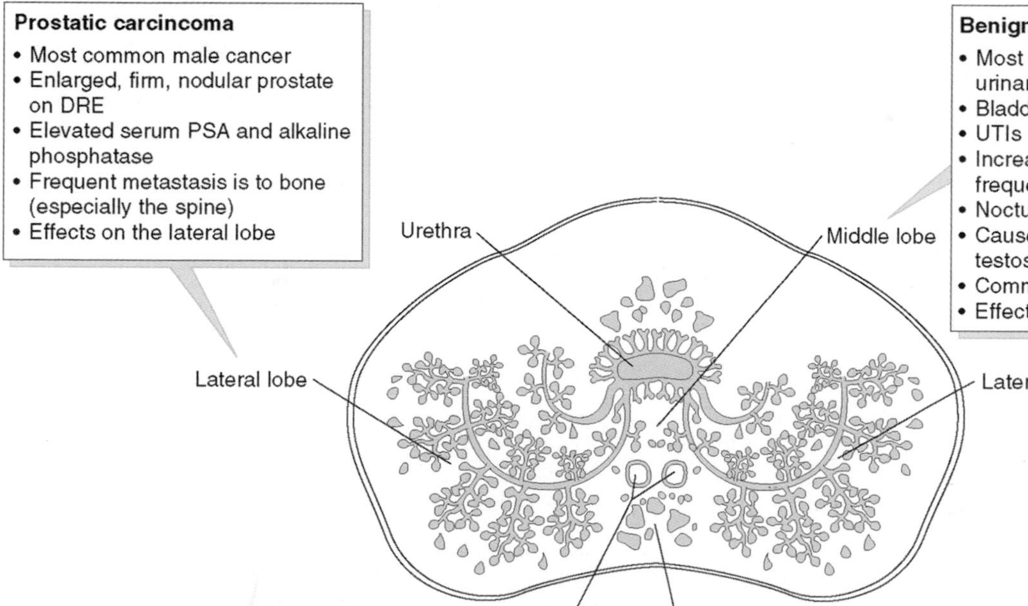

Prostatic carcincoma
• Most common male cancer
• Enlarged, firm, nodular prostate on DRE
• Elevated serum PSA and alkaline phosphatase
• Frequent metastasis is to bone (especially the spine)
• Effects on the lateral lobe
Benign prostatic hyperplasia
• Most common cause of male urinary tract obstruction
• Bladder distention or hypertrophy
• UTIs
• Increased residual volume and frequency
• Nocturia, difficulty initiating stream
• Caused by age-related increase in testosterone and estrogen
• Common after 40 years of age
• Effects on middle lobe
Urethra
Middle lobe
Lateral lobe
Lateral lobe
Ejaculatory ducts
Posterior lobe

TESTICULAR PATHOLOGY

Anatomic disorders of the testis occur more often in young children, whereas the infectious and neoplastic diseases are more likely to occur in the young adult, sexually active population. Routine testicular examinations can often prevent and detect serious complications. When detected early, testicular neoplasms are one of the most curable cancers.

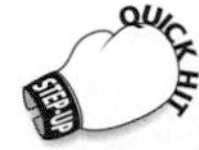

BPH is not a precancerous disorder, and it cannot be accurately diagnosed by measuring prostate-specific antigen (PSA).

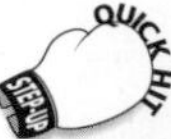

Prostate cancer is the second most common cause of cancer death in males. The leading cause is lung cancer.

The digital rectal examination is essential because many of the male pelvic organs can be assessed. When the examining finger is introduced into the rectum, anal tone (S_2S_4 innervation) can be evaluated. Anteriorly, from inferior to superior, lies the lower border of the prostate, the posterior aspect of the prostate, and the bladder, if distended.

I. Testicular disorders (Table 8-10)

II. Testicular neoplasms (Table 8-11)

TABLE 8-10 Testicular Disorders

Disorder	Clinical Features
Hydrocele	• **Serous fluid** collects in the tunica vaginalis • Caused by **patency** between the peritoneal cavity and the tunica vaginalis
Hematocele	• **Blood** collects in the tunica vaginalis • Usually caused by **trauma**
Varicocele	• **Engorgement of the veins** of the spermatic cord • Most noticeable when patient is standing
Spermatocele	• Epididymal cyst containing **sperm**
Cryptorchidism	• **Failure** of one or both of the testes to **descend** • Increased incidence of **germ cell testicular cancer** such as seminoma and embryonal carcinoma (see testicular neoplasms [Table 8-11]) • Failure of descent leads to testicular **atrophy**, **sterility**, and increased risk of **germ-cell neoplasia**
Testicular torsion	• **Twisting** of the spermatic cord • If untreated, will result in **testicular necrosis**
Orchitis	• Testicular infection and inflammation • May be viral or bacterial in origin • Can lead to **sterility if bilateral**
Epididymitis	• **Inflammation and infection** of the epididymis • Most often caused by ***Neisseria gonorrhoeae, Chlamydia trachomatis,*** *Escherichia coli*, and *Mycobacterium tuberculosis*

TABLE 8-11 Testicular Neoplasms

Neoplasm	Site of Origin; Morphology	Clinical Features
Seminoma	Germ cell; arranged in lobules or nests	Malignant; incidence highest in 35- to 40-year-olds; painless enlargement of testis; **most common germ cell tumor;** similar to dysgerminoma of the ovary; radiosensitive and curable
Embryonal carcinoma	Germ cell; variable morphology with papillary convolutions	Malignant; highest incidence in men in their 20s; more aggressive than seminomas; very common in mixed tumors
Yolk sac tumor (endodermal sinus tumor)	Germ cell; anastomosing cords; malignant; presents with pain or metastasis; similar to ovarian tumor; peak incidence in childhood (infants to 3 years of age); **increased AFP**	
Teratoma	Two or more embryonic layers; **multiple tissue types** such as cartilage, epithelium, liver, and muscle	Malignant; occurs at any age, but more common in children; mature: heterogeneous tissue in organoid fashion; immature: incompletely differentiated
Mixed germ cell tumor	Variable	Malignant; aggressive; more than one neoplastic pattern; **most common**
Leydig cell tumor (interstitial)	Testicular stroma; intracytoplasmic **Reinke crystals**	Benign; produces androgens, estrogens, or corticosteroids; often seen with **precocious puberty** or gynecomastia; similar to ovarian Sertoli–Leydig cell tumor
Sertoli cell tumor	Testicular stroma; forms cordlike structures	Benign; minor endocrine abnormalities; similar to ovarian Sertoli–Leydig cell tumor
Choriocarcinoma	Trophoblastic cells; villous structures resembling placenta	Malignant; hemorrhagic; **β-hCG elevated;** peaks in early adulthood

HUMAN IMMUNODEFICIENCY VIRUS

I. Etiology (Figure 8-12)

FIGURE 8-12 **Replication of the human immunodeficiency virus and its effect**
gp, glycoprotein; HIV, human immunodeficiency virus; mRNA, messenger ribonucleic acid; snRNP, small nuclear ribonucleoprotein particle.

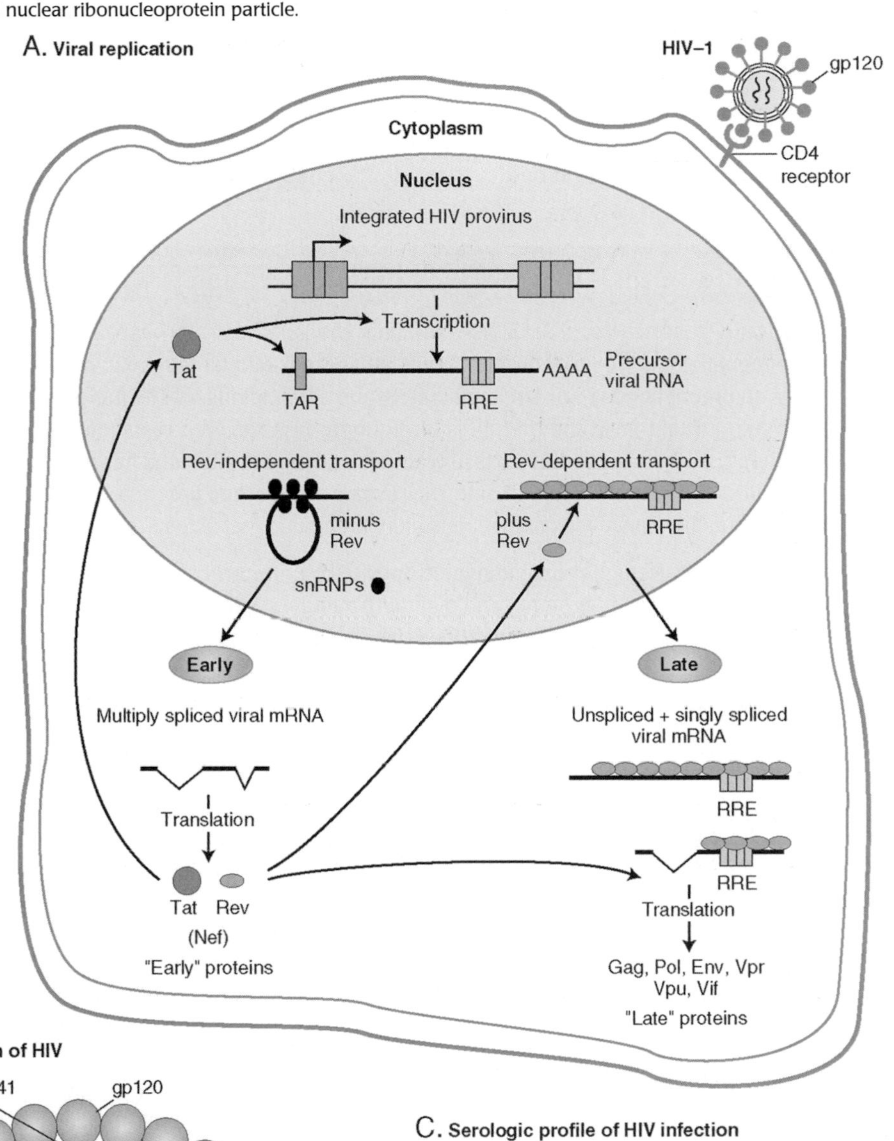

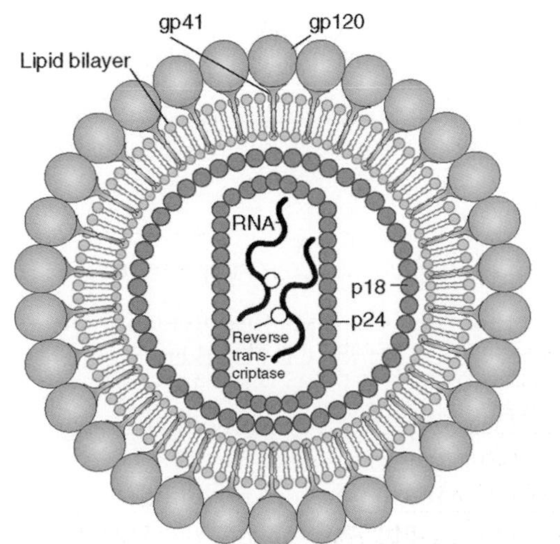

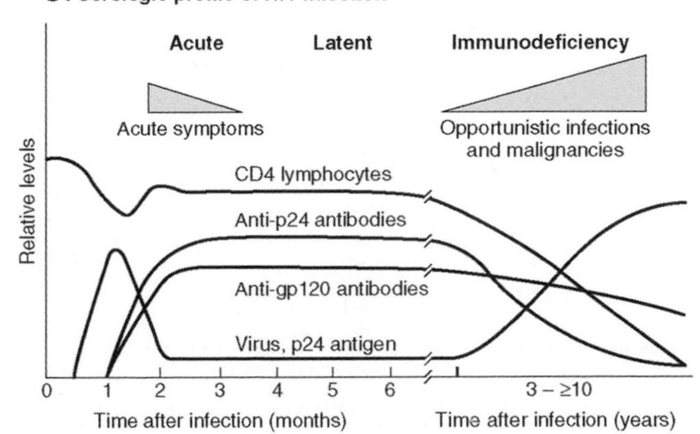

A. HIV-1 (more common) or HIV-2 **retrovirus**
B. Transmitted by
   1. Sexual contact
   2. **Intravenous (IV) drug** abusers sharing needles
   3. Contact with bodily fluids (blood, semen, breast milk, etc.)
   4. Mother to fetus (transplacentally)
C. Not transmitted through
   1. Casual contact
   2. Toilet seats
   3. Kissing
   4. Mosquitoes
D. Occupational risk to healthcare workers is low. A needle stick with an HIV-positive patient's blood carries a **0.3% chance of transmission.**

Clinical Vignette 8-2

Clinical Presentation: A 55-year-old male presents to his primary care physician with the chief complaint of **frequent urination** that has increased over the past few months. Although he feels an **urgent need to urinate immediately,** the patient finds that he has a **weak urinary stream** with **intermittent flow** and that he is **straining to urinate,** with resulting feeling of **incomplete emptying.** Also, the patient reports of **waking to urinate** at night and has noted **some blood in his urine** lately. Rectal examination deferred reveals an enlarged prostate with no nodules palpable. Otherwise, the physical examination is benign and the vital signs are stable.

Differential: Benign prostatic hypertrophy (BPH), urethral strictures, urinary tract infection, bladder cancer, bladder stone, and bladder trauma. Lower urinary tract symptoms can be best remembered by the mnemonic **WISE FUN. WISE** refers to the obstructive symptoms: **W**eak urinary stream, **I**ntermittent flow, **S**training to urinate, and incomplete **E**mptying. **FUN** refers to the irritative symptoms: **F**requency, **U**rgency, and **N**octuria. BPH can present with any of these lower urinary tract symptoms and also hematuria. Urethral strictures can also result in obstructive symptoms, urinary tract infection (UTI) in irritative symptoms, and bladder cancer/stones/trauma in hematuria.

Laboratory Studies: Urinalysis and **urine culture** should be obtained to rule out urinary tract infection. Also, **ultrasound** is useful for determining the bladder and prostate size but is not commonly used in initial evaluation of uncomplicated cases. More precise measurements of prostate can be made via **transrectal ultrasound,** which is indicated in select patients.

Management: An **α-blocker** relaxes the prostatic smooth muscle and is the first-line treatment for BPH. The most common side effect is dizziness. A **5α-reductase** inhibitor (finasteride) reduces symptoms by reducing the volume of the prostate. If pharmacologic therapy is unsuccessful, **transurethral resection of the prostate** is the gold standard surgical procedure for the treatment of BPH. Open radical prostatectomy is a cancer operation and is ***not*** indicated for benign prostatic obstruction.

II. Pathology

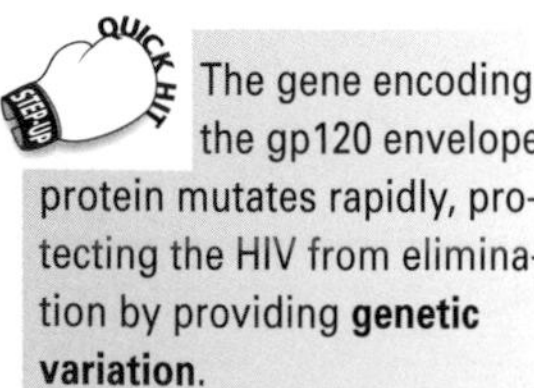

The gene encoding the gp120 envelope protein mutates rapidly, protecting the HIV from elimination by providing **genetic variation.**

A. Primary infection
   1. Transmitted virus infects **T-helper lymphocytes** (CD4) via the interaction of viral proteins **gp120** and **gp41** with each other and the CD4 marker (Figure 8-12 and Table 8-12).
   2. The virus also infects macrophages and monocytes (proposed portal of entry into the central nervous system).
   3. Viremia is accompanied by the "**acute retroviral syndrome**" (a flulike illness).
   4. The first month is the **window period** as p24 antigen is not yet detectable in the blood (patient is contagious).

TABLE 8-12 HIV Proteins and Function

Gene	Product and Function
gag	Viral core proteins p17 and p24
pol	Protease, integrase, reverse transcriptase, and RNAse H
env	gp120 and gp41
tat	Transcriptional transactivator (increases gene expression); essential for replication
rev	Transition from early to late gene expression; protein transport from nucleus to cytoplasm; essential for replication
nef	Transcriptional silencer; may produce latent infection
vif	Viral infectivity gene; cell-to-cell transmission
vpu	Viral protein U; viral particle export
vpr	Viral protein R; activates viral and cellular promoters

B. Chronic infection
  1. Immune response lowers viral blood counts but active replication persists.
  2. No clinical symptoms for up to 10 years (latent period).
  3. CD4 count steadily declines.
  4. Near end of the latent period, constitutional symptoms develop
    a. Weight loss
    b. Fever
    c. Night sweats
    d. Adenopathy

C. Acquired immunodeficiency syndrome (AIDS)
  1. Defined as a **CD4 count of ≤200 cells/mL** coupled with the presence of certain **opportunistic** infections
  2. Infections typically seen with AIDS
    a. ***Pneumocystis carinii* pneumonia** (80%)
    b. **Kaposi sarcoma** (human herpes virus [HHV]-8)
    c. B-cell lymphoma (brain and bone marrow)
    d. *Toxoplasma gondii* (brain tissue infection)
    e. CMV (leads to retinitis)
    f. *Cryptococcus neoformans* (meningeal infection)
    g. *Mycobacterium avium-intracellulare* (MAI)
    h. Tuberculosis (TB)
    i. *Candida albicans* (thrush, esophagitis)
    j. *Cryptosporidium* (chronic diarrhea)

D. Epidemiology
  1. In the United States, during the 1980s, the infection first spread among **male homosexuals.**
  2. **IV drug abusers** and **hemophiliacs** (before tests were developed to screen blood) were the next populations affected.
  3. **Heterosexual** transmission is rising in the United States and is now the leading cause of infection in Africa.

E. Laboratory diagnosis
  1. **The enzyme-linked immunosorbent assay (ELISA) test** for antibodies lends a presumptive diagnosis (screening test).
  2. This must be confirmed by the **Western blot** test, which demonstrates antibodies to gp41 or p24 (Figure 8-12).

III. Treatment (Table 8-13)

TABLE 8-13 Therapeutic Agents in HIV

Therapeutic Agent (common name, if relevant) [trade name, where appropriate]	Class—Pharmacology and Pharmacokinetics	Indications	Side or Adverse Effects	Contraindications or Precautions to Consider; Notes
Saquinavir (SQV), ritonavir (RTV), indinavir (IDV), nelfinavir, amprenavir	**Protease inhibitor**—protease responsible for final step of viral proliferation; inhibits protease in progeny virons → assembly of nonfunctional viruses	**HAART**	**GI irritation (nausea and diarrhea), hyperglycemia, lipodystrophy, thrombocytopenia (indinavir)**	**All protease inhibitors ending in—navir; metabolism occurs by CYP450**
Zidovudine (ZDV, formerly AZT)	**Nucleoside reverse transcriptase inhibitor**—inhibits viral reverse transcriptase → prevents integration of DNA copy of viral genome into host DNA	**HAART; HIV pregnant female** to reduce fetal transmission	**Neutropenia, anemia** (megaloblastic anemia), **peripheral neuropathy, pancreatitis, and lactic acidosis**	**Effects of bone marrow suppression such as neutropenia and anemia can be reduced by the addition of GM-CSF**
Didanosine (ddI)	**Nucleoside reverse transcriptase inhibitor—competitive inhibitor of deoxythymidine triphosphate** → incorporated into the viral DNA by reverse transcriptase →terminates viral DNA synthesis (lacks 3′-hydroxyl group) → prevents integration of DNA copy of the viral genome into the host DNA	**HAART**	**Neutropenia, anemia, peripheral neuropathy, pancreatitis, and lactic acidosis**	
Zalcitabine (ddC)	**Nucleoside reverse transcriptase inhibitor—2′,3′-dideoxyadenosine analog**→ incorporated into the viral DNA by reverse transcriptase →terminates viral DNA synthesis (lacks 3′-hydroxyl group) → prevents integration of DNA copy of viral genome into host DNA	**HAART**	**Neutropenia, anemia, peripheral neuropathy, pancreatitis, and lactic acidosis**	
Stavudine (d4T)	**Nucleoside reverse transcriptase inhibitor—thymidine analog**→ incorporated into the viral DNA by reverse transcriptase →terminates viral DNA synthesis → prevents integration of DNA copy of the viral genome into the host DNA	**HAART**	**Neutropenia, anemia, peripheral neuropathy, pancreatitis, and lactic acidosis**	**Good CNS penetration**

(continued)

TABLE 8-13 Therapeutic Agents in HIV *(Continued)*

Therapeutic Agent (common name, if relevant) [trade name, where appropriate]	Class–Pharmacology and Pharmacokinetics	Indications	Side or Adverse Effects	Contraindications or Precautions to Consider; Notes
Lamivudine (3TC)	**Nucleoside reverse transcriptase inhibitor—cytidine analog** → inhibits viral reverse transcriptase → prevents integration of DNA copy of the viral genome into the host DNA	**HAART**	**Neutropenia, anemia, peripheral neuropathy, pancreatitis, and lactic acidosis**	
Abacavir (ABC)	**Nucleoside reverse transcriptase inhibitor—guanosine analog** → inhibits viral reverse transcriptase → prevents integration of DNA copy of the viral genome into the host DNA	**HAART**	**Neutropenia, anemia, peripheral neuropathy, pancreatitis, and lactic acidosis**	
Nevirapine, efavirenz, and delaviridine	**Non-nucleoside reverse transcriptase inhibitor**—binds viral reverse transcriptase and inhibits the movement of protein domains → terminates viral DNA synthesis → prevents integration of viral genome into the host DNA	**HAART**; noncompetitive inhibitors of reverse transcriptase	**Neutropenia, anemia, peripheral neuropathy, and rash**	**Effects of bone marrow suppression such as neutropenia and anemia can be reduced by the addition of GM-CSF**
Enfuvirtide	**Fusion inhibitor**—binds viral gp41 subunit → inhibits conformation change (required for fusion with CD4 cell) → blocks vital entry and replication	**Patients on antiretroviral therapy with persistent viral replication**	**Hypersensitivity reactions; reaction at injection site; bacterial pneumonia**	**Used in combination with other antiretroviral drugs**

A. Agents used in the treatment of HIV include **protease inhibitors**, **nucleoside reverse transcriptase inhibitors**, **nonnucleoside reverse transcriptase inhibitors**, and **fusion inhibitors**.

B. **Combination therapy** has drastically improved HIV treatment by forestalling the development of resistance to medication and is referred to as **highly active antiretroviral therapy (HAART)**.
   1. Two reverse transcriptase inhibitors and a protease inhibitor are often combined.
   2. Therapy should be initiated before compromise of the immune system occurs.
   3. The most common "cocktail" used is a combination of zidovudine (a nucleoside reverse transcriptase inhibitor), lamivudine (a nucleoside reverse transcriptase inhibitor), and indinavir (a protease inhibitor).
   4. Ideally, therapy should be based on the virus strain isolated from the patient.

PSYCHOSOCIAL DEVELOPMENT

TIMELINE OF THE DEVELOPMENTAL STAGES OF LIFE (Figure 8-13)

FIGURE 8-13 **Stages of development**
ECT, electroconvulsive therapy; m, month old; y, years of age.

	Infancy (0–1 y)	Toddler (1–3 y)	School age (3–11 y)	Adolescence (11–20 y)	Early adulthood (20–40 y)	Middle adulthood (40–60 y)	Late adulthood (60–80 y)
Freud	Oral	Anal	Phallic-oedipal (3–6 y); latency (6–11 y)	Genital			
Erikson	Trust vs. mistrust	Autonomy vs. shame and doubt	Initiative vs. guilt (3–6 y); industry vs. inferiority	Identity vs. role confusion	Intimacy vs. isolation	Generativity vs. stagnation	Ego integrity vs. despair
Piaget	Sensorimotor (0–2 y)	Preoperational (2–7 y)	Concrete operations (7–11 y)	Formal operations			
Characteristics	Reflexes: • Palmer grasp (0–2 m) • Rooting (0–3 m) • Babinski (0–12 m) Milestones: • Turn over (5 m) • Sit (6 m) • Walk (12 m)	Terrible two's ("no"); band-aid (2–4 y); parallel play (2–4 y); balance on one foot (2 y); climb stairs (3 y)	Cooperative play (4–7 y); conservation of mass (7–11 y); button clothes (4 y); throw a ball (4 y);	First menstruation (11 y); first ejaculation (13 y); peer pressure	New family; children; role in society solidified; period of reassessment	Height of career; mid-life crises; menopause (45–55 y)	Depression (ECT); women outlive men by 6–8 y; Kübler-Ross (stages of grief and dying) • Denial • Anger • Bargaining • Depression • Acceptance

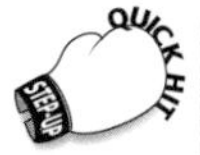

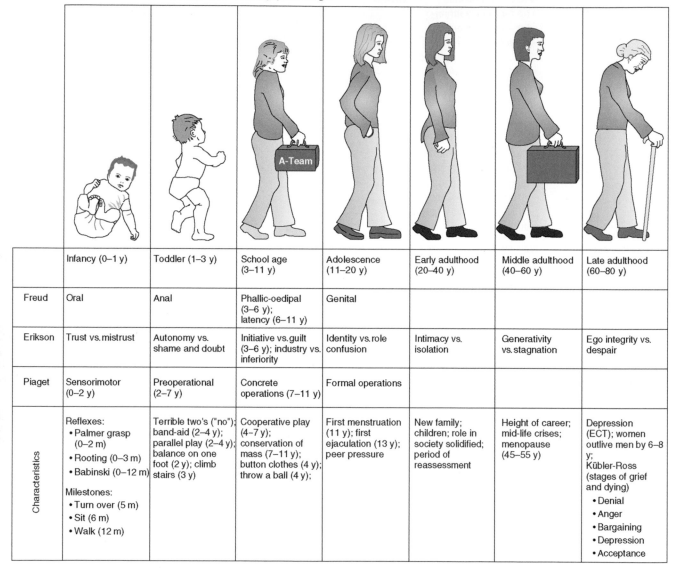

The Minnesota Multiphasic Personality Inventory (MMPI) is the most commonly used objective personality test while the **Rorschach** test is the major projective test of personality. Intelligence is measured by the **Stanford–Binet** scale as an intelligence quotient (IQ) and is relatively stable throughout life.

THE FAMILY UNIT AND RELATED CONCEPTS

I. The family cycle

A. Phase 1: **Marriage**
1. Statistically, married couples are mentally and physically healthier than unmarried couples.
2. Over half of all marriages end in divorce.

B. Phase 2: **Child-rearing**
1. Children raised in single-parent families have higher rates of depression, drug abuse, suicide, and criminal activity.
2. Children from divorced families are more likely to become divorced themselves later in life.

C. Phase 3: **Children leave home**
D. Phase 4: **Physical decline** and final distribution of goods

II. Postpartum depression

A. Up to 50% of all women develop a short-lived depression after giving birth (postpartum blues).
B. Etiology
   1. Change in hormone levels
   2. Increased responsibility
   3. Fatigue
C. Major depression is seen in 5% to 10% of all women after childbirth.

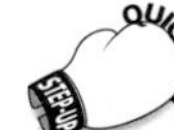

Depression is defined as a 2-week course marked by four of the following eight criteria: (a) anhedonia, (b) increased or decreased sleep, (c) feelings of guilt, (d) decreased energy level, (e) inability to concentrate (f) changes in appetite, (g) psychomotor retardation, and (h) suicidal ideation.

III. Attachment of the child to the mother

A. **Anaclitic depression:** sustained absence of mother when child is between 6 and 12 months of age leads to a withdrawn and unresponsive infant.
B. **Harlow** showed that monkeys raised in **isolation** do not develop normally
   1. Males are more affected than females.
   2. Recovery is not possible if isolation lasts longer than 6 months.
C. **Bowlby** showed that **physical contact** between the mother and the child is crucial to development.
D. **Spitz** observed that children **without proper mothering** are slow to develop and have a greater number of medical problems.
E. **Mahler** documented the development as a process in which the infant **separates** from the mother
   1. Normal autistic phase (0 to 1 month): infant has little interaction
   2. Symbiotic phase (15 months): infant is close to mother
   3. Separation–individuation phase (5 to 16 months): child realizes individuality and begins to explore the environment

IV. Child abuse

A. It includes physical abuse, sexual abuse, and emotional neglect.
B. Risk factors
   1. Substance abuse by parents
   2. Poverty
   3. Marital problems or single-parent home
C. Physical abuse is marked by numerous fractures, bruises, subdural hematomas, or burns (at various stages of healing).
D. Sexual abuse of children is marked by trauma to the genitalia, sexually transmitted diseases, or urinary tract infections.
E. Abuse predisposes the child to posttraumatic stress disorder (PTSD), dissociative disorders, depression, anorexia, phobias, and personality disorders.
F. Physician intervention is necessary and obligatory.

V. Family therapy

A. Involves all members of a family even though only one person might have a problem
B. Identifies dysfunctional behavior and encourages communication and problem solving
C. Based on the concept that the family system is composed of subsystems in which boundaries are established and mutual accommodation occurs

SEXUALITY

I. Gender

A. **Gender identity** is an individual's sense of being male or female whereas **gender role** is the expression of one's gender.
B. Sexual orientation is a physical preference for one or both genders (heterosexual, homosexual, and bisexual).

C. Psychological factors play a role in gender identity and sexual orientation
   1. **Transsexual:** a person who has the sense of being in the wrong-sex body and has a strong desire to correct it
   2. **Homosexual:** a person who has a sexual preference for same-sex individuals
   3. **Transvestite:** a man who dresses in women's clothing for pleasure, usually heterosexual

MNEMONIC

To remember the four phases of normal sexual response, think **EXPLORE: EX**citation, **PL**ateau, **O**rgasm, and **RE**solution.

II. Sexual dysfunction

A. Premature ejaculation (early climax without reaching plateau phase) is the **most common** male sexual disorder.

B. The most common sexual dysfunction in women is **sexual arousal disorder** in which lubrication cannot be maintained throughout the sexual act.

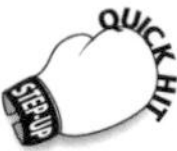

Penile erection is achieved via two crucial steps: (a) parasympathetic-mediated relaxation of arterioles to the penis and (b) mechanical compression of the venous outflow channels.

C. Impotence (in men)
   1. Failure to achieve erection or ejaculation
   2. Usually has an organic component but may be psychogenic (e.g., caused by stress or anxiety)
      a. It is often related to alcohol abuse.
      b. It may also result from medical problems such as diabetes or illicit drug use.
      c. Psychogenic cause can be confirmed by observing erections during rapid eye movement (REM) sleep.

D. Vaginismus (in women)
   1. Spasm in the outer third of the vagina
   2. Difficulty during intercourse or pelvic examination
   3. Often results from rape, incest, or abuse

E. Paraphilias (Table 8-14)

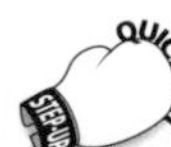

Pedophilia is the **most common** paraphilia and needs to be reported to the authorities on discovery by the physician if the patient acts on this desire.

TABLE 8-14 Paraphilias

Category	Description (How Sexual Pleasure is Derived)
Exhibitionism	Exposing one's genitalia
Fetishism	Inanimate objects (e.g., women's high-heeled shoes or undergarments)
Frotteurism	Furtively rubbing genitalia against a woman (e.g., pushing up against a woman in a crowded subway)
Necrophilia	Corpses
Pedophilia	Children
Masochism	Receiving physical or psychological pain and humiliation
Sadism	Inducing physical or psychological pain and humiliation in others
Transvestic fetishism	Wearing women's clothing (such men are still attracted to women)
Voyeurism	Furtively watching individuals engaged in intercourse or seductive activities
Zoophilia	Animals

Clinical Vignette 8-3

Clinical Presentation: A 45-year-old man presents to his primary care physician for his yearly physical examination. His past medical history is significant for **diabetes, hypertension,** and **hypercholesterolemia.** He has been keeping physically fit with **lengthy bike rides.** He has not cut back on his tobacco usage and smokes 0.5 pack per day × 5 years. As you review the systems, he tells you that he has had **increasing difficulty achieving a firm erection.** He denies any **recent penile or perineal trauma, surgery, or radiation.** Vital signs: $T = 97.4°F$; RR = 20 breaths/min; **BP** = 150/90 mm Hg; and HR = 85 bpm.

(continued)

Clinical Vignette 8-3 *(Continued)*

Differentials: Erectile dysfunction (ED) from vascular, neurologic, iatrogenic, traumatic, or psychogenic origin. It is important to note the bolded items in this patient's history are the risk factors for ED.

Laboratory Studies: Direct injection of prostaglandin E_1 into the corpora should result in a normal erection within minutes if the penile vasculature is normal. **Nocturnal penile tumescence testing** is useful in distinguishing psychogenic from organic impotence. Inadequate nocturnal erections suggest organic dysfunction while normal erection during rapid eye movement (REM) sleep suggests psychogenic etiology. Given his diabetic history, formal **neurologic testing** may be needed.

Management: All patients with ED should be given an empiric trial of **sildenafil** as long as they do not have any contraindications. Contraindications include use of nitrates, active cardiac disease, or hypertension. **Phosphodiesterase inhibitors** such as sildenafil increase cyclic guanosine monophosphate (cGMP), which relaxes the smooth muscle surrounding the penile arterioles with resulting dilation of vasculature and erection. Patients with ED refractory to therapy with oral phosphodiesterase inhibitors should be referred to urology for other therapies such as **vacuum constriction device, prostaglandin E_1 injections,** and surgical placement of a **penile prosthesis.**

RAPE

I. An act of sexual aggression in which the penis penetrates the outer vulva.

II. Rapists tend to be male and tend to rape women of their own race

A. Roughly, half of the assailants are Black and half are White.
B. Use of weapons and alcohol is common.
C. Rapists are usually young (younger than 25 years of age).
D. Rapes are under-reported (usually only 39% of total)
   1. Victims are generally 15 to 30 years of age.
   2. Rape usually occurs inside the woman's home by an individual whom she knows.
E. Rape usually results in rape trauma syndrome, which involves emotional lability for more than 1 year
   1. Group therapy and support are important treatment modalities.
   2. PTSD may occur even after treatment
      a. PTSD occurs in a subgroup of individuals exposed to trauma.
      b. Usually develops in adolescents or young adults.

SUICIDE

I. Third-leading cause of death in persons 15 to 24 years of age and eighth leading cause of death in the United States.

II. Women attempt suicide three times more often than men, but men are four times more successful owing to the lethality of the method used.

III. Gay and lesbian youths have a threefold increased risk of suicide because of increased societal pressures and stigmata.

IV. Marriage reduces the risk of suicide.

V. Professional women may be at an increased risk for suicide.

VI. Suicide risk should be assessed during the mental status examination

A. Patients with a suicide **plan** are at higher risk.
B. Indications for hospitalization include impulsiveness, lack of social support, and a plan.

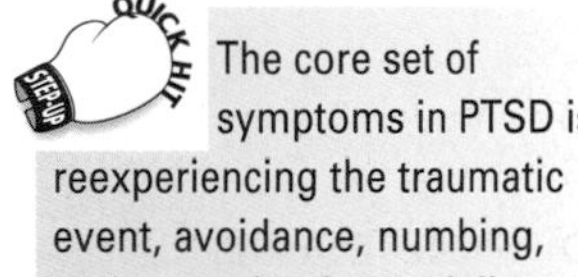

The core set of symptoms in PTSD is reexperiencing the traumatic event, avoidance, numbing, and arousal or hypervigilance.

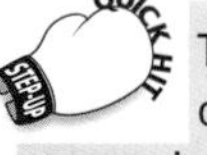

The death of a child or the suicide of a spouse is the most severe psychological stressor.

Divorced White males older than 65 years of age, who have a plan and are taking three or more medications, have the highest risk of suicide.

Taking oral contraceptives provides other benefits such as decreased risk of dysmenorrheal, iron deficiency anemia, ectopic pregnancy, benign breast disease, endometrial cancer, ovarian cysts, ovarian cancer, and postmenopausal hip fracture.

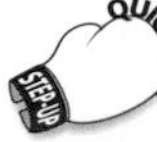

Tamoxifen, a competitive inhibitor of estrogen at the estrogen receptor, can be used to treat advanced breast cancer and certain types of endometrial cancer in postmenopausal women. It can lead to the regression of estrogen-stimulated tumors in some cases.

THERAPEUTIC AGENTS FOR THE REPRODUCTIVE SYSTEM

(Table 8-15)

TABLE 8-15 Therapeutic Agents for the Reproductive System

Therapeutic Agent (common name, if relevant) [trade name, where appropriate]	Class—Pharmacology and Pharmacokinetics	Indications	Side or Adverse Effects	Contraindications or Precautions to Consider; Notes
Hormone antagonists				
Finasteride [Proscar]	**Antiandrogen—5α-reductase inhibitor** → decreases the conversion of testosterone to dihydrotestosterone	**Benign prostatic hyperplasia;** male pattern baldness		
Flutamide [Eulexin]	**Antiandrogen**—nonsteroidal, competitive androgen receptor blocker	**Metastatic prostate cancer**		
Ketoconazole [Nizoral]	**Antiandrogen**—inhibits ergosterol (steroid) synthesis → inhibits adrenal and gonadal steroid synthesis; also prevents cell membrane formation	**Prostate carcinoma; fungal infections**	Nausea; vomiting; diarrhea; rash; headache; anorexia; thrombocytopenia; gynecomastia; hepatotoxic	**Inhibits cytochrome P-450**
Spironolactone [Aldactone]	**Antiandrogen**—inhibits steroid binding	**Hirsutism in women, acne in women**; hyperaldosteronism, hypokalemia, hypertension, edema, and CHF	Gynecomastia; breast pain; hyperkalemia; impotence; menstrual irregularities	
Mifepristone (RU-486)	**Antiprogesterone** —synthetic steroid, progesterone receptor blocker → blocks the effects of progesterone → myometrium contraction	**Termination of intrauterine pregnancy**	**Heavy bleeding; uterine cramping;** GI effects (nausea, vomiting, and anorexia)	Controversial "Morning after" drug
Anastrozole [Arimidex]	Aromatase inhibitor	**Breast cancer** in postmenopausal women	Hot flashes; nausea; vomiting	Can be used in ER positive or hormone receptor unknown breast cancer
Hormone agonists				
Methyltestosterone [Android, Virilon]	**Androgen**—androgen receptor agonist	**In males: hypogonadism, delayed puberty** (promotes secondary sex characteristics), impotence; **In females: estrogen receptor positive breast cancer**	**Masculinization (hirsutism); testicular atrophy;** prostate hyperplasia; prostate cancer; impotence; **stunted growth** (premature epiphyseal plate closure), hyperlipidemia	Decrease testicular testosterone leading to Leydig cell inhibition and gonadal atrophy

(continued)

THE REPRODUCTIVE SYSTEM

TABLE 8-15 Therapeutic Agents for the Reproductive System *(Continued)*

Therapeutic Agent (common name, if relevant) [trade name, where appropriate]	Class—Pharmacology and Pharmacokinetics	Indications	Side or Adverse Effects	Contraindications or Precautions to Consider; Notes
Ethinyl estradiol, DES, mestranol	**Estrogen**—bind estrogen receptor	**In females: Hypogonadism, ovarian failure,** menstrual abnormalities; **In males: androgen dependent prostate cancer**	**Endometrial cancer; bleeding; thrombosis**	Used in combination with progestin in patients with intact uterus given increased risk of endometrial cancer with unopposed estrogen therapy; females exposed to DES in utero-increased risk of **vaginal clear cell adenocarcinoma**
Progesterone, norethindrone, levonorgestrel [Plan B], norgestimate, desogestrel, gestodene	**Progesterone**—bind progesterone receptors	**Endometrial cancer;** amenorrhea; abnormal uterine bleeding; **prevention of pregnancy**		Also used to prevent endometrial hyperplasia in postmenopausal women taking estrogen
Partial agonists and antagonists				
Clomiphene [Clomid]	**Selective estrogen receptor modulator**—binds estrogen receptors in pituitary → prevents normal feedback inhibition, increases LH and FSH release from the pituitary → stimulates ovulation	**Infertility—stimulates ovulation; PCOS**	**Hot flashes; ovarian enlargement; multiple gestation pregnancy; visual disturbances**	
Tamoxifen [Nolvadex]	**Selective estrogen receptor modular—competitively binds estrogen receptors; breast (estrogen antagonist):** prevents proliferation of estrogen receptor positive tumor cells; **endometrium (partial agonist); bone (agonist):** decreases bone turnover, increases bone density	**Treats estrogen-dependent breast cancer in postmenopausal women;** reduces contralateral breast cancer; osteoporosis prevention	**May increase the risk of endometrial cancer; hot flashes**; flushing	
Raloxifene [Evista]	**Selective estrogen receptor modulator—breast (estrogen antagonist); endometrium (estrogen antagonist):** prevents the proliferation of endometrium; **bone (estrogen agonist):** decreases bone turnover, increases bone density; **cardiovascular (estrogen agonist):** decreases LDL	**Osteoporosis; breast cancer**	**Hot flashes;** sinusitis; weight gain; muscle pain; leg cramps; **increased risk of blood clots**	Unlike estrogen, raloxifene **does not decrease HDL**

(continued)

TABLE 8-15 Therapeutic Agents for the Reproductive System *(Continued)*

Therapeutic Agent (common name, if relevant) [trade name, where appropriate]	Class–Pharmacology and Pharmacokinetics	Indications	Side or Adverse Effects	Contraindications or Precautions to Consider; Notes
Other				
Leuprolide [Lupron]	**GnRH analog**—agonist (when given pulsatile), antagonist (when given continuously)	**Infertility** (given pulsatile); **prostate cancer** (given continuous); **uterine fibroids;** PCOS; endometriosis; precocious puberty	Nausea; vomiting; antiandrogen effects (testicular atrophy)	
Sildenafil [Viagra], vardenafil	**Phosphodiesterase type 5 inhibitor (cGMP-specific)**— increased cGMP → smooth muscle relaxation → increased blood flow in the corpus cavernosum → penile erection	**Erectile dysfunction**	**Abnormal vision** (impaired blue-green color vision); **UTIs; cardiovascular events; priapism; dyspepsia;** headache; flushing	Risk of hypotension (fatal) in a patient taking nitrates
Misoprostol [Cytotec]	**Prostaglandin—PGE_1 analog** → cervical dilation; uterine contractions	**Induction of labor;** termination of pregnancy		
Dinoprostone	Prostaglandin—PGE_2 analog → cervical dilation; uterine contraction	Induction of labor; termination of pregnancy		
Ritodrine, terbutaline	β agonist → uterine relaxation	Inhibits preterm labor		
Combination Oral contraceptives	**Combination of estrogen and progesterone— estrogen** → inhibits midcycle surge of gonadotropin secretion → prevents ovulation; **progesterone** →alters endometrium cervical mucus, tube motility, and peristalsis → less suitable for sperm penetration and implantation	**Contraception; acne; hirsutism; PCOS**		Contraindicated in patients with stroke or prior thromboembolic event, estrogen dependent tumor, pregnancy, hypertriglyceridemia, **heavy smokers;** avoid use in women with migraines and poorly controlled hypertension
Hormone replacement therapy	**Combination of estrogen and progesterone**	**Menopause** (relief of symptoms); osteoporosis; vulvar/vaginal atrophy; hypoestrogenism (hypogonadism)	Possible increased risk of **stroke**	Combination of progesterone and estrogen is used because **unopposed estrogen increases the risk of endometrial cancer**

ER, estrogen receptor; GnRH, gonadotropin-releasing hormone; PCOS, polycystic ovarian syndrome.

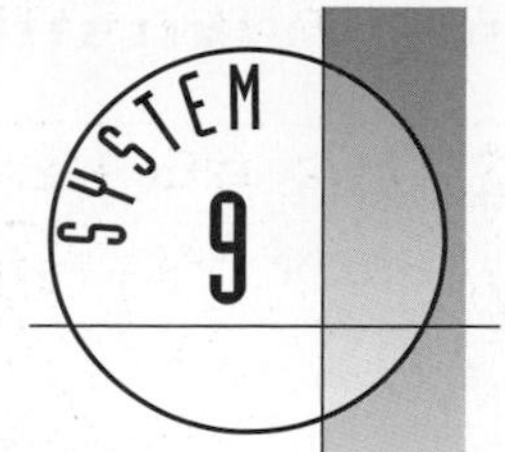

The Musculoskeletal System

DEVELOPMENT

I. Bone formation

A. **Endochondral bone**
   1. Forms over a cartilage frame
   2. Becomes the **long bones** of the skeleton (e.g., **femur**)

B. **Membranous bone**
   1. Forms without a cartilage frame
   2. Becomes the **flat bones** of the skeleton (e.g., bones of the cranium)

II. Skeletal muscle

A. It derives from **somites.**
B. Each somite produces its own **myotome.**
C. Each somite produces its own **dermatome.**

III. Pharyngeal arches

Begin to develop in the **fourth week** and originate from **neural crest cells.**

A. **Arch 1**
   1. Innervated by the mandibular branch of the trigeminal nerve (**cranial nerve [CN] V**)
   2. Gives rise to the following muscles
      a. Muscles of mastication (temporalis, masseter, lateral pterygoid, medial pterygoid)
      b. Two tensor muscles (tensor veli palatini, tensor tympani)
      c. Two other muscles (mylohyoid, anterior belly of the digastric)
   3. Gives rise to the following skeletal structures
      a. Malleus
      b. Incus
   4. Gives rise to the following ligamentous structures
      a. Anterior ligament of malleus
      b. Sphenomandibular ligament

B. **Arch 2**
   1. Innervated by the facial nerve (**CN VII**)
   2. Gives rise to the following muscles
      a. Muscles of facial expression (orbicularis oculi, orbiculare oris, buccinator)
      b. Three other muscles (stylohyoid, stapedius, and the posterior belly of the digastric)
   3. Gives rise to the following skeletal structures
      a. Greater cornu of hyoid bone
      b. Inferior portion of the body of hyoid bone

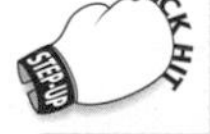

All the intrinsic muscles of the pharynx, except the cricothyroid, are innervated by the recurrent laryngeal branches of the vagus nerve. Consequently, bilateral injury to the recurrent laryngeal nerves leaves the cricothyroid unopposed, and the vocal cords become tense and adducted.

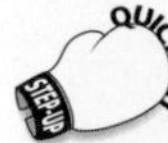

Of all the intrinsic muscles of the larynx (posterior cricoarytenoid, lateral cricoarytenoid, arytenoid, thyroarytenoid, cricothyroid, transverse arytenoid, oblique arytenoid, and vocal muscle), the posterior cricoarytenoid muscle is the only muscle that **abducts** the vocal cords.

C. **Arch 3**
   1. Innervated by the glossopharyngeal nerve (CN IX)
   2. Gives rise to the stylopharyngeus muscle
   3. Gives rise to the following skeletal structures
      a. Greater cornu of the hyoid bone
      b. Lower portion of the body of hyoid bone

D. **Arch 4**
   1. Innervated by the vagus nerve (pharyngeal and superior laryngeal branches of CN X)
   2. Gives rise to the following muscles
      a. Cricothyroid muscle
      b. All the muscles of the soft palate and pharynx except the stylopharyngeus muscle (arch 3) and tensor veli palatini (arch 1)

E. **Arch 6**
   1. Innervated by the vagus nerve (recurrent laryngeal branch of CN X)
   2. Gives rise to the intrinsic muscles of the larynx except the cricothyroid

F. **Arch 4 and Arch 6** fuse to give rise to the thyroid, cricoids, arytenoids, corniculate, and cuneiform cartilages.

Among the most common bacteria found on the skin are *Staphylococcus epidermidis* and various species of *Corynebacterium* and *Propionibacterium.*

IV. Skin (Figure 9-1)

A. Stratum basale is actively mitotic, and gives rise to the other four layers.
B. Epidermis forms from **ectoderm** and dermis forms from mesoderm.
C. Melanocytes contain melanin pigment and are derived from neural crest.
D. Skin renews every 2 to 3 weeks.
E. Function
   1. Barrier to infection
   2. Thermoregulation
   3. Protection from desiccation
F. Two types of skin
   1. Thick skin (e.g., palms and soles of feet)
      a. Stratum basale (deepest layer)
      b. Stratum spinosum
      c. Stratum granulosum
      d. Stratum lucidum
      e. Stratum corneum (most superficial layer)
   2. Thin skin (e.g., face, genitalia, and back of hands): stratum lucidum is absent in thin skin (although it has all the other layers).

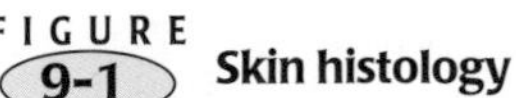

FIGURE 9-1 **Skin histology**

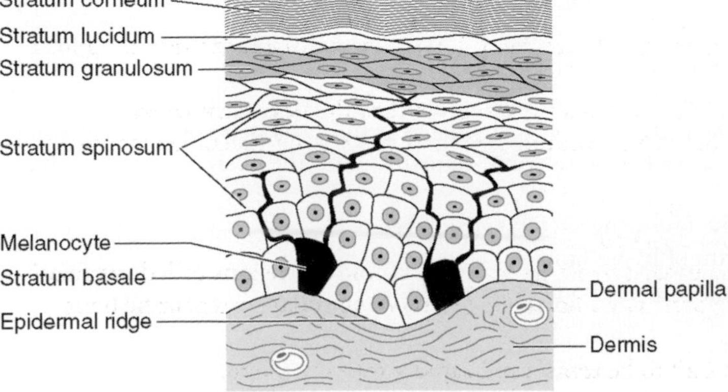

THE MUSCULOSKELETAL SYSTEM

BONE FUNCTION AND METABOLISM (Figure 9-2)

FIGURE 9-2 **Bone histology**

(Adapted with permission from Damjanov IM. Histology: A Color Atlas and Textbook. Baltimore, MD: Williams & Wilkins, 1996:422.)

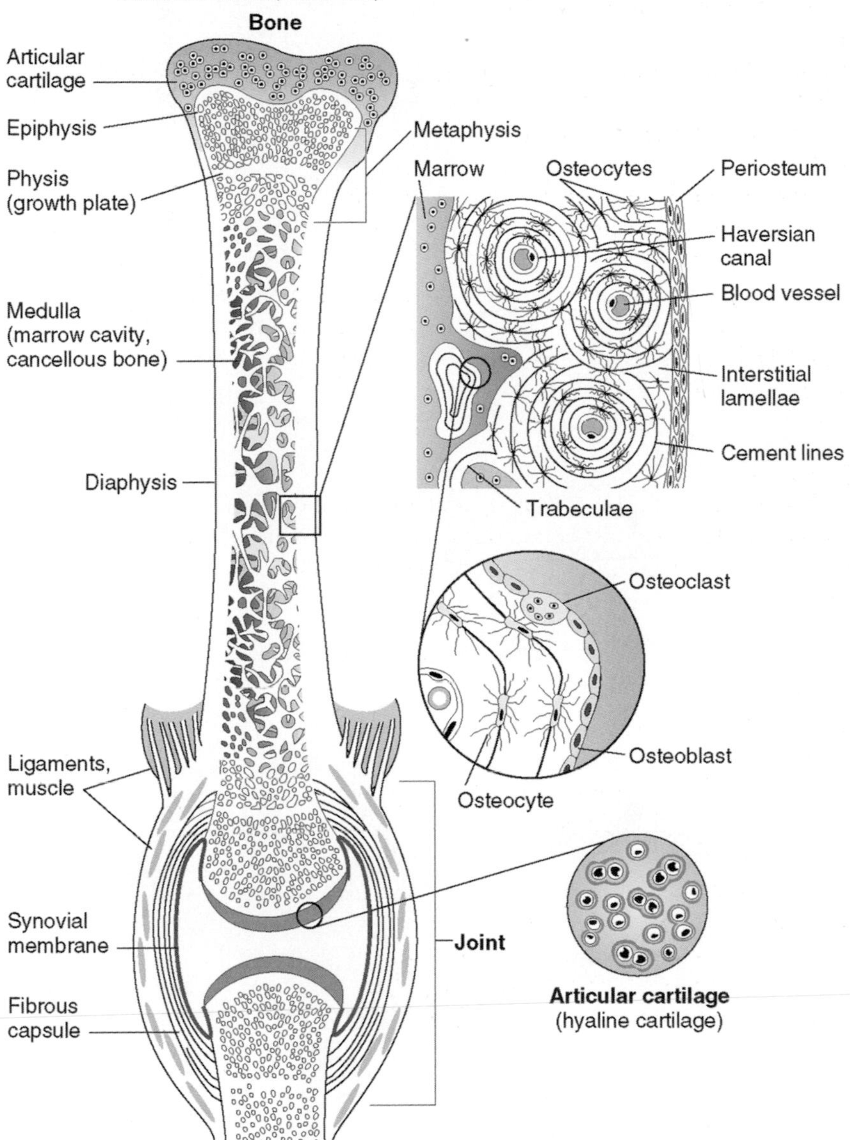

I. Osteoblasts

A. They synthesize type I collagen and bone matrix proteins to form an unmineralized osteoid (Figure 9-3).

B. Calcium (Ca^{2+}) and phosphate are deposited on the cartilaginous matrix to form mineralized bone.

C. Blood supply goes to osteoblasts via vessels within the **haversian canals.**

D. When osteoblasts become surrounded by bone matrix they become **osteocytes.**

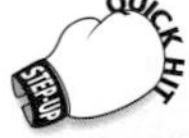

Exogenous estrogen administration (hormone replacement therapy) slows the rate of bone loss that occurs after menopause by stimulating osteoblasts via estrogen receptors.

II. Osteocytes

A. Occupy a space called lacuna.

B. Communicate with other osteocytes via cytoplasmic extensions called canaliculi.

C. Are influenced by parathyroid hormone **(PTH)** to stimulate osteoclastic bone resorption.

D. Resorption allows Ca^{2+} to be transferred rapidly into the blood.

E. Are not directly involved in bone resorption.

FIGURE 9-3 **Collagen synthesis**

DNA, deoxyribonucleic acid; mRNA, messenger RNA; RER, rough endoplasmic reticulum. (Adapted from Champe PC, Harevey RA. Lippincott's Illustrated Reviews: Biochemistry. 2nd Ed. Philadelphia, PA: Lippincott-Raven. 1994:41. Used by permission of Lippincott, Williams & Wilkins.)

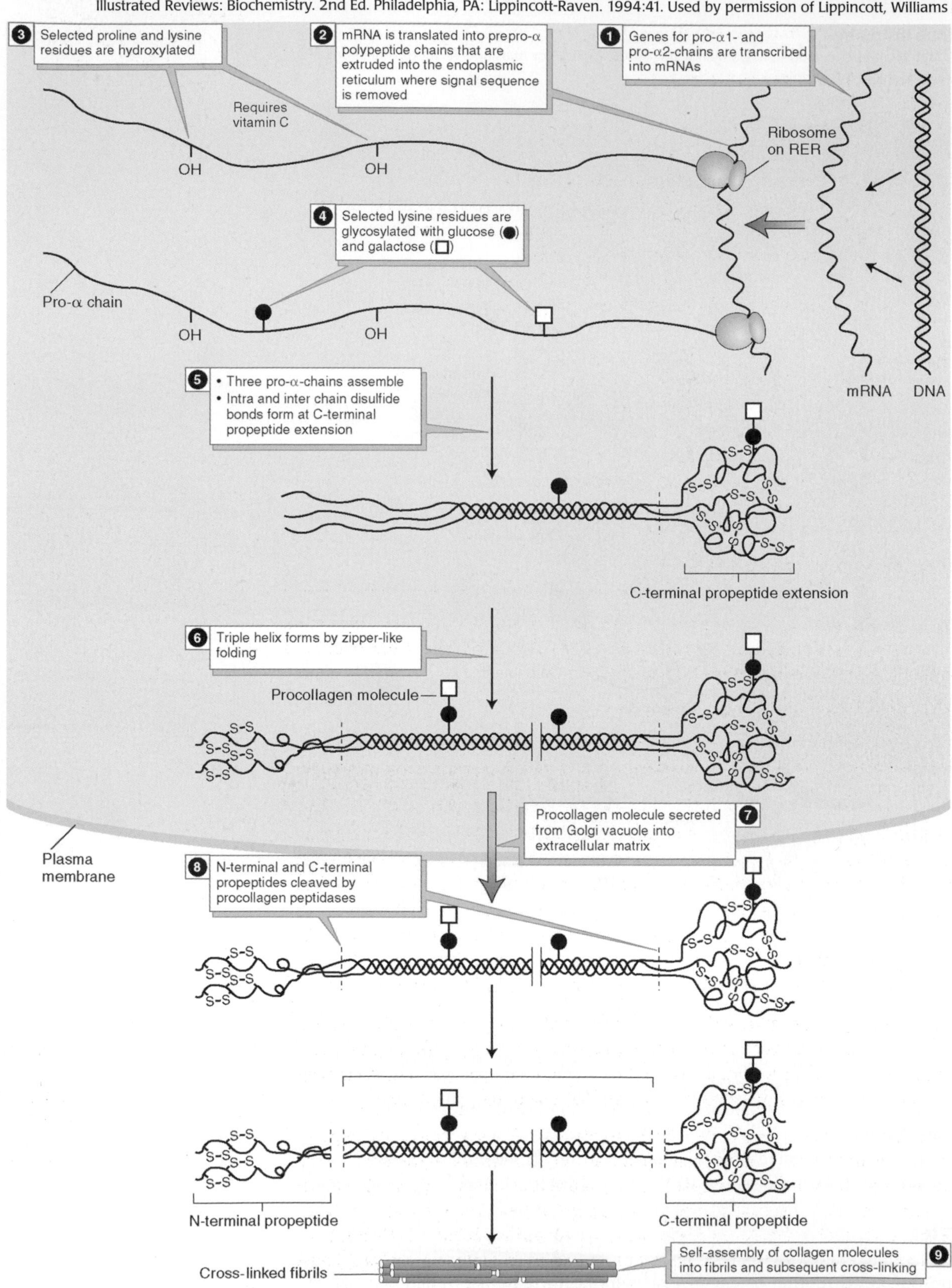

III. Osteoclasts

A. Multinucleated cells formed from monocytes that are responsible for bone resorption
B. Contain acid phosphatase
C. Resorb bone under influence of **PTH**

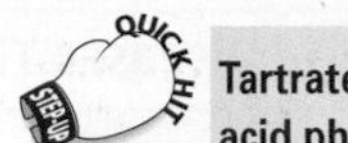

Tartrate-resistant acid phosphatase (TRAP) is used as an indicator of osteoclast activity and also as a marker for hairy cell leukemia.

IV. Hormonal control (also see System 7)

A. **Parathyroid hormone**
   1. Release is stimulated by hypocalcemia and hyperphosphatemia
   2. Stimulates osteoclastic activity causing osteolysis and release of Ca^{2+} from bone
   3. Promotes the reabsorption of Ca^{2+} in the distal tubule of the kidney
   4. Inhibits phosphate (PO_4^{3-}) reabsorption in the proximal tubule of the kidney
   5. Converts vitamin D to its active form, 1,25-dihydroxycholecalciferol
   6. Raises blood calcium and lowers blood phosphate

B. **Calcitonin**
   1. Inhibits osteoclasts, which inhibits bone resorption
   2. Lowers blood calcium

C. **Vitamin D**
   1. Assists PTH in the resorption of bone
   2. Increases Ca^{2+} absorption from the intestine
   3. Increases Ca^{2+} reabsorption from the kidney
   4. Increases PO_4^{3-} reabsorption from the kidney
   5. Raises blood calcium and phosphate
   6. Has net effect on bone growth

BONE, CARTILAGE, AND JOINT DISEASE

In the healthy adult, bone mass peaks between 20 and 25 years of age. Peak bone mass is typically higher in males and Blacks. Bone diseases can adversely affect the mass and strength of the skeleton, predisposing the patient to fractures.

- **Diseases That Affect Bone Formation** (Table 9-1)

Clinical Vignette 9-1

Clinical Presentation: A 4-year-old child with the chief complaint of "belly pain" is brought to the emergency department by his mother. As you begin his physical examination, you note that the child is short for his age and that there are multiple ecchymoses on his lower extremities. The mother reports that her son bruises easily. A head, ears, eyes, nose, and throat examination shows multiple dental caries and blue sclera. Physical examination shows that the abdomen is soft, nontender, and nondistended. There are normoactive bowel sounds. The patient is without organomegaly or masses. T = 98.6°F; HR = 80 bpm; RR = 18 breaths/min; BP = 100/80 mm Hg.

Differentials: Osteogenesis imperfecta (OI), child abuse, child neglect. Short stature, multiple ecchymoses, and dental caries can be seen in each of the listed differentials. However, blue sclera is a characteristic finding of OI. Also, child abuse can be differentiated from OI based on nonskeletal manifestations such as retinal hemorrhage, intracranial bleeding, and splenic trauma.

Diagnostic Workup: **Radiographs** should be obtained of the skull, chest, long bones, and pelvis, looking for **type of fracture** as well as **osteopenia** (seen in OI). Diaphyseal fractures (break in the midshaft of long bone) and metaphyseal fractures (appear as corner chip of bone edge) suggest child abuse. In addition to multiple fractures, osteopenia would be seen on radiograph in OI. In child abuse, serial plain films should show healing and remineralization. In OI, fractures continue to occur in protective custody. In difficult cases, **collagen synthesis analysis** would show abnormal findings in OI.

Management: Medical therapy of OI is supportive, and in some cases, surgical interventions are done to improve weight bearing.

TABLE 9-1 Diseases That Affect Bone Formation

Disease	Etiology	Clinical Features
Osteitis fibrosa cystica (von Recklinghausen disease of bone)	Caused by increased levels of **PTH;** primary or secondary hyperparathyroidism	Cystic spaces in the bone that are lined with osteoclasts; often colored brown owing to hemorrhage, hence the name **"brown tumor of bone"**
Achondroplasia (dwarfism)	Caused by failure of long bones to elongate because of narrow epiphyseal plates and sealing of these plates with the metaphysis; **autosomal dominant** disease; **most common cause of dwarfism;** linked to activating mutation in gene for fibroblast growth factor-3 receptor	Short limbs; normal-size head and trunk
Osteogenesis Imperfecta ("brittle bone disease")	Group of gene mutations that cause **defective Type I collagen synthesis;** most common type of mutation is **autosomal dominant**	Multiple fractures occur with only minor trauma; **blue sclera;** deformities of teeth and skin; deafness
Osteopetrosis ("marble bone disease")	**Defective osteoclasts** cause a decrease in reabsorption leading to **increased bone density;** the most severe form is autosomal recessive	Multiple **fractures** despite increased density; narrowing of marrow spaces causes anemia; narrowing of other cavities causes blindness, deafness, and cranial nerve compression
Paget disease of bone	Increased osteoblastic and osteoclastic activity by an unknown cause; occurs most commonly in the elderly; may involve one or more bones	**Skeletal deformities;** complications include bone pain owing to fracture, multiple arteriovenous (AV) shunts in bone causing high output cardiac failure, hearing loss as a result of thickening of bony structures in ear; may lead to osteosarcoma; Increased levels of serum alkaline phosphatase; three phases of disease: • Osteolytic phase—resorption owing to osteoclasts • Mixed phase—osteoclastic and osteoblastic activity leads to a **mosaic pattern** in the bone • Late phase—increase in bone density as a result of osteoblastic activity

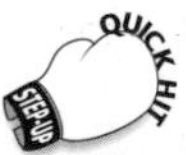

QUICK HIT **Gardner syndrome** is an autosomal dominant disorder characterized by multiple colonic polyps associated with other tumors such as osteomas of the skull, fibromas, thyroid cancer, epidermoid cysts, and sebaceous cysts.

QUICK HIT In osteosarcoma, a "sunburst" appearance on radiography is due to calcified streaks that radiate from a tumor. Codman's triangle is due to peristeum lifting away from the bone due to an underlying tumor.

METABOLIC AND INFECTIOUS SKELETAL DISEASE (Table 9-2)

I. Bisphosphonates

The bisphosphonates, which include alendronate, pamidronate, and etidronate inhibit osteoclast-mediated bone resorption by binding to hydroxyapatite. The bisphosphonates are most commonly used to prevent or treat postmenopausal osteoporosis, but can also be used for Paget disease and steroid-induced osteoporosis.

II. Tumors of bone and cartilage (Table 9-3)

Tumors of the bone and cartilage, although rare, occur most commonly in the lower extremities of young males. Metastases are more common than primary tumors of the bone. Tumors of the prostate, breast, and lung account for 80% of bone metastases.

III. Arthritic joint disease (Table 9-4)

The etiology of arthritic joint diseases is not well understood. For this reason, treatment is often palliative rather than curative.

TABLE 9-2 Metabolic and Infectious Bone Disease

Disease	Etiology	Clinical Features
Osteoporosis	**Primary:** ***Type I:*** postmenopausal, with excess loss of trabecular bone; ***Type II:*** men and women >70 years of age, with loss of trabecular and cortical bone **Secondary:** Physical inactivity, increased parathyroid levels, hypercortisolism, hyperthyroidism, vitamin D deficiency, hypocalcemia	**Bone mineral density** is 2.5 or more standard deviations **below** normal; **decrease in bone mass** leads to fractures (especially of the weight-bearing bones of the spine); radiolucent bone seen on radiograph; DEXA scan positive
Scurvy	Lack of vitamin C intake; defective **proline and lysine hydroxylation** in collagen synthesis (Figure 9-3)	Impaired bone formation and lesions result; painful subperiosteal hemorrhage; osteoporosis; bleeding gums; poor wound healing
Rickets (children); osteomalacia (adults)	Impaired calcification of bone because of deficiency of vitamin D; if caused by renal disease, termed "renal osteodystrophy"	**Children:** Skeletal malformations Craniotabes (thinned and softened bones of the skull) Late fontanelle closure Decreased height Rachitic rosary (costochondral junction thickening resembling string of beads) Pigeon breast owing to a protruding sternum **Adults:** Fractures Radiolucency on radiography
Avascular necrosis	Death of osteocytes and fat necrosis via the following mechanisms: vascular compression, vascular interruption (fracture), thrombosis (sickle cell disease, caisson disease), vessel injury	Joint pain; osteoarthritis; sites include head of the femur, shoulder, knee
Pyogenic osteomyelitis	Infection of bone most often caused by ***Staphylococcus aureus;*** routes of infection include hematogenous, extension from adjacent infection, open fracture or surgery	Acute febrile illness; pain; tenderness; usually affects metaphysis of distal femur, proximal tibia, and proximal humerus; forms sequestrum and involucrum
Tuberculous osteomyelitis	Tuberculous infection spreads to bone from elsewhere in body	Seen in hips, long bones, hands, feet, and vertebrae **(Pott disease)**

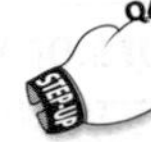
Osteoporosis versus Osteopenia: osteoporosis is a loss of bone that predisposes to fractures; osteopenia is detectable loss of bone via resorption.

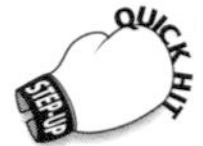
Dual-energy x-ray absorptiometry (DEXA) scan is the gold standard for diagnosis of osteoporosis.

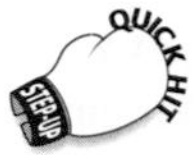
Osteochondrosis is avascular necrosis of epiphysis sites in children. **Legg-Calvé-Perthes disease** is avascular necrosis of the femoral head in children and often presents with limp. **Osgood–Schlatter disease** is an inflammation at the insertion site of the patellar tendon on the tibial apophysis.

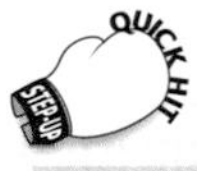
The most common cause of avascular necrosis is steroid-induced vascular compression, most commonly occurring in the femoral head.

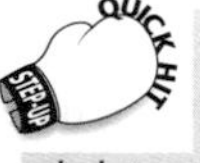
The most common malignancy of the skeleton are metastatic tumors.

The most common bone sarcoma in children is an osteosarcoma, followed by Ewing sarcoma.

TABLE 9-3 Tumors of Bone and Cartilage

Tumor	Morphology	Clinical Features
Osteochondroma	Benign bone tumor; **most common benign tumor;** originates in metaphysis of long bones; growth of mature bone (exostosis) with a cartilaginous cap	Most common in men younger than 25 years of age; usually occurs on the lower end of the femur or upper end of the tibia
Giant cell tumor	Benign bone tumor; spindle-shaped cells with multinuclear giant cells; most commonly occur in the epiphysis of the distal femur or proximal tibia	Most common in women 20–55 years of age; has **"soap bubble"** appearance on radiograph; usually occurs on the lower end of the femur or upper end of the tibia
Osteoma	Benign bone tumor; mature bone (dense tissue)	Most common in men; affects skull or facial bones; protrudes from surface; associated with Gardner syndrome
Osteoid osteoma	Benign bone tumor; **nidus** rimmed by osteoblasts and surrounded by vascular, spindled stroma; <2 cm in diameter	Most common in men 20–30 years of age; occurs near the ends of the tibia and femur; painful due to excess prostaglandin E2 production; radiolucent **nidus** is seen on radiograph

(continued)

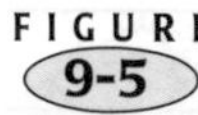

FIGURE 9-5 **Nerve damage and regeneration**
CNS, central nervous system; PNS, peripheral nervous system.

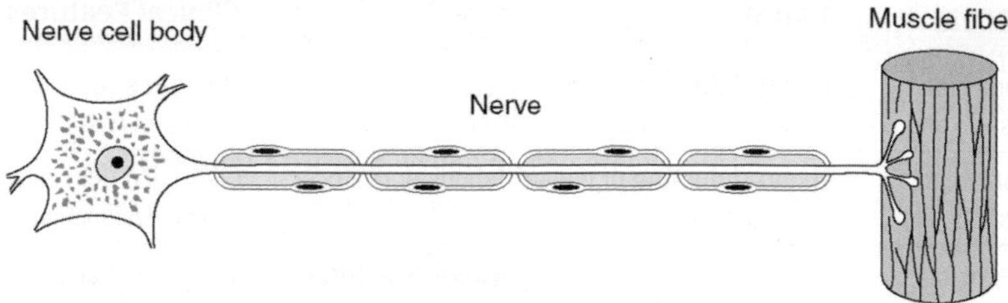

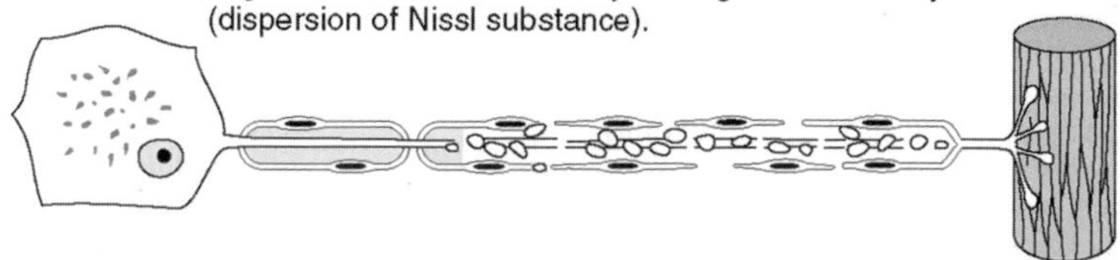

Nerve damage causes some degeneration of the distal segment. The nerve cell body undergoes chromatolysis (dispersion of Nissl substance).

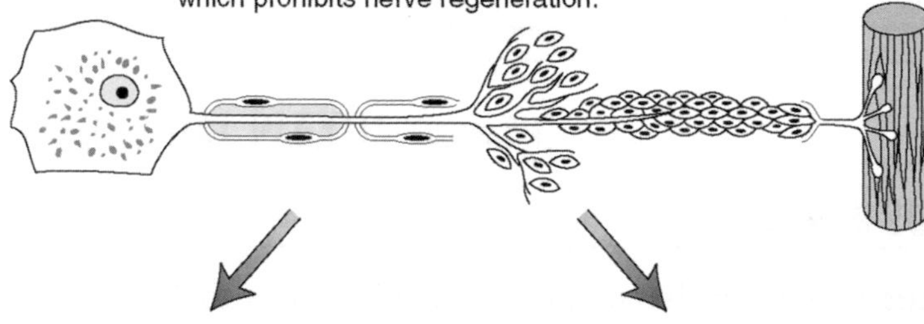

The muscle continues to atrophy for 3 weeks. In the PNS, Schwann cells proliferate and help direct the regenerating neuron. In the CNS, astrocyte proliferation forms a scar, which prohibits nerve regeneration.

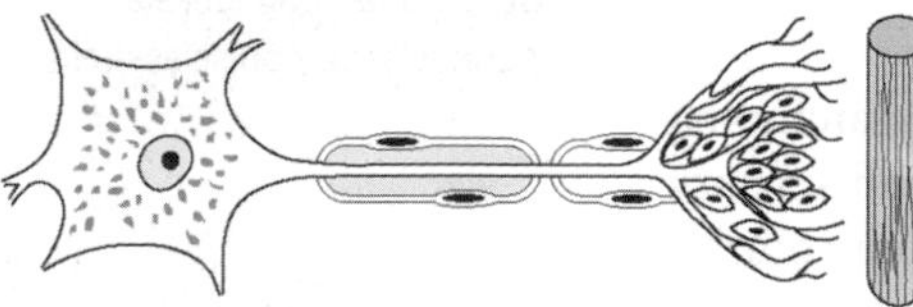

If the nerve fibers do not find the degenerating segment, a neuroma is formed.

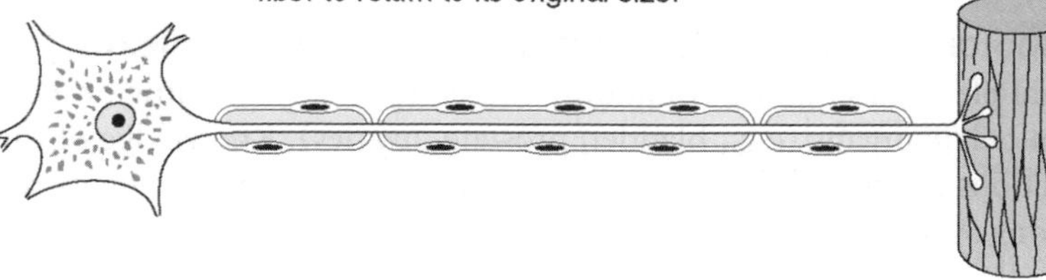

Successful nerve regeneration allows the muscle fiber to return to its original size.

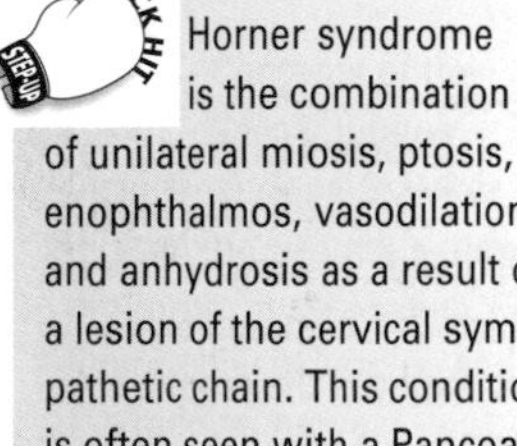

QUICK HIT: Horner syndrome is the combination of unilateral miosis, ptosis, enophthalmos, vasodilation, and anhydrosis as a result of a lesion of the cervical sympathetic chain. This condition is often seen with a Pancoast tumor.

QUICK HIT: The radial nerve is also involved in lateral epicondylitis (tennis elbow).

depletion of liver **glutathione** levels may occur, resulting in hepatic necrosis as a result of the excess *N*-acetyl-*p*-benzoquinoneimine (NAPQI). Treatment for acetaminophen overdose is aerosolized ***N*-acetylcysteine which regenerates the depleted levels of glutathione.**

III. Nonsteroidal anti-inflammatory drugs (NSAIDs)

NSAIDs are similar to acetaminophen in that they have **antipyretic** and **analgesic** properties. In addition, these agents have **anti-inflammatory** effects. NSAIDs act by inhibiting cyclooxygenase (COX) enzymes (Figure 9-7).

A. **Aspirin**, the most common NSAID, blocks prostaglandin synthesis from arachidonic acid in the hypothalamus and in peripheral tissue which provides its antipyretic, antiplatelet, analgesic, and anti-inflammatory benefits. Unlike other NSAIDs, its inhibitory effect on COX enzymes is irreversible.

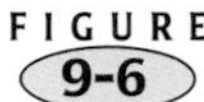

Lumbosacral plexus
L, lumbar vertebra; S, sacral vertebra; T, thoracic vertebra.

A. **The Lumbar Plexus**

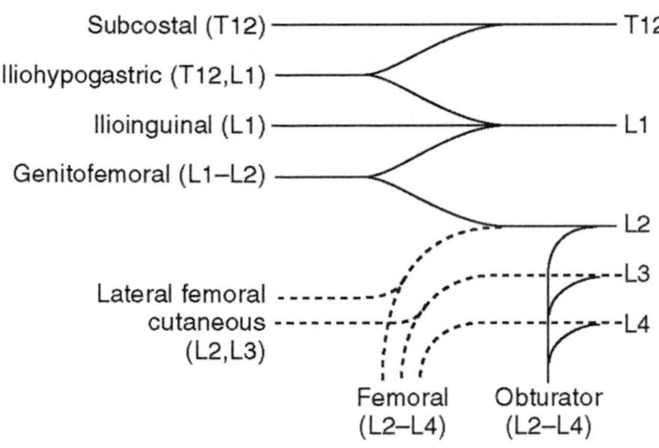

B. **The Sacral Plexus**

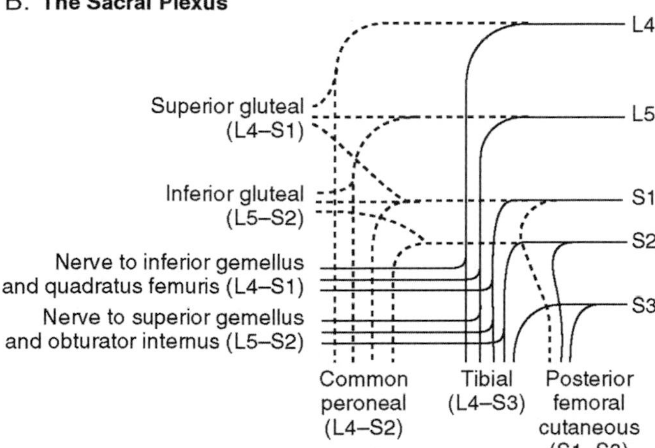

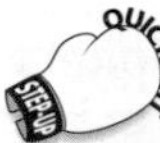

All the nerves of the sacral plexus and the pudendal nerve (S2–S4) emerge from the pelvis through the greater sciatic foramen below the piriformis muscle except the superior gluteal nerve, which passes above the piriformis.

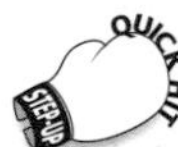

Acute gout treatment includes **indomethacin** (NSAIDs) and **colchicine**. Chronic gout treatment includes **probenecid** (inhibits tubular reabsorption of urate) and **allopurinol** (xanthine oxidase inhibitor).

Administration of aspirin to children with chickenpox increases the risk of Reye syndrome. Acetaminophen and other NSAIDs are a viable alternative for pain and fever associated with chickenpox.

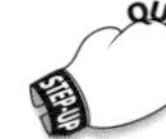

Drugs such as carbamazepine, rifampin, and isoniazid can increase the action of liver enzymes, thus increasing the metabolism and reducing the effectiveness of acetaminophen.

TABLE 9-8 Segmental Nerve Functions of the Lumbosacral Plexus

Spinal Nerve	Muscle Innervation	Muscle Test	Sensory Function
L1	Cremaster	Cremasteric reflex	Inguinal region
L2	Iliopsoas	Hip flexion	Upper anteromedial thigh
L3	Medial thigh Quadriceps femoris	Hip adduction Knee extension	Lower anteromedial thigh
L4	Tibialis anterior	Ankle dorsiflexion	Anteromedial leg
L5	Extensor hallucis longus	Great toe extension	Anterolateral leg, medial dorsal foot, plantar region of great toe
S1	Gastrocnemius, soleus Posterior thigh Gluteus maximus	Ankle plantarflexion Hip extension, knee flexion Power hip extension, external rotation	Heel region, plantar foot, lateral dorsal foot
S2	Gastrocnemius, soleus Foot intrinsics	Ankle plantarflexion Abduction and adduction of toes	Posterior upper thigh and leg
S3–S4	External anal sphincter Bulbospongiosus	External anal sphincter tone Bulbospongiosus reflex	Circumanal and perineal region

TABLE 9-9 Peripheral Nerve Functions of the Sacral Plexus

Nerve	Muscle Innervation	Muscle Test	Sensory Function
Genitofemoral	Cremaster	Cremasteric reflex	Skin below middle of inguinal ligament
Lateral femoral cutaneous	None	None	Skin of lateral thigh
Femoral	Anterior thigh (quadriceps)	Knee extension	Skin of anteromedial thigh and leg
Obturator	Medial thigh	Hip adduction	Hip joint and medial skin of knee
Superior gluteal	Gluteus medius, gluteus minimus	Hip abduction and internal rotation	None
Inferior gluteal	Gluteus maximus	Power hip extension and external rotation	None
Posterior femoral cutaneous	None	None	Skin of posterior thigh and upper leg
Superficial peroneal	Lateral leg	Foot eversion	Skin of anterolateral leg and dorsum of foot
Deep peroneal	Anterior leg	Ankle dorsiflexion, foot inversion, metatarsophalangeal joint extension	Skin of dorsum of web space between great and second toes
Tibial	Posterior thigh Gastrocnemius, soleus Deep posterior leg Planar muscles	Hip extensions, knee flexion, foot inversion, toe flexion	Skin of posterior leg and plantar foot

TABLE 9-10 Other Traumatic Injuries

Injury	Description
Anterior cruciate ligament (ACL) tear	Positive **anterior drawer sign** (lower leg pulled forward with knee flexed); often manifests as **"terrible triad"** (i.e., torn medial collateral ligament, medial meniscus damage, and torn ACL) which occurs due to a force to the knee directed laterally to medially
Clavicle fracture	**Middle third** of clavicle; upward displacement of proximal fragment due to the sternocleidomastoid muscle; downward displacement of distal fragment; severe pain
Compartment syndrome	Fascial sheets separate the limbs into anterior and posterior compartments; hemorrhage into these compartments owing to crush injury or fracture, results in **compression of neurovascular structures** and further complications; emergent fasciotomy is needed
Inversion sprain of ankle	**Most common ankle injury;** results from forced inversion; stretches or tears lateral ligaments (especially the **anterior talofibular**)
Scaphoid fracture	Tenderness in the anatomical snuffbox; may lead to **avascular necrosis** if left untreated; easily missed on radiographs
Scoliosis	Complex lateral deviation and torsion of the spine; may be idiopathic or congenital, or may result from a short leg, hip displacement, or polio
Shoulder separation	Downward displacement of the clavicle as a result of laxity of the acromioclavicular and coracoclavicular ligaments
Subacromial bursitis	Inflammation of the subacromial bursa; **most common bursitis** in the body
Tennis elbow (lateral epicondylitis)	Sprain of radial collateral ligament (lateral epicondyle); pain on wrist extension and forearm supination
Golfers elbow (medial epicondylitis)	Overuse of the pronator teres, palmaris longus, and flexor carpi radialis; causes sprain of their tendinous insertion on the anterior medial epicondyle; pain on wrist flexion
Waddling gait	Limp caused by superior gluteal nerve injury affecting gluteus medius and gluteus minimus; inability to abduct thigh; results in **Trendelenburg sign**

FIGURE 9-7 **Mechanism of action of nonsteroidal anti-inflammatory drugs (NSAIDs)**
ASA, aspirin; COX, cyclooxygenase; PG, prostaglandin; TX, thromboxane.

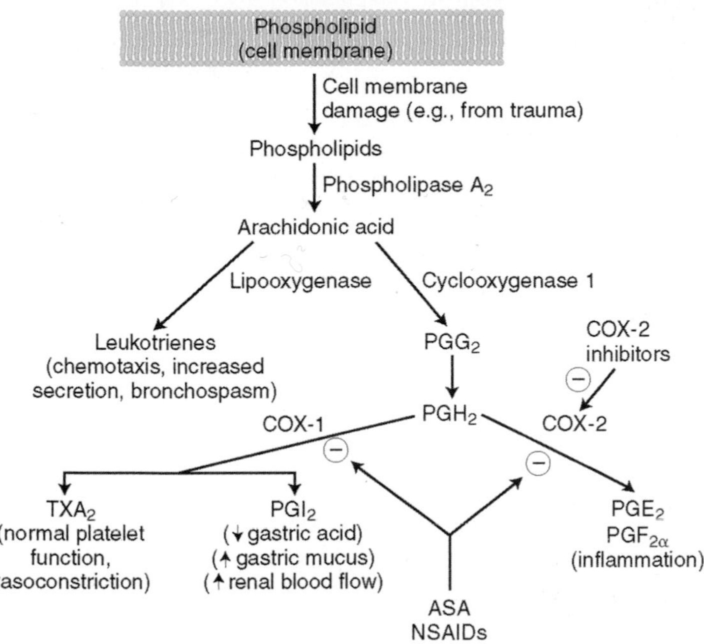

B. A major adverse effect of aspirin and NSAIDs (e.g., ibuprofen, indomethacin, naproxen, diclofenac, ketorolac) is increased risk of **GI bleeding.** By blocking prostaglandin synthesis, NSAIDs may result in GI ulcers and hemorrhage. Prostacyclin (PGI2) inhibits gastric acid secretion, whereas prostaglandin (PG) E2 and PGF2a help synthesize protective mucus in the stomach and small intestine. **COX-2 inhibitors**, including **celecoxib** and **rofecoxib**, may be indicated in patients who have a history of GI conditions; these NSAIDs are more specific for the inflammatory mediators (Figure 9-7).

IV. Opioids

Opioids are useful for severe pain that is uncontrolled by NSAIDs. Opioids exert their effects by interacting with protein receptors in the central nervous system (CNS) and by inhibiting G proteins and adenylyl cyclase in the peripheral nervous system. Each family of opioid receptors—μ, κ, σ, and δ—has its own set of properties and binding potency, which correlates with the amount of analgesia provided. The μ receptors primarily mediate analgesia.

The strong agonists of the various receptor families are **morphine, meperidine, methadone, fentanyl,** and **heroin**. Moderate agonists include codeine and propoxyphene. Some of these agents can produce extreme states of euphoria and become drugs of abuse because of their binding affinity and their intrinsic effects on the CNS. Methadone, which induces less euphoria and has a longer duration of action, is often used to provide controlled withdrawal from addiction to agents such as morphine and heroin.

Opioid overdose can lead to respiratory depression, depression of the cough reflex, pinpoint pupils, constipation, bronchoconstriction, diaphoresis, and urinary retention. Naloxone and naltrexone reverse the adverse effects of opioids. A rapid-acting drug, naloxone, displaces the receptor-bound opioid agents. Its effects are short-lived (approximately 2 h). However, naltrexone works for up to 48 h.

(text continues on page 266)

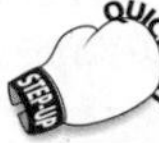
It is believed that prostaglandin E2 (PGE2) sensitizes the nerve endings to the action of bradykinin, histamine, and other chemical mediators.

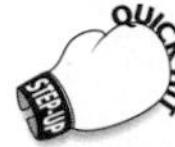
Because of the irreversible effect of aspirin on thromboxane production in platelets, it can be used as an anticoagulant. A daily low dose of aspirin has a cardioprotective effect in men.

The anatomic snuffbox is bounded dorsally by the extensor pollicis longus and on the palmar side by the extensor pollicis brevis and the abductor pollicis longus, with the scaphoid and the trapezium bones creating the base.

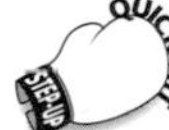
The artery supplying the scaphoid first goes distally then curves proximally, making the proximal aspect of the scaphoid susceptible to avascular necrosis.

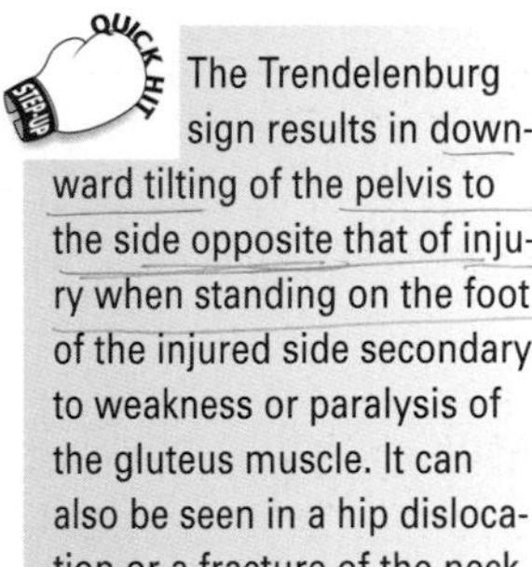
The Trendelenburg sign results in downward tilting of the pelvis to the side opposite that of injury when standing on the foot of the injured side secondary to weakness or paralysis of the gluteus muscle. It can also be seen in a hip dislocation or a fracture of the neck of the femur.

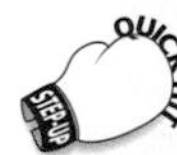
In vitro, the hypocoagulable state is caused by antibodies that react with the cardiolipin test substrate. However, this reaction does not occur in vivo as the SLE patient is prone to excessive clotting, not excessive bleeding. Xerostomia and xerophthalmia alone are characteristic of **sicca syndrome,** which is also autoimmune in nature.

TABLE 9-11 Therapeutic Agents for Pain

Therapeutic Agent (common name, if relevant) [trade name, where appropriate]	Class–Pharmacology and Pharmacokinetics	Indications	Side or Adverse Effects	Contraindications or Precautions to Consider; Notes
Acetaminophen [Tylenol]	Analgesic, antipyretic—reversibly inhibits cyclooxygenase centrally (inactivated peripherally), prostaglandin inhibitor, **not anti-inflammatory**	Pain; fever	Liver toxicity in high doses **(high levels deplete glutathione)**	**Overdose treated with** *N*-acetyl-cysteine (regenerates glutathione); unlike aspirin, **can be used in children, gout, peptic ulcer, and patients with platelet dysfunction**
Acetylsalicylic acid (aspirin)	**Anti-inflammatory, antipyretic, analgesic**—acetylates COX irreversibly	Articular, musculoskeletal pain; chronic pain; **maintenance therapy for preventing clot formation**	GI distress, **GI ulcers; inhibits platelet aggregation;** causes **hypersensitivity reactions (rash)**; reversible hepatic dysfunction	**Contraindicated** for **children** with the flu or chicken pox (leads to **Reye syndrome**), **gouty patients**
Ibuprofen [Advil, Motrin]	**NSAID—reversibly inhibits cyclooxygenase** (both COX-1 and COX-2) → decreases prostaglandin synthesis	**Inflammation; pain**	GI distress, **GI ulcers;** coagulation disorders; aplastic anemia metabolic abnormalities; hypersensitivity; renal damage	
Naproxen [Naprosyn, Aleve]	**NSAID—reversibly inhibits cyclooxygenase** (both COX-1 and COX-2) → decreases prostaglandin synthesis	Inflammation; pain	GI distress, **GI ulcers;** coagulation disorders; aplastic anemia metabolic abnormalities; hypersensitivity; renal damage	
Indomethacin [Indocin]	**NSAID—reversibly inhibits cyclooxygenase** (both COX-1 and COX-2) → decreases prostaglandin synthesis	Acute gout, closes patent ductus arteriosus	GI distress, **GI ulcers;** coagulation disorders; aplastic anemia metabolic abnormalities; hypersensitivity; renal damage	
Ketorolac [Toradol]	**NSAID—reversibly inhibits cyclooxygenase** (both COX-1 and COX-2) → decreases prostaglandin synthesis; relieves pain and reduces swelling	**Postoperative pain;** severe pain	GI distress, **GI ulcers;** coagulation disorders; aplastic anemia metabolic abnormalities; hypersensitivity; renal damage	
Celecoxib [Celebrex]	**NSAID—selectively inhibits COX-2**	Rheumatoid arthritis, osteoarthritis; pain, inflammation	**Increased risk of thrombosis, sulfa allergy, less toxic to GI mucosa**	COX-2 selectivity reduces inflammation while minimizing GI adverse effects (ulcers).

(continued)

TABLE 9-11 Therapeutic Agents for Pain *(Continued)*

Therapeutic Agent (common name, if relevant) [trade name, where appropriate]	Class–Pharmacology and Pharmacokinetics	Indications	Side or Adverse Effects	Contraindications or Precautions to Consider; Notes
Colchicine	**Antigout—depolymerizes microtubules → inhibits leukocyte chemotaxis, degranulation, phagocytosis, and secretion of inflammatory mediators;** decreases LTB_4	**Acute** gout	Nausea; **diarrhea;** vomiting; abdominal cramps	**Contraindicated** in **elderly and feeble patients** and in patients with **GI disturbances, cardiac anomalies,** or **renal problems**
Probenecid [Benemid]	**Antigout—small dose inhibits uric acid secretion; large dose inhibits uric acid reabsorption** (e.g., promotes excretion) of uric acid	**Chronic gout**	**Rash; GI disturbances; drowsy**	Do not use in acute gout
Allopurinol [Zyloprim]	Antigout—**competitive inhibitor of xanthine oxidase** → decreases **conversion of xanthine to uric acid**	**Chronic gout** (caused by renal obstruction or impairment or overproduction); **rheumatic arthritis**	Rash; fever; GI problems; hepatotoxicity; inhibition of the metabolism of other drugs; enhance effect of azathioprine	Do not use in acute gout. Used in lymphoma and leukemia to prevent tumor lysis associated urate nephropathy
Etanercept	Recombinant form of human TNF receptor → binds TNF → decreases inflammatory response	Rheumatoid arthritis, psoriasis, ankylosing spondylitis	**Infections**	
Infliximab	Anti-TNF antibody → binds TNF → decreases inflammatory response	Rheumatoid arthritis, ankylosing spondylitis, Chron disease	**Infections,** reactivation of latent tuberculosis	
Morphine [MS Contin, MSIR, Roxanol]	**Opioid agonist**—converted to more potent morphine-6-glucose	Severe pain; general anesthetic; antitussive; antidiarrheal	Respiratory depression; histamine release; constipation; nausea; miosis	
Meperidine [Demerol]	**Opioid agonist**	**Pain;** acute migraine attacks	**CNS excitation at high doses;** histamine release	**Contraindicated in patients with MAOI** (results in hyperpyrexia)
Fentanyl	**Opioid agonist**	**Pain;** general anesthetic	Prolonged recovery; nausea	
Codeine	**Opioid agonist**	**Pain;** antitussive	**Constipation**	
Oxycodone [Roxicodone]	**Partial opioid agonist** at μ receptor	Severe pain; general anesthetic	Respiratory depression; constipation; nausea	
Hydromorphone [Dilaudid]	Opioid agonist	**Pain;** antitussive	Respiratory depression; constipation; nausea	
Methadone	**Opioid agonist**—synthetic	Maintenance therapy for **heroin addiction**	Respiratory depression; histamine release; constipation; nausea; miosis	
Tramadol [Ultram]	Analgesic—similar to opioid agonist	Chronic pain of **osteoarthritis**	Nausea, vomiting, constipation, drowsiness	

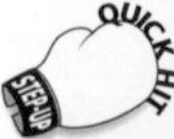
Opioids can also be used as effective medications to combat diarrhea and cough.

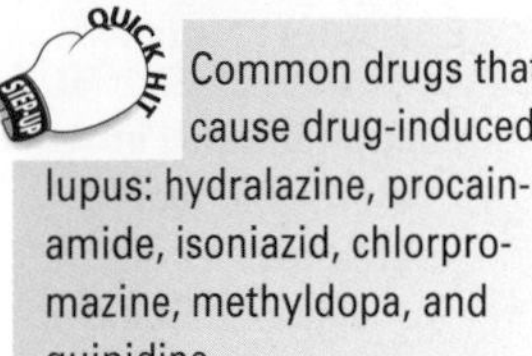
Common drugs that cause drug-induced lupus: hydralazine, procainamide, isoniazid, chlorpromazine, methyldopa, and quinidine.

The embryonal type of rhabdomyosarcoma is related to sarcoma botryoides, resulting in a "bunch of grapes" appearance (see System 8: The Reproductive System).

MUSCLE FUNCTION AND DYSFUNCTION (Figure 9-8)

I. Comparison of muscle fibers (Table 9-12)

A. **Smooth muscle** plays a significant role in the maintenance of the lumens of the respiratory and GI tracts, and blood vessels. **Cardiac muscle** contracts the heart and propels blood through the vasculature.

B. **Skeletal muscle fiber types** (Table 9-13)

Skeletal muscle maintains posture and produces movement. Muscle can be divided into **two subtypes** with differing physiologic roles.

II. Muscle tumors (Table 9-14)

Pathology of muscles can take many forms. Metabolic dyscrasias, which can be induced or inherited, are far more common than neoplasms.

III. Other neuromuscular disorders (Table 9-15)

IV. Neuromuscular blocking agents

Neuromuscular blocking agents, which are most often encountered in the operating room, are used to produce the flaccid paralysis that is essential for many procedures, such as abdominal operations and joint replacements. These drugs affect the muscles of the body in

FIGURE 9-8 **Myocyte contraction**
ADP, adenosine diphosphate; ATP, adenosine triphosphate; Ca^{2+}, calcium; Pi, inorganic phospate; T, troponin.

A. **The cross-bridge cycle of skeletal muscle.**

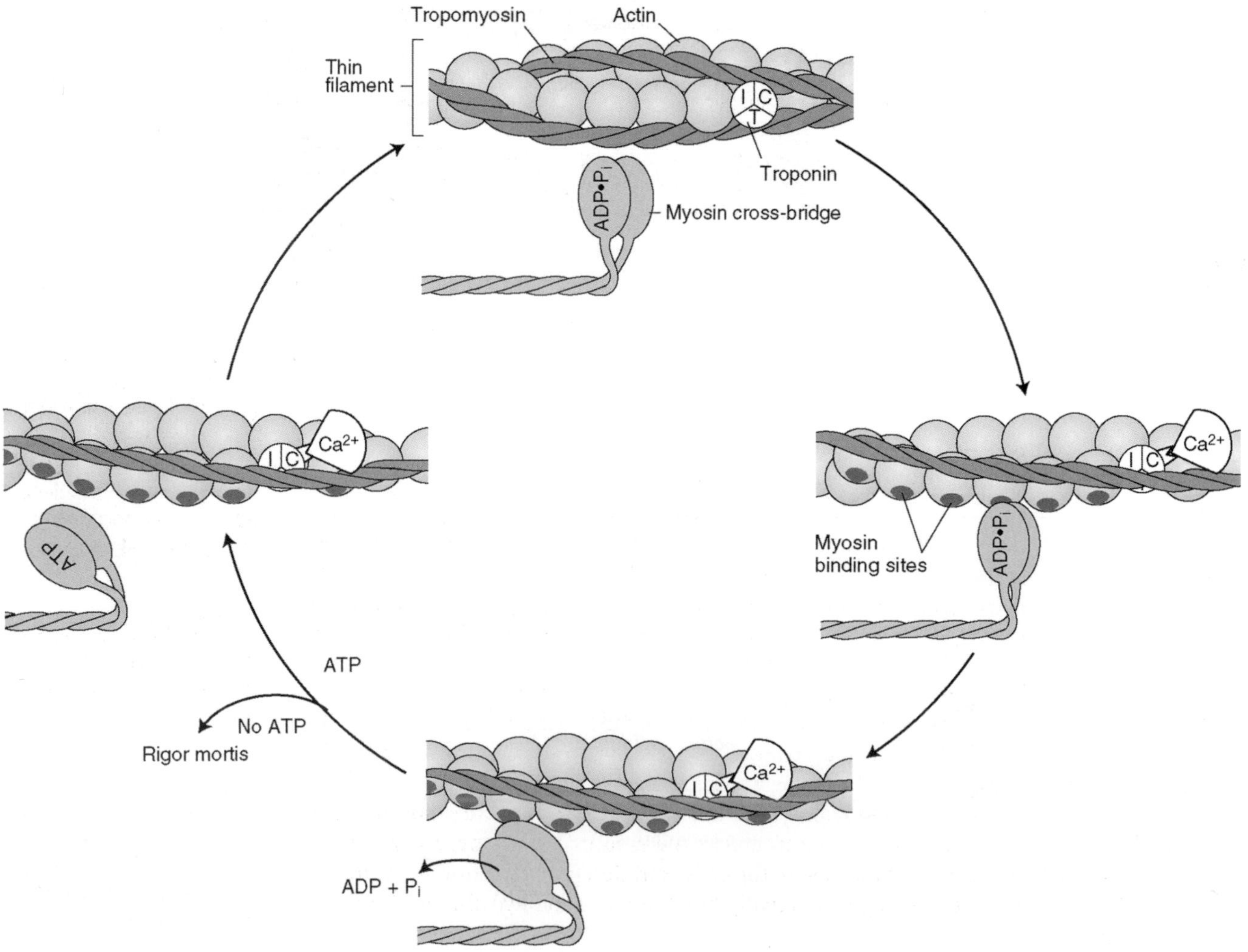

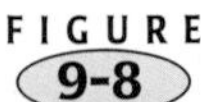

B. **Gross, histologic, microscopic anatomy of skeletal muscle.**

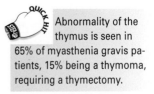

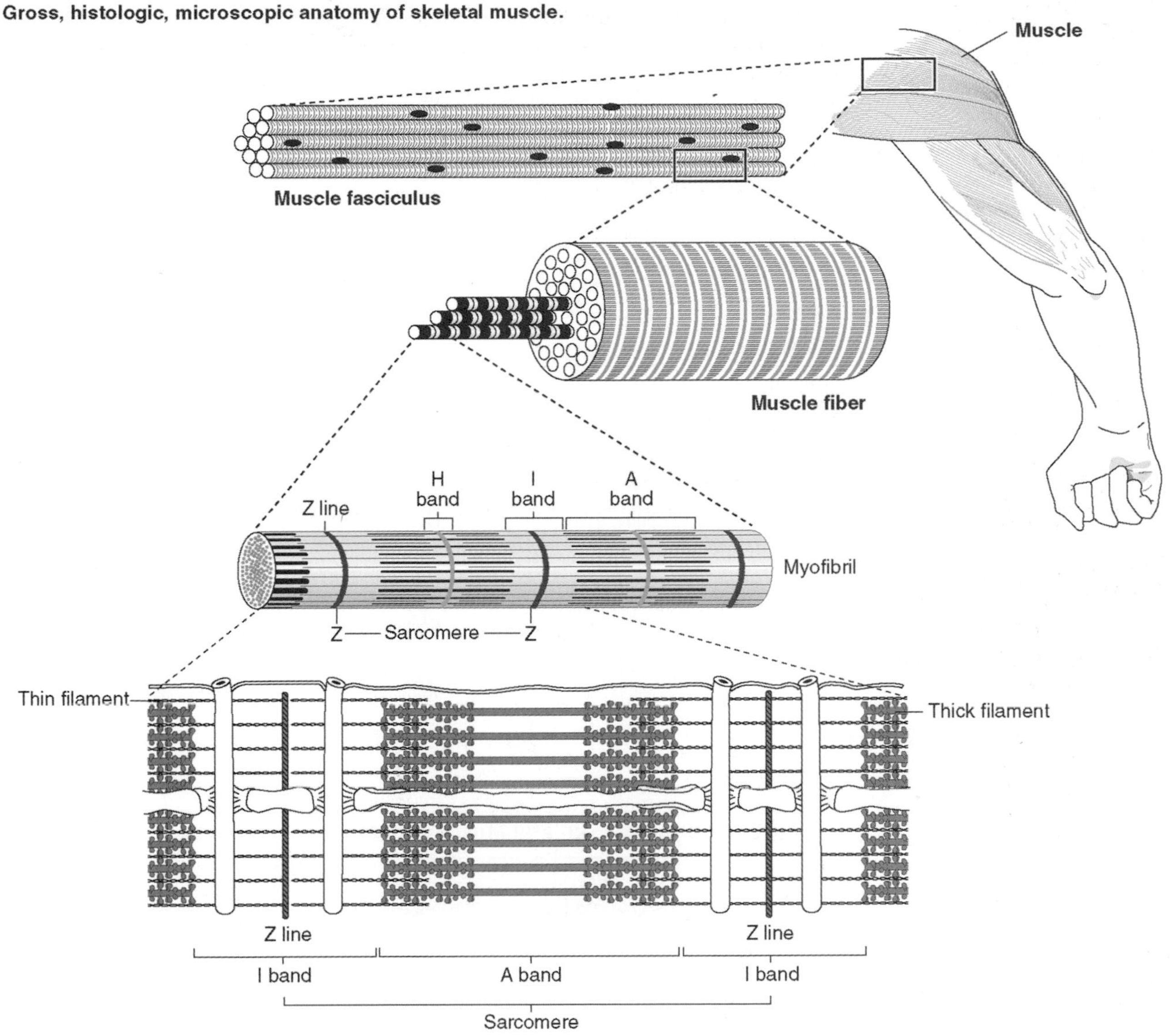

a typical order. The small, fast-twitch muscles of the face and eyes are the first to be paralyzed, followed by the muscles of the hand, limbs, and trunk. The intercostal muscles and the diaphragm are the last to be affected. As the effects of neuromuscular blockers wear off, the muscles regain function in the reverse order.

Neuromuscular blocking agents can be categorized in several ways. The most useful system divides them into central-acting and neuromuscular endplate (NMEP) blockers. The NMEP blockers can be further divided into depolarizing and nondepolarizing agents.

Centrally acting neuromuscular blocking drugs include diazepam and baclofen. **Diazepam**, a benzodiazepine, acts at γ-aminobutyric acid (GABA) receptors in the CNS. **Baclofen**, another GABA mimetic, also acts in the CNS to decrease muscle tone. Peripherally acting drugs include curare, succinylcholine, and dantrolene.

Curare acts as a nicotinic antagonist at the motor endplate to produce muscle relaxation. At low doses, this agent binds to and blocks the nicotinic receptor, a competitive blockade that can be overcome by increasing the concentration of acetylcholine. At higher doses, curare and the curare-like agents actually block ion channels at the NMEP (noncompetitive block).

QUICK HIT: Dantrolene, which acts by inhibiting the release of calcium from the sarcoplasmic reticulum, is used in the treatment of malignant hyperthermia.

QUICK HIT: Becker muscular dystrophy is similar to Duchenne muscular dystrophy, but is much less severe.

QUICK HIT: Abnormality of the thymus is seen in 65% of myasthenia gravis patients, 15% being a thymoma, requiring a thymectomy.

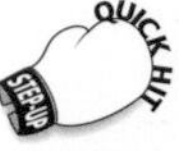
Pseudohypertrophy is initially caused by muscle hypertrophy. Then as atrophy ensues, an increase in fat and connective tissue deposition occurs.

The miosis seen in opioid overdose is a result of stimulation of the Edinger-Westphal nucleus of the oculomotor nerve, which leads to enhanced parasympathetic stimulation of the eye.

MNEMONIC

Remember the number of nuclei in muscle cells by simply noting **one** heart in the body and **one** nucleus per heart muscle cell; **many** skeletal muscles, so **many** nuclei per skeletal muscle fiber. Also, **location** of nucleus mirrors **location** in human body. The heart is in the center of the body and the nucleus is centrally located. Skeletal muscles predominate in the periphery of the body and the nuclei are at the periphery.

Increased anion gap metabolic acidosis may also be caused by salicylate poisoning, alcohol intoxication, acute renal failure, diabetic ketoacidosis, and aspirin ingestion. Normal anion gap metabolic acidosis is caused by diarrhea and renal tubular acidosis.

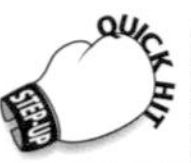
Becker Muscular Dystrophy is a less common and less severe variant of Duchenne muscular dystrophy that involves the same gene (Xp21) and the dystrophin protein.

TABLE 9-12 Comparison of Muscle Fibers

Category	Smooth Muscle Fiber	Cardiac Muscle Fiber	Skeletal Muscle Fiber
Nuclei	Centrally located single nucleus	Centrally located single nucleus	Peripherally located multiple nuclei
Banding	No distinct bands	Distinct bands	Distinct bands
Z-line (convergence actin filaments)	None; dense bodies present	Present	Present
Transverse (T) tubules (membrane invaginations)	None	At Z-line; diads	At A–I junction; triads
Junctional communication	Gap junctions	Intercalated disks	None
Neuromuscular junction	None	None	Present
Regeneration	High	None	Some
Calcium source	Sarcoplasmic reticulum; extracellular	Sarcoplasmic reticulum; extracellular	Sarcoplasmic reticulum
Mechanism of calcium release	IP_3 (inositol-1,4,5-triphosphate)	Calcium-induced	Depolarization of T tubule
Calcium-binding protein	Calmodulin	Troponin	Troponin

TABLE 9-13 Types of Skeletal Muscle Fiber

Category	Type 1	Type 2
Action	Sustained force; weight-bearing muscles	Sudden movement; directed action
Lipid stores	Abundant	Few
Glycogen stores	Few	Abundant
Energy utilization	Aerobic; many mitochondria	Anaerobic; few mitochondria; easily fatigued
Twitch	Slow	Fast
Color	Red (owing to blood supply)	White

Succinylcholine, the only depolarizing neuromuscular blocking agent, acts by binding to and activating the nicotinic receptor of the NMEP. In phase 1 block, a wave of fasciculations rapidly pass over the patient as the drug is administered. The drug then remains attached to the nicotinic receptor and is not broken down by acetylcholinesterase. In phase 2 block, the membrane of the NMEP repolarizes, the muscles relax, and the succinylcholine continues to block the nicotinic receptor. Plasma cholinesterase quickly breaks down the drug, and its duration of action is only a few minutes. The rapid onset and short duration of action of succinylcholine make it ideal for use during rapid-sequence endotracheal intubation and electroconvulsive therapy.

TABLE 9-14 Muscle Tumors

Category	Leiomyoma	Leiomyosarcoma	Rhabdomyosarcoma
Morphology	Benign; elongated nuclei; whorled bundles of smooth muscle cells; no larger than 2 cm	Malignant; "cigar-shaped" nuclei dense bodies	Malignant; embryonal, alveolar, and pleomorphic types; rhabdomyoblast is diagnostic cell
Location	Smooth muscle; **uterus**	Smooth muscle; skin; deep soft tissues	Skeletal muscle; head and neck; genitourinary tract; retroperitoneum
Immunohistochemistry	Antibodies to actin and desmin	Antibodies to vimentin, actin, and desmin	Antibodies to vimentin, actin, desmin, and myoglobin
Prognosis	Indolent course; easily cured	Variable; prognosis worse with increased size	Aggressive; treat with surgery, radiation, chemotherapy
Notes	Afflicts women more often than men; **most common tumor in women**	Uncommon	**Most common soft-tissue sarcoma of childhood** and adolescence

TABLE 9-15 Other Neuromuscular Disorders

Disorder	Etiology	Clinical Features	Notes
Lactic acidosis	Shock; sepsis; methanol poisoning; metformin toxicity; liver failure; diabetic ketoacidosis	Increased serum lactate; **metabolic acidosis;** increased anion gap	May lead to coma or death
Myasthenia gravis	Acetylcholine receptor **autoantibodies at the neuromuscular junction;** linked to HLA-DR3; associated with thymus disorders	Muscle weakness with use; ptosis; manifests itself in facial, ocular, and limb muscles; proximal muscles affected first	Four times more common in women; diagnosis includes the edrophonium (Tensilon) test; anticholinesterase (e.g., edrophonium) improves condition
Duchenne muscular dystrophy	**X-linked recessive;** deficiency in **dystrophin** leading to lack of actin stabilization	Progressive; proximal muscle weakens, beginning with the pelvic girdle and extending to the shoulder girdle; **pseudohypertrophy** of muscles (e.g., calf); positive Gowers maneuver; leads to death via respiratory or cardiac failure	Increased serum creatine kinase and lactate dehydrogenase; Clinical symptoms usually appear by age 5 with wheelchair dependence by the end of the first decade of life and death in the 20s
Mitochondrial myopathy	Transmitted via mitochondrial DNA (mtDNA); non-Mendelian inheritance	**Ragged red fibers** seen on muscle biopsy; proximal muscle weakness	**Maternal** mode of transmission

V. Muscle glycogen storage disorders (Figure 9-9)

THE INGUINAL CANAL (Figure 9-10)

I. The inguinal canal (Table 9-16)

II. Hernias (Table 9-17)

(text continues on page 272)

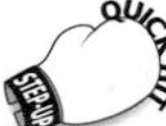

When succinylcholine is used in combination with halothane, it can cause malignant hyperthermia in certain predisposed individuals. Treatment of this condition, which is characterized by severe, prolonged muscle contractions, involves the use of dantrolene and cooling blankets.

FIGURE 9-9 **Muscle glycogen storage disorders**

(Adapted from Champe PC, Harevey RA. Lippincott's Illustrated Reviews: Biochemistry. 2nd Ed. Philadelphia, PA: Lippincott-Raven, 1994:140. Used by permission of Lippincott, Williams & Wilkins.)

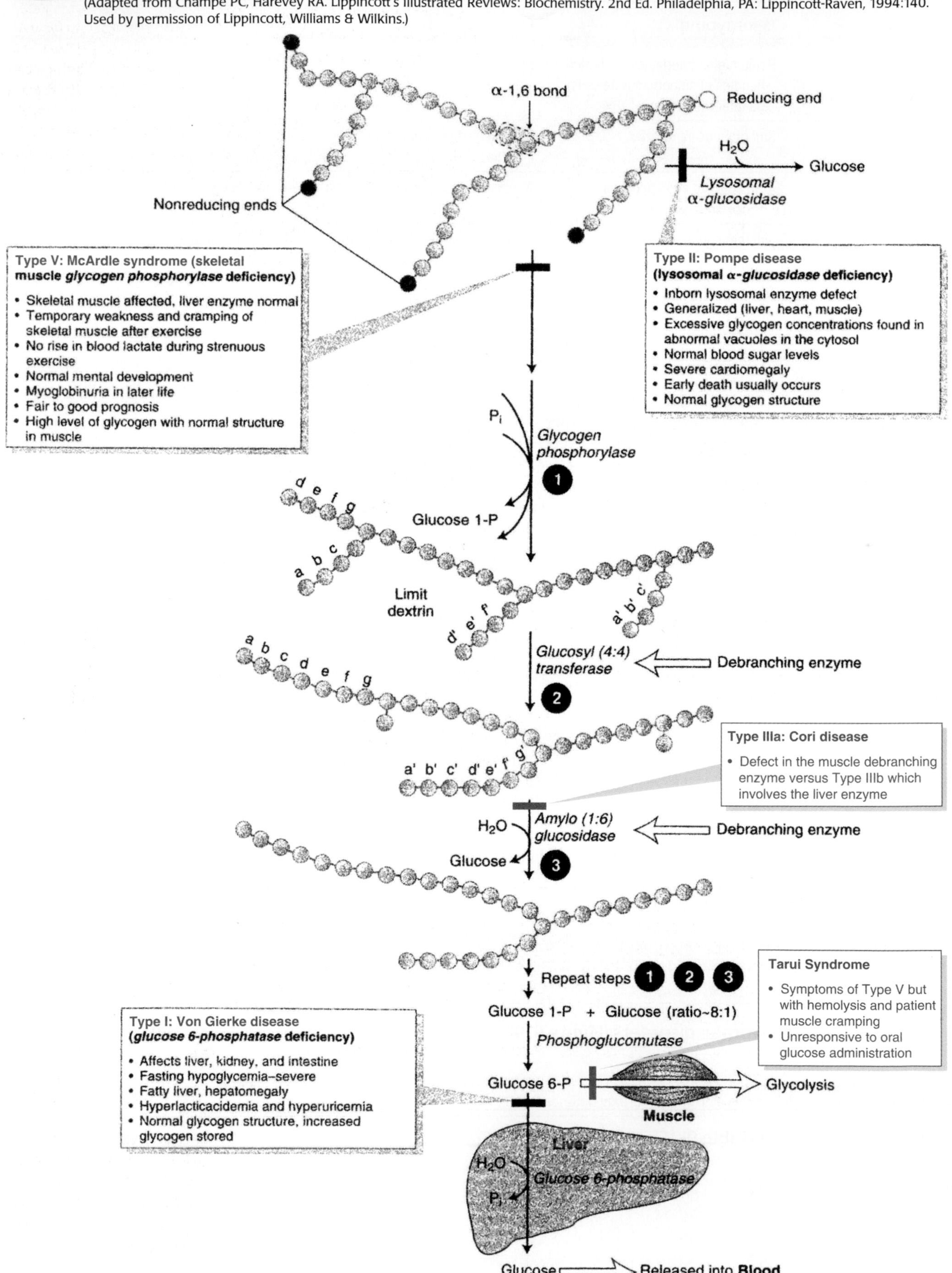
α-1,6 bond
Reducing end
Nonreducing ends
H_2O
Glucose
Lysosomal α-glucosidase
Type V: McArdle syndrome (skeletal muscle glycogen phosphorylase deficiency)
• Skeletal muscle affected, liver enzyme normal
• Temporary weakness and cramping of skeletal muscle after exercise
• No rise in blood lactate during strenuous exercise
• Normal mental development
• Myoglobinuria in later life
• Fair to good prognosis
• High level of glycogen with normal structure in muscle
Type II: Pompe disease (lysosomal α-glucosidase deficiency)
• Inborn lysosomal enzyme defect
• Generalized (liver, heart, muscle)
• Excessive glycogen concentrations found in abnormal vacuoles in the cytosol
• Normal blood sugar levels
• Severe cardiomegaly
• Early death usually occurs
• Normal glycogen structure
P_i
Glycogen phosphorylase
1
Glucose 1-P
Limit dextrin
Glucosyl (4:4) transferase
2
Debranching enzyme
Type IIIa: Cori disease
• Defect in the muscle debranching enzyme versus Type IIIb which involves the liver enzyme
H_2O
Amylo (1:6) glucosidase
Glucose
3
Debranching enzyme
Repeat steps 1 2 3
Glucose 1-P + Glucose (ratio~8:1)
Phosphoglucomutase
Tarui Syndrome
• Symptoms of Type V but with hemolysis and patient muscle cramping
• Unresponsive to oral glucose administration
Type I: Von Gierke disease (glucose 6-phosphatase deficiency)
• Affects liver, kidney, and intestine
• Fasting hypoglycemia–severe
• Fatty liver, hepatomegaly
• Hyperlacticacidemia and hyperuricemia
• Normal glycogen structure, increased glycogen stored
Glucose 6-P
Glycolysis
Muscle
Liver
H_2O
Glucose 6-phosphatase
P_i
Glucose
Released into Blood

FIGURE 9-10 **The inguinal canal**

The inguinal canal contains the ilioinguinal nerve (sensory to the anterior aspect of labia or scrotum), spermatic cord in males (vas deferens, testicular artery, pampiniform plexus, genital branch of the genitofemoral nerve), and the round ligament of the uterus in females.

TABLE 9-16 The Inguinal Canal

Border	Anatomic Composition
Superior	Falx inguinalis: internal abdominal oblique (IAO) and transversus abdominis muscles
Inferior	Inguinal ligament
Anterior	External abdominal oblique (EAO) aponeurosis; IAO and transversus abdominis muscles laterally
Posterior	Transversalis fascia; falx inguinalis medially

Littre hernia is a groin hernia containing a Meckel diverticulum.

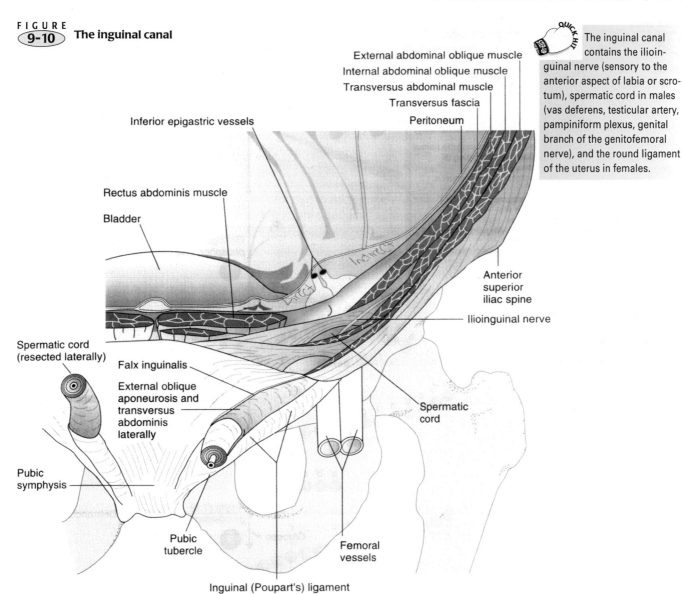

Hesselbach triangle is formed from the border of the rectus abdominis medially, inferior epigastric artery laterally, and the inguinal ligament inferiorly.

MNEMONIC

Remember MCARLES syndrome: **M**yoglobinuria; **C**ramping after exercise; **A**ccumulated glycogen; **R**ecessive inheritance; **D**eficiency of muscle glycogen phosphorylase; **L**actate levels fail to rise; **E**levated creatinine kinase; **S**keletal muscle only.

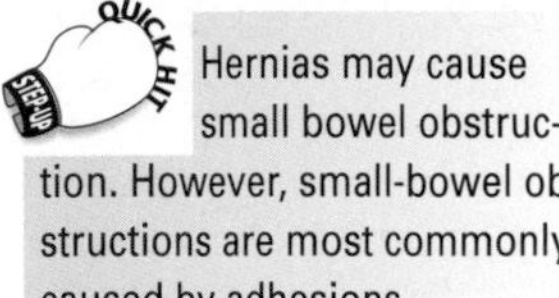

Hernias may cause small bowel obstruction. However, small-bowel obstructions are most commonly caused by adhesions.

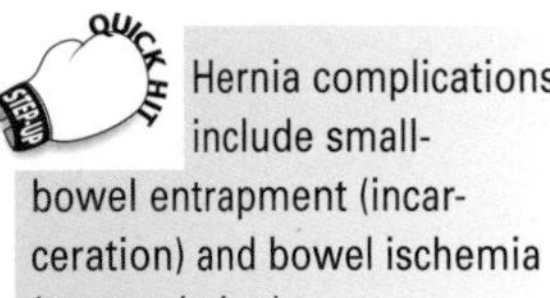

Hernia complications include small-bowel entrapment (incarceration) and bowel ischemia (strangulation).

A lack of pigment, such as in albinism, predisposes one to a variety of skin disorders including actinic keratosis, basal cell carcinoma, squamous cell carcinoma, and malignant melanoma.

TABLE 9-17 Hernias

Hernia	Pathology	Clinical Features	Diagnosis
Direct inguinal hernia	Parietal peritoneum passes directly through abdominal wall (through the **Hesselbach** triangle)	More common in older males	Medial to inferior epigastric artery; located above pubic tubercle
Indirect inguinal hernia	Parietal peritoneum passes through internal inguinal ring and follows the inguinal canal; failure of the processus vaginalis to close properly	**Most common** type; occurs in young adult males more frequently than in females	Lateral to inferior epigastric artery; located above and medial to pubic tubercle; hernia sac may enter the scrotum in males
Femoral hernia	Parietal peritoneum passes through the femoral canal	More common in older females	Located below and lateral to pubic tubercle

SKIN DISORDERS (Table 9-18)

Skin disorders are often characterized by pruritus, inflammation, and irritability. Skin lesions that are suggestive of malignancy demonstrate asymmetry, irregular borders, variations in color, and increasing size.

- **Skin Cancers and Premalignant Conditions** (Table 9-19)

TABLE 9-18 Skin Disorders

Disorder	Description
Keloid scarring	• **Excessive scarring** that occurs after minor trauma • Results in raised, firm lesions on the skin • Occurs more frequently in Blacks • Genetic predisposit ion is a factor
Xanthomas	• Accumulation of foam-filled histiocytes within the dermis • Often associated with **hyperlipidemia** or lymphoproliferative disorders • Often found on the Achilles tendon, the extensor tendons of the fingers, and the eyelids
Seborrheic keratosis	• Common **benign neoplasm** in the elderly • Raised papules and plaques that appear to be "pasted on"
Albinism	• **Lack of melanin pigment** production • Ocular type limited to eyes; X-linked • Oculocutaneous type involves the skin, eyes, and hair; autosomal recessive; lack of tyrosinase enzyme, which converts tyrosine to DOPA (3,4-dihydroxyphenylalanine)
Hemangiomas	• Large-vessel malformation composed of masses of blood-filled channels • **Port-wine stain** birthmarks are the most common manifestation • Cavernous hemangiomas are a subset with large cavernous vascular spaces that can occur in von Hippel-Lindau disease

TABLE 9-19 Skin Cancers and Premalignant Conditions

Disorder	Description
Acanthosis nigricans	• A thickening and **hyperpigmentation** of the axilla, neck, and groin region • Benign type—several causes (e.g., diabetes mellitus) • Malignant type—is an important marker of an underlying visceral **adenocarcinoma**
Actinic keratosis	• A series of dysplastic changes that occur before the onset of **squamous cell carcinoma** • A buildup of keratin caused by excessive exposure to sunlight leads to a **"warty"** appearance • Higher incidence in lightly pigmented individuals
Squamous cell carcinoma	• Malignant tumor of the skin associated with excessive exposure to sunlight (UV rays) leading to DNA damage, immunosuppresion, or xeroderma pigmentosum • Rarely metastasizes • Characterized by ulcerated, scaling nodules • Appears microscopically as islands of neoplastic cells with **whorls of keratin** ("pearls") and cells with atypical nuclei at all levels of the epidermis
Basal cell carcinoma	• **Most common skin tumor** • Appears grossly as a pearllike papule on sun-exposed areas • Appears histologically as a dark cluster with **palisading peripheral cells** • Almost never metastasizes
Malignant melanoma	• Aggressive tumor that arises from melanocytes (neural crest origin) • Associated with excess exposure to sunlight, immunosuppresion, and xeroderma pigmentosum • Two growth patterns: • **Benign radial manner** (growth within skin layer) • **Aggressive vertical manner** (growth through deeper layers) • Associated with the S-100 tumor marker

MNEMONIC

MElanoma is more likely to **ME**tastasize. Basal and squamous cell carcinoma hardly ever metastasize.

MNEMONIC

Use ABCDE to identify nevi with poorer prognostic value: **A**symmetry; **B**order irregular; **C**olor irregular; **D**iameter greater than 0.5 cm; **E**levation irregular.

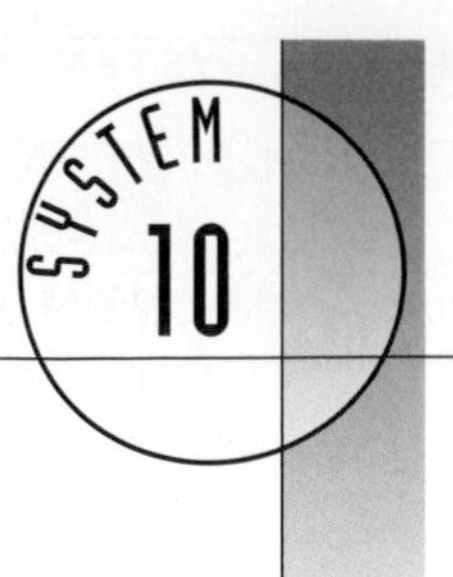

The Hematopoietic and Lymphoreticular System

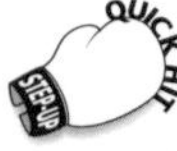

Hematopoiesis expands into fetal sites in times of hematologic stress (e.g., sickle cell anemia).

Neutrophils are hypersegmented (six to seven segments) in megaloblastic anemia.

MNEMONIC

To remember the concentrations of the WBCs, think "Never Let Monkeys Eat Bananas."
Neutrophils (65%)
Lymphocytes (25%)
Monocytes (8%)
Eosinophils (3%)
Basophils (<1%)

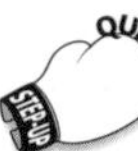

Slow-reacting substance of anaphylaxis (SRS-A) is comprised of leukotriene C_4 and leukotriene D_4 which bronchoconstrict, vasoconstrict, and increase vascular permeability.

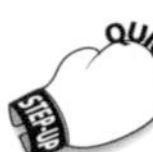

Eosinophilia occurs in response to trematodes (also called flukes), including schistosomes, *Clonorchis sinensis*, and *Paragonimus westermani*, or cestodes (also called tapeworms), including *Taenia solium, Taenia saginata, Diphyllobothrium latum*, and *Echinococcus granulosus*.

DEVELOPMENT

I. Hematopoiesis timetable

A. **Week 3: Embryonic visceral mesoderm** gives rise to **angioblasts.**
B. **First trimester: Yolk sac** produces red blood cells (RBCs).
C. **Second trimester: Liver and spleen** produce RBCs.
D. **Third trimester: Central and peripheral skeletons** produce RBCs.
E. **Adulthood: Axial skeleton (vertebral bodies, sternum, ribs, and pelvis)** produces RBCs.

II. Hemoglobin structure

A. Normal **hemoglobin** consists of four protein subunits and four heme prosthetic groups.
B. **Fetal hemoglobin** consists of Hemoglobin F that is composed of two alpha and two gamma subunits, $\alpha_2\gamma_2$. Fetal hemoglobin has a higher affinity for oxygen.
C. **Adult hemoglobin** mostly consists of **Hemoglobin A** that is made up of two alpha and two beta subunits, $\alpha_2\beta_2$. A small quantity of Hemoglobin A_2 may also be found in adult blood consisting of two alpha and two delta chains, $\alpha_2\delta_2$.

THE CELLS (Table 10-1)

The hematopoietic lymphoreticular system is composed of a multitude of cells. Most of these cells can be found circulating in the bloodstream, although a few are found within peripheral tissues.

THE ORGANS OF THE LYMPHORETICULAR SYSTEM

I. Thymus

A. It is derived from the **third pharyngeal pouch.**
B. The cortex contains thymocytes (immature T lymphocytes).
C. The medulla contains mature T lymphocytes and **Hassall corpuscles** (whorl-like bodies that contain keratin). As T lymphocytes mature, they express T-cell receptors and CD receptors. T lymphocytes that recognize "self" undergo apoptosis, whereas those that recognize "nonself" undergo clonal expansion.

II. Lymph nodes (Figure 10-1)

A. It is derived from **mesenchymal cells.**
B. **Outer cortex** contains B lymphocytes.

TABLE 10-1 The Cells of the Hematopoietic–Lymphoreticular System

Cell	Relative Amounts	Life Span	Morphology		Functions	Secretion	Notes
Neutrophils (PMNs)	40%–75% of WBCs, Band form 3%–5% of WBCs	Less than 7 days	Multilobed nucleus, azurophilic granules (lysosomes)	Neutrophil	Phagocytic, acute inflammatory response	**Myeloperoxidase**, lysozyme, lactoferrin, hydrolytic enzymes	Lysosomes contain lysozyme and myeloperoxidase, which are **bactericidal**
Basophils	<1% of WBCs	Years	Bilobate, basophilic	Basophil	Allergies	Heparin, histamine, SRS-A	**Bind IgE** antibody to their membrane
Eosinophils	1%–6% of WBCs	Less than 2 weeks in connective tissues	Bilobed, azurophilic granules	Eosinophil	Phagocytic for Ag–Ab complexes, **antiparasitic**, inactivated histamine and SRS-A	Histaminase, arylsulfatase	Large numbers found in lamina propria of GI tract
Mast cells	Found in connective tissue	9–18 months	Basophil-like, round nucleus	Mast cell	Bind IgE; mediate **type I hypersensitivity** reaction	ECF, histamine, leukotrienes, heparin, tryptase	**Cromolyn sodium** prevents degranulation by stabilizing membrane
Macrophages	Found **only in tissues,** not in the blood	Extended life in tissues	Ameboid	Macrophage	Phagocytize bacteria, RBCs, and damaged cells; APC	IL-1, **IL-2,** TNF-α	Activated by LPS and INF-γ
Monocytes	3%–9% of WBCs	Less than 3 days in the blood	Large kidney-shaped nucleus	Monocyte	Differentiate into macrophages and osteoclasts	IL-1, IL-6	Chemotactically **attracted to sites of inflammation**
T lymphocytes	15%–18% of WBCs, 75% of lymphocytes	Years	Basophilic, large nucleus, scant cytoplasm	Large T-lymphocyte	**Cell-mediated immune response**	IL-2, IL-3, IL-4, IL-5, IL-6, INF-γ, TNF-α, TNF-β	Originate in bone marrow, mature in thymus
B lymphocytes	5%–7% of WBCs, 25% of lymphocytes	Months	Basophilic, large nucleus, scant cytoplasm; plasma cell has clock-faced chromatin distribution	Plasma cell	**Humoral immune response**	INF-α	Differentiate into plasma cells (produce large amounts of Ab specific to an Ag) and long-lived memory cells
Erythrocytes	5 × 10^6/mL in men, 4.55 × 10^6/mL in females	120 days	**Anucleate, biconcave disc** (allows for large surface area to volume ratio)	Erythrocyte	Gas exchange		Anaerobic metabolism exclusively, membrane contains chloride bicarbonate antiport
Platelets	250,000–400,000/mL	7–10 days	Irregularly shaped, membrane bound, anucleate, extremely small	Platelets	Prevention of bleeding by **clot formation**	Histamine, PDGF, serotonin, TXA_2, clotting factors, thrombospondin (thromboglobulin)	Disorders of number or function can result in bleeding

Ag–Ab, antigen–antibody; APC, antigen-presenting cell; ECF, eosinophilic chemotactic factor; GI, gastrointestinal; Ig, immunoglobulin; IL, interleukin; INF, interferon; LPS, lipopolysaccharide; RBC, red blood cell; SRS-A, slow-reacting substance of anaphylaxis; TNF, tumor necrosis factor; TXA_2, thromboxane A_2; WBC, white blood cell.

MNEMONIC

To remember the causes of eosinophilia, think NAACP:
Neoplastic
Asthma
Allergies
Connective tissue disorders
Parasites

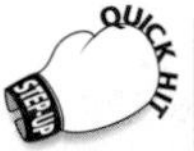

QUICK HIT The erythrocyte relies on glucose for energy, 90% is metabolized anaerobically to lactate and 10% by the HMP shunt.

QUICK HIT Adrenocorticotropin, steroids, estrogens, and androgens cause involution of the thymus.

QUICK HIT **Virchow (sentinel) nodes** are supraclavicular nodes often enlarged by metastasis from gastric carcinoma.

FIGURE 10-1 **The lymph node**

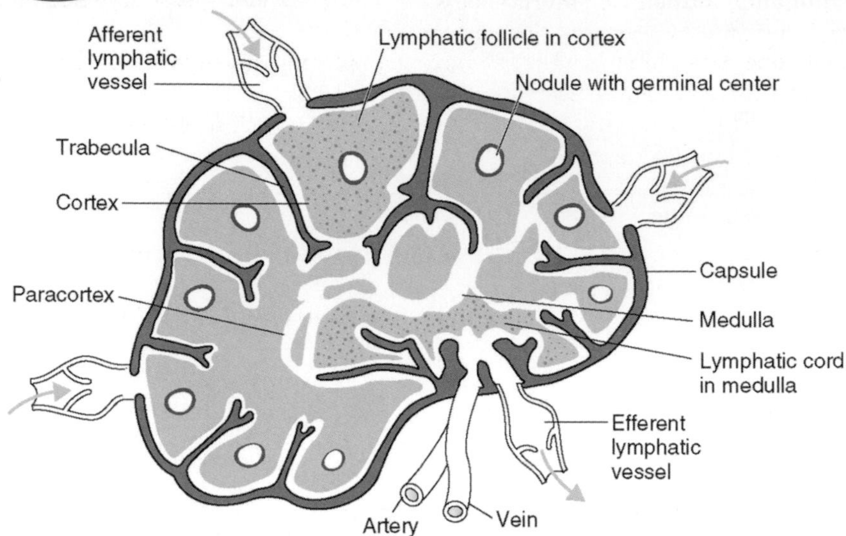

C. **Inner cortex** (also called the paracortex) contains T lymphocytes and is thymic dependent.
D. **Medulla** contains B lymphocytes, plasma cells, and macrophages.

III. Lymph

A. It is the fluid that returns lipids, proteins, and water-soluble substances to the circulation via the lymphatic vessels.
B. The **left side of the head**, **the left thorax**, **the left upper limb**, and **everything below the diaphragm** drain into the **thoracic duct**. This duct terminates at the junction of the left subclavian and left internal jugular veins.
C. The **right upper quadrant of the body** (right side of the head, right upper limb, and right thorax) empties into the **great vessels of the right side**.

IV. Spleen (Figure 10-2)

FIGURE 10-2 **The spleen**

CA, central artery; Cap, capillary; PALS, periarteriolar lymphatic sheaths; T, trabeculae; Tv, trabecular vein; WP, white pulp. (From Ross MH, Romrell LJ, Kaye GI. Histology: A Text and Atlas. 3rd Ed. Baltimore, MD: Williams & Wilkins, 1995:365. Used by permission of Lippincott, Williams & Wilkins.)

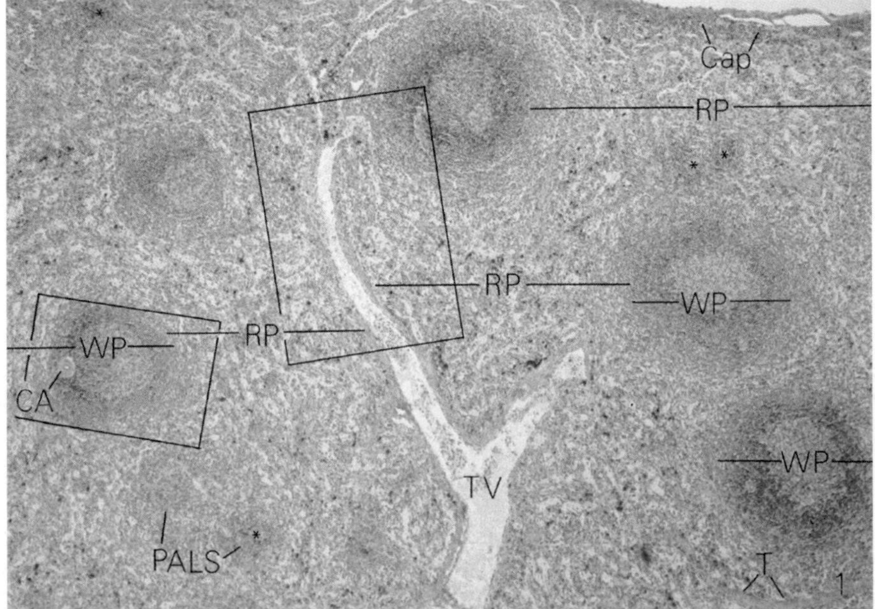

A. It is derived from **mesenchyme** beginning in the 5th week.
B. **White pulp**: B lymphocytes surround the central artery and T lymphocytes are arranged into periarteriolar lymphatic sheaths (PALS).
C. **Marginal zone**: It is the zone where blood meets spleen parenchyma; antigen-presenting cells (APCs) and macrophages are present.
D. **Red pulp**: It contains splenic (Billroth) cords separated by sinusoids and also has plasma cells, macrophages, lymphocytes, and RBCs.

V. Liver

A. **Endoderm** of the foregut (**hepatic diverticulum**) grows into the surrounding **mesoderm (septum transversum)**.
B. Hepatic cords from diverticulum, arranged around umbilical and vitelline veins, form **hepatic sinusoids**.
C. It produces **fetal hemoglobin** (HbF) during the second trimester.
D. It produces **clotting factors** of coagulation cascade.
E. It can function to sequester and break down RBCs if spleen is removed.

VI. Gut-associated lymphatic tissue

A. Found in **tonsils**, **Peyer patches** of the jejunum, **appendix**, and cecum
B. **M cells**: present antigens to lymphocytes and secrete IgA

RED BLOOD CELL PHYSIOLOGY (Figure 10-3)

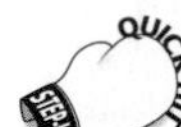

Carbon monoxide poisoning causes hypoxic injury to the basal ganglia and results in a cherry-red color of the skin and viscera. The treatment is 100% oxygen.

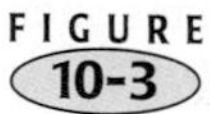

FIGURE 10-3 **RBC physiology**

Cl^-, chloride; CO_2, carbon dioxide; H^+, hydrogen ion; HCO_3^-, bicarbonate; H_2O, water; HCO_3^-, carbonic acid.

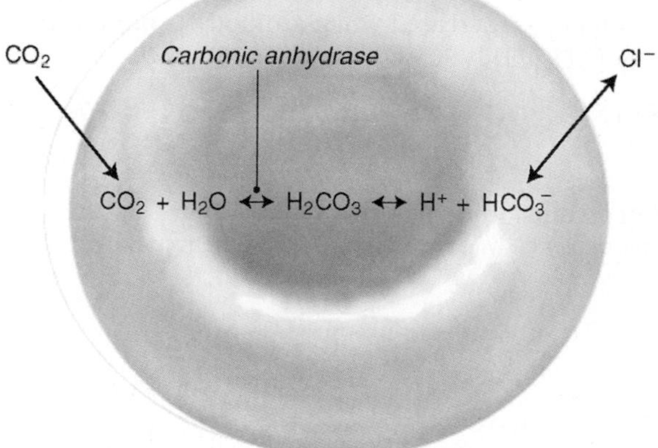

- **Hemoglobin–Oxygen Dissociation Curve (Figure 10-4)**

RBCs deliver oxygen to tissues and carry carbon dioxide (CO_2) to the lungs. In the tissues, CO_2 diffuses into the RBC, combines with water via **carbonic anhydrase** (CA), and produces carbonic acid. This dissociates into hydrogen ions and bicarbonate. The **bicarbonate leaves** the RBC in exchange for chloride (**chloride shift**). In the lungs, this process is reversed. Thus, **bicarbonate in the plasma** is the **major route** for CO_2 transport to the lungs.

Deoxyhemoglobin exists in the **tense state** which resists oxygen binding. Binding of the first oxygen molecule requires considerable energy and precipitates a conformational change from the tense state to the relaxed state. Binding of further oxygen molecules requires less energy (**positive cooperativity**). Certain factors affect hemoglobin affinity for oxygen (Figure 10-4). Hemoglobin binds with carbon monoxide 200-fold more readily than with oxygen. The presence of carbon monoxide on one of the four heme sites causes the oxygen to bind with greater affinity. This makes it difficult for the hemoglobin to release the oxygen to the tissues and causes the hemoglobin oxygen dissociation curve to shift to the left. Therefore, increased levels of carbon monoxide can lead to severe hypoxemia while maintaining a normal PO_2.

FIGURE 10-4 **Hemoglobin–oxygen dissociation curve**
2,3-DPG, 2,3-diphosphoglycerate; HbF, fetal hemoglobin; PCO_2, partial pressure of carbon dioxide; pH, hydrogen ion concentration; PO_2, partial pressure of oxygen; temp, temperature. Left shift: Hgb molecules have more affinity for O_2; Right shift: Hgb molecules have less affinity for O_2.

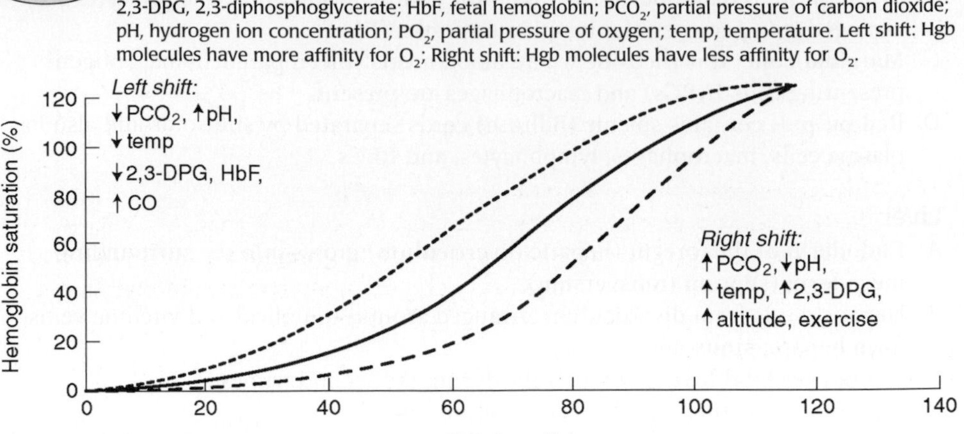

MNEMONIC

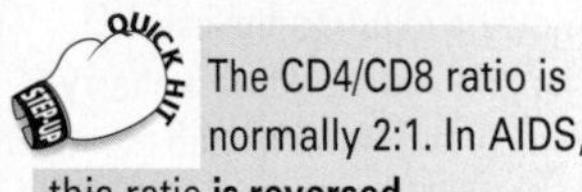

To remember which T cells interact with which MHC, think of the "=8" rule: 2 × 4 = 8 and 1 × 8 = 8; thus, MHC **II** goes with CD**4** and MHC **I** goes with CD**8**.

The CD4/CD8 ratio is normally 2:1. In AIDS, this ratio **is reversed**.

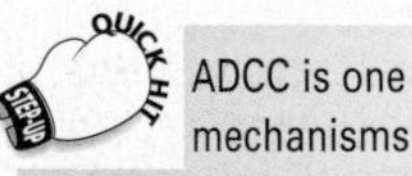

ADCC is one of the mechanisms by which type II hypersensitivity reactions can occur. Other mechanisms are complement-fixing antibodies (e.g., Goodpasture syndrome) and anticell-surface-receptor antibodies (e.g., Grave disease).

LYMPHOCYTE DIFFERENTIATION

T-helper (Th) lymphocytes recognize **major histocompatibility complex (MHC) class II** with **CD4 proteins** on their membranes. They participate in the cellular response to **extracellular** antigens (e.g., bacteria). Cytotoxic T lymphocytes (T-cyt) **recognize MHC class I with CD8 proteins** on their membranes. T-cyt cells are involved in the immune response to **intracellular** antigens (e.g., viruses and obligate intracellular organisms such as Chlamydiae or Rickettsiae). Natural killer (NK) cells are a form of T lymphocytes that do not pass through the thymus for maturation. As one of the body's innate defenses, NK cells kill **tumor cells and virus-infected** cells by secreting cytotoxins (perforins). They do not require antibodies to kill but their potency is increased when antibody is present (i.e., antibody-dependent cellular cytotoxicity [ADCC]).

- T-Cell Differentiation (Figure 10-5)

FIGURE 10-5 **T-cell differentiation and effect on other immune cells**
IL, interleukin; INF-f, interferon-f; T-cyt, cytotoxic T lymphocytes; Th, T-helper lymphocytes.

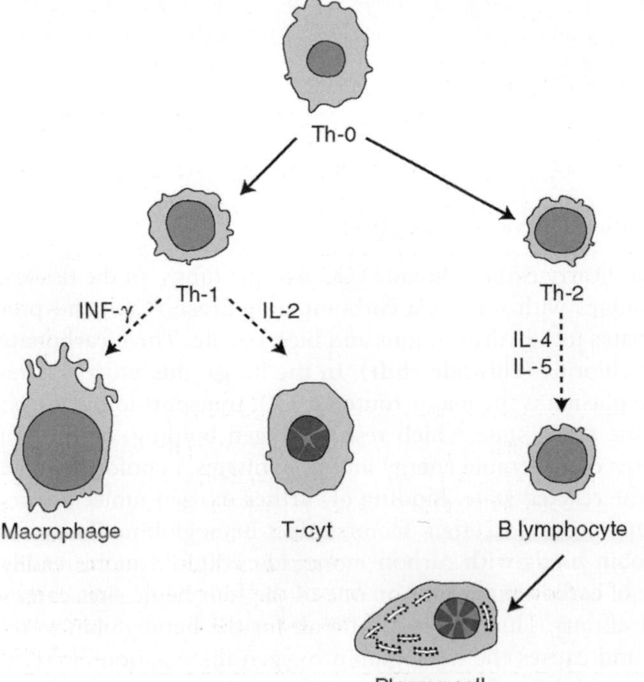

IMMUNOGLOBULINS

I. Characteristics

A. Structure
1. Immunoglobulins are glycoproteins consisting of two identical **heavy (H) chains** and two identical **light (L) chains** linked by **disulfide bonds** in a "Y" shape.
2. **Variable regions** exist on both the L and H chains.
3. The **H chain** is composed of **Fc** and **Fab** fragment. The **L chain** is composed of **Fab** fragment only. The **Fab** is the **antigen-binding fragment**. The **Fc** fragment is **constant** and in the case of IgM and IgG, it is **complement-binding**. It also contains a **carboxy terminal** and **carbohydrate side chains**.

B. **Antibody diversity** is created by
1. Random recombination of the VJ (L chain) or VDJ (H chain) genes
2. Random combination of H chains with L chains
3. Somatic hypermutation
4. Addition of nucleotides to DNA during recombination by terminal deoxynucleotidyl transferase

C. **Antibody functions**
1. **Opsonization** in which the antibody promotes phagocytosis
2. **Neutralization** in which the antibody prevents bacterial adherence to cells and membranes
3. **Complement activation** in which antibody activates complement, enhancing opsonization and lysis

D. **Allotype, Isotype, and Idiotype**
1. **Allotypes** are Ig epitopes that are different among the members of the same species. It is secondary to polymorphisms in the constant portion of the H chain or L chain. When trying to find appropriate transplant donors, allotypes are matched.
2. An **isotype** is an Ig epitope that is common to a single class of immunoglobulins. For example, IgG, IgM, and IgA are different isotypes of Ig. It is determined by the constant region of the H chain.
3. An **idiotype** is an Ig epitope that is specific for a given antigen. It is determined by the antigen-binding site contributed by the variable and hypervariable regions.

MNEMONIC

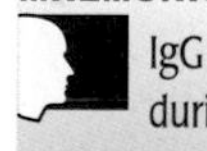

IgG crosses the placenta during Gestation.

MNEMONIC

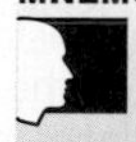

IMmunoGlobulin: IgM is released first, followed by IgG.

II. Types (Table 10-2)

TABLE 10-2 Immunoglobulin (Ig) properties

	IgM	IgG	IgE	IgA	IgD
Percentage of total Ig	9%	75% (most abundant)	0.004% (least abundant)	15%	0.2%
Structure	Monomer or pentamer Pentamer held together by J chain	Monomer	Monomer	Monomer or dimer Dimer held together by J chain (secretory piece)	Monomer
Function	Fixes complement, Antigen receptor on B cell surface, **Primary response**	Fixes complement Opsonizes bacteria **Crosses the placenta** Neutralizes bacterial toxins and viruses **Secondary response**	Allergic response **(type I hypersensitivity)** Binds to basophils and mast cells (induces release of mediators) Antihelminthic (by activating eosinophils)	Found in **secretions** Prevents bacterial and viral attachment to mucous membranes Does not fix complement Picks up secretory component from epithelial cells before secretion	Unknown May be antigen receptor on B cell surface

COMPLEMENT SYSTEM (Figure 10-6)

I. Function of complement

A. Causes **lysis** of target cell
B. Defends against **Gram-negative bacteria**

FIGURE 10-6 **Complement pathway**
(Adapted with permission from Bhushan V, Le T, Amin C. First Aid for the USMLE Step 1. Stamford, CT: Appleton & Lange, 1999:207).

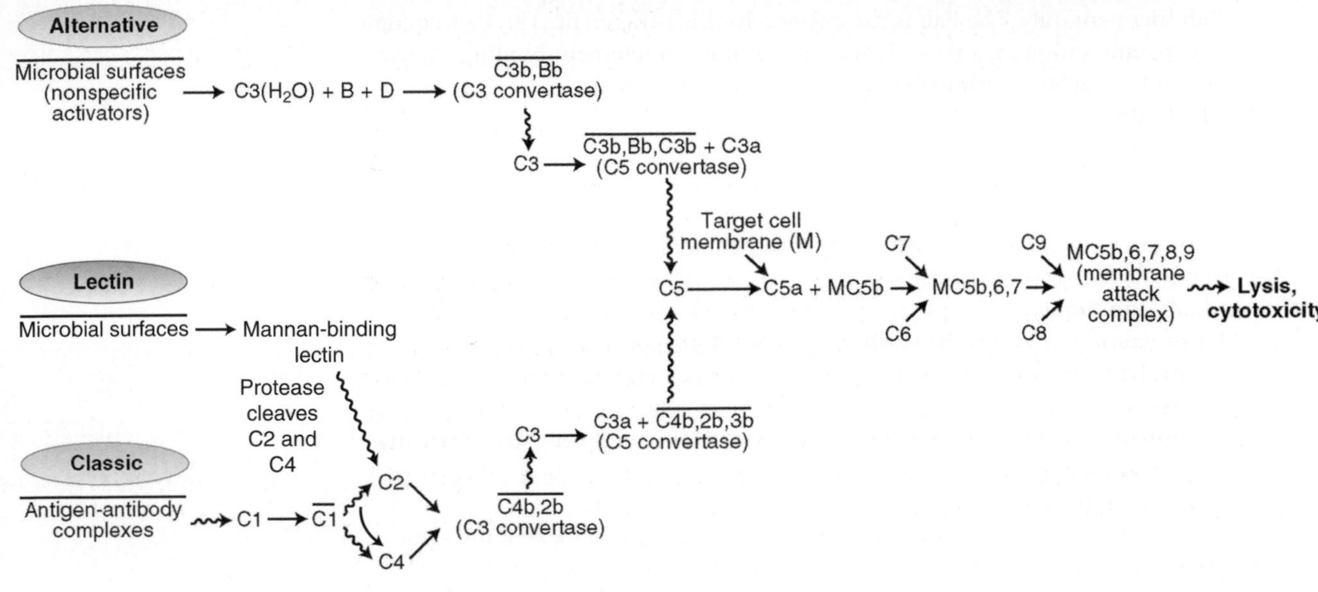

Complement
Complement defends against Gram-negative bacteria. Activated by Ig**G** or Ig**M** in the **classic** pathway, and activated by toxins (including endotoxin), aggregated IgA, or other conditions in the alternative pathway.

II. Activation of pathways

A. IgG and IgM activate the **classic pathway**
  1. The activation is initiated by antigen–antibody complexes.
  2. The first step of activation involves formation of the complex by C1, C2, and C4.
B. Antigens activate the **alternative pathway**
  1. The activation is initiated by microbial surfaces and aggregated IgA.
  2. The first step of activation involves C3.
C. Mannose chains on bacteria activate the **lectin pathway**
  1. The activation is initiated by mannose-binding lectin (MBL) and associate protease binding to mannose residues.
  2. The first step of activation involves the MBL–mannose complex activating proteases that activate C4 and C2 which then go on to activate the rest of the classical pathway.

QUICK HIT: The membrane attack complex (MAC) has only one component each of C5b, C6, C7, and C8 but has numerous C9 components.

MNEMONIC
Remember that **C3a** activates **a**cute inflammation whereas **C3b b**inds **b**acteria (opsonization).

III. Properties of complement cascade components

A. **C1**: only component not made in liver (made in gastrointestinal [GI] epithelium)
B. C1–C4: involved in viral neutralization
C. **C3b**: involved in opsonization
D. C3a: produces anaphylatoxin I

E. **C5a**: produces anaphylatoxin II, neutrophil, and macrophage chemotaxis
F. **C5b–C9**: also known as the MAC
G. **C1 inhibitor**: deficiency of this component leads to hereditary angioedema
H. Table 10-3 discusses alterations in the complement cascade (complement deficiencies)

TABLE 10-3 Complement Deficiencies

Disease	Defect	Significant Features
Hereditary angioedema	Decreased C1 (first component of complement) inhibitor	Increased capillary permeability; edema
PNH	Deficiency of DAF; increased complement activation	Complement-mediated hemolysis; brown urine in the morning; **decreased LAP**

MNEMONIC

Decreased leukocyte alkaline phosphatase (LAP) is also seen in chronic myelogenous leukemia (CML).

IV. Deficiencies of C1, C3, C5, C6, C7, and C8 lead to increased bacterial infections. C1 deficiency results in hereditary angioedema. C3 deficiency causes increased susceptibility to *Staphylococcus aureus* and severe, recurrent sinus and respiratory infections. C6, C7, and C8 deficiencies lead to *Neisseria gonorrhoeae* infection and meningitis. Manifestations of C2 and C4 deficiencies resemble autoimmune diseases such as systemic lupus erythematosus (SLE). C2 deficiency is the most common complement deficiency. Deficiency of decay accelerating factor (DAF) leads to complement-mediated lysis of erythrocytes and paroxysmal nocturnal hemoglobinuria.

V. Cytokines (Table 10-4)

Cytokines are hormones that have a low molecular weight and are involved in cell-to-cell communication. Human recombinant cytokines are useful in the management of neoplasms, transplant rejection, and to stimulate the growth of various cell lines in cases of bone marrow suppression (Table 10-5).

TABLE 10-4 Cytokines

Cytokine	Secreted by	Function
IL-1	Macrophages	Endogenous **pyrogen;** stimulates T cells
IL-2	T-helper cells	Activates T-helper and T-cytotoxic cells
IL-3	Activated T cells	Stimulates the growth and differentiation of bone marrow stem cells
IL-4	T-helper cells	Stimulates the growth of B cells; increases IgE and IgG
IL-5	T-helper cells	Differentiation of B cells; increases IgA
IL-10	T-helper cells	Inhibits the development of Th-1 cells; inhibits INF-γ production
IL-12	Macrophages	Promotes Th-1 cell development; stimulates INF-γ production
IFN-α	Virus-infected leukocytes	Produces ribonuclease that degrades viral mRNA inhibiting viral protein synthesis
IFN-β	Virus-infected fibroblasts	Produces ribonuclease that degrades viral mRNA inhibiting viral protein synthesis
INF-γ	T-helper cells	Stimulates macrophages and NK cells; increases MHC expression; stimulates phagocytosis and killing
Tumor necrosis factor	Macrophages	At low concentrations, activates neutrophils and increases IL-2 receptor synthesis; at high concentrations, mediates septic shock and results in tumor necrosis
Transforming growth factor	T cells, B cells, and macrophages	Inhibits the growth and activities of T cells; enhances collagen synthesis; dampens the immune response

IL, interleukin; INF, interferon; MHC, major histocompatibility complex; NK, natural killer; Th, T-helper.

TABLE 10-5 Recombinant cytokines

Therapeutic Agent (common name, if relevant) [trade name, where appropriate]	Class—Pharmacology and Pharmacokinetics	Indications	Side or Adverse Effects	Contraindications or Precautions to Consider; Notes
Aldesleukin (Proleukin)	Human recombinant **interleukin-2**	**Metastatic renal cell carcinoma, metastatic melanoma, AML**		
Erythropoietin (EPO) (Procrit, Epogen)	**Colony-stimulating factor**	**Anemias (especially in renal failure); AIDS**	Hypertension	
Filgrastim (Neuopogen)	**Granulocyte–macrophage colony- stimulating factor**	**Recovery of bone marrow (e.g., chemotherapy induced neutropenia)**		
Sargramostim (Leukine)	**Granulocyte–macrophage colony- stimulating factor**	**Recovery of bone marrow (e.g., bone marrow transplant failure)**	Hypertension	
Interferon α-2a (Roferon A), **α-2b** (Intron A), **and α-n3** (Alferon-N)	Antiviral—decreases protein synthesis	**Genital warts; chronic hepatitis B and C; AIDS-related Kaposi sarcoma; laryngeal papillomatosis; hairy cell leukemia; malignant melanoma**	**Flulike symptoms; tachycardia; fever; neutropenia; headache; somnolence; malaise**	
Interferon β-1a (Avonex, Rebif)	Antiviral—decreases protein synthesis	**Multiple sclerosis**	**Flulike symptoms**, headache; fatigue; fever; pain; chills; depression	
Interferon γ-1b (Actimmune)	Antiviral—decreases protein synthesis	**Chronic granulomatous disease**	Fever; headache; chills; fatigue	
Oprelvekin (Neumega)	**Interleukin-11** stimulates multiple stages of **thrombopoiesis** increasing the platelet production	**Thrombocytopenia**		
Thrombopoietin	Recombinant human thrombopoietin	**Thrombocytopenia**		

mTOR, mammalian target of rapamycin.

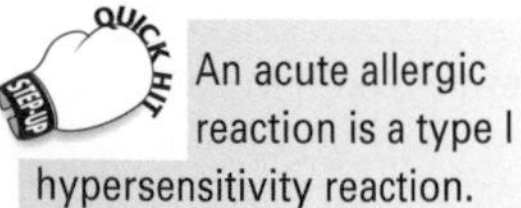

An acute allergic reaction is a type I hypersensitivity reaction.

HYPERSENSITIVITY REACTIONS

I. There are four types of hypersensitivity reactions. They vary in onset of symptoms, severity, and mechanism (Table 10-6).

II. Transplant rejection.

III. Timeline (Figure 10-7).

TABLE 10-6 Hypersensitivity reactions

Reaction Type	Description	Example
Type 1 **(anaphylaxis)**	Mediated by **IgE** antibody bound to mast cells or basophil antigens cross-link antibody Release of **histamine,** SRS-A, eosinophilic chemotactic factor, and platelet-activating factor p-tryptase, leukotrienes	Anaphylaxis Allergic rhinitis (hay fever) Asthma Wheal and flare
Type 2 (cytotoxic)	Antibody-dependent cellular cytotoxicity Antibody produced to specific cell-surface antigens IgM- and IgG-mediated lysis via complement Immunofluorescence, stains smooth, linear Abs staining in biopsy	Rh incompatibility Goodpasture syndrome Myasthenia gravis Hemolytic anemia Idiopathic thrombocytopenic purpura Rheumatic fever Grave disease Bullous pemphigoid
Type 3 (immune-complex)	**Antigen–antibody complexes** induce inflammatory response Deposition of complexes in tissue	**Arthus reaction** **Serum sickness** Glomerulonephritis Rheumatoid arthritis SLE Polyarteritis nodosum
Type 4 (delayed or cell-mediated)	**Helper (CD4) Th1 lymphocyte-mediated** Response is delayed (from hours to days) Predominantly mononuclear cell infiltration	Tuberculin (PPD) test GVHD Contact dermatitis Type I diabetes mellitus Multiple sclerosis Guillain–Barre syndrome Hashimoto thyroiditis

PPD, purified protein derivative; Rh, rhesus (factor); SLE, systemic lupus erythematosus; SRS-A, slow-reacting substance of anaphylaxis.

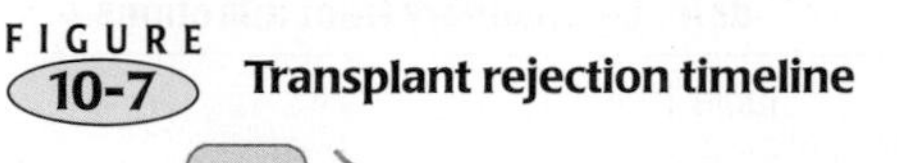

FIGURE 10-7 Transplant rejection timeline

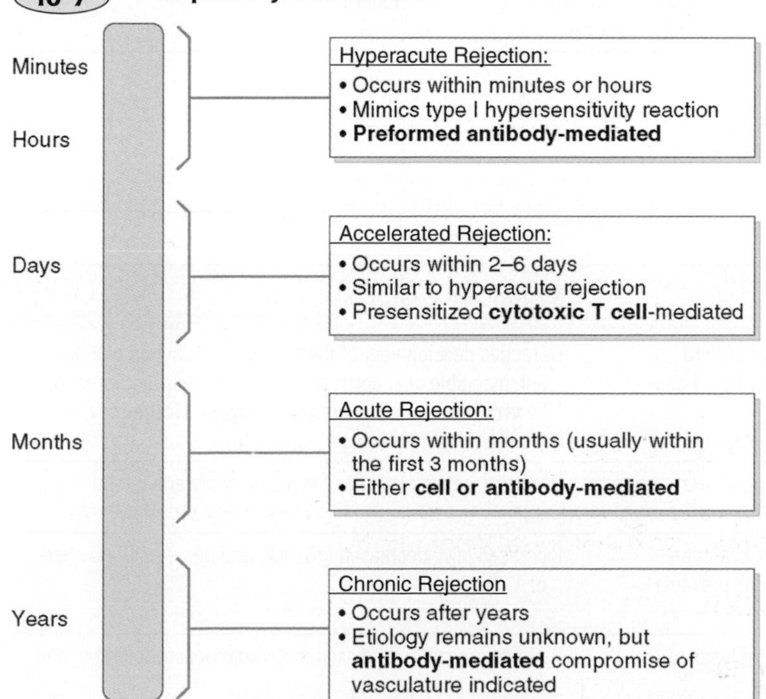
Minutes
Hours
Days
Months
Years
Hyperacute Rejection:
• Occurs within minutes or hours
• Mimics type I hypersensitivity reaction
• Preformed antibody-mediated
Accelerated Rejection:
• Occurs within 2–6 days
• Similar to hyperacute rejection
• Presensitized cytotoxic T cell-mediated
Acute Rejection:
• Occurs within months (usually within the first 3 months)
• Either cell or antibody-mediated
Chronic Rejection
• Occurs after years
• Etiology remains unknown, but antibody-mediated compromise of vasculature indicated

MNEMONIC

Use **ACID** to help remember immunology of each hypersensitivity reaction:
Anaphylactic: Type I
Cytotoxic: Type II
Immune complex disease: Type III
Delayed hypersensitivity (cell mediated): Type IV.

MNEMONIC

Remember poison **IV**y causes type **IV** hypersensitivity.

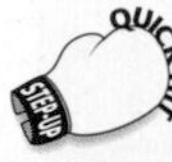

Radioimmunosorbent test (RIST) is a radioimmunoassay (RIA) that measures total IgE. A radioallergosorbent test (RAST) is an RIA that determines specific IgE concentration. Both the RIST and RAST can be used to measure IgE concentration to predict anaphylactic response.

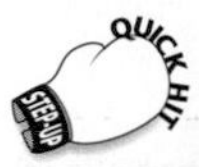

Serum sickness is more common than an Arthus reaction.

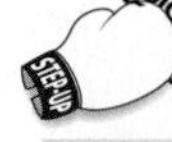

Graft-versus-host disease (GVHD) is caused by donor lymphocytes attacking recipient cells. It is characterized by elevated IgE, elevated bilirubin and liver enzymes, and skin lesions. It is seen commonly in bone marrow transplants.

Candida albicans causes thrush.

MNEMONIC

Remember the features of DiGeorge syndrome by thinking of it as the disease of Ts:
Third and fourth branchial pouch absent
Thymic aplasia
T-cells absent
Twenty-Two chromosome deletion
Tetany: ParaThyroid (decreased PTH results in hypocalcemia).

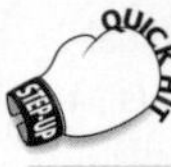
Treat hyper-IgM syndrome with pooled γ-globulin.

Measles, a paramyxovirus, results in a T-cell deficiency.

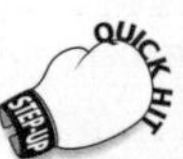
Severe combined immunodeficiency (SCID) caused by adenosine deaminase (ADA) deficiency was one of the first diseases successfully treated with gene therapy.

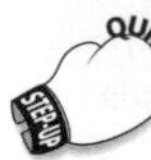
Interferon-γ (INF-γ) is used to treat chronic granulomatous disease (CGD).

IMMUNODEFICIENCIES

I. Diseases affecting the immune system leave the individual prone to infection. The immune system can be affected on any level and at any time—from its development to its most distal signaling mechanisms.

II. Congenital B-cell deficiencies (Table 10-7).

III. Congenital T-cell deficiencies (Table 10-8).

IV. Congenital combined T- and B-cell deficiencies (Table 10-9).

V. Plasma cell abnormalities (Table 10-10).

VI. Phagocyte deficiencies (Table 10-11).

VII. Acquired immunodeficiencies (Table 10-12).

TABLE 10-7 Congenital B-cell Deficiencies

Disease	Defect	Significant Features
X-linked agammaglobulinemia (of Bruton)	Lack of maturation of B cells, secondary to lack of tyrosine kinase gene	Absence of plasma cells, serum IgG; recurrent **pyogenic infections** beginning after 6 months; a common congenital B cell disease; lymphoid tissue has **poorly defined germinal centers**
Selective IgA deficiency	Lack of maturation of B cells; failure of gene switching in H chain	**Most common congenital B cell defect; 1 in 700 newborns has this defect; pulmonary tract infections**
Common variable immunodeficiency	Failure of terminal B cell differentiation	Table 10-8

TABLE 10-8 Congenital T-cell deficiencies

Disease	Defect	Significant Features
Thymic aplasia (DiGeorge syndrome)	Deficiency of development of third and fourth branchial pouches; T-cell defect	Defective development of the thymus, parathyroid glands, ear, mandible, and aortic arch; leads to recurrent infections by **viral and fungal organisms; hypocalcemia** from low parathyroid hormone leads to tetany
Chronic mucocutaneous candidiasis	Lack of T-cell response to *Candida*	Recurrent candidal skin and mucous membrane infections
Hyper IgM syndrome	Mutation in CD4+ helper T-cell interaction with CD40 on B cell prevents class switching	Increased IgM; decreased IgG, IgA, and IgE; normal numbers of T and B cells
Ig-12 receptor deficiency	Deficiency in Ig-12 receptor leads to decreased Th1 response	Patients present with disseminated mycobacterial infections

TABLE 10-9 Congenital combined T- and B-cell deficiencies

Disease	Defect	Significant Features
SCID	**Autosomal recessive** (defect in tyrosine kinase zeta-associated protein [ZAP]-70 or adenosine deaminase deficiency); X-linked forms (interleukin [IL]-2 receptor defect)	Susceptible to recurrent bacterial, viral, fungal, and protozoal infections
Wiskott–Aldrich syndrome	IgM response to capsule polysaccharide (e.g., pneumococcus) is weak	**Eczema, thrombocytopenia, and recurrent infections;** becomes notable in first year of life
Ataxia–telangiectasia	IgA deficiency and lymphopenia	**Autosomal recessive;** becomes noticeable in first 2 years of life; ataxia (cerebellar dysfunction), telangiectasia, recurrent infections, and thymic aplasia

TABLE 10-10 Plasma Cell Abnormalities

Disease	Etiology	Clinical Features	Notes
Multiple myeloma	Clonal plasma cell tumor	**Lytic, punched-out bone lesions,** especially in the skull; hyperglobulinemia; **Bence Jones proteinuria**	**Rouleaux formation** ("stack of coins" appearance)
Waldenström macroglobulinemia	Excessive production of IgM by lymphoid cells	Slowly progressive course; usually in men older than 50 years of age; platelet function abnormal; hyperviscosity syndrome	No bone lesions (which differentiates this from multiple myeloma)
Benign monoclonal gammopathy	Increased production of monoclonal antibodies from an unknown origin	Asymptomatic; occurring in older individuals	Monoclonal spike without Bence Jones proteinuria (vs. multiple mycloma)

TABLE 10-11 Phagocyte Deficiencies

Disease	Defect	Significant Features
Chronic granulomatous disease (CGD)	Neutrophils **lack NADPH oxidase**	**X-linked** (some autosomal recessive); no oxidative burst in macrophages; B and T cells normal; opportunistic infections (e.g., *Staphylococcus aureus, Aspergillus*, enteric Gram-negative rods)
Chédiak–Higashi syndrome	Failure of neutrophils to empty lysosomes	**Autosomal recessive;** recurrent pyogenic infections (e.g., *Staphylococcus, Streptococcus*)
Job syndrome	T-helper lymphocytes fail to produce INF-g	Eczema; increase in Th-2 (Figure 10-5) leads to an increase in IgE, causing increased histamine release
Leukocyte adhesion deficiency	Defect in adhesion protein LAF-1	Pyogenic infections early in life; poor phagocytosis

INF-γ, interferon-γ; LAF-1, leukocyte-activating factor-1; NADPH, nicotinamide adenine dinucleotide phosphate; Th, T-helper.

TABLE 10-12 Acquired Immunodeficiencies

Disease	Defect	Significant Features
Common variable hypogammaglobulinemia	Acquired or congenital (unknown) B-cell defects	Recurrent pyogenic bacterial infections (e.g., *Pneumococcus, H. influenzae*); decreased IgG production
AIDS	**HIV virus infects CD4 cells and macrophages**	Opportunistic infections (e.g., ***Mycobacterium avium-intracellulare,*** *Cryptococcus neoformans,* ***Pneumocystis carinii,*** and *Candida albicans*); increased tumors (e.g., Kaposi sarcoma)

IMMUNOSUPPRESSANTS (Table 10-13)

TABLE 10-13 Immunosupressants

Therapeutic Agent (common name, if relevant) [trade name, where appropriate]	Class–Pharmacology and Pharmacokinetics	Indications	Side or Adverse Effects	Contraindications or Precautions to Consider; Notes
Cyclosporine (Sandimmune)	Binds **cyclophilins** → complex inhibits **calcineurin** → prevents production of **IL-2, IL-3, and IFN**-f → inhibits **T-helper cell** activity	**Transplant rejection; selected autoimmune disorder**	**Nephrotoxic;** hepatotoxic; hypertension; **increased incidence of viral infection and lymphoma**	Nephrotoxicity preventable with mannitol diuresis
Tacrolimus (FK506) (Prograf)	Binds to **FK-binding protein** (T-cell transcription factor) → Inhibits **calcineurin** → inhibits **IL-2** synthesis and T-cell signal transduction → inhibits **T-cell** activity	**Transplant rejection**	**Nephrotoxic; neurotoxic (peripheral neuropathy); hyperglycemia; hypertension; pleural effusion;** GI disturbances	Potent immunosuppressant
Azathioprine (Imuran)	**Purine antagonist**; Antimetabolite precursor of **6-mercaptopurine** → inhibits nucleic acid synthesis and metabolism → toxic to **proliferating lymphocytes**; blocks both CMI and humoral response	**Transplant (esp. kidney);** acute glomerulonephritis; renal component of lupus; rheumatoid arthritis; hemolytic anemia	**Bone marrow supression;** rash; fever; nausea; vomiting; hepatotoxicity; malignancy; GI intolerance	Metabolized by xanthine oxidase, **toxic effects may be increased by allopurinol**
Muromonab (OKT3)	**Monoclonal antibody** that binds CD3 on T lymphocytes → blocks cellular interaction with CD3 protein responsible for T-cell signal transduction	Acute rejection of **renal transplants**	**Cytokine release syndrome;** hypersensitivity reaction	
Sirolimus (Rapamycin)	Binds to mTOR → inhibits response to **IL-2** → inhbits **T-cell proliferation**	Immunosupression after **kidney transplantation** (in combination with cyclosporine and corticosteroids)	**Hyperlipidemia, thrombocytopenia, and leukopenia**	
Mycophenolate mofetil (Cellcept)	Inhibits de novo **guanine synthesis** → blocks **lymphocyte production**	Prevents rejection after **organ transplantation**; myasthenia gravis	Hypertension; hyperglycemia; hypercholesterolemia; leucopenia; thrombocytopenia	
Daclizumab (Zenapax)	Monoclonal antibody with high affinity for the **IL-2 receptor** on activated T cells → **prevents T-cell activation**	**Prevents rejection after kidney transplantation**		Decreased incidence of opportunistic infections when compared with other immunosupressants

THROMBOSIS AND THE CLOTTING CASCADE (Figure 10-8)

Thrombosis is the intravascular coagulation of blood and involves the interaction of platelets, coagulation proteins, and endothelial cells. With intact endothelium, a balance exists between prothrombotic (platelet-derived thromboxane A_2 [TXA_2]) and antithrombotic (endothelium-derived prostaglandin I2 [PGI2]) mediators. With damaged endothelium, exposed collagen causes adhesion of platelets through glycoprotein receptors and **von Willebrand factor (vWF)**. This adhesion triggers platelet release of adenosine diphosphate (ADP), serotonin, histamine, platelet-derived growth factor (PDGF), and TXA_2, resulting in primary plug formation and cessation of bleeding. Stabilization of the primary plug (formation of the secondary plug) is mediated by fibrin and factor XIIIa, a result of activation of the clotting cascade.

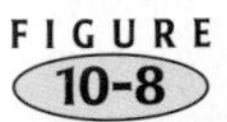

FIGURE 10-8 **Thrombosis and the clotting cascade**
Ca^{2+}, calcium; HMW-K, high-molecular-weight kininogen; PL, phospholipid.

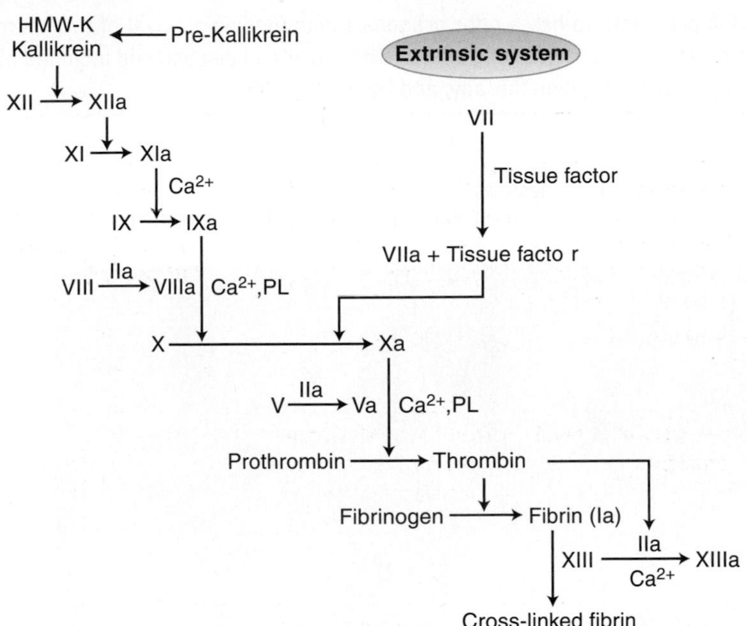

Factor XIa in the presence of Ca^{2+} activates factor IX. Factor IXa requires Ca^{2+} and a phospholipid to activate factor X. Activated factor X requires Ca^{2+}, phospholipid, and factor Va to activate prothrombin to thrombin. Thrombin and Ca^{2+} activate factor XIII that promotes the cross-linking of fibrin.

- **Key Players in Inhibition of Coagulation**

α1-antitrypsin	Inhibits factor XIa
α2-macroglobulin	Inhibits serine proteases
Antithrombin III	Inhibits factor Xa and thrombin
Inhibitor of the first component	Inhibits factor XII and kallikrein of complement (C1 INH)
Heparin cofactor II	Inhibits thrombin
Protein C	Inactivates factors Va and VIIIa
Protein S	Is a cofactor for protein C

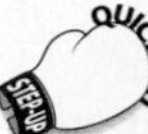

Aspirin functions as an antithrombotic agent by permanently acetylating cyclooxygenase (COX), thereby inhibiting TXA_2 production. TXA_2 triggers the aggregation of platelets. Aspirin also inhibits prostaglandin formation, but unlike platelets, endothelium can synthesize new COX.

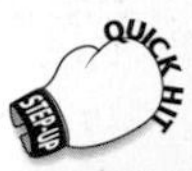

Factors II, VII, IX, and X and **proteins C and S require vitamin K** for their synthesis and are produced in the liver.

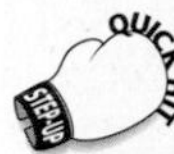

Partial thromboplastin time (**PTT**) measures the **intrinsic system.** Therapeutic drug monitoring of heparin is measured using PTT. Heparin overdose is treated with intravenous protamine sulfate.

P prothrombin time (**PT**) measures the **extrinsic system.** Therapeutic drug monitoring of warfarin is measured using PT. Warfarin overdose is treated with the administration of vitamin K. In acute cases of hemorrhage, fresh frozen plasma may be given to quickly reverse the effects of warfarin.

Vitamin K is administered to newborns in the United States to prevent hemorrhagic diseases.

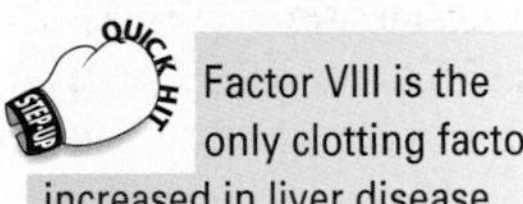

Factor VIII is the only clotting factor increased in liver disease.

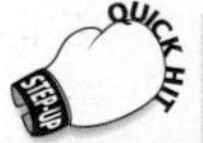

Factor XIII is the only clotting factor that is not a serine protease.

Osteolytic lesions are secondary to the release of osteoclast-activating factor by the neoplastic plasma cells.

Clinical Vignette 10-1

Clinical Presentation: A 65-year-old male presents to his primary care physician complaining of **bad back pains** for the past several months aggravated by **walking or bending over.** Yesterday, he fell on his right arm while shoveling snow. Patient has no past medical or surgical history, but the patient was recently hospitalized for a **kidney stone.** Physical examination reveals tenderness to palpation over the thoracic and lumbar spine. No splenomegaly or lymphadenopathy. Plain films of the spine show several **lytic lesions in the vertebral bodies at L3–L4 levels.** Plain films of the right upper extremity show lytic lesions in the diaphysis and a **fracture line.**

Differentials: Fibromyalgia, herniated disk (nerve root impingement), osteoarthritis, metastatic bone lesion, and multiple myeloma. The lytic lesions, pathologic fractures, and kidney stones (evidence of hypercalcemia) suggest multiple myeloma.

Laboratory Studies: In addition to the **lytic lesions on the plain film** (Figure 10-9A), **serum and urine electrophoresis** showing M-protein spike would support a diagnosis of multiple myeloma. To confirm a diagnosis of multiple myeloma, a **bone marrow biopsy** showing 10% plasma cells (Figure 10-9B) would need to be performed. A **complete blood count (CBC) showing mild anemia** and **electrolytes showing hypercalcemia and renal insufficiency** are also findings seen in multiple myeloma.

Management: Multiple myeloma has a poor prognosis with median survival of few months without treatment. Treatment is reserved for patients with advanced disease and includes chemotherapy (alkylating agents), radiation therapy, and transplantation.

FIGURE 10-9 **Multiple Myeloma (A) Lytic lesions**

(Reproduced with permission from Rubin E, Farber JL. Pathology. 3rd Ed. Philadelphia, PA: Lippincott Williams & Wilkins, 1999.)

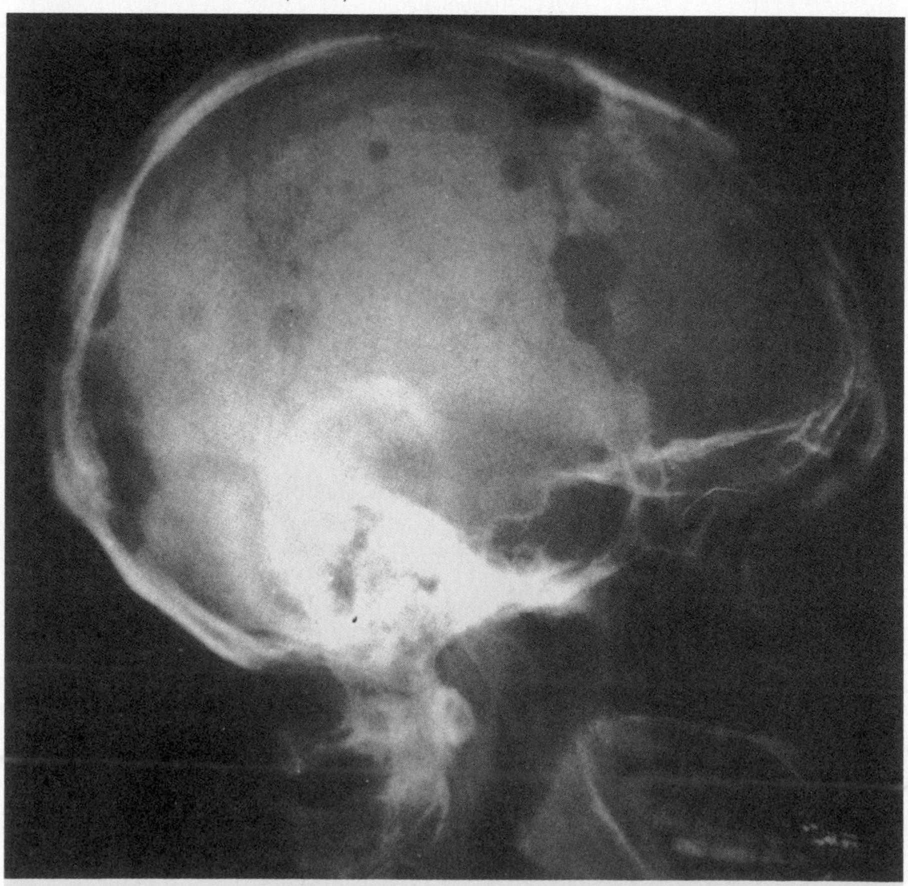

(A)

FIGURE 10-9 **(B) Plasma cells *(Continued)***

(Reproduced with permission from Anderson SC. Anderson's Atlas of Hematology. Wolters Kluwer Health/Lippincott Williams & Wilkins, 2003.)

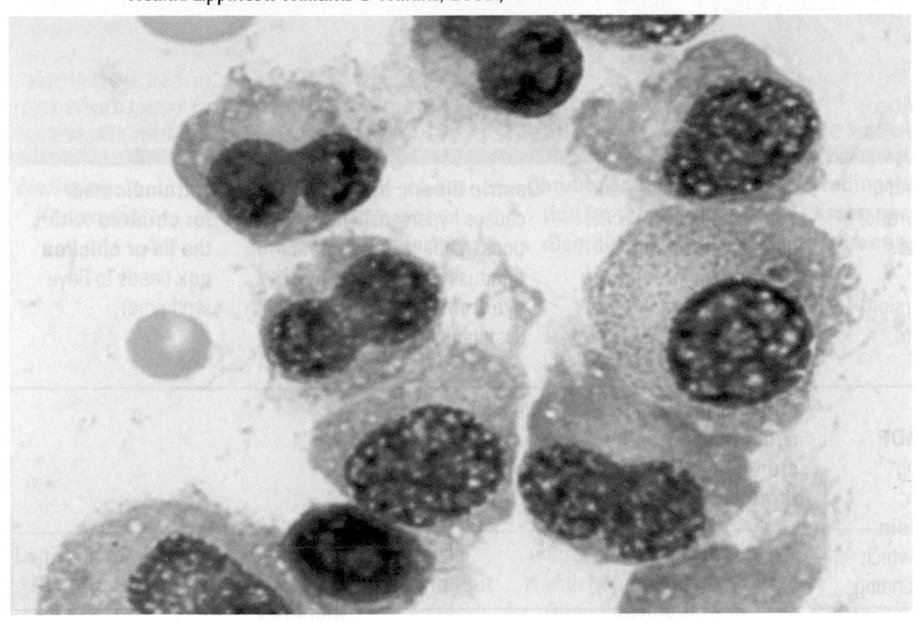

(B)

ANTITHROMBOTIC THERAPEUTIC AGENTS

I. Platelet inhibitors (Figure 10-10) (Table 10-14)

Aspirin inhibits thromboxane-mediated platelet aggregation, ticlopidine and clopidogrel block platelet ADP receptors, and argatroban and hirudin inhibit thrombin directly.

FIGURE 10-10 **Inhibition of platelet aggregation pathways**

Aspirin inhibits thromboxane-mediated platelet aggregation, ticlopidine and clopidogrel block platelet ADP receptors, and argatroban and hirudin inhibit thrombin directly. ADP, adenosine diphosphate; TXA_2, thromboxane A_2; vWF, von Willebrand factor.

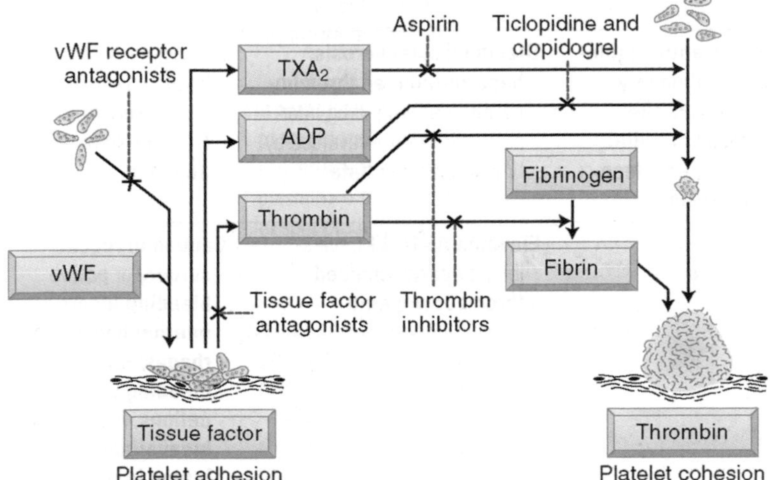

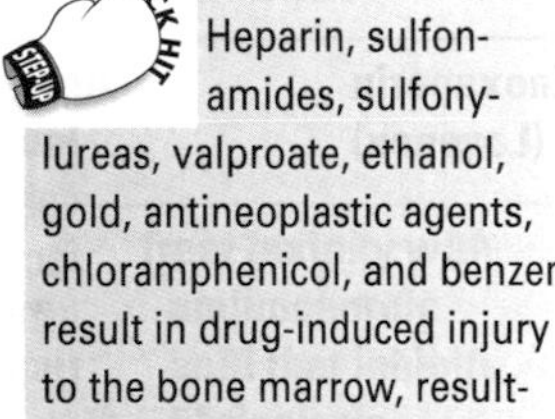

Heparin, sulfonamides, sulfonylureas, valproate, ethanol, gold, antineoplastic agents, chloramphenicol, and benzene result in drug-induced injury to the bone marrow, resulting in a decreased platelet production.

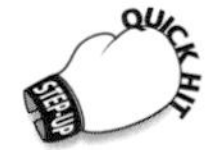

Aspirin, ticlopidine, and clopidogrel work globally to reduce the risk of thrombotic occlusion and thromboembolism, regardless of the anatomic site.

A. Aspirin
1. Irreversibly acetylates **platelet COX**
2. Results in disruption of TXA_2-dependent platelet aggregation
3. Leads to less platelet hemostasis
4. Can be used in acute myocardial infarctions (MIs) or prophylactically to reduce the likelihood of platelet-mediated vascular occlusion

(text continues on page 292)

B. Ticlopidine and clopidogrel
   1. Irreversible **blockage of platelet ADP receptors**
   2. Can be used for the same clinical scenarios in which aspirin has failed
   3. Are at least as safe as aspirin in terms of side effects

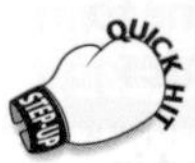

Low-molecular-weight heparins (LMWHs) such as enoxaparin and dalteparin are much more convenient than standard intravenous heparin therapy as they require no PPT monitoring and are administered subcutaneously. Uses for LMWHs include postsurgical prophylaxis against DVT and the treatment of venous thromboembolism. However, the use of LMWHs is limited in patients with renal failure.

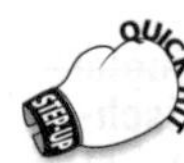

The effect of heparin is determined by measuring the activated PTT (aPTT). The effect of warfarin is determined by measuring the PT.

II. Anticoagulants (Table 10-14)

A. Heparin
   1. Binds to antithrombin III.
   2. Greatly **enhances the ability of antithrombin III to inhibit coagulation proteases, primarily thrombin.**
   3. Is useful in a variety of situations in which anticoagulation is necessary
      a. Deep venous thrombosis (DVT) or pulmonary embolism
      b. Brain attack (thrombotic occlusion)
      c. MI
      d. Others
   4. Leads to **heparin-induced thrombocytopenia or thrombosis**, a notable side effect that occurs in 1% to 3% of patients. A heparin-platelet factor 4 antibody is the cause.
   5. Reversal by protamine sulfate.

B. Warfarin (Coumadin)
   1. **Impairs vitamin K metabolism**
      a. Low levels of vitamin K prevent γ-carboxylation of **clotting factors II, VII, IX, and X.**
      b. Lack of γ-carboxylation leads to **hypofunctional clotting factors II, VII, IX, and X.**
   2. Is used in a variety of clinical scenarios in which oral anticoagulation is required
      a. Atrial fibrillation
      b. Prosthetic valves
      c. DVT or pulmonary embolism
      d. Postoperative anticoagulation
      e. Hypercoagulable states
   3. Use requires care because excessive anticoagulation can lead to hemorrhage
   4. Reversal by Vitamin K and Factor VIIa

III. Thrombolytics (Table 10-14)

A. **Convert plasminogen to plasmin**, which disrupts vascular clot formation
B. Are useful in acute MI, acute ischemic stroke, acute arterial thromboembolic occlusion, severe DVT, and pulmonary embolism
C. Include tissue plasminogen activator (t-PA), streptokinase, urokinase, and anistreplase
   1. t-PA leads to the most rapid lysis of the clot and results in less systemic fibrinolysis.
   2. However, t-PA is also the most expensive.
D. Require careful monitoring because of **increased risk of abnormal bleeding**

IV. Direct thrombin inhibitors (Table 10-14)

A. **Do not require antithrombin III for activity**
B. Allow for more efficient inhibition of clot-bound fibrin
C. Include hirudin (lepirudin) and argatroban
D. Are currently under study for use in venous thrombosis, heparin-induced thrombocytopenia, hemodialysis, arterial thrombosis (angioplasty, unstable angina), and other conditions

COAGULATION DISORDERS (Table 10-15)

Abnormalities of the coagulation cascade, endothelial cells, or platelets can lead to inappropriate bleeding or clot formation. These coagulopathies can be manifested as symptomatology involving skin, joints, vasculature, or internal organs.

TABLE 10-15 Coagulation Disorders

Disease	Etiology	Clinical Features	Notes
DIC	Multifactorial; causes include sepsis, trauma, and neoplasms	**Thrombocytopenia; diffuse hemorrhage;** microthrombus formation; schistocytes	Activation of factors V, VIII, and protein C
vWD	**Autosomal dominant** disorder	Impaired platelet adhesion; **decreased factor VIII** (vWF binds factor VIII in the blood); **increased bleeding time**	**Most common hereditary bleeding disorder;** similar deficiency diseases include Bernard–Soulier disease and Glanzmann thrombasthenia
Hemophilia A	**X-linked** factor VIII deficiency	Bleeding into muscle, subcutaneous tissues, and joints	**Most common type of hemophilia;** variable penetrance
Hemophilia B (Christmas disease)	**X-linked** factor IX deficiency	Bleeding into muscle, subcutaneous tissues, and joints	Presentation is identical to hemophilia A
ITP	**Antiplatelet antibodies**	Thrombocytopenia	Follows upper respiratory tract infection in children and is self-limiting; chronic in purpura (ITP) adults
TTP	Idiopathic systemic disease	Hyaline occlusions and microangiopathic hemolytic anemia leading to schistocytes; **classic pentad:** anemia, thrombocytopenia, renal failure, neurologic changes, and fever	May cause neurologic abnormalities

MNEMONIC

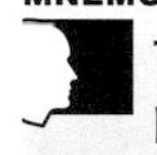

To remember the classic pentad of TTP, think **FAT RN:**
Fever
Anemia
Thrombocytopenia
Renal failure
Neurologic changes

I. vWF deficiency versus hemophilia A (Table 10-16)

II. Clotting time algorithm (Table 10-17)

TABLE 10-16 von Willebrand Factor (vWF) Deficiency versus Hemophilia A

	vWF Deficiency	Hemophilia A
Factor VIII: coagulant activity	↓	↓
vWF level	↓	Normal
Ristocetin[a] cofactor activity	↓	Normal
Ristocetin[a] aggregation	↓	Normal
Bleeding time	↑	Normal
Inheritance	**Autosomal dominant**	**X-linked**

[a]An antibiotic not used for clinical disease, has platelet aggregation properties.

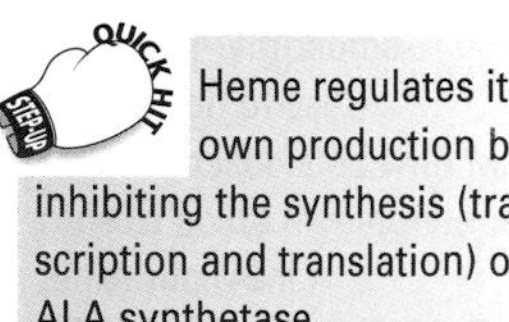

Heme regulates its own production by inhibiting the synthesis (transcription and translation) of ALA synthetase.

TABLE 10-17 Clotting time algorithm

	PT Normal	PT Prolonged
PTT normal	Factor XIII deficiency	Factor VII deficiency
PTT prolonged	Factor VIII, IX, and XI deficiencies in patients with bleeding; factor XII, prekallikrein, and HMW-K deficiencies in patients without bleeding	Common pathway deficiency: factor V, X, II, and I; severe hepatic diseases; DIC

DIC, disseminated intravascular coagulation; HMW-K, high-molecular-weight kininogen; PT, prothrombin time; PTT, partial thromboplastin time.

Heme keeps the translational initiation complex active on the ribosome which increases the production of globin.

TABLE 10-18 Hodgkin versus non-Hodgkin Disease

Hodgkin Disease	Non-Hodgkin Disease
Number of **Reed–Sternberg cells** (binucleated giant cells) proportional to severity	Malignant neoplasm of lymphocytes (85% B cell, 15% T cell) within lymph nodes (especially periaortic)
Causes inflammation, fever, diaphoresis **(night sweats), leukocytosis,** hepatosplenomegaly, and pruritus	Causes painless peripheral lymphadenopathy
Usually affects **young men** (peak incidence in adolescents)	Usually affects White men younger than 65 years of age
Often curable	Nodular type has better prognosis than diffuse
More reactive lymphocytes signal better prognosis	Small cell type has better prognosis than large cell
Rye classifications (low- to high-grade)	**Working classification** (low- to high-grade)
Lymphocytic predominance (least common; best prognosis; L/H variant of RS cells; "popcorn" cells)	Small lymphocytic cell (B cell; elderly; indolent course; chronic lymphocytic leukemia related)
Mixed cellularity (most frequent, numerous RS cells)	Follicular small cell (cleaved B cell; elderly; most **common non-Hodgkin lymphoma t[14;18],** expression of *bcl-2* oncogene)
Nodular sclerosis (collagen banding, lacunar cells) (predominantly in **women;** fibrous bands in lymph nodes; lacunar cells; often found in the mediastinum)	Large cell (elderly and children; usually B cell)
Lymphocytic depletion (worst prognosis; rare necrosis and fibrosis of lymphocytic tissue)	Lymphoblastic (T cell; children; **mediastinal mass** progressing to ALL)
	Small, noncleaved (**[Burkitt]** B cell, Epstein–Barr virus infection; **"starry-sky"** appearance; related to B-cell **acute lymphocytic leukemia; t[8;14],** expression of *c-myc* oncogene)
	Cutaneous T cell (*Mycosis fungoides;* Pautrier microabscesses; Sézary syndrome; skin lesions)
	Mantle cell lymphoma (B cells; poor prognosis)

TABLE 10-19 Classification of Leukemia

Acute Myeloblastic	Acute Lymphoblastic	Chronic Myeloid	Chronic Lymphocytic
Myeloblasts; defect in maturation beyond myeloblast or promyelocyte stage; **Auer rods;** predominantly affects **adults;** poor prognosis	Small lymphoblasts; decreased cytoplasm; predominantly affects **children;** responsive to therapy	t(9;22) results in **Philadelphia chromosome** (BCR–ABL); leukocytosis; **decreased leukocyte alkaline phosphatase;** Splenomegaly; onset at **35–55** years of age; ends in blastic crisis	Usually B cells; "smudge cells" in smear; WAIHA; hypogammaglobulinemia; lymphadenopathy; hepatosplenomegaly; more common in **men older than 60** years of age

TABLE 10-20 Classification of Anemia

Microcytic (MCV <80)	Normocytic (MCV 80–100)	Macrocytic (MCV >100)
Iron deficiency	Aplastic anemia	Liver disease
Lead poisoning	Acute blood loss	Vitamin B_{12} deficiency
Sickle cell	Hemolytic anemia	Folate deficiency
Chronic disease		
Sideroblastic		
Thalassemia		

MCV, mean cell volume.

C. Sickle cell disease (sickle cell hemoglobin or hemoglobin S [HbS])
   1. It is primarily seen in **Blacks**.
   2. The homozygous form is most severe.
   3. Severe hemolytic anemia is seen.
   4. It leads to painful crises, organ infarction (**autosplenectomy**), and strokes.
   5. Aplastic crises occur, usually provoked by viral infection (usually parvovirus B19).
   6. Patients are especially susceptible to infection by **encapsulated bacteria** (*Streptococcus pneumoniae* and *Haemophilus influenzae*) and osteomyelitis caused by *Salmonella*.
   7. Sickle cells and Howell–Jolly bodies are seen in peripheral blood smear.
   8. Treatment is with **hydroxyurea** to increase HbF.

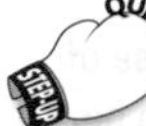

In sickle cell disease, the sixth amino acid of the β-chain of hemoglobin is changed from glutamate to valine. Sickling only occurs when the RBCs are **deoxygenated.** Oxygenated HbS RBCs function normally.

MNEMONIC

Remember the encapsulated bacteria by the phrase "**S**ome **N**asty **K**illers **H**ave **S**ome **C**apsule **P**rotection":
***S**treptococcus pneumoniae*
***N**eisseria meningitidis*
***K**lebsiella pneumoniae*
***H**aemophilus influenza*
***S**almonella typhi*
***C**ryptococcus neoformans*
***P**seudomonas aeruginosa.*

D. Chronic disease
   1. Anemia is seen in chronic disease states such as cancer and autoimmune disease.
   2. It is the second most common anemia.
   3. **TIBC is reduced (ferritin is increased).**
   4. Low serum iron but high iron stores in the bone marrow are observed.

E. Sideroblastic anemia
   1. Iron stain reveals ringed sideroblasts.
   2. TIBC is reduced and serum iron is increased.
   3. RBC count is reduced.

F. Thalassemia
   1. This is a group of genetic disorders, all in some way deficient in α- or β-globin chain synthesis.
   2. **β-Thalassemia is more common** (especially in people of Mediterranean origin)
      a. The homozygous form, called thalassemia major (also known as Mediterranean or Cooley anemia), causes splenomegaly, bone distortions, hemosiderosis, and increased HbF, and it is fatal in childhood.
      b. The heterozygous form of β-thalassemia (thalassemia minor) causes a minor anemia but has no effect on the life span.
   3. α-Thalassemia is caused by a deletion in one or more of the four α-globin genes; loss of all four genes is incompatible with life.

II. Normocytic anemias

A. Aplastic anemia
   1. Dysfunctional or deficient multipotent myeloid stem cells lead to pancytopenia.
   2. It is caused by viruses, chemicals, radiation, or renal failure (via decreased erythropoietin), or may be idiopathic.
   3. Drugs causing aplastic anemia include **NSAIDs**, **benzene**, and **chloramphenicol**.
   4. Symptoms include fatigue, pallor, mucosal bleeding, and petechia as a result of thrombocytopenia.
   5. Neutropenia occurs, leading to frequent infections.
   6. **Fat infiltration** into hypocellular marrow occurs.

B. Anemia caused by acute blood loss
   1. Leads to a **transient normocytic** anemia (however, chronic bleeding can lead to iron deficiency and hence microcytic anemia)
   2. May appear macrocytic because of increased reticulocyte release from bone marrow 7 to 10 days later

C. Hemolytic anemias
   1. Increased RBC destruction leads to an increase in unconjugated bilirubin, hemoglobinemia, hemoglobinuria, and hemosiderosis and decreased serum haptoglobin.
   2. Increase in reticulocytes occurs because of additional erythropoiesis.

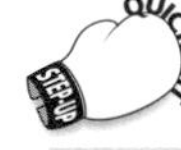

ABO transfusion reactions are almost always a result of clerical (human) error.

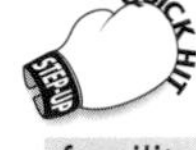

Spherocytes are characterized by osmotic fragility in hypotonic solution.

FIGURE 10-14 Approach to anemia

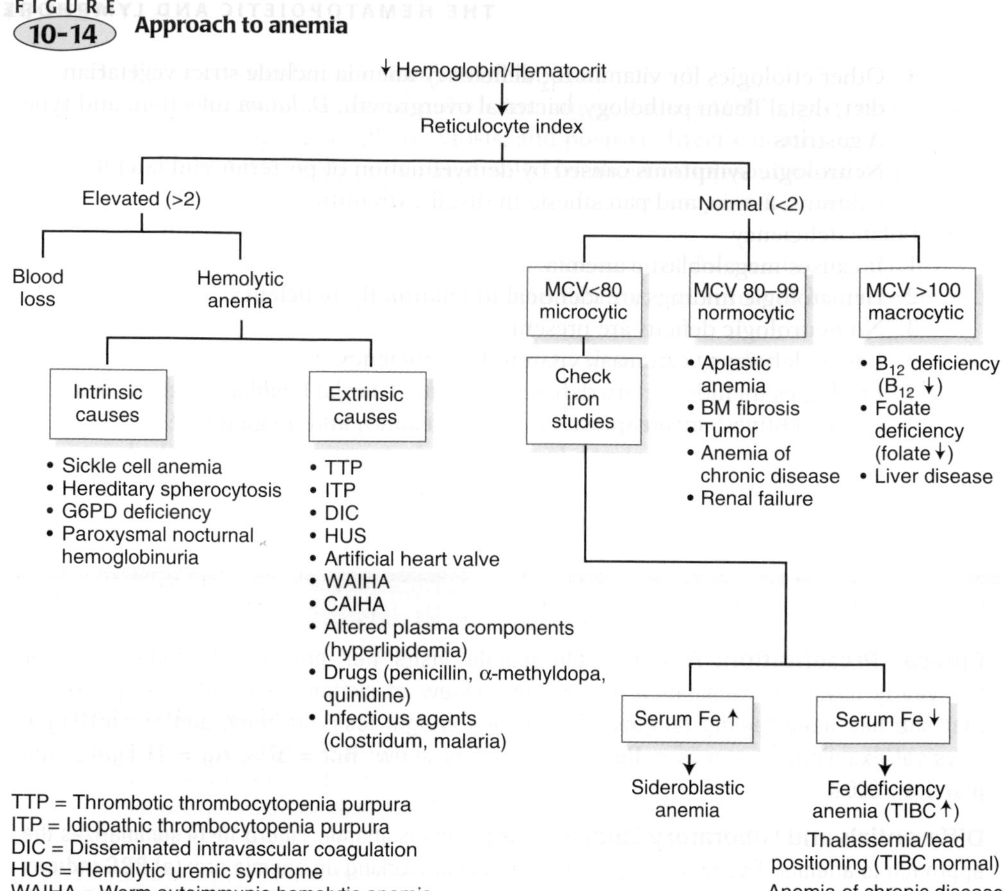

QUICK HIT: Spur cells occur in liver disease and are caused by the reticuloendothelial system "biting" the RBCs.

TABLE 10-21 Approach to Laboratory Blood Studies

Blood Lab Study	Definition	Notes
Hemoglobin	Concentration of Hg in 100 mL of blood	**Increased:** severe dehydration, erythrocytosis, polycythemia, severe burn, shock, COPD, CHF, high altitudes, drugs (gentamicin, methyldopa) **Decreased:** hyperthyroidism, leukemia, liver disease, hemolytic reaction, overhydration, pregnancy, drugs (acetaminophen, antineoplastic agents, chloramphenicol, hydralazine, MAOI, nitrites, penicillin, tetracycline, sulfonamide)
Hematocrit	Percentage of RBCs in a volume of whole blood. Not reliable immediately after blood loss or blood transfusion	**Increased:** severe dehydration, erythrocytosis, polycythemia, severe burns, shock, high altitudes **Decreased** (defined as anemia): hyperthyroidism, leukemia, liver disease, hemolytic reactions, pregnancy, and causes of macrocytic, normocytic, and microcytic anemia (see below)
MCV	Represents volume of single RBC; indicator of cell size	**Increased** (>100) (defined as macrocytic anemia): vitamin B_{12} deficiency, folate deficiency, liver disease, alcoholism **Decreased** (<80) (defined as microcytic anemia): iron deficiency, thalassemia, anemia of chronic disease, lead poisoning, sideroblastic anemia, hemolytic anemias
MCHC	Represents average concentration of Hgb in RBC	**Increased:** spherocytosis
MCH	Represents average weight of Hgb in RBCs; confirms accuracy of MCV value	**Increased:** macrocytic anemia (see above) **Decreased:** microcytic anemia (see above)
Reticulocyte count	Reticulocyte is nonnucleated immature RBC formed in bone marrow; increased values indicate accelerated erythropoiesis	**Increased:** hemolytic anemias, sickle cell disease, pregnancy, splenectomy, hemorrhage **Decreased:** aplastic anemia, chronic infection, radiation therapy

COPD, chronic obstructive pulmonary disease; CHF, congestive heart failure; Hgb, hemoglobin; MAOI, monoamine oxidase inhibitor; MCV, mean cell volume; MCH, mean corpuscular hemoglobin; MCHC, mean corpuscular hemoglobin concentration; RBC, red blood cell.

TABLE 10-22 Peripheral Blood Smear Findings

Peripheral Blood Smear	Conditions Associated
Hypersegmented neutrophils (Figure 10-13)	Folate/B_{12} deficiency
Basophilic stippling of RBCs	Lead poisoning
Echinocytes (Burr cells)	Uremia
Spherocytes	Spherocytosis
Microspherocytes	Coombs hemolysis
Schistocytes (fragmented cells, helmet cells) (Figure 10-10)	Disseminated intravascular coagulation, TTP, HUS
Poikilocytes (irregularly shaped cells)	Thalassemia
Target cells	Liver disease, thalassemia
Acanthocytes (spur cells)	Liver disease, abetalipoproteinemia
Sickle cells	Sickle cell anemia
Howell–Jolly bodies	Asplenia
Heinz bodies	Glucose-6-phosphate dehydrogenase deficiency
Teardrop cells	Myeloid metaplasia with myelofibrosis
Sideroblast (ring of small basophilic granules in the periphery of RBC)	Sideroblastic anemia

TABLE 10-23 Differential for Platelet Destruction

Lab Study	DIC	HUS	TTP	ITP
Blood smear	Schistocytes	Schistocytes	Schistocytes	Normal
PT/PTT	Markedly increased	Normal or mildly increased	Normal or mildly increased	Normal
Fibrin-split products	Increased	Normal	Normal	Normal
Fibrinogen	Decreased	Normal	Normal	Normal
Notes	Platelets trapped in fibrin mesh deposited in blood vessels	***Escherichia coli*** implicated in pathogenesis; usually occurs in **children**	Idiopathic	Autoimmune: autoantibody-mediated platelet destruction; follows URI in children
	Risk factors: sepsis, traumas, obstetrical complication, cancer	Symptoms: anemia, thrombocytopenia, acute renal failure, **bloody diarrhea, abdominal pain, seizures**	**Classic Pentad:** anemia, thrombocytopenia, renal failure, **neurologic changes, fever**	

DIC, disseminated intravascular coagulation; HUS, hemolytic uremic syndrome; ITP, idiopathic thrombocytopenic purpura; TTP, thrombotic thrombocytopenic purpura; URI, upper respiratory infection.

TABLE 10-24 Differential for Microcytic Anemia

Lab Study	Iron-deficiency anemia	Thalassemia or Lead Poisoning	Anemia of Chronic Disease	Sideroblastic Anemia
Serum Fe	Low	Low	Low	**High**
Serum Ferritin	Low	Normal/high	Normal/high	High
TIBC	High	Normal	Low	Normal/high

MNEMONIC

To remember the findings of TIBC in iron deficiency and chronic disease, use **TIBC**: **T**op = **I**ron, **B**ottom = **C**hronic disease. TIBC levels are high **(top)** in iron-deficiency anemia and low **(bottom)** in chronic disease.

TABLE 10-25 Chemotherapeutics *(Continued)*

Therapeutic Agent (common name, if relevant) [trade name, where appropriate]	Class–Pharmacology and Pharmacokinetics	Indications	Side or Adverse Effects	Contraindications or Precautions to Consider; Notes
Cytarabine	**S phase specific antimetabolite—inhibits DNA polymerase**	**AML**	Leukopenia; thrombocytopenia; megaloblastic anemia	
Cyclophosphamide [Cytoxan]	**Cell cycle nonspecific agent—alkylating agent** → crosslinks DNA strands → decreases DNA synthesis and prevents cell division → destroys proliferating lymphoid cells; alkylates the resting cells; potent immunosuppressant	**Transplant rejection; rheumatic arthritis; non-Hodgkin's lymphoma; breast and ovarian carcinoma**	**GI and bone marrow toxicity; hemorrhagic cystitis** (can be partially prevented by mesna)	Requires bioactivation by liver
Ifosfamide	**Cell cycle nonspecific agent—alkylating agent** → crosslinks DNA strands → decreases protein and DNA synthesis → prevents cell division	**Testicular cancer**	**GI and bone marrow toxicity; hemorrhagic cystitis** (can be partially prevented by mensa)	Requires bioactivation by liver
Carmustine, lomustine, semustine, streptozocin	**Cell cycle nonspecific agent (Nitrosureas)—alkylating agent** → crosslinks DNA and RNA strands	**Brain tumors** (including **glioblastoma multiforme**)	**CNS toxicity** (dizziness, ataxia)	**Crosses blood brain barrier to CNS;** requires bioactivation
Cisplastin	**Cell cycle nonspecific agent—alkylating agent** → crosslinks DNA and RNA strands	**Bladder, testicular, ovarian, and lung carcinomas**	**Nephrotoxicity; acoustic nerve damage**	
Busulfan	**Cell cycle nonspecific agent—alkylating agent** → crosslinks DNA and RNA strands	**Chronic myelogenous leukemia**	**Pulmonary fibrosis; hyperpigmentation**	
Doxorubicin [Adriamycin]	**Cell cycle nonspecific agent—oxidizes free radicals → intercalates into DNA →** breaks DNA; affects plasma membrane	**Hodgkin's lymphoma; myeloma;** sarcoma; solid tumors of breast, ovary, and lung	Cardiac changes resulting in cumulative **cardiotoxicity**, myelosuppression, alopecia, and toxic extravasation	Part of the **A**BVD combination regimen for Hodgkin lymphoma
Daunorubicin [DaunoXome, Cerubidine]	**Cell cycle nonspecific agent—oxidizes free radicals → intercalates into DNA** → breaks DNA; affects plasma membrane	**Hodgkin lymphoma; myeloma;** sarcoma; solid tumors of breast, ovary, and lung	Cardiac changes resulting in cumulative **cardiotoxicity**, myelosuppression, alopecia, and toxic extravasation	Part of the **A**BVD combination regimen for Hodgkin lymphoma
Dactinomycin [Cosmegen]	**Cell cycle nonspecific agent—crosslinks DNA and intercalates into DNA**	**Wilms tumor; Ewing sarcoma; rhabdomyosarcoma**	**Skin eruptions; hyperkeratosis; myelosuppression**	

(continued)

TABLE 10-25 Chemotherapeutics *(Continued)*

Therapeutic Agent (common name, if relevant) [trade name, where appropriate]	Class–Pharmacology and Pharmacokinetics	Indications	Side or Adverse Effects	Contraindications or Precautions to Consider; Notes
Bleomycin [Blenoxane]	**G2 phase specific agent—induces formation of free radicals** that bind, intercalate, and cut DNA	**Testicular cancer; Hodgkin disease**	**Pulmonary fibrosis**; fever; **blistering; stomatitis**; hypersensitivity reactions (anaphylaxis)	**Minimal myelosupression;** part of the A**B**VD regimen for Hodgkin lymphoma
Hydroxyurea [Hydrea]	**S phase specific agent—binds ribonucleotide reductase** → inhibits formation of DNA	**Melanoma; CML; sickle cell disease**	**Nausea; vomiting; bone marrow suppression**	
Etoposide	**G2 phase specific—inhibits topoisomerase II → increases DNA degradation**	**Small cell carcinoma of the lung** and prostate; testicular carcinoma	**Myelosuppression;** nausea; vomiting; **alopecia**	
Prednisone [Deltasone]	**Glucocorticoid—inhibits protein synthesis**; reduces lymph node and spleen size; **inhibits cell cycle activity of lymphoid cells; lyses T cells; suppresses antibody, prostaglandin, and leukotriene synthesis; blocks monocyte production of IL-1**	**CLL, Hodgkin's lymphoma**, rheumatic arthritis; **autoimmune disorders; allergic reaction; asthma; organ transplantation (esp. during rejection crisis)**	**Osteoporosis; Cushingoid reaction; psychosis; hyperglycemia; immunosuppression, infection; hypertension; cataracts; acne; peptic ulcers**	Part of the MOP**P** regimen for Hodgkin lymphoma
Tamoxifen [Nolvadex]	**Selective estrogen receptor modular—competitively binds estrogen receptors**; **breast (estrogen antagonist)**: prevents proliferation of estrogen receptor positive tumor cells; **endometrium (partial agonist)**; bone (agonist): decreases bone turnover and increases bone density	**Treats estrogen-dependent breast cancer in postmenopausal women;** reduces contralateral breast cancer; osteoporosis prevention	**May increase the risk of endometrial cancer; hot flashes**; flushing	
Raloxifene [Evista]	**Selective estrogen receptor modulator—breast (estrogen antagonist); endometrium (estrogen antagonist):** prevents proliferation of endometrium; **bone (estrogen agonist):** decreases bone turnover and increases bone density; **cardiovascular (estrogen agonist):** decreases LDL	**Osteoporosis; breast cancer**	**Hot flashes**; sinusitis; weight gain; muscle pain; leg cramps; **increased risk of blood clots**	Unlike estrogen, raloxifene **does not decrease HDL**

(continued)

TABLE 10-25 Chemotherapeutics *(Continued)*

Therapeutic Agent (common name, if relevant) [trade name, where appropriate]	Class–Pharmacology and Pharmacokinetics	Indications	Side or Adverse Effects	Contraindications or Precautions to Consider; Notes
Trastuzumab [Herceptin]	**Monoclonal antibody against HER-2;** binds to tumor cells over expressing HER-2 → mediates antibody-dependent cytotoxicity → destruction of tumor cells	**Metastatic breast cancer**	**Cardiotoxicity**	
Imatinib [Gleevec]	**Tyrosine kinase inhibitor—inhibits BCR–ABL tyrosine kinase** (abnormal product of **Philadelphia chromosome** in CML) → blocks proliferation → induces apoptosis in BCR–ABL positive cell lines and fresh leukemic cells	**CML**, GI stromal tumors	**Fluid retention**	
Vincristine [Oncovin]	**M phase specific (vinca alkaloid)—depolymerizes microtubules** → mitotic spindle cannot form	**Hodgkin lymphoma; Wilms tumor; choriocarcinoma; acute leukemia**	**Peripheral neuritis; areflexia;** paralytic ileus	Part of the M**O**PP regimen for Hodgkin lymphoma
Vinblastine [Velban]	**M phase specific (vinca alkaloid)—depolymerizes microtubules** → mitotic spindle cannot form	**Hodgkin lymphoma; Wilms tumor; choriocarcinoma**	**Bone marrow suppression**	
Paclitaxel [Taxol]	**M phase specific (taxol)—polymerizes microtubules** → mitotic spindle cannot break down → anaphase cannot occur	**Ovarian and breast cancer**	**Myelosupression; hypersensitivity**	

M phase, mitotic phase; G1 phase, synthesis of components needed for DNA synthesis; S phase, DNA synthesis phase; G2 phase, synthesis of components needed for mitosis; HER-2, Human epidermal growth factor receptor 2 protein; AML, acute myelogenous leukemia, CML; chronic myelogenous leukemia; ALL, acute lymphoblastic leukemia; CLL, chronic lymphoblastic leukemia.

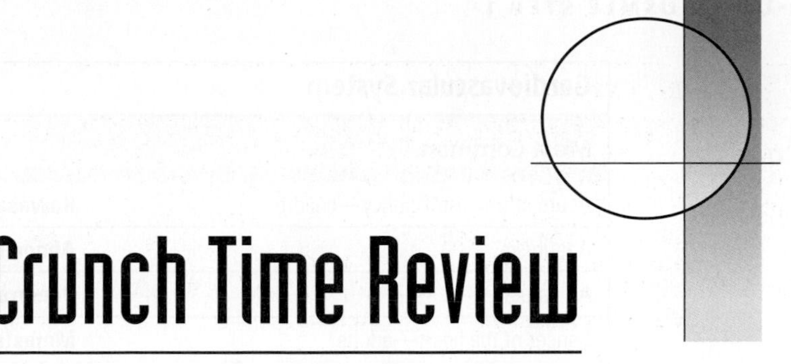

Crunch Time Review

The following pages contain high yield information designed for review in the days just preceding the Step 1 examination.

MOST COMMON

Often on the USMLE exam, the student finds two responses that could potentially answer a question. The NBME is testing the student to identify the more common of the two responses; for example, the more common cause, site, or type. Below is a high yield summary of the most common characteristics of the various disorders listed in this text.

Nervous System	
Most Common...	
Aneurysm of Circle of Willis	**Anterior communicating artery; bitemporal hemianopsia**
Blindness	**Diabetic retinopathy**
Blindness—preventable	***Chlamydia trachomatis***
Bacterial meningitis—elderly	***Streptococcus pneumoniae***
Bacterial meningitis—newborns	***E. coli***
Bacterial meningitis—toddlers	***Haemophilus influenza* type b**
Bacterial meningitis—young adults	***Neisseria meningitidis***
Cancer of the brain—child	**Medulloblastoma (cerebellum)**
Cancer of the brain—adult	**Astrocytoma (including glioblastoma multiforme),** then metastasis, meningioma, schwannoma
Dementia	1. **Alzheimer's** 2. Multi-infarct dementia
Demyelinating disease	**Multiple sclerosis**
Location of adult brain tumors	**Above tentorium**
Location of childhood brain tumors	**Below tentorium** (Mnemonic: Children are short, they cannot reach above the tentorium)
Mental retardation	1. **Down syndrome or Fragile X** 2. Fetal alcohol syndrome
Motor neuron disease	**Amyotrophic lateral sclerosis (ALS)**
Viral encephalitis	**HSV**

Cardiovascular System

Most Common...	
Acute mitral insufficiency—children	**Kawasaki disease**
Aneurysm	**Abdominal aorta**
AV fistula	**Penetrating knife wound**
Cancer of the heart—adults	**Metastases**
Cancer of the heart—primary—adults	**Myxoma "Ball Valve"**
Cancer of the heart—primary—kids	**Rhabdomyoma**
Cardiomyopathy	**Dilated (congestive) cardiomyopathy**
Cause of acute endocarditis	***Staphylococcus aureus***
Cause of subacute endocarditis	***Streptococcus viridans***
Congenital cardiac anomaly	**Ventricular septal defect** (membranous > muscular)
Congenital early cyanosis	**Tetralogy of Fallot**
Coronary artery thrombosis	**Left anterior descending**
Death in HTN	1. **Acute mitral insufficiency** 2. Lenticulostriate stroke 3. Renal failure (benign nephrosclerosis)
Death in the United States	**Ischemic heart disease**
Heart murmur	**Mitral valve prolapsed**
Heart valve in bacterial endocarditis	**Mitral**
Heart valve in bacterial endocarditis in IV drug users	**Tricuspid**
Heart valve involved in rheumatic fever	**Mitral** > Aortic
Hypertension	1. **Essential (95%)** 2. Renal disease
Hypertension—children	**Renal disease;** cystic disease, Wilms tumor
Hypertension—young women	**Oral contraceptives**
Myocarditis	**Coxsackie B virus**
Right heart failure	**Left heart failure**
Secondary hypertension	**Renal disease**
Sites of atherosclerosis	**Abdominal aorta** > coronary > popliteal > carotid
Vasculitis (of medium and small arteries)	**Temporal arteritis**

Respiratory System

Most Common...	
Cause of pneumonia in debilitated, hospitalized patient	***Klebsiella***
Cause of epiglottitis	***Haemophilus influenza*** **type b**
Cause of IV drug user bacteremia/pneumonia	***Staphylococcus aureus***
Cause of opportunistic infection of AIDS	***Pneumocystis carinii*** **is most common overall**
Death in Alzheimer patients	**Pneumonia**
Fatal genetic defect in Caucasians	**Cystic fibrosis**
Pneumonia—community—typical	1. ***Streptococcus pneumoniae*** 2. *H. influenza* 3. *Klebsiella*
Pneumonia—hospital acquired	1. ***Klebsiella*** 2. ***Pseudomonas*** 3. ***E. coli***
Pneumonia—community—atypical	1. ***Mycoplasma*** 2. *Legionella*
Pulmonary HTN	**COPD**
SIADH	**Small cell carcinoma of the lung**
Tracheoesophageal fistula	**Lower esophagus communicates with trachea, upper esophagus ends in blind pouch**

Gastrointestinal System

Most Common...	
Bug in food poisoning	***Staphylococcus aureus***
Bug in GI tract	1. ***Bacteroides*** 2. *E. coli*
Cancer of the appendix	**Carcinoid—rarely metastasizes**
Cancer of the esophagus	**Leiomyoma**
Cancer of the esophagus—malignant	**Squamous cell carcinoma (60%)** > adenocarcinoma (40%)
Cancer of the liver	**Metastasis;** lung > GI
Cancer of the liver—primary, benign	**Cavernous hemangioma**
Cancer of the liver—primary	**Hepatocellular carcinoma**
Cancer of the mouth	**Squamous cell carcinoma or mucoepidermoid carcinoma**
Cancer of the mouth—upper lip	**Basal cell carcinoma**
Cancer of the nasal cavities	**Squamous cell carcinoma**
Cancer of the pancreas	**Adenocarcinoma** (usually in the head of pancreas)
Cancer of the salivary glands	**Pleomorphic adenoma**
Cancer of the small bowel	**Carcinoid**—frequent metastasis from ileum
Cancer of the spleen—benign	**Cavernous hemangioma**
Cancer of the stomach	**Gastric adenocarcinoma** (intestinal type or diffuse type)
Cirrhosis	**Alcohol**
Congenital GI anomaly	**Meckel diverticulum**
Diarrhea—children	**Rotavirus**
Dietary deficiency	**Iron**
GI obstruction	1. **Adhesions** 2. Indirect inguinal hernia
Intussusception	**Terminal ileum into cecum**
Liver disease	**Alcoholic liver disease**
Liver infection	**Viral hepatitis—HVA**
Lysosomal storage disease	**Gaucher disease**
Portal hypertension	**Cirrhosis**
Protozoal diarrhea	***Giardia***
Site of diverticula	**Sigmoid colon**
Surgical emergency	**Acute appendicitis**
Worm infection in the United States	1. **Pinworm** 2. Ascaris

Renal System

Most Common...	
Amyloidosis	**Immunologic** (Bence Jones protein in multiple myeloma is also called the amyloid light chain)
Death in SLE patients	Lupus nephropathy type IV (diffuse proliferative)
End-stage renal disease	**Diabetes**
Glomerulonephritis	**IgA nephropathy (aka Berger's)**
Nephrotic syndrome—adults	**Membranous glomerulonephritis**
Nephrotic syndrome—kids	**Minimal change disease**
Renal failure	**Acute tubular necrosis**

Endocrine System

Most Common...	
Addison disease	1. **Autoimmune** 2. Infection
Cancer of the adrenal medulla—adults	**Pheochromocytoma**
Cancer of the adrenal medulla—kids	**Neuroblastoma**
Cancer of the pituitary	1. **Prolactinoma** 2. Somatotropic "acidophilic" adenoma
Cancer of the thyroid	**Papillary carcinoma**
Congenital adrenal hyperplasia	1. **21-Hydroxylase deficiency** 2. 11-hydroxylase deficiency
Cushing's	1. **Exogenous steroid therapy** 2. Primary ACTH tumor 3. Adrenal adenoma 4. Ectopic ACTH tumor
Enzyme deficiency	**21 hydroxylase—95% of congenital adrenal hyperplasia**
Hypercalcemia	**Hyperparathyroidism**
Hyperparathyroidism—primary	1. **Solitary adenomas** 2. Parathyroid hyperplasia 3. Parathyroid carcinoma
Hyperparathyroidism—secondary	**Hypocalcemia due to chronic renal failure**
Hyperthyroidism	**Graves disease**
Hypopituitarism—adults	**Nonfunctioning pituitary adenoma**
Hypopituitarism—kids	**Craniopharyngioma**
Hypothyroidism	**Hashimoto thyroiditis**
Peripheral neuropathy	**Diabetes mellitus**
Thyroid disease	**Goiter**

Reproductive System	
Most Common...	
Breast mass (premenopausal)	**Fibrocystic change (premenopausal)**
Breast mass (postmenopausal)	**Breast carcinoma**
Cancer in gynecologic—malignancy	**Endometrial carcinoma**
Cancer in men	**Prostate carcinoma**
Cancer in women	**Leiomyoma (fibroids)**
Cancer in women—malignant	**Breast carcinoma**
Cancer of the breast	**Infiltrating ductal adenocarcinoma**
Cancer of the ovary—benign	**Serous cystadenoma**
Cancer of the ovary—malignant	**Serous cystadenocarcinoma**
Cancer of the placenta—benign	**Cavernous hemangioma**
Cancer of the testicles	**Seminoma**
Cancer that invades the female GU tract	**Endometrial adenocarcinoma**
Cause of PID	***Neisseria gonorrhoeae* or *Chlamydia***
Chromosomal disorder	**Down syndrome**
Hernia	**Indirect**
Opportunistic infection in AIDS	***Pneumocystis carinii***
Sexually transmitted disease	***Chlamydia***

Musculoskeletal System	
Most Common...	
Bacterial arthritis in young Adults	***N. gonorrhea***
Cancer of the bone	**Metastases from breast and prostate**
Cancer of the bone—primary—adults	**Multiple myeloma**
Cancer of the connective tissue—benign	**Lipoma**
Cancer of the skin	**Basal cell carcinoma**
Carpal bone dislocation	**Lunate**
Carpal bone fx	**Scaphoid**
Disk herniation	**L4–L5**

The Hematopoietic and Lymphoreticular System	
Most Common...	
Cancer—leukemia—14 y old	**ALL**
Cancer—leukemia—60 y old	**CLL**
Cancer—leukemia—15–39 y old	**AML**
Cancer—leukemia—40–60 y old	**CML**
Cancer in infancy	**Hemangioma**
Cancer in children	1. **Leukemia**
	2. Medulloblastoma of cerebellum
Cancer; malignant lymphoma in children	**Burkitt lymphoma**
Cancer; site of metastasis	**Regional lymph nodes**
Cancer; site of metastasis (2nd most common)	**Liver**
Cancer; genetic alteration	**p53**
Hereditary bleeding disorder	**von Willebrand Disease**
Single gene disorder	**Thalassemia**
Type of hodgkin lymphoma	**Mixed cellularity versus lymphocytic predominance, lymphocytic depletion, and nodular sclerosis**
Type of nonhodgkin lymphoma	**Follicular, small cleaved**

QUICK LISTS

The following Quick Lists contain high yield information organized by basic science subject.

Physiology

Quick List: Important Formulas

	Formula	Notes
Cardiac output	CO = Rate of O_2 Consumption/ (Arterial O_2 Content – Venous O_2 Content) CO = SV × HR	SV = Stroke volume HR = Heart rate
Mean arterial pressure	MAP = CO × TPR MAP = 1/3 SBP + 2/3 DBP	CO = Cardiac output TPR = Total peripheral resistance SBP = Systolic blood pressure DBP = Diastolic blood pressure
Stroke volume	EDV – ESV	EDV = End diastolic volume ESV = End systolic volume
Ejection fraction	SV/EDV × 100	SV = Stroke volume EDV = End diastolic volume
Resistance	$8\eta L/\pi r^4$	η = Viscosity L = length r = radius
Net filtration pressure	$(P_C - P_I) - (\pi_C - \pi_I)$	P_C = Hydrostatic capillary pressure P_I = Hydrostatic interstitial pressure π_C = Osmotic capillary pressure π_I = Osmotic interstitial pressure
Glomerular filtration rate	$GFR = K_f (P_{GC} - P_{BS}) - (\pi_{GC} - \pi_{BS})$ $GFR = C_{inulin} = U_{inulin} \times V/P_{inulin}$	K_f = filtration constant P_{GC} = Hydrostatic pressure in glomerular capillaries P_{BS} = Hydrostatic pressure in Bowman's space π_{GC} = Osmotic pressure in glomerular capillaries π_{BS} = Osmotic pressure in Bowman's space C_{inulin} = Clearance of PAH U_{inulin} = Urine concentration of PAH V = Urine flow rate P_{inulin} = Plasma concentration of PAH
Effective renal plasma flow	$C_{PAH} = U_{PAH} \times V/P_{PAH}$	C_{PAH} = Clearance of PAH U_{PAH} = Urine concentration of PAH V = Urine flow rate P_{PAH} = Plasma concentration of PAH
Renal blood flow	RPF/(1– Hct)	RPF = Renal plasma flow Hct = Hematocrit
Filtration fraction	GFR/RPF	GFR = Glomerular filtration rate RPF = Renal plasma flow
Free water clearance	$C_{H_2O} = V - C_{osm}$, where $C_{osm} = U_{osm}\ V/P_{osm}$	C_{H_2O} = Clearance of water U_{osm} = Urine osmolarity P_{osm} = Plasma osmolarity V = Urine flow rate

Biostatistics

Quick List: Important Formulas

	Formula
Sensitivity	TP/(TP + FN)
Specificity	TN/(TN + FP)
Positive predictive value	TP/(TP + FP)
Negative predictive value	TN/(TN + FN)
Prevalence	TP + FN/(TP + FP +TN + FN) Generally calculated by incidence × duration of disease
Incidence	Generally calculated by number of new cases/susceptible population
Relative risk	RR = [TP/(TP + FP)]/ [FN/(FN + TN)]
Attributable risk	AR = [TP/(TP + FP)] – [FN/(FN + TN)]

Genetics

Quick List: Inherited diseases

Mode of inheritance	Diseases
Autosomal dominant diseases	Adult polycystic kidney disease, familial hypercholesterolemia, Marfan syndrome, Neurofibromatosis type 1, Neurofibromatosis type 2, Tuberous sclerosis, von Hippel–Lindau disease, Huntington disease, Familial adenomatous polyposis, Hereditary spherocytosis, Achondroplasia
Autosomal recessive diseases	Cystic fibrosis, albinism, alpha1-antitrypsin deficiency, phenylketonuria, thalassemias, sickle cell anemia, glycogen storage disease, mucopolysaccharidoses (except Hunter disease), sphingolipidoses (except Fabry disease), infant polycystic kidney disease, hemochromatosis
X-linked dominant diseases	Hypophosphatemic rickets
X-linked recessive diseases	Bruton's agammaglobulinemia, Wiskott–Aldrich syndrome, Fragile X syndrome, G6PD deficiency, ocular albinism, Lesch–Nyhan syndrome, Duchenne muscular dystrophy, Hemophilia A and B, Fabry disease, Hunter syndrome
Mitochondrial disease	Leber hereditary optic neuropathy, mitochondrial myopathies
Trisomies	Down syndrome (Chromosome 21), Edward syndrome (Chromosome 18), Patau syndrome (Chromosome 13)
Trinucleotide repeat diseases	Huntington diease, myotonic dystrophy, Friedreich ataxia, fragile X syndrome

Pharmacology

Quick List: Important Formulas

	Formula	Notes
Volume of distribution	Total drug in body/plasma concentration	
Clearance	Rate of elimination of drug/plasma concentration	
Half life	0.7 × Volume of distribution/Clearance	
Loading dose	Target plasma concentration × Volume of distribution/Bioavailability	Bioavailability = 1, when medication given IV
Maintenance dose	Target plasma concentration × Clearance/Bioavailability	Bioavailability = 1, when medication given IV

Quick List: Important Drug Side Effects based on Organ System (*Figure 1*)

FIGURE 1 **Important drug side effects based on organ system**

SKIN
1. Photosensitivity-sulfonamides, amiodarone, tetracycline
2. Lupus like syndrome–hydralazine, isoniazid, procainamide, phenytoin

VASCULAR
1. Facial flushing–niacin, verapamil, nifedipine, diltiazem, adenosine, vancomycin

CARDIAC
1. Coranary vasospasm-cocaine, sumatriptan
2. Dilated cardiomyopathy-doxorubicin, daunorubicin
3. Torsades des pointes–antiarrhythmics (sotalol, quinidine), cisapride

PULMONARY
1. Cough-ACE inhibitors
2. Pulmonary fibrosis–bleomycin, busulfan, amiodarone

HEPATOBILIARY
1. Hepatitis–isoniazid
2. Hepatic necrosis–halothane, valproic acid, acetaminophen
3. Acute cholestatic hepatitis-erythromycin, azithromycin, clarithromycin

HEMATOPOIETIC
1. Agranulocytosis-clozapine, carbamazepine, colchicine, propylthoiuracil, methimazole
2. Aplastic anemia-chloramphenicol, benzene, NSAIDS, propythiouracil, methimazole
3. Hemolytic anemia (direct Coombs-positive)-methyldopa
4. Hemolytic anemia in G6PD-deficient patients-isoniazid, sulfonamide, primaquine, aspirin, ibuprofen, nitrofurantoin
5. Gray baby syndrome-chloramphenicol
6. Thrombosis-oral contraceptives

GENITOURINARY
1. Interstitial nephritis-methicillin, NSAIDS
2. Hemorrhaghic cystitis-cyclophosphamide, ifosfamide
3. Fanconi's syndrome expired tetracycline

INTESTINAL
1. Pseudomembrane colitis-clindamycin, ampicilin

MUSCULOSKELETAL
1. Osteoporosis-corticosteroids, heparin
2. Gout-furosemide, thiazide diuretic
3. Tendonitis, tendon rupture, cartilage damage-fluroquinolones
4. Gingival hyperplasia-phenytoin

ENDOCRINE
1. Adrenocortical insuffuciency-glucocorticoid withdrawal
2. Gynecomastia-spironolactone, digitalis, cimetidine, alcohol (chronic use), estrogens, ketoconazole
3. Hot flashes- tamoxifen, clomiphene
4. Diabetes insipidus-lithium, demeclocyline

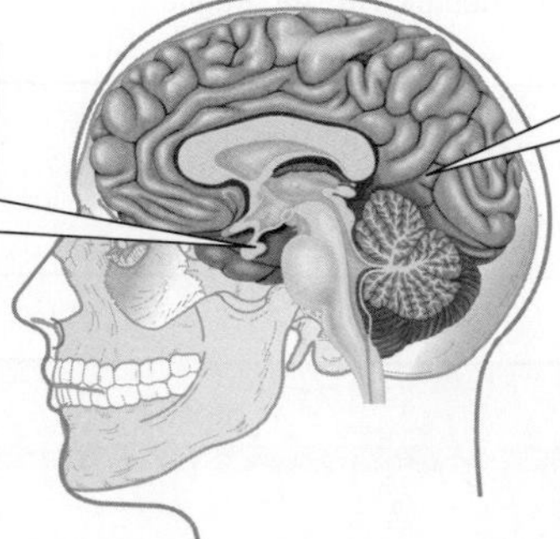

NERVOUS SYSTEM
1. Seizures- buproprion, imipenem/cilastin
2. Tardive dyskinesia-antipsychotics
3. Reaction with alcohol intake (headache, nausea, vomiting, flushing)-metronidazole, specific cephalosporins, procarbazine, sulfonylureas (1st generation)
4. Neurotoxicity/neptrotoxicity-polymyxins
5. Ototoxicity/nephrotoxicity-cisplatin, furosemide, bumetanide, ethacrynic acid, gentamicin, neomycin, tobramycin, amikacin

Quick List: Drugs to Avoid in Pregnancy

Drug	Reason
Atorvastatin	Congenital defects, termination of pregnancy
ACE inhibitors (captopril, enalapril, fosinopril, lisinopril, and quinapril)	Fetal renal malformations
Aminoglycosides	Ototoxicity
Chloramphenicol	Gray baby syndrome
Erythromycin	Acute cholestatic hepatitis (mother), Embyrotoxic (clarithromycin)
Fluroquinolones	Cartilage damage
Griseofulvin	Teratogenic
Methysergide	Oxytocic effects
Metronidazole	Mutagenesis
Ribavirin	Teratogenic
Sulfonamides	Kernicterus
Tetracyclines	Discolored teeth, inhibition of bone growth
Warfarin	Teratogenic

Quick List: CYP-450 Interactions

Effect	Agent	Notes
Inhibitors	Isoniazid, sulfonamides, cimetidine, ketoconazole, erythromycin, grapefruit juice	
Inducers	Quinidine, barbiturates, phenytoin, rifampin, griseofulvin, carbamazepine, St. John's wort	While induction is the more important effect, quinidine can both induce and inhibit different isoforms of CYP-450

Quick List: Antidotes

Toxic agent	Treatment
Acetaminophen	*N*-acetylcysteine
Amphetamine	Ammonium chloride (acidify urine)
Anticholinesterases	Atropine, pralidoxime
Anticholinergic	Physostigmine salicylate
Antimuscarinic	Physostigmine salicylate
Arsenic	Dimercaprol (BAL), sucimer, Penicillamine
Benzodiazepines	Flumazenil
Beta blockers	Glucagon
Carbon monoxide	100% oxygen, hyperbaric oxygen
Copper	Penicillamine
Cyanide	Nitrite, hydroxocobalamin, thiosulfate
Digitalis	Stop digoxin, normal potassium, lidocaine, anti-dig Fab fragments, Mg^{2+}
Ethylene glycol (antifreeze)	Ethanol, dialysis, fomepizole
Gold	Dimercaprol (BAL), sucimer, Penicillamine
Heparin	Protamine
Iron	Deferoxamine
Lead	CaEDTA, dimercaprol, succimer, penicillamine
Mercury	Dimercaprol (BAL), sucimer
Methemoglobin	Methylene blue
Methanol	Ethanol, dialysis, fomepizole
Opioids	Naloxone/natrexone
Organophosphates	Atropine, pralidoxime
Salicylate	Sodium bicarbonate (alkalinize urine)
Streptokinase	Aminocaproic acid
Tricyclic antidepressants	Sodium bicarbonate (serum alkalinization)
tPA	Aminocaptoic acid
Warfarin	Vitamin K, fresh frozen plasma

Microbiology

Quick List: Buzzwords for Microbiological Infections

Clinical characteristics	Organism
Branching rods in oral infections	*Actinomyces israeli*
Chancroid	*Haemophilus ducreyi*
Clue cells	*Gardenella vaginitis*
Cold agglutinins	*Mycoplasma pneumoniae*
Currant jelly sputum	*Klebsiella*
Dog or cat bite	*Pasteurella multocida*
Erythema chronicum migrans	Lyme disease
Ghon focus	Primary tuberculosis
Jarisch–Herxheimer reaction	Syphillis—treatment of an asymptomatic patient results in rapid lysis leading to symptoms
Negri bodies	Rabies
Owl's eye	CMV
Pediatric infection	*Haemophilus influenzae*
Pneumonia in cystic fibrosis or burn infections	*Pseudomonas aeruginosa*
Rash on palms or soles	Rocky Mountain Spotted fever, Secondary syphillis
Roth spots in retina	Endocarditis
Slapped cheeks	Erythema infectiosum
Splinter hemorrhages in finger nails	Endocarditis
Strawberry tongue	Scarlet fever
Suboccipital lymphadenopathy	Rubella
Sulfur granules	*Actinomyces israeli*
Traumatic open wound	*Clostridium perfringens*
Tabes dorsales	Tertiary syphillis
Thumb sign on lateral X-ray	Epiglottis (usually with *Haemophilus influenzae*)
Urethritis, conjunctivitis, arthritis	Reiter syndrome

Quick List: Gram Stain Characteristics of Various Bacteria

Gram Stain Characteristics	Organisms
Gram positive cocci	*Staphylococcus* (catalase +), *Streptococcus* (catalase –), *Enterococcus* (catalase –)
Gram positive rods	*Clostridium* (anaerobe), *Corynebacterium, Listeria, Bacillius*
Gram negative cocci	*Neisseria*
Gram negative coccoid rods	*Haemophilus influenzae, Pasteurella, Brucella, Bordetella pertussis*
Gram negative rods	**Lactose fermenters:** *Klebsiella* (fast*), *E. coli* (fast), *Enterobacter* (fast), *Citrobacter* (slow*), *Serratia* (slow) **Lactose nonfermenter:** *Shigella* (oxidase –), *Salmonella* (oxidase –), *Proteus* (oxidase –), *Pseudomonas* (oxidase +)

*Fast fermenter, Slow fermenter.

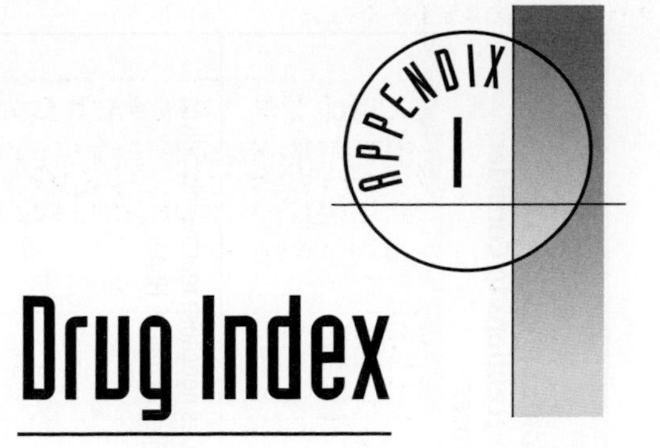

Drug Index

The therapeutic agents shown in boldface type are those that are often emphasized in the classroom and the clinic. Particular attention should be paid to the information about these agents.

Therapeutic Agent (common name, if relevant) [trade name, where appropriate]	Class–Pharmacology and Pharmacokinetics	Indications	Side or Adverse Effects	Contraindications or Precautions to Consider; Notes
Abacavir (ABC)	**Antiviral, nucleoside reverse transcriptase inhibitor—guanosine analog →** inhibits viral reverse transcriptase → prevents integration of DNA copy of viral genome into host DNA	**AIDS (Used in HAART)**	**Neutropenia, anemia, peripheral neuropathy, pancreatitis, and lactic acidosis**	
Acarbose [Precose]	**Hypoglycemic agent, α-glucosidase inhibitor**—inhibits intestinal brush border enzyme α-glucosidase→ delays sugar hydrolysis and glucose absorption from gut → decreases **postprandial hyperglycemia**	Oral treatment for **NIDDM (type II diabetes)** postprandially	**Flatulence,** cramps, diarrhea; may reduce absorption of iron	Does not cause reactive hypoglycemia; decreases HbA1c
Acebutolol [Sectral]	Antiarrhythmic (class II)—antihypertensive; β-blocker	Hypertension; PVCs		Cardioselective; intrinsic sympathomimetic activity (useful in treating patients with hypertension who also have bradycardia)
Acetaminophen [Tylenol]	Analgesic, antipyretic—reversibly inhibits cyclooxygenase centrally (inactivated peripherally), prostaglandin inhibitor, **not anti-inflammatory**	Pain; fever	Liver toxicity in high doses **(high levels deplete glutathione)**	**Overdose treated with *N*-acetylcysteine** (regenerates glutathione); **unlike aspirin, can be used in children, gout, peptic ulcer, and patients with platelet dysfunction**
Acetazolamide [Diamox]	**Carbonic anhydrase inhibitor, diuretic—inhibits carbonic anhydrase on PCT and DCT,** which prevents HCO_3^- reabsorption; lose Na^+, HCO_3^-, and K^+ in urine	**Glaucoma; high altitude; metabolic alkalosis; alkalinization of urine; epilepsy**	**Hyperchloremic metabolic acidosis, sulfa drug allergy,** neuropathy, and ammonium toxicity	**Weak diuretic because other sites further downstream along the nephron can compensate for sodium loss;** causes decreased secretion of HCO_3^- in aqueous humor
Acetylcholine	**Muscarinic and nicotinic agonist**	**Eye surgery (miotic)**	**Increased parasympathetic/cholinergic stimulation** (**MNEMONIC: DUMBELS**—**D**iarrhea/**D**ecreased BP, **U**rination, **M**iosis, **B**ronchoconstriction, **E**xcitation of skeletal muscle, **L**acrimation, **S**alivation)	Contraindicated for patients with **peptic ulcer, asthma, hyperthyroidism, or parkinsonism**

Acetylsalicylic acid (aspirin)	**Anti-inflammatory, antipyretic, analgesic**—acetylates COX irreversibly	Articular, musculoskeletal pain; chronic pain; **maintenance therapy for preventing clot formation**	GI distress, **GI ulcers; inhibits platelet aggregation;** causes **hypersensitivity reactions (rash);** reversible hepatic dysfunction	**Contraindicated** for **children** with flu or chicken pox (leads to **Reye syndrome**) and **gouty patients**
ACTH (corticotropin)	Increases production of steroids by the adrenal cortex	Test adrenal function in adrenocortical insufficiency		**Increased cortisol indicates pituitary defect; unchanged cortisol indicates adrenal defect**
Acyclovir [Zovirax]	**Antiviral—guanosine analog;** monophosphorylated by **viral thymidine kinase;** triphosphorylated form **inhibits viral DNA polymerase**	**HSV, VZV, EBV, CMV** (at high doses); **HSV-induced mucocutaneous genital lesions** and **encephalitis**	**Side effects depend on the route of administration: IV—neurotoxicity, renal problems, tremor Oral—diarrhea,** headache **Topical—local skin irritation**	**Resistant forms lack thymidine kinase**
Adenosine [Adenocard]	**Antiarrhythmic —increases potassium efflux → hyperpolarizes cell**	**Diagnosis and treatment of AV nodal arrhythmias**	**Flushing, hypotension, and chest pain**	Very short acting
Albendazole [Albenza]	Antihelminthic—blocks glucose uptake, resulting in eventual depletion of the parasite's energy stores	*Ascaris* (roundworm), *Ancylostoma* (hookworm), *Trichuris* (whipworm), *Strongyloides*; **cysticercosis, hydatid disease**	**Teratogenic; embryotoxic;** mild nausea, vomiting, and dizziness	Contraindicated in pregnant patients
Albuterol [Proventil, Ventolin]	**Bronchodilation—β_2 agonist, leads to relaxation of smooth muscle**	Asthma; COPD; bronchitis	**Tremor, tachycardia, arrhythmia**, headache, nausea, and vomiting	
Alcohol (EtOH)	Acts at **$GABA_a$ receptor**	Sedative; hypnotic; depressive action on brain; **indicated for methanol and ethylene glycol overdose**	**Intoxication (in order of increasing BAL):** fine motor, coordination, ataxia, lethargy, coma, and respiratory depression; **Withdrawal:** nausea, diaphoresis, delirium tremens, and seizures; **Fetal alcohol syndrome:** mental retardation, growth deficiencies, microcephaly, and smooth philtrum; **Chronic effects of alcoholism:** decreased liver function; Wernicke–Korsakoff syndrome, dilated cardiomyopathy, gynecomastia, and testicular atrophy	Benzodiazepines used for withdrawal symptoms; intoxication treated by thiamine, glucose, folic acid, and multivitamins
Aldesleukin [Proleukin]	Recombinant cytokine—human recombinant interleukin-2	**Metastatic renal cell carcinoma, metastatic melanoma, AML**		
Alendronate [Fosamax]	Bone stabilizer—bisphosphonate; **pyrophosphate analog;** reduces hydroxyapatite crystal formation, growth, and dissolution, which reduces bone turnover	**Hypercalcemia of malignancy; Paget disease; osteoporosis; hyperparathyroidism**	**Pill-induced esophagitis**	

Therapeutic Agent (common name, if relevant) [trade name, where appropriate]	Class–Pharmacology and Pharmacokinetics	Indications	Side or Adverse Effects	Contraindications or Precautions to Consider; Notes
Allopurinol [Zyloprim]	**Antigout—competitive inhibitor of xanthine oxidase;** converted to oxypurinol by xanthine oxidase, which also produces uric acid → allopurinol and oxypurinol inhibit xanthine oxidase → decreased uric acid production	**Chronic gout therapy;** lymphoma, leukemia (prevents tumor lysis associated urate nephropathy), and uric acid stones; rheumatic arthritis	Rash; fever; GI problems; hepatotoxicity; inhibition of the metabolism of other drugs; enhances the effect of azathioprine	Should not be used to treat acute gout; inhibition of the metabolism of other drugs; enhances the effect of azathioprine
Alprazolam [Xanax]	Antianxiety—intermediate acting benzodiazepine	**Panic attack; phobia; MNEMONIC:** AL PRAYS when he's in fear	Sedation	Respiratory depression if taken with alcohol
Alprostadil [Vasoprost]	Impotency therapy; **prostaglandin E_1 agonist**	**Impotency; maintains patent ductus arteriosus**	Penile pain; prolonged erection; flushing, bradycardia, tachycardia, hypotension, and apnea	
Aluminum hydroxide	**Antacid**—buffers gastric acid by raising the pH; **antidiarrheal—delays gastric empyting**	Peptic ulcer, gastritis, esophageal reflux, and diarrhea	**Constipation,** hypophosphatemia, muscle weakness, **osteodystrophy,** seizures, **and hypokalemia**	Can affect the **absorption, bioavailability,** or **urinary excretion** of drugs by changing **gastric pH, urinary pH,** or **gastric emptying**
Amantadine [Symmetrel]	**Antiviral—antiparkinsonian; inhibits** fusion of lysosomes; inhibits viral penetration and uncoating; increases release of endogenous dopamine	**Influenza A** (prophylaxis and treatment); **Parkinson disease**	**CNS effects** (ataxia, dizziness, slurred speech, nervousness, and seizure); **anticholinergic;** orthostatic hypotension; **livedo reticularis** (skin rash)	Mechanism of viral resistance is mutated M2 protein
Amicar (EACA)	Competitive inhibition of plasminogen activation	Inhibits fibrinolysis; promotes thrombosis		Oral administration
Amikacin [Amikin]	**Antibiotic—aminoglycoside,** protein synthesis inhibitor; **irreversibly binds 30S ribosome** subunits; **bacteriostatic** at low concentration; **bactericidal** at high concentration	**Broad-spectrum:** Gram-negative rods; good for **bone** and **eye** infections; *Proteus, Pseudomonas, Enterobacter, Klebsiella, E. coli*	**Ototoxicity; renal toxicity; neuromuscular blockade;** nausea; vomiting; vertigo; allergic skin rash; superinfections	Does not cover anaerobes
Amiloride [Midamor]	Potassium sparing diuretic—binds to intracellular aldosterone steroid receptors in **collecting tubules;** blocks induction of Na^+ channels and Na^+/ATPase synthesis and blocks Na^+ channels directly; lose Na^+ and Cl^- in urine	Hyperaldosteronism, potassium depletion, congestive heart failure	**Hyperkalemic metabolic acidosis, gynecomastia** (spironolactone), and antiandrogen effects	Results in decreased secretion of K^+ and H^+, which can lead to **hyperkalemic metabolic acidosis**; often given in combination with a thiazide
Aminoglutethimide [Cytadren]	Antineoplastic—aromatase inhibitor; cytochromic P450 inhibitor that catalyzes the rate limiting step of adrenal steroid synthesis	Breast cancer; Cushing syndrome	GI and neurological side effects; transient maculopapular rash	Do not cover anaerobes because oxidative metabolism is required for uptake of these drugs

Aminoglycosides	Antibiotic—**irreversibly binds 30S ribosome** subunits; **bacteriostatic** at low concentration; **bactericidal** at high concentration	**Broad-spectrum:** Gram-negative rods; good for **bone** and **eye** infections; *Proteus, Pseudomonas, Enterobacter, Klebsiella*, and *E. coli*	**Ototoxicity; renal toxicity; neuromuscular blockade;** nausea; vomiting; vertigo; allergic skin rash; superinfections	Examples include gentamycin, neomycin, and streptomycin
Amiodarone [Cordarone]	**Antiarrhythmic (class III)—K^+-channel blocker**	**Ventricular/supraventricular arrhythmias**	Bradycardia; heart block/failure; **pulmonary fibrosis; photodermatitis**	**Also functions as class IA, II, and IV**
Amitriptyline **[Elavil]**	Tricyclic antidepressants –inhibit **reuptake** of NE and 5-HT at neuronal synapses	Major depression, panic disorder; sedative; prophylaxis for migraines	Sedation, **alpha blocking effects** (orthostatic hypotension), **anticholinergic** (tachycardia, dry mouth, and urinary retention), hallucinations (in elderly), and confusion (elderly); overdose toxicity results in **convulsions, coma, cardiotoxicity** (arrhythmias), respiratory depression, and hyperpyrexia	
Amobarbital [Amytal sodium]	Sedative—hypnotic; barbiturate; prolongs IPSP duration for GABA receptor	Antiepileptic; cerebral edema; anesthetic	Sedation, respiratory depression	
Amodiaquine	Antimalarial—uncertain mechanism	Suppression and treatment of acute attacks	Headache; GI and visual disturbances; pruritus; prolonged therapy may lead to retinopathy	
Amoxapine	Tricyclic antidepressants—inhibit **reuptake** of NE and 5-HT at neuronal synapses	Major depression, panic disorder	Sedation, **alpha blocking effects** (orthostatic hypotension), **anticholinergic** (tachycardia, dry mouth, and urinary retention), hallucinations (in elderly), and confusion (elderly); overdose toxicity results in **convulsions, coma, cardiotoxicity** (arrhythmias), respiratory depression, and hyperpyrexia	
Amoxicillin	**Antibiotic—β-lactam, penicillin derivative,** cell wall inhibitor; same mechanism as penicillin; distinguished by activity against **Gram-negative rods**; bactericidal	Gram positive cocci, Gram-positive rods, Gram-negative cocci, and **Gram-negative rods—extended spectrum**: *E. coli, Proteus, Salmonella, Shigella*, and *H. influenzae*	**Hypersensitivity reaction; pseudomembrane colitis; rash when given to mononucleosis patients**	Not effective against penicillinase resistant staphylococcus, **combined with clauvulanic acid** (pencillinase inhibitor) to enhance spectrum; amoxicillin is used as an oral agent and ampicillin as IV agent
Amoxicillin/ Clavulanic acid [Augmentin]	**Antibiotic—clavulanic acid inhibits β-lactamase**			
Amphetamine	**Stimulant—releases NE, dopamine,** and 5-HT	**Narcolepsy; attention-deficit disorder; weight reduction**	**Dilated pupils; psychosis; hallucinations;** increased BP; **MNEMONIC:** AmFATamines = FAT eyes	Contraindicated with MAOI; metabolized by liver

Therapeutic Agent (common name, if relevant) [trade name, where appropriate]	Class–Pharmacology and Pharmacokinetics	Indications	Side or Adverse Effects	Contraindications or Precautions to Consider; Notes
Amphotericin B [Fungizone]	**Antifungal—binds to cell membrane sterols** (esp. ergosterol); forms pores in membrane; fungicidal	**Wide spectrum fungal coverage: *Candida, Histoplasma, Cryptococcus, Blastomyces, Aspergillus, Coccidioides, Sporothrix*, and *Mucor***	**Impairment of renal function; hypersensitivity; flushing; fever; chills;** hypotension; **convulsions;** thrombophlebitis; anemia; arrhythmias	**Does not enter CNS;** poor GI absorption, so given IV; administered intrathecal for meningitis
Ampicillin	**Antibiotic—β-lactam, penicillin derivative,** cell wall inhibitor; same mechanism as penicillin; distinguished by activity against **Gram-negative rods**; bactericidal	Gram-positive cocci, Gram-positive rods, Gram-negative cocci, and **Gram-negatives rods—extended spectrum**: *E. coli, Proteus, Salmonella, Shigella*, and *H. influenzae*	**Hypersensitivity reaction; pseudomembrane colitis; rash, when given to mononucleosis patients**	Not effective against penicillinase resistant staphylococcus, **combined with clauvulanic acid** (penicillinase inhibitor) to enhance spectrum; amoxicillin is used as oral agent and ampicillin as IV agent
Amprenavir	**Antiviral, protease inhibitor—** protease responsible for final step of viral proliferation; inhibits protease in progeny virons → assembly of nonfunctional viruses	**AIDS (Used in HAART)**	**GI irritation (nausea, diarrhea), hyperglycemia, and lipodystrophy**	**All protease inhibitors end in -navir; metabolism occurs by CYP450**
Amrinone [Inocor]	Inotropic agent—**phosphodiesterase inhibitor;** increases contractility via increase in intracellular Ca^{2+}	Acute CHF heart failure	**Thrombocytopenia,** arrhythmias, hepatotoxicity, and gastrointesinal disturbances	Rarely used today because of the side effects
Anastrozole [Arimidex]	Aromatase inhibitor	**Breast cancer** in postmenopausal women	Hot flashes, nausea, and vomiting	Can be used in ER positive or hormone receptor unknown breast cancer
Anistreplase (APSAC) [Eminase]	**Thrombolytic—plasminogen activator**	Lysis of clots	Hemorrhage	Active compound via deacylation by esterase
Anthraquinones	**Simulant laxative**—reduces absorption of electrolytes and water from gut	Constipation		
α_2-Antiplasmin	Inhibits fibrinolysis			
Aprotinin [Trasylol]	Hemostatic agent—antiplasmin activator	Inhibits fibrinolysis; promotes thrombosis		
Asparaginase [Elspar]	Antineoplastic—deprives cells of asparagines	Cancer	Fever; mental depression; coma; hepatotoxicity	
Aspart [Novolog]	**Rapid acting insulin—***see mechanism for insulin*	**Diabetes mellitus** (typically **Type 1**), **hyperkalemia, and stress induced hyperglycemia**	**Hypoglycemia** (diaphoresis, vertigo, and tachycardia); insulin allergy; insulin antibodies; lipodystrophy	

Atenolol [Tenormin]	Antihypertensive—β_1 **blocker**	Hypertension; angina	Bradycardia, heart block, fatigue, impotence, **masks signs of hypoglycemia in diabetics**	**Cardioselective**
Atorvastatin [Lipitor]	**Lipid-lowering agent—HMG-CoA reductase inhibitor,** inhibits synthesis of cholesterol precursor mevalonate; **decreases LDL, increases HDL, and decreases TG**	**High LDL, preventative after thrombotic event (e.g., MI and stroke)**	Reversible increase in LFTs, myositis	**Contraindicated in pregnancy** or lactating women and children; **increased incidence of rhabdomyolysis when taken with fibric acid, niacin, cyclosporine, and erythromycin**
Atracurium [Tracrium injection]	**Nondepolarizing** neuromuscular blocker			Minimal histamine release
Atropine	**Reversible cholinergic muscarinic blocker**	Dries salivary secretions; Parkinson disease; peptic ulcer; diarrhea; GI spasm; bladder spasm; COPD; asthma; cholinomimetic poisoning; antidiarrheal; antiemetic; high dose: vasodilation as a result of histamine release; mydriasis and cyclopegia (thorough fundus exam, accurate refraction)	Dry mouth; hyperthermia; mydriasis; tachycardia; hot and flushed skin; agitation; delirium; **MNEMONIC: Dry as a bone (dry mouth), hot as a hare (inhibition of sweating), red as a beet (tachycardia, cutaneous vasodilation), blind as a bat (blurring vision), mad as a hatter (hallucinations and delirium)**	Contraindicated in patients with glaucoma and elderly men with BPH
Aurothioglucose [Solganal]	Antirheumatic—gold salt	Rheumatic arthritis	Skin eruption; itching; toxic nephritis; bone marrow suppression	
Aurothiomalate	Antirheumatic—gold salt	Rheumatic arthritis	Skin eruption; itching; toxic nephritis; bone marrow suppression	
Azathioprine [Imuran]	Immunosuppressant—**purine antagonist;** inhibits nucleic acid metabolism; blocks both CMI and humoral response	**Transplant** (esp. kidney); **acute glomerulonephritis; renal component of lupus; rheumatoid arthritis**	Bone marrow depression; rash; fever; nausea; vomiting; hepatotoxicity; malignancy; GI intolerance	**Metabolized by xanthine oxidase**
Azithromycin	**Antibiotic—macrolide,** protein synthesis inhibitor; binds to the 23S RNA of the 50S ribosome subunits → blocks translocation → prevents protein synthesis; bacterostatic	**First choice for cell wall–deficient bugs: *Mycoplasma, Rickettsia, Chlamydia, Legionella*; *Corynebacterium diphtheria*;** Gram-positive cocci (*Streptococcus*)	GI discomfort, **acute cholestatic hepatitis, eosinophilia, skin rashes;** increases the concentration of **oral anticoagulants** and theophyllines	Can be used in patients with **streptococcal infections** and **pencillin allergies**
Azlocillin	Antibiotic—β-lactam	*Pseudomonas; Proteus*		IV or IM (cannot be given PO because extremely unstable in gastric acid)
Aztreonam [Azactam]	**Antibiotic—monocyclic β-lactam,** cell wall inhibitor; same mechanism as penicillin (binds to PBP3); bactericidal	**Gram-negative bacteria, esp. *Pseudomonas, Klebsiella, Serratia,* and *Enterobacteriacaea*; no activity against Gram-positives or anaerobes**	Skin rash, GI distress (nausea, vomiting, etc.)	**Does not cross-react with penicillin; synergistic with aminoglycosides;** can be used in patients with **penicillin allergies** and **renal insufficiency who cannot take aminoglycosides**

Therapeutic Agent (common name, if relevant) [trade name, where appropriate]	Class–Pharmacology and Pharmacokinetics	Indications	Side or Adverse Effects	Contraindications or Precautions to Consider; Notes
Bacitracin	Antibiotic—**inhibits cell wall formation; bactericidal**	**Gram-positive** bacteria	**Nephrotoxic**	Topical only
Baclofen [Lioresal]	Skeletal muscle relaxant—**GABA mimetic;** works at the $GABA_b$ receptor	**Muscle spasms;** tetanus contractions; orthopedic manipulation		
BCNU (carmustine)	Antineoplastic—**DNA alkylation**	Cancer	Delayed bone marrow suppression; lung and kidney damage	
Beclomethasone	Corticosteroids—inhibit leukotriene synthesis → reduces inflammation and leads to bronchodilation	Asthma; COPD	**Osteoporosis; Cushingoid reaction; psychosis; glucose intolerance; infection; hypertension; cataracts**	
Benserazide	Antiparkinsonian—inhibits decarboxylase (L-DOPA to dopamine) in periphery	Parkinson disease		
Benztropine [Cogentin]	**Antiparkinsonian—muscarinic blocker; H_1 blocker**	Parkinson disease	Sedation, urinary retention, dry mouth, constipation, and mental confusion	Less effective than levodopa in Parkinson disease
Bephenium hydroxynaphthoate	Antihelmintic—cholinergic agonist causing contraction, then relaxation in worm	Necator and Ancylostoma (hookworms)	Vomiting	
Betamethasone	Glucocortcoid	**Induction of surfactant synthesis in premature infants**		One of two steroids to cross placenta
Bethanechol [Urecholine, Duvoid]	**Muscarinic agonist**	**Atony of bladder; paralytic ileus; MNEMONIC:** **B**ethanechol stimulates the **b**ladder and **b**owel	**D**iarrhea/**D**ecreased BP, **U**rination, **M**iosis, **B**ronchoconstriction, **E**xcitation of skeletal muscle, **L**acrimation, **S**alivation/**S**weating— **MNEMONIC: DUMBELS**	**Contraindicated in patients with peptic ulcer, asthma, hyperthyroidism, and Parkinson disease**
Bisacodyl [Ducolax]	**Stimulant laxative**; increases peristalsis	Constipation	Electrolyte imbalances (chronic use); gastric irritation	
Bis-chloroethylamines (nitrogen mustards) [Mustargen]	Antineoplastic—**DNA alkylation and cross-linking**	Cancer	Nausea; vomiting; bone marrow suppression; alopecia; teratogenicity; carcinogenicity	
Bismuth [Pepto-Bismol]	**Cytoprotectant—binds to ulcer base → protection; allows bicarbonate ion secretion to reestablish pH gradient in the mucous layer**	**Traveler's diarrhea,** peptic ulcer disease		

Black widow spider venom	**Presynaptic neuromuscular junction blocker—overstimulates ACh release**			
Bleomycin [Blenoxane]	**Antineoplastic—binds, intercalates, and cuts DNA**	**Cancer; testicular cancer and Hodgkin disease**	**Pulmonary fibrosis;** fever; blistering; stomatitis; hypersensitivity reactions (anaphylaxis)	
Botulinum [Botox, Dysport]	**Neuromuscular blocker—presynaptic neuromuscular junction blocker; prevents ACh release**	Wrinkles, muscle spasm	Paralysis	
Bretylium [Bretylol]	Antiarrhythmic (class III)—K^+-channel blocker; prolongs ventricular action potential, effective refractory period, and blocks NE release	Arrhythmias; refractory ventricular fibrillation and ventricular tachycardia during cardiac arrest	Orthostatic hypotension; nausea; vomiting	
Bromocriptine [Parlodel]	Antiparkinsonian—**agonist at D_2; partial antagonist at D_1**	**Parkinson disease; hyperprolactinemia; acromegaly** (paradoxical effect—releases growth hormone from normal pituitary)	**Inhibits prolactin release;** hallucination, delirium, nausea, vomiting, cardiac arrhythmia, postural hypotension, and erythromelagia	
Buclizine	Antiemetic	Sedation; parkinsonism		
Budesonide [Rhinocort]	Intranasal glucocorticoids—decrease cytokine synthesis, downregulate inflammatory response in the nasal mucosa	Nasal congestion, allergic rhinitis	Local irritation of nasal mucosa, epistaxis	
Bumetanide [Bumex]	Loop diuretic—inhibits $Na^+/K^+/2Cl^-$ reabsorption in the Loop of Henle	CHF; diuresis; pulmonary edema; acute hypercalcemia; acute hyperkalemia; acute renal failure	Ototoxicity; interstitial nephritis; hyperuricemia; acute hypovolemia; hypokalemia; metabolic alkalosis; hyperglycemia; hypocalcemia; hypomagnesmia	
α-Bungarotoxin	Postsynaptic neuromuscular junction blocker; irreversibly binds nicotinic receptor		Paralysis	Component of snake venom
Bupivacaine	Anesthetic—blocks Na^+ channel intracellularly	Local anesthetic	Sleepiness; light-headedness; myocardial depression; hypotension; visual/audio disturbances; restlessness; nystagmus; shivering; tonic–clonic convulsions; death	
Buprenorphine [Buprenex]	Opioid analog—mixed agonist/antagonist action	Treatment of opioid/cocaine dependence	Respiratory depression, sedation, and nausea/vomiting	
Buproprion [Wellbutrin, Zyban]	**Antidepressant—unknown mechanism; thought to be an agonist at D_2, 5-HT**	Major depression, **smoking cessation**	Tachycardia, insomnia, headache, and seizure (especially bulimic patients)	Does not have sexual side effects such as those occurring with SSRIs

Therapeutic Agent (common name, if relevant) [trade name, where appropriate]	Class–Pharmacology and Pharmacokinetics	Indications	Side or Adverse Effects	Contraindications or Precautions to Consider; Notes
Buspirone [BuSpar]	Antidepressant—partial agonist at serotonin receptors	Generalized anxiety		**2 weeks for effects to become apparent**
Caffeine [NoDoz]	Stimulant—**adenosine receptor blocker;** stimulates CNS and cardiac muscle; relaxes smooth muscle; produces diuresis; increases cerebrovascular resistance	**Acute migraine attack**	Crosses placenta and into breast milk	**Avoid in peptic ulcer patients** because it stimulates gastric mucosal secretions
Calcitonin [Calcimar, Miacalcin]	Hypocalcemic agent—antiosteoporotic agent; **lowers plasma Ca^{2+} and phosphate;** inhibits bone and kidney reabsorption	**Hypercalcemia; Paget disease; osteoporosis**		
Calcium carbonate [TUMS, Caltrate]	**Antacid**—buffers gastric acid by raising pH	Peptic ulcer, gastritis, esophageal reflux, and calcium deficiency	**Hypercalcemia, rebound acid increase, and hypokalemia**	**Can affect the absorption, bioavailability, or urinary excretion of drugs by changing gastric pH, urinary pH, or gastric emptying**
Calcium citrate	Dietary Ca^{2+} supplement	Ca^{2+} deficiency		
Calcium gluconate	Dietary Ca^{2+} supplement	Ca^{2+} deficiency		
Calcium lactate	Dietary Ca^{2+} supplement	Ca^{2+} deficiency		
Captopril [Capoten]	Antihypertensive—ACE inhibitor → inhibits conversion of angiotensin I to II → decreases angiotensin II levels → prevents vasoconstriction from angiotensin II	Hypertension; CHF; post-MI agent; vasodilator	**Hyperkalemia, cough** (persistent dry), **angioedema,** taste changes, orthostatic hypotension, proteinuria, renal failure (in bilateral renal artery stenosis), neutropenia, and rash	Contraindicated in pregnancy (fetal renal malformation)
Carbachol [Isopto carbachol]	Antiglaucoma agent—muscarinic cholinergic agonist, works on both muscarinic and nicotinic receptors	Miotic; glaucoma	**DUMBELS** (see Acetylcholine)	Contraindicated in patients with peptic ulcer, asthma, hyper-thyroid, and Parkinson disease
Carbamazepine [Tegretol]	Antiepileptic—prolongs inactivated state of Na^+ channels; decreases release of glutamate (and other excitatory neurotransmitters)	Epilepsy (partial and **tonic–clonic** (drug of choice); **trigeminal neuralgia** (drug of choice)	**Agranulocytosis, liver toxicity (check LFTs), and aplastic anemia**	**Induces** cytochrome **P450**
Carbenicillin	**Antibiotic—β-lactam, penicillin derivative,** cell wall inhibitor; same mechanism as penicillin; distinguished by activity against ***Pseudomonas***; bactericidal	**Extended spectrum**–*Pseudomonas*; *Proteus*, and *Enterobacter* species	**Hypersensitivity reactions,** decreased platelet function	Not effective against penicillinase resistant staphylococcus, **combined with clauvulanic acid** (pencillinase inhibitor) to enhance spectrum; **resistant to β-lactamase;** administered IV

Carbidopa [Sinemet]	Antiparkinsonian—inhibits decarboxylase (l-DOPA to dopamine) **in periphery, does not cross BBB**	**Parkinson's disease; used with levodopa,** which reduces metabolism of dopamine in periphery and increases its availability in CNS, especially effective for bradykinesia	**Treatment efficacy declines with progression of disease** due to a decrease in healthy dopaminergic neurons required for levodopa's MOA	
Carboplatin [Paraplatin]	Antineoplastic—**cross-links DNA**	Ovarian cancer	Bone marrow suppression and anemia	Contains platinum
Carboprost [Prostin]	Abortive agent—PGF_{2a}	Therapeutic abortion	Nausea; vomiting; diarrhea	
Carvedilol	**Antihypertensive,** antiarrhythmic (class II)— α- and β-blocker	**Hypertension, angina, MI, and antiarrythmic**	**Impotence, asthma, bradycardia,** AV block, heart failure, sedation, and sleep alterations	
Caspofungin	**Antifungal**—inhibits cell wall synthesis	Invasive aspergillosis or *Candida*	GI irritation, flushing	Administered IV
Castor oil	**Stimulant laxative**—reduces absorption of electrolytes and water from gut; active component is ricinoleic acid	Constipation; labor induction		
Celecoxib [Celebrex]	**NSAID—selectively inhibits COX-2**	Rheumatoid arthritis, osteoarthritis; pain, inflammation	**Increased risk of thrombosis, sulfa allergy, and less toxic to GI mucosa**	COX-2 selectivity reduces inflammation while minimizing GI adverse effects (ulcers)
Cephalosporin	**Antibiotic—β-lactam,** cell wall inhibitor; same mechanism as penicillin, **from first generation to third generation:** a. **Gram-positive** coverage **decreases** b. **Gram-negative** coverage **increases** c. **CNS penetration increases** d. β-lactamase **resistance increases**; bactericidal	**First generation: Gram + cocci and PEcK** (*Proteus mirabilis*, ***E.** coli*, and ***K**lebsiella*); **Second generation:** same as 1st generation + **HENPEcK** (***H.** flu*, ***E**nterobacter*, and ***N**eisseria*); **Third generation: cephalosporins are used for meningitis, *Klebsiella*, Lyme disease, and Gram-negative bacteria**	**Hypersensitivity reaction; pain at injection site; nephrotoxicity; intolerance to alcohol** (cefamandole, cefotetan, moxalactam, and cefoperazone); **hypothrombinemia** (cefamandole, cefoperazone, and moxalactam, due to vitamin K inhibition); **thrombophlebitis; positive Coombs' test**	**First generation:** cefazolin, cephalexin; **second generation:** cefaclor, cefoxitin, and cefuroxime; **third generation:** cef**tri**axone, cefoperazone, and ceftazidime; **fourth generation:** cefepime; **Pseudomonas coverage:** ceftazidime, cefoperazone, and cefepime; **cross-hypersensitivity with penicillins occurs in 5%–10% of patients**
Chloral hydrate	Anesthetic agent	Sedative (in children); hypnotic	Bitter taste, GI distress	Inexpensive
Chlorambucil [Leukeran]	Antineoplastic—DNA **alkylation and cross-linking**	Cancer	Nausea, vomiting, bone marrow suppression (mild), alopecia, teratogenicity, carcinogenicity, and **pulmonary fibrosis**	
Chloramphenicol [Chloromycetin]	**Antibiotic—protein synthesis inhibitor; inhibits 50S peptidyl transferase activity; bacteriostatic,** but bactericidal vs. *Haemophilus influenzae* and *Neisseria meningitides*	Meningitis (*H. influenza, N. meningitidis, and S. pneumoniae*); typhoid fever; *Salmonella*; *Rickettsia* (Rocky Mountain spotted fever in children); Bacteroides	**Fatal aplastic anemia; bone marrow suppression; gray baby syndrome** (cyanosis, vomiting, green stools, and vasomotor collapse due to insufficient glucorindase in neonatal liver)	Interactions with phenytoin, warfarin, or coumadin; inhibits cytochrome P450; used to treat serious infections after other antibiotics have failed given side effects

Therapeutic Agent (common name, if relevant) [trade name, where appropriate]	Class–Pharmacology and Pharmacokinetics	Indications	Side or Adverse Effects	Contraindications or Precautions to Consider; Notes
Chlordiazepoxide [Libritabs]	Long-acting benzodiazepine; antianxiety; enhances GABA; increases IPSP amplitude	Sedative; hypnotic; antianxiety; antiepileptic, alcohol withdrawal		
Chlorguanide	Antimalarial—inhibits dihydrofolate reductase	**Prophylaxis for falciparum** malaria; **suppression** of **vivax** malaria	Minor GI upset	
Chloroquine phosphate [Aralen]	Antimalarial—uncertain mechanism	**Suppression of malaria** and treatment of **acute** attack; **amebiasis; Clonorchis; rheumatoid arthritis; SLE**	Headache; GI disturbances; visual disturbances; **pruritus;** prolonged therapy may lead to **retinopathy**	
Chlorpheniramine [Chlor-Trimeton]	Antihistamine—H_1 blocker	Allergies; **motion sickness**	Sedation; CNS depression; atropine-like effects; allergic dermatitis; blood dyscrasias; teratogenicity; acute antihistamine poisoning	
Chloroprocaine	Anesthetic—block Na^+ channel intracellularly	Local anesthetic	Sleepiness; light-headedness; visual/audio disturbances; restlessness; nystagmus; shivering; tonic–clonic convulsions; death	
Chlorpromazine [Thorazine]	Antiemetic, antipsychotic— phenothiazines; blocks D_2, α_1, and H_1 receptors	Antipsychotic; antiemetic; hiccups	**Extrapyramidal** (dystonia, akinesia, akathisia,and tardive dyskinesia), **anticholinergic** (dry mouth, constipation), **alpha blockade** (hypotension), **histamine** (sedation); toxicity results in neuroleptic malignant syndrome (rigidity, myoglobinuria, autonomic instability, and hyperpyrexia)	Atropine-like effects fairly common
Chlorpropamide [Diabinese]	**Hypoglycemic agent, first generation sulfonylurea**—closes potassium channel in β-cell membrane → reduces K^+ efflux, increases Ca^{2+} influx → increases secretion of insulin	Oral treatment for **NIDDM (type II diabetes)**	**Hypoglycemia;** GI disturbances; muscle weakness; mental confusion	
Cholestyramine [Questran]	Lipid-lowering agent—**bile acid resins** act by binding bile acids in the small intestine, forming insoluble complexes that are excreted; decreased bile acids stimulate the liver to increase conversion of cholesterol to bile acids, increasing hepatic LDL receptors, decreasing serum LDL	Reduction of cholesterol	Steatorrhea; constipation; impairment of absorption of drugs/vitamins	**Inhibits warfarin absorption**

Chorionic gonadotropin [Pregnyl]	Infertility therapy—LH-like in action	Treats infertility; induces ovulation; induces masculinization in infertile men; diagnostic for cryptorchidism in young boys		
Cimetidine [Tagamet]	**H_2 blocker—blocks histamine H_2 receptors reversibly → decreases proton secretion by parietal cells**	**Peptic ulcer disease, gastritis, esophageal reflux**	**Gynecomastia, impotence**, decreased libido in males, **confusion, dizziness, and headaches**	**Crosses placenta; decreases renal excretion of creatinine; P-450 inhibitor**
Ciprofloxacin [Cipro]	**Antibiotic—Quinolone, DNA synthesis inhibitor; inhibits DNA gyrase** (topoisomerase II) and **topoisomerase IV** → blocks DNA synthesis; bactericidal	**Gram-negative infections** (esp. UTI and bone): *Pseudomonas*, Enterobacteriaceae, and *Neisseria*; **Gram-positive infections:** (staphylococci); **intracellular**: **Legionella**	**GI disturbances; headache; dizziness; phototoxicity; cartilage damage (children, fetus); tendonitis** and **tendon rupture (adults); myalgias (children)**	May elevate theophylline to toxic levels, causing seizure
Cisapride [Propulsid]	**GI stimulant—prokinetic; increases acetylcholine release at myenteric plexus** → increases esophageal tone, gastric/duodenal contractility (improves colon transit time)	Constipation	**Torsades des pointes**	Rarely used; interacts with **erythromycin, ketocaonazole, nefazodone, and fluconazole** to produce **Torsades des pointes**
Cisplatin [Platinol]	Antineoplastic—cross-links DNA	Cancer	Bone marrow and renal toxicity; **cystitis; peripheral neuropathy; ototoxicity;** alopecia (severe)	
Citalopram	Selective serotonin reuptake inhibitors—inhibit **reuptake** of 5-HT at neuronal synapses	Major depression, OCD, anorexia,and bulimia	Inhibits liver enzymes, nausea, agitation, **sexual dysfunction** (anorgasmia), and dystonic reactions	Contraindicated with **MAOIs** secondary to **serotonin syndrome** (hyperthermia, muscle rigidity, and cardiovascular collapse); allows time for antidepressant effect, usually takes 2–3 weeks
Clarithromycin	**Antibiotic—Macrolide**, protein synthesis inhibitor; binds to the 23S RNA of the 50S ribosome subunits → blocks translocation → prevents protein synthesis; bacterostatic	**First choice for cell wall–deficient bugs: *Mycoplasma, Rickettsia, Chlamydia*, and *Legionella*; *Corynebacterium diphtheria;*** Gram-positive cocci (*Streptococcus*)	GI discomfort, **acute cholestatic hepatitis, eosinophilia,** and **skin rashes;** increases concentration of **oral anticoagulants** and theophyllines	Can be used in patients with **streptococcal infections** and **pencillin allergies**
Clavulanic acid	β-lactamase inhibitor; synergistic with penicillins			
Clindamycin [Cleocin]	**Antibiotic—protein synthesis inhibitor; binds to 50S subunits →** blocks peptide bond formation; bacteriostatic or bactericidal depending on concentration, site, and organism	**Gram-positive bacteria (*Streptococcus, Pneumococcus,* and *Staphylococcus*); treats anaerobic** infections (*Bacteroides fragilis, Clostridium perfringens*)	Severe diarrhea; **potentially fatal pseudomembranous colitis caused by *Clostridium difficile***	
Clofazimine [Lamprene]	Antibiotic—antileprosy; unknown mechanism	*Mycobacterium leprae*	Turns skin red-brown or black	

Therapeutic Agent (common name, if relevant) [trade name, where appropriate]	Class–Pharmacology and Pharmacokinetics	Indications	Side or Adverse Effects	Contraindications or Precautions to Consider; Notes
Clofibrate [Atromid-S]	Lipid-lowering agent—**upregulates lipoprotein lipase (periphery) → increases TG clearance; decreases LDL, increases HDL, and decreases TG**	**Increased TG, increased LDL**	Myositis, increased LFTs; increased risk of GI and liver cancer; potentiates anticoagulant drugs; gallstones; mild GI disturbances	
Clomiphene [Clomid]	**Selective estrogen receptor modulator**—binds estrogen receptors in pituitary → prevents normal feedback inhibition, increases LH and FSH release from pituitary → stimulates ovulation	**Stimulates ovulation in infertility, PCOS**	**Hot flashes, ovarian enlargement, multiple gestation pregnancy, and visual disturbances**	
Clomipramine	Tricyclic antidepressants—inhibit **reuptake** of NE and 5-HT at neuronal synapses	Major depression, OCD, and panic disorder	Sedation, **alpha blocking effects** (orthostatic hypotension), **anticholinergic** (tachycardia, dry mouth, and urinary retention), hallucinations (in elderly), and confusion (elderly); overdose toxicity results in **convulsions, coma, cardiotoxicity** (arrhythmias), respiratory depression, and hyperpyrexia	
Clonazepam [Klonopin]	**Antiepileptic—benzodiazepine**	**Epilepsy (absence of seizures)**		
Clonidine [Catapres]	**Antihypertensive—c**entrally acting sympathetic agent (α_2 agonist) → decreases sympathetic outflow from CNS → decreases peripheral resistance	**Hypertension; smoking withdrawal; heroin and cocaine withdrawal**	Drowsiness; **dry mouth; rebound hypertension after abrupt withdrawal**	
Clotrimazole [Lotrimin, Mycelex]	Antifungal—inhibits ergosterol synthesis, preventing cell membrane formation	**Topical use against yeasts, dermatophytes, ringworm, fungi, mold, and oral candidiasis in AIDS**	Burning, itching, and redness when used topically; thrombophlebitis; nausea; vomiting; anaphylaxis when used IV	
Cloxacillin [Cloxapen]	**Antibiotic—β-lactam; penicillinase-resistant**	***Staphylococcus* infections**		
Clozapine **[Clozaril]**	Atypical antipsychotic—blocks D_4, α_1, 5-HT, muscarinic receptors	Schizophrenia, useful for positive and negative symptoms	Agranulocytosis, **Extrapyramidal** (occurs at a lower rate than typicals), **anticholinergic** (dry mouth, constipation), **alpha blockade** (hypotension), **histamine** (sedation); toxicity results in neuroleptic malignant syndrome (occurs at a lower rate than typicals)	Second-line agent used for refractory schizophrenia; weekly blood counts for patients on this agent due to agranulocytosis

Cocaine	**CNS stimulant—blocks NE, 5-HT, and dopamine reuptake**	**Local anesthetic**	**Vasoconstriction; hypertension; nasal mucus ischemia**	
Codeine	**Opioid agonist**	**Pain;** antitussive	**Constipation**	Converted to morphine 10%
Colchicine	Anti-inflammatory—interrupts **microtubule formation**, thereby interfering with normal mitosis and inhibiting WBC migration and phagocytosis	Acute gout therapy	Diarrhea (common)	Contraindicated in elderly and feeble patients and in patients with GI disturbances, cardiac anomalies, or renal problems
Colestipol [Colestid]	Lipid-lowering agent—**bile acid resin,** impedes fat absorption; **lowers LDL;** binds cholesterol metabolites	Reduction of cholesterol	Steatorrhea; constipation; impaired absorption of drugs and vitamins	
Corticotropin-releasing hormone (CRH)	Increases ACTH production by anterior pituitary	Used in diagnosis of Cushing syndrome		
Cortisol (hydrocortisone) [Hydrocortone, Nutracort]	**Glucocorticoid—induces new protein synthesis; increases gluconeogenesis and lipolysis; reduces peripheral glucose use; catabolic effect on muscle, bone, skin, fat, and lymph tissue; anti-inflammatory; immunosuppressant**	**Adrenal insufficiency; congenital adrenal hyperplasia; diagnosis of pituitary-adrenal disorder; reduces inflammation (esp. chronic); leukemia; decreases hypercalcemia**	**Iatrogenic Cushing syndrome; redistribution of fat; acne; insomnia; weight gain; hypokalemia; decrease in skeletal muscle; osteoporosis; hyperglycemia; ulcers; psychosis; cataracts; increased susceptibility to infections; growth suppression in children**	
Cosyntropin [Cortrosyn]	ACTH analog—increases production of steroids by adrenal	Used in diagnosis of adrenocortical insufficiency		
Cromolyn [Nasalcrom, Gastrocrom]	**Antiasthmatic—p**revents release of mediators from mast cells → prevents bronchoconstriction and inflammation	Asthma prophylaxis	**Laryngeal edema (rare)**	Not used during acute exacerbation
Cyanocobalamin (Anacobin)	Supplies vitamin B_{12}	B_{12} deficiency		
Cyclobenzaprine [Flexeril]	Centrally acting muscle relaxant	Muscle spasms; tetanus contractions; orthopedic manipulation	Antimuscarinic effects	
Cyclophosphamide [Cytoxan]	Immunosuppressant—**alkylating agent; destroys proliferating lymphoid cells; alkylates resting cells**	**Transplant rejection; rheumatic arthritis**	GI and bone marrow toxicity; **hemorrhagic cystitis**	
Cycloserine [Seromycin]	Antibiotic—analog of D-alanine; interferes with cell wall synthesis	Mycobacterium	Psychotic reactions	
Cyclosporine [Sandimmune]	Immunosuppressant—**inhibits T-helper cell activity; inhibits IL-2, IL-3, and IFN-γ formation by T-helper cells**	**Transplant rejection**	**Nephrotoxic; hepatotoxic; hypertension; increased incidence of viral infection and lymphoma**	

Therapeutic Agent (common name, if relevant) [trade name, where appropriate]	Class–Pharmacology and Pharmacokinetics	Indications	Side or Adverse Effects	Contraindications or Precautions to Consider; Notes
Cyproheptadine [Periactin]	Antihistamine—antipruritic; 5-HT_3 agonist; histamine blocker	Decreases diarrhea in carcinoid tumors; decreases dumping syndrome	Weight gain	
Cytosine arabinoside [Cytosar-U]	Antineoplastic—inhibits DNA replication and RNA polymerization; competitive inhibitor of dCTP; inhibits chain elongation	Cancer; AML	Severe myelosuppression; stomatitis; alopecia	
Dacarbazine (DTIC-Dome)	Antineoplastic—DNA alkylation; strand breakage; inhibits nucleic acid and protein synthesis	Cancer		
Dactinomycin [Cosmegen]	Antineoplastic—cross-links DNA; intercalates into DNA	Cancer	Skin eruptions; hyperkeratosis	
Danazol [Danocrine]	**Testosterone derivative—weak agonist for androgen, progesterone, and glucocorticoid receptors**	**Endometriosis and fibrocystic disease**	**Masculinization in females; gynecomastia** in males	
Dantrolene [Dantrium]	**Noncentrally acting muscle relaxant—decreases Ca^{2+} from sarcoplasmic reticulum**	**Malignant hyperthermia**	**Hepatotoxic**	
Dapsone [Dapsone]	Antibiotic—related to sulfonamides	*Mycobacterium leprae*	GI disturbances; hemolysis; methemoglobinemia	
Daunorubicin [DaunoXome, Cerubidine]	Antineoplastic**—oxidizes free radicals; breaks DNA; intercalates into DNA;** affects plasma membrane	Cancer	Cardiac changes resulting in cumulative **cardiotoxicity**	
Deferoxamine [Desferal]	**Metal chelator**	**Acute toxicity of iron**	**Hypotensive shock; neurotoxic if long-term use**	
Delaviridine	**Antiviral, non-nucleoside reverse transcriptase inhibitor—**binds viral reverse transcriptase and inhibits movement of protein domains → terminates viral DNA synthesis → prevents integration of viral genome into host DNA	**AIDS (Used in HAART)**	**Neutropenia, anemia, peripheral neuropathy, and rash**	**Effects of bone marrow suppression such as neutropenia and anemia can be reduced by the addition of GM-CSF**
Desflurane [Suprane]	Anesthetic	General anesthetic	Irritating to airway	

Desipramine [Norpramin]	Tricyclic antidepressants—inhibit **reuptake** of NE and 5-HT at neuronal synapses	Major depression, panic disorder, and anxiety	Sedation, **alpha blocking effects** (orthostatic hypotension), **anticholinergic** (tachycardia, dry mouth, and urinary retention), hallucinations (in elderly), and confusion (elderly); overdose toxicity results in **convulsions, coma, cardiotoxicity** (arrhythmias), respiratory depression, and hyperpyrexia	Desipramine is the least sedating of the TCA
Desmopressin (DDAVP)	**Antidiuretic—synthetic analog of ADH,** recruits water channels to luminal membrane in collecting duct	Antidiuresis; central (pituitary) diabetes insipidus	Overhydration; allergic reaction; larger doses result in pallor, diarrhea, and hypertension; coronary constriction; chronic rhinopharyngitis	**Synthetic analog to vasopressin; intranasal administration**
Desogestrel	**Progesterone**—binds progesterone receptors	**Endometrial cancer,** amenorrhea, abnormal uterine bleeding, and **prevention of pregnancy**		Also used to prevent endometrial hyperplasia in postmenopausal women taking estrogen
Dexamethasone [Decadron, Maxidex]	**Corticosteroid—reduces lymph node and spleen size; inhibits cell cycle activity of lymphoid cells; lyses T cells; suppresses antibody, prostaglandin, and leukotriene synthesis; blocks monocyte production of IL-1**	**Antiemetic; autoimmune disorders; allergic reactions; asthma; organ transplantation (esp. during rejection crisis); test for etiology of hypercortisolism**	Insomnia; epigastric disturbances; **Cushingoid reaction; psychosis; glucose intolerance; infection; hypertension; cataracts**	
DHEA	Androgen and estrogen precursor	Acne; hair loss; hirsutism; deepening of voice		
Diazepam [Valium]	**Antianxiety, benzodiazepine—enhances GABA; increases IPSP amplitude**	**Sedative; hypnotic; antianxiety; antiepileptic (status epilepticus, grand mal)**	**Sedation**	
Diazepam-binding inhibitor (DBI)	Benzodiazepine receptor antagonist			
Diazoxide	**K^+ channel opener**—hyperpolarizes and relaxes vascular smooth muscle	**Hypertension**	Hypoglycemia (reduces insulin release); hypotension	
Diclofenac [Cataflam, Voltaren]	NSAID—enteric-coated			
Dicloxacillin [Dynapen, Pathocil]	**Antibiotic—β-lactam, penicillin derivative,** cell wall inhibitor; same mechanism as penicillin; distinguished by activity against **penicillinase-producing *Staphylococcus*;** bactericidal	**Staphylococcus infections** (except MRSA)	**Hypersensitivity reactions;** interstitial nephritis (methicillin)	Penicillinase resistant; MRSA is resistant to methicillin because of altered penicillin binding protein target site

Therapeutic Agent (common name, if relevant) [trade name, where appropriate]	Class–Pharmacology and Pharmacokinetics	Indications	Side or Adverse Effects	Contraindications or Precautions to Consider; Notes
Dicyclomine [Bentyl]	Antimuscarinic	Bladder/GI spasm; decreases acid in ulcer		
Didanosine [ddA, Videx]	**Antiviral, nucleoside reverse transcriptase inhibitor—competitive inhibitor of deoxythymidine triphosphate** → incorporated into viral DNA by reverse transcriptase →terminates viral DNA synthesis (lacks 3′-hydroxyl group) → prevents integration of DNA copy of viral genome into the host DNA	**AIDS (Used in HAART)**	**Neutropenia, anemia, peripheral neuropathy, pancreatitis, and lactic acidosis**	
Diethylcarbamazine [Hetrazan]	Antihelmintic—sensitizes helminths	Filariasis to phagocytosis by macrophages	Headache; malaise; joint pain; anorexia; death of filaria causes: swelling and edema of skin, enlarged lymph nodes, hyperpyrexia, and tachycardia	
Digitoxin [Crystodigin]	Inotropic agent—cardiac glycoside; increases cardiac contractility	Severe left ventricular systolic dysfunction; antiarrhythmic	Progressive dysrhythmia; anorexia; nausea; vomiting; headache; fatigue; confusion; blurred vision; altered color perception; halos around dark objects	Contraindicated in patients with right-sided heart failure, diastolic failure; Wolff–Parkinson–White syndrome; ECG changes: increases PR, decreases QT, depresses ST, and inverts T
Digoxin [Lanoxin]	**Inotropic agent—cardiac glycoside; inhibits Na/K/ATPase → indirect inhibition of Na^+/Ca^{2+} exchanger → increases Ca^{2+} → increases cardiac contractility**	**Severe left ventricular systolic dysfunction** (increases contractility); **atrial fibrillation** (decreases conduction at AV node and depresses SA node)	**Progressive dysrhythmia;** anorexia; nausea; vomiting; headache; fatigue; **confusion; blurred vision; altered color perception; halos around dark objects**	Contraindicated in patients with right-sided heart failure, diastolic failure; **ECG changes: increases PR, decreases QT, depresses ST, and inverts T; toxicities of digoxin are increased by renal failure** (decreases excretion), **hypokalemia** (potentiates drug's effects), and **quinidine** (decreases clearance, displaces digoxin)
Diiodohydroxyquin [Yodoxin]	Antiprotozoal—direct action	Amebae	Subacute myelo-optic neuropathy	
Diltiazem [Cardizem, Dilacor]	**Antiarrhythmic (class IV)—Ca^{2+}-blocker**	**Angina; AV nodal arrhythmia; decreases blood pressure**		
Dimenhydrinate [Dramamine]	Antivertigo—antiemetic; H_1-blocker	Emesis; dizziness		
Dimercaprol [British antilewisite]	Metal chelator	Arsenic, mercury, or cadmium poisoning	Hypertension; tachycardia; headaches; nausea; vomiting; pain at injection site	

Dinoprostone [Cervidil, Prepidil]	Prostaglandin—PGE_2 analog → cervical dilation, uterine contraction	Induction of labor, termination of pregnancy		
Diphenhydramine [Benadryl]	**Antihistamine—antiemetic; muscarinic blocker; H_1-blocker (first generation)**	**Allergic reactions; asthma; motion sickness; antiemetic; insomnia**	Sedation; CNS depression; **atropine-like effects; allergic dermatitis; blood dyscrasias; teratogenicity;** acute antihistamine poisoning	Rarely used as antiparkinsonian agent
Disopyramide [Norpace]	Antiarrhythmic (class IA)—Na^+-channel blocker	Wolff–Parkinson–White syndrome	Heart failure	Contraindicated in patients with sick sinus syndrome
Disulfiram [Antabuse]	**Antialcoholic agent—inhibits aldehyde dehydrogenase**	**Alcoholism**	**Tachycardia; hyperventilation; nausea**	
Dobutamine [Dobutrex]	**Inotropic agent—β-agonist; positive inotropic effects on the heart and vasodilation**	**Acute** heart failure; **increases cardiac output**		
Docusate	**Stool softener;** by emulsifying stool, makes passage of stool easier	Constipation	Skin rash	
Doxazosin [Cardura]	Antihypertensive—α_1-blocker	Hypertension		
Doxepin [Sinequan]	Tricyclic antidepressants—inhibit **reuptake** of NE and 5-HT at neuronal synapses	Major depression, panic discrder, and potent antihistamine	Sedation, **alpha blocking effects** (orthostatic hypotension), **anticholinergic** (tachycardia, dry mouth, and urinary retention), hallucinations (in elderly), and confusion (elderly); overdose toxicity results in **convulsions, coma, cardiotoxicity** (arrhythmias), respiratory depression, and hyperpyrexia	
Doxorubicin [Adriamycin]	Antineoplastic—oxidizes free radicals; breaks DNA; intercalates into DNA; affects plasma membrane	Cancer	Cardiac changes resulting in cumulative cardiotoxicity	
Dronabinol [Marinol]	Antiemetic—unknown mechanism; binds cannabinoid receptors and inhibits vomiting center in medulla	Antiemetic, appetite stimulant in AIDS patients	Dry mouth; dizziness; inability to concentrate; disorientation; anxiety; tachycardia; depression; paranoia; psychosis	THC derivative
Echothiophate [Phospholine Iodide]	Antiglaucoma—inhibits cholinesterase; nicotinic receptor stimulator; irreversible	Closed-angle glaucoma	Open-angle glaucoma	
Edetate calcium disodium (calcium EDTA) [Calcium disodium versenate]	Metal chelator	Lead toxicity	Nephrotoxic	
Edrophonium [Enlon, Tensilon]	**Cholinesterase inhibitor**	**Diagnosis of myasthenia gravis; emergency anesthetic**		

Therapeutic Agent (common name, if relevant) [trade name, where appropriate]	Class–Pharmacology and Pharmacokinetics	Indications	Side or Adverse Effects	Contraindications or Precautions to Consider; Notes
Efavirenz	Antiviral, non-nucleoside reverse transcriptase inhibitor—**binds viral reverse transcriptase and inhibits movement of protein domains → terminates viral DNA synthesis → prevents integration of viral genome into host DNA**	**AIDS (Used in HAART)**	Neutropenia, anemia, peripheral neuropathy, and rash	Effects of bone marrow suppression such as neutropenia and anemia can be reduced by the addition of GM-CSF
Emetine	**Antiprotozoal—causes degeneration of nucleus and reticulation of cytoplasm; directly lethal**	**Severe amebic infection**	Diarrhea; nausea; vomiting; abdominal pain; cardiac effects: hypotension, precordial pain, ECG changes	
Enalapril [Vasotec]	**Antihypertensive**—ACE inhibitor → inhibits conversion of angiotensin I to II → decreases angiotensin II levels → prevents vasoconstriction from angiotensin II	Hypertension, CHF, post-MI agent, vasodilator	**Hyperkalemia, cough** (persistent dry), **angioedema,** taste changes, orthostatic hypotension, proteinuria, renal failure (in bilateral renal artery stenosis), neutropenia, and rash	Contraindicated in pregnancy (fetal renal malformation)
Encainide	Antiarrhythmia (class IC)—Na^+-channel blocker	Wolff–Parkinson–White syndrome		No antimuscarinic action; no effect on action potential
Enflurane [Ethrane]	Anesthetic agent	General anesthetic	Seizure	Abnormal ECG or seizures
Enfuvirtide	**Antiviral, fusion inhibitor**—binds viral gp41 subunit → inhibits conformation change (required for fusion with CD4 cell) → blocks vital entry and replication	**AIDS (used in patients on antiretroviral therapy with persistent viral replication)**	**Hypersensitivity reactions, reaction at injection site, and bacterial pneumonia**	**Used in combination with other antiretroviral drugs**
Enoxaparin [Lovenox]	Low-molecular-weight heparin; enhances **inhibition of factor Xa and thrombin by increasing antithrombin III activity** (preferentially increases the inhibition of factor Xa)	Prophylaxis of thrombosis	**Elevated AST/ALT (reversible); heparin-associated thrombocytopenia**	Caution in recent surgery or active bleeding ulcers or internal hemorrhages; fewer bleeding complications, more bioavailable, and longer half-life than unfractionated heparin; no requirement for monitoring
Ephedrine	Bronchodilation—mixed adrenergic agonist	Stimulates NE release; antitussive; myasthenia gravis	Increases BP	
Epinephrine	Adrenergic agonist	Acute asthma; anaphylactic shock		Activates both α and β receptors, but is preferential for β

Eplerenone	**Potassium sparing diuretic**—binds to intracellular aldosterone steroid receptors in **collecting tubules**; blocks induction of Na^+ channels and Na^+/ATPase synthesis; loss of Na^+, Cl^- in urine	Hyperaldosteronism, potassium depletion, and congestive heart failure	**Hyperkalemic metabolic acidosis**, **gynecomastia** (spironolactone), and antiandrogen effects	Like spironolactone but more selective for mineralocorticoid receptors; results in decreased secretion of K^+ and H^+, which can lead to **hyperkalemic metabolic acidosis**; often given in combination with a thiazide
Epoprostenol [Flolan]	**Prostacyclin—increases cardiac index and stroke volume; decreases pulmonary vascular resistance and mean systemic pressure**	**Pulmonary hypertension**		
Ergotamine [Ergomar]	**Antimigraine—vasoconstriction**	**Acute attack of migraine**	**Gangrene** as a result of vasoconstriction	**Contraindicated in pregnant patients or patients with cardiovascular disease or coronary artery disease**
Erythromycin [E-Mycin]	**Antibiotic—Macrolide,** protein synthesis inhibitor; binds to the 23S RNA of the 50S ribosome subunits → blocks translocation → prevents protein synthesis; bacterostatic	**First choice for cell wall–deficient bugs: *Mycoplasma, Rickettsia, Chlamydia,* and *Legionella*; *Corynebacterium diphtheria;*** Gram-positive cocci (*Streptococcus*)	GI discomfort, **acute cholestatic hepatitis, eosinophilia,** and **skin rashes;** increases concentration of **oral anticoagulants** and theophyllines	Can be used in patients with **streptococcal infections** and **pencillin allergies**
Erythropoietin (EPO) [Procrit, Epogen]	**Colony-stimulating factor**	**Anemia (especially in renal failure); AIDS**	**Hypertension**	
Esmolol [Brevibloc]	**Antiarrhythmic (class II)—β_1-selective blocker**	**Blocks the effect of catecholamines on heart; decreases the activity of nodal tissue; slow sinus rate; depresses AV conduction**	**Asthma; negative inotropic agent**	Short duration
Estrogen [Estratab, Premarin]	**Growth and development of female organs; linear bone growth; epiphyseal closure; endometrial growth; maintains responsiveness of breasts, uterus, and vagina; inhibits bone resorption; increases hepatic production of α_2-globulins, coagulation factors II, VII, IX, and X, and HDL; decreases antithrombin III and cholesterol**	**Osteoporosis; contraception; can be used in combination with progesterone**	**Small increased incidence of breast and endometrial cancers; blood clots; may lead to sodium and water retention; nausea; breast tenderness; hyperpigmentation; increased risk of bleeding, gallbladder disease, migraines, hypertension**	
Etanercept	Recombinant form of human TNF receptor → binds TNF → decreases inflammatory response	Rheumatoid arthritis, psoriasis, and ankylosing spondylitis	**Infections**	

Therapeutic Agent (common name, if relevant) [trade name, where appropriate]	Class–Pharmacology and Pharmacokinetics	Indications	Side or Adverse Effects	Contraindications or Precautions to Consider; Notes
Ethacrynic acid [Edecrin]	Phenoxyacetic acid derivative diuretic—prevents cotransport of Na^+, K^+, and Cl^- in **thick ascending limb;** loss of Na^+, Cl^-, Ca^{2+}, and K^+ in urine	**Diuresis in patients with sulfa drug allergy**	**Ototoxicity, hypokalemic metabolic alkalosis,** and dehydration	**Can be given to patients with sulfa drug allergy,** hyperuricemia, and acute gout
Ethambutol [Myambutol]	Antibiotic—unknown mechanism	Mycobacterium	**Optic neuropathy (red-green color blindness);** tolerance develops	
Ethosuximide	Antiepileptic—**decreases Ca^{2+} conduction**	Epilepsy **(absence seizures)**		
Ether	**Anesthetic agent**	**General anesthetic**	Fire/explosion	No longer used
Ethinyl estradiol	**Estrogen**—binds estrogen receptor	**In females: hypogonadism, ovarian failure,** and menstrual abnormalities; In males: **androgen dependent prostate cancer**	**Endometrial cancer, bleeding, and thrombosis**	Used in combination with progestin in patients with intact uterus given increased risk of endometrial cancer with unopposed estrogen therapy; females exposed to DES in utero increased risk of **vaginal clear cell adenocarcinoma**
Etidocaine [Duranest]	Anesthetic agent—blocks Na^+ intracellularly	Local anesthetic	Sleepiness; light-headedness; visual/audio disturbances; restlessness; nystagmus; shivering; tonic–clonic convulsions; death; greater toxicity than other local anesthetics	
Etidronate [Didronel]	Bone stabilizer—pyrophosphate analog; reduces hydroxyapatite crystal formation, growth, and dissolution, which reduces bone turnover	Hypercalcemia of malignancy; Paget disease; osteoporosis; hyperparathyroidism		
Etomidate [Amidate]	Anesthetic agent	Induces stage 3 anesthesia	Painful injection; myoclonic movements	
Etretinate	Vitamin A analog	Severe acne; psoriasis		
Exenatide [Byetta]	Hypoglycemic agent—**incretin mimetic;** mimics the actions of GLP-1; increases secretion of insulin; slows absorption of glucose from gut; reduces action of glucagon (decreasing hepatic gluconeogenesis)	Oral treatment for **NIDDM** (type II diabetes)	**Hypoglycemia;** GI disturbances: nausea, vomiting, diarrhea, and abdominal discomfort; decreased appetite	

Ezetimibe [Zocor]	Antihyperlipidemia; **cholesterol absorption blocker**—prevents cholesterol reabsorption at brush border in small intestine; **decreases LDL; no effect on HDL or TG**	**Increased LDL; hypertrigyceridemia;** cardiac event risk reduction	**Increases LFT (rarely); myopathy;** hepatotoxicity; pancreatitis; abdominal symptoms	
Famotidine [Pepcid]	**H_2 blocker—reversibly blocks histamine H_2 receptors → reduces gastric acid secretion**	**Peptic ulcer disease, gastritis, and esophageal reflux**	**Gynecomastia;** rare: confusion, dizziness, and headaches	**Crosses placenta; milder side effect profile** than cimetidine and ranitidine
Fenofibrate	**Lipid lowering agent—upregulates lipoprotein lipase (periphery) → increases TG clearance; decreases LDL, increases HDL, and decreases TG**	**Increased TG, increased LDL**	Myositis, increased LFTs	Reduces TG more than other agents
Fentanyl	**Opioid agonist**	**Pain;** general anesthetic	Prolonged recovery; nausea	
Fexofenadine hydrochloride [Allegra]	Antihistamine			
Filgrastim [Neuopogen]	**Granulocyte-macrophage colony-stimulating factor**	**Recovery of bone marrow (e.g., chemotherapy induced neutropenia)**		
Finasteride [Proscar]	**Antiandrogen—5α reductase inhibitor** → decreases the conversion of testosterone to dihydrotestosterone	**Benign prostatic hyperplasia,** male pattern baldness		
Flecainide [Tambocor]	**Antiarrhythmic (class IC)—Na^+-channel blocker**			
Fluconazole [Diflucan]	**Antifungal—inhibits ergosterol synthesis,** preventing cell membrane formation	**Cryptococcal meningitis; oral candidiasis in AIDS**	**Abdominal pain; nausea**	
Flucytosine [Ancobon]	Antifungal—competitive inhibitor of thymidylate synthetase; impairs DNA synthesis	*Candida*; *Cryptococcus*; *Aspergillus*	Nausea; vomiting; diarrhea; rash; bone marrow and liver toxicity; enterocolitis	Imported in the fungus via permease
Fludrocortisone [Florinef]	Mineralocorticoid—aldosterone analog	Used with cortisol in adrenal insufficiency		
Flumazenil [Romazicon]	Benzodiazepine receptor antagonist	Alcohol abuse; anxiety		IV only
Flunarizine [Sibelium]	Weak Ca^{2+}-channel blocker	Prophylaxis for migraine		
Fluoride	Stabilizes hydroxyapatite crystal structure; stimulates new growth of bone (unknown mechanism)		Nausea; vomiting; neurologic symptoms; arthralgias; arthritis	Stains teeth in toxic amounts

Therapeutic Agent (common name, if relevant) [trade name, where appropriate]	Class–Pharmacology and Pharmacokinetics	Indications	Side or Adverse Effects	Contraindications or Precautions to Consider; Notes
5-Fluorouracil (5-FU)	Antineoplastic—**inhibits thymidylate synthetase; inhibits RNA synthesis**	**Colon and breast cancer**	**Delayed toxicity: nausea, oral and GI ulcers, and bone marrow depression**	
Fluoxetine **[Prozac]**	Selective serotonin reuptake inhibitors—inhibit **reuptake** of 5-HT at neuronal synapses	Major depression; OCD; anorexia; bulimia; anxiety	Inhibits liver enzymes, nausea, agitation, **sexual dysfunction** (anorgasmia), and dystonic reactions	Contraindicated with **MAOIs** secondary to **serotonin syndrome** (hyperthermia, muscle rigidity, and cardiovascular collapse); allows time for antidepressant effect, usually takes 2–3 weeks
Fluphenazine [Prolixin]	Antipsychotic—phenothiazine; blocks D_2, α_1, and H_1 receptors	Psychosis	**Extrapyramidal** (dystonia, akinesia, akathisia, and tardive dyskinesia), **anticholinergic** (dry mouth, constipation), **alpha blockade** (hypotension), and **histamine** (sedation); toxicity results in neuroleptic malignant syndrome (rigidity, myoglobinuria, autonomic instability, and hyperpyrexia)	**Extrapyramidal** side effects are more common
Flurazepam [Dalmane]	Benzodiazepine—enhances GABA; increases IPSP amplitude	Sedative; hypnotic; antianxiety; antiepileptic		
Flutamide [Eulexin]	**Antiandrogen**—nonsteroidal, competitive androgen receptor blocker	**Metastatic prostate cancer**		
Fluticasone [Flonase]	Intranasal glucocorticoids—decrease cytokine synthesis, downregulate inflammatory response in the nasal mucosa	Nasal congestion, allergic rhinitis	Local irritation of nasal mucosa, epistaxis	
Fluvastatin [Lescol]	Lipid-lowering agent—inhibits HMG-CoA reductase; lowers LDL	Hyperlipidemia (especially type II)	Liver toxicity; myopathy; mild GI disturbances	Contraindicated in pregnant or lactating women and children
Fluvoxamine [Luvox]	Antidepressant—SSRI	Anxiety; obsessive-compulsive disorder		
Foscarnet [Foscavir]	**Antiviral**—non-nucleoside inhibitor of DNA polymerase	**CMV retinitis (resistant to ganciclovir), HSV (resistant to acyclovir)**	Hypocalcemia; CNS, cardiac, and **renal toxicity**; anemia	**Does not require activation by viral kinase**
Fosinopril [Monopril]	Antihypertensive—ACE inhibitor → inhibits conversion of angiotensin I to II → decreases angiotensin II levels → prevents vasoconstriction from angiotensin II	Hypertension, CHF, post-MI agent, and vasodilator	**Hyperkalemia, cough** (persistent dry), **angioedema,** taste changes, orthostatic hypotension, proteinuria, renal failure (in bilateral renal artery stenosis), neutropenia, and rash	Contraindicated in pregnancy (fetal renal malformation)

Furosemide [Lasix]	Loop diuretic— prevents cotransport of Na^+, K^+, and Cl^- in **thick ascending limb**; loss of Na^+, Cl^-, Ca^{2+}, and K^+ in urine	**Hypertension; congestive heart failure;** cirrhosis, nephrotic syndrome, **pulmonary edema,** hypercalcemia	**Potassium wasting, metabolic alkalosis,** hypotension, dehydration, ototoxicity, nephritis, and gout	Do not give in patients with **sulfa drug allergy**; rapid onset and short duration of action, which is ideal for relieving acute edema
Gabapentin [Neurontin]	Antiepileptic—blocks Na^+ channels	Add-on drug for epilepsy		
Ganciclovir [Cytovene]	**Antiviral—guanosine analog;** inhibits viral DNA polymerase	**CMV (esp. CMV retinitis in AIDS)**	**Bone marrow suppression** (leukopenia, neutropenia, and thrombocytopenia); **renal impairment; seizures**	**Resistance from lack of thymidine kinase or mutation of viral DNA polymerase; more toxic than acyclovir**
Gemfibrozil	**Lipid-lowering agent—upregulates lipoprotein lipase (periphery) → increases TG clearance; decreases LDL, increases HDL, and decreases TG**	**Increased TG, increased LDL**	Myositis, increased LFTs; potentiates **anticoagulant drugs**; gallstones; mild GI disturbances	Reduces TG more than other agents; contraindicated in patients with impaired renal or hepatic function and pregnant or lactating women
Gentamicin [Garamycin]	**Antibiotic—aminoglycoside,** protein synthesis inhibitor; **irreversibly binds 30S ribosome subunits; bacteriostatic** at low concentration; **bactericidal** at high concentration	**Broad-spectrum:** Gram-negative rods; good for **bone** and **eye** infections; *Proteus, Pseudomonas, Enterobacter, Klebsiella*, and *E. coli*	**Ototoxicity; renal toxicity; neuromuscular blockade;** nausea; vomiting; vertigo; allergic skin rash; superinfections	
Gestodene	**Progesterone**—binds progesterone receptors	**Endometrial cancer,** amenorrhea, abnormal uterine bleeding, and **prevention of pregnancy**		Also used to prevent endometrial hyperplasia in postmenopausal women taking estrogen
Glargine [Lantus]	**Long-acting insulin**—*see mechanism for insulin*	**Diabetes mellitus** (typically **Type 1**)	**Hypoglycemia** (diaphoresis, vertigo, and tachycardia); insulin allergy; insulin antibodies; lipodystrophy	
Glimepiride [Diabinese]	**Hypoglycemic agent, second generation sulfonylurea**—closes potassium channel in pancreatic β-islet cell membrane → reduces K^+ efflux, increases Ca^{2+} influx → increases secretion of insulin	Oral treatment for **NIDDM (type II diabetes)**	**Hypoglycemia;** GI disturbances; muscle weakness; mental confusion; weight gain	Not useful in Type 1 DM because requires some islet function

Therapeutic Agent (common name, if relevant) [trade name, where appropriate]	Class–Pharmacology and Pharmacokinetics	Indications	Side or Adverse Effects	Contraindications or Precautions to Consider; Notes
Glipizide [Glucotrol]	**Hypoglycemic agent, second generation sulfonylurea**—closes potassium channel in pancreatic β-islet cell membrane → reduces K^+ efflux, increases Ca^{2+} influx → increases secretion of insulin	Oral treatment for **NIDDM (type II diabetes)**	**Hypoglycemia;** GI disturbances; muscle weakness; mental confusion; weight gain	Not useful in Type 1 DM because requires some islet function
Glyburide [DiaBeta, Micronase]	**Hypoglycemic agent, second generation sulfonylurea**—closes potassium channel in pancreatic β-islet cell membrane → reduces K^+ efflux, increases Ca^{2+} influx → increases secretion of insulin	Oral treatment for **NIDDM (type II diabetes)**	**Hypoglycemia;** GI disturbances; muscle weakness; mental confusion; weight gain	Not useful in Type 1 DM because requires some islet function
Glyceryl guaiacolate [Fenesin]	**Expectorant—increases bronchial secretions**	**Promotes cough**		
Glycopyrrolate [Robinul]	**Antimuscarinic**	**Bladder/GI spasm; decreases acid in ulcer**		Quaternary amine
GnRH	**Controls release of FSH, LH**	**Stimulates pituitary function**		
Gonadorelin [Lutrepulse]	**Analog of GnRH—controls release of FSH, LH**	**Stimulates pituitary function**		
Griseofulvin [Fulvicin, Grifulvin, Grisactin]	**Antifungal—inhibits cell mitosis by disrupting mitotic spindles; binds to tubulin**	**Dermatophytes (esp. *Trichophyton rubrum*)**	**Headache; mental confusion; rash; GI irritation; hepatotoxic; photosensitivity; carcinogenic; teratogenic**	Increases **cytochrome P450** and warfarin metabolism
Growth hormone (somatotropin) [Somatrem]	**Synthetic analog of growth hormone—causes liver to produce insulinlike growth factors (somatomedins)**	Replacement therapy in children with **growth hormone deficiency, Turner syndrome; burn victims**		
Growth hormone-releasing hormone (GH-RH)	**Synthetic analog of GHRH—stimulates the release of GH**	Dwarfism	Pain at injection	
Guaifenesin [Robutussin]	Expectorant—thins mucus and lubricates irritated respiratory tract	Cough associated with common cold and minor upper respiratory tract infections		Does not suppress cough reflex
Guanethidine [Ismelin]	**Antihypertensive**—interferes with norepinephrine release	**Severe hypertension**	Orthostatic hypotension, exercise hypotension, impotence, and diarrhea	**Contraindicated in patients taking TCAs**

Haloperidol **[Haldol]**	**Antipsychotic**—butyrophenone; blocks D_2 and α_1 receptors	**Schizophrenia, psychosis, acute mania, and Tourette syndrome**	**Extrapyramidal** (dystonia, akinesia, akathisia, and tardive dyskinesia), **endocrine** (galactorrhea), **anti-cholinergic** (dry mouth, constipation), **alpha blockade** (hypotension), and **histamine** (sedation); prolonged QT syndrome; toxicity results in neuroleptic malignant syndrome (rigidity, myo-globinuria, autonomic instability, and hyperpyrexia)	Extrapyramidal side effects are more common; neuroleptic malignant syndrome is treated with dantrolene and dopamine agonists
Haloprogin [Halotex]	**Antifungal—unknown mechanism; fungistatic**	**Topical for tinea pedis**		
Halothane	**Anesthetic agent**	**General anesthetic**	**Hepatotoxic; malignant hyper-thermia (with succinylcholine); arrhythmia**	**Contraindicated in adults**
Heparin	**Increases PTT by joining with antithrombin III**	**Deep vein thrombosis; pulmonary thrombosis**	**Overdose reversed by IV protamine sulfate;** osteoporosis	**Fast-acting; does not cross placenta**
Heroin	**Metabolized to morphine**			**More lipid-soluble than morphine**
Hexamethonium	Nicotinic ganglionic blocker	Hypertensive emergency	Severe orthostatic hypotension, blurred vision, constipation, and sexual dysfunction	
Hydralazine [Apresoline]	**Antihypertensive**—increases cGMP → smooth muscle relaxation → vasodi-lates arterioles → afterload reduction	**Severe hypertension, congestive heart failure**	**Compensatory tachycardia,** fluid retension, **lupuslike syndrome**	**First line therapy for hypertension in pregnancy,** used with methyl-dopa; contraindicated in angina/CAD because of compensatory tachycardia
Hydrochlorothiazide [Esidrix, HydroDIURIL]	Thiazide diuretic—inhibits transport of Na^+ and Cl^- into the cells of DCT	**Hypertension, congestive heart failure,** idiopathic hypercalciuria, and nephrogenic diabetes insipidus	**Hypokalemia, metabolic alkalosis, mild hyperlipidemia, hyperuri-cemia,** malaise, **hypercalcemia,** hyperglycemia, and hyponatremia	Do not give in patients with sulfa drug allergy
Hydrocodone [Bancap-HC]	Opioid agonist	Antitussive; analgesic		
Hydromorphone [Dilaudid]	Opioid agonist	Antitussive; analgesic	Respiratory depression; constipation; nausea	
Hydroxychloroquine [Plaquenil]	Antiprotozoal—antirheumatic	Rheumatic arthritis; malaria	Ocular toxicity (blurred vision)	Contraindicated in patients with psoriasis
Hydroxyurea [Hydrea]	**Antineoplastic—binds ribonucle-otide reductase; inhibits formation of DNA**	**Melanoma; chronic myelogenous leukemia; sickle cell disease**	Nausea; vomiting; bone marrow suppression	

Therapeutic Agent (common name, if relevant) [trade name, where appropriate]	Class–Pharmacology and Pharmacokinetics	Indications	Side or Adverse Effects	Contraindications or Precautions to Consider; Notes
Ibuprofen [Advil, Motrin]	**NSAID—reversibly inhibits cyclooxygenase** (both COX-1 and COX-2) → decreases prostaglandin synthesis	**Inflammation; pain**	GI distress, **GI ulcers;** coagulation disorders; aplastic anemia metabolic abnormalities; hypersensitivity; renal damage	
Ibutilide [Corvert]	Antiarrhythmic (class III)—K^+-channel blocker	Terminates atrial fibrillation and flutter	Prolongs QT interval	
Idazoxan	Antihypertensive—α_2-blocker			
Idoxuridine [Herplex Liquifilm]	Antiviral—thymidine analog; inhibits DNA polymerase; inhibits DNA synthesis	Topical for HSV keratitis	Local irritation; allergic contact keratitis	
Ifosfamide [IFEX]	Antineoplastic—DNA alkylation and cross-linking	Cancer	Cystitis; nephrotoxicity; nausea; vomiting; bone marrow suppression; alopecia; teratogenicity; carcinogenicity	
Imipenem [Primaxin] **cilastin**	**Antibiotic—Carbapenem,** cell wall inhibitor; same mechanism as penicillin; bactericidal	**Broad spectrum—Gram-positive cocci** (MSSA and *Streptococcus*), **Gram-negative rods** (*Pseudomonas* and *Enterobacter* sp.), **anaerobes,** dormant bacteria	Hypersensitivity reaction, **seizure,** confusion state, and superinfection (pseudomembrane colitis)	Significant side effects limit use to when other drugs have failed or life-threatening infections; always administered with cilastin (inhibits renal dihydropeptidase) to reduce inactivation in renal tubules
Imipramine [Tofranil]	Tricyclic antidepressants—inhibit **reuptake** of NE and 5-HT at neuronal synapses	Major depression, nocturnal enuresis, and panic disorder	Sedation, **alpha blocking effects** (orthostatic hypotension), **anticholinergic** (tachycardia, dry mouth, and urinary retention), hallucinations (in elderly), and confusion (in elderly); overdose toxicity results in **convulsions**, **coma**, **cardiotoxicity** (arrhythmias), respiratory depression, and hyperpyrexia	
Indecainide	Antiarrhythmic (class IC)—Na^+-channel blockers			No antimuscarinic action; no effect on action potential
Indinavir [Crixivan]	**Antiviral, protease inhibitor**—protease responsible for final step of viral proliferation; inhibits protease in progeny virons → assembly of nonfunctional viruses	**AIDS (Used in HAART)**	**GI irritation (nausea, diarrhea), hyperglycemia, lipodystrophy, thrombocytopenia**	**All protease inhibitors ending in navir; metabolism occurs by CYP450**

Indomethacin [Indocin]	**Anti-inflammatory, NSAID**—reversibly inhibits cyclooxygenase **(both COX-1 and COX-2) → decreases prostaglandin synthesis**	**Acute gout therapy; closes PDA**	**GI distress,** GI ulcers; **coagulation disorders; aplastic anemia metabolic abnormalities; hypersensitivity; renal damage**	
Infliximab	Anti-inflammatory—**monoclonal antibody that binds TNF → inhibits proinflammatory effects of TNF**	Crohn disease**, rheumatoid arthritis, and** ankylosing spondylitis	**Infections, fever, hypotension, and** reactivation of latent tuberculosis	
Insulin, Regular [Humulin R, Novolin R]	**Short acting insulin—Liver:** promotes glucose storage as glycogen, increases trigylceride synthesis; **Muscle:** facilitates protein and glycogen synthesis; **Adipose tissue:** improves triglyceride storage by activating plasma lipoprotein lipase; reduces circulating free fatty acids	**Diabetes mellitus (**typically **Type 1), hyperkalemia, and stress induced hyperglycemia**	**Hypoglycemia** (diaphoresis, vertigo, and tachycardia); insulin allergy; insulin antibodies; lipodystrophy	
Interferon alfa-2a [Roferon A], alfa-2b [Intron A], and alfa-n3 [Alferon-N]	**Antiviral—glycoproteins—block viral RNA, DNA, and protein synthesis**	**Genital warts; chronic hepatitis B and C; AIDS-related Kaposi sarcoma; laryngeal papillomatosis; hairy cell leukemia**	**Flulike symptoms; neutropenia**	
Interfon beta-1a [Avonex, Rebif]	**Antiviral—glycoproteins—block viral RNA, DNA, and protein synthesis**	**Multiple sclerosis**	**Flulike symptoms; neutropenia**	
Interferon gamma-1b [Actimmune]	**Antiviral—glycoproteins—block viral RNA, DNA, and protein synthesis**	**NADPH oxidase deficiency**	**Flulike symptoms; neutropenia**	
Ipratropium [Atrovent]	Bronchodilator—muscarinic antagonist; competitively blocks muscarinic receptors → prevents bronchoconstriction	Asthma; COPD		
Isocarboxazid [Marplan]	Monoamine oxidase inhibitors—inhibit **degradation** of NE and 5-HT at neuronal synapses	**Atypical depression** (with hypersomnia, anxiety, sensitivity to rejection, and hypochondriasis)	**Hypertensive episodes** with ingestion of tyramine-containing foods or beta agonists, hyperthermia, and convulsions	Contraindicated with **SSRIs** and **meperidine** secondary to **serotonin syndrome** (hyperthermia, muscle rigidity, and cardiovascular collapse)
Isoflurane	Anesthetic	General anesthetic		Best muscle relaxant, most widely used
Isoniazid [INH, Nydrazid]	**Antibiotic**—inhibits synthesis of mycolic acids	***Mycobacterium* treatment (*M. tuberculosis and M. kansasii*); *M. tuberculosis prophylaxis***	**Peripheral and CNS effects as a result of pyridoxine deficiency; liver damage; hemolytic anemia in G-6-PD deficiency; SLE-like syndrome**	Pyridoxine (Vitamin B_6) can prevent neurotoxicity

Therapeutic Agent (common name, if relevant) [trade name, where appropriate]	Class–Pharmacology and Pharmacokinetics	Indications	Side or Adverse Effects	Contraindications or Precautions to Consider; Notes
Isoproterenol [Isuprel]	Bronchodilator—β-agonist (nonselective), relaxes bronchial smooth muscle through β_2 receptor activity	Asthma	Tachycardia (β_1 receptor activity)	
Isosorbide dinitrate [Isordil]	Antianginal—stimulates the synthesis of cGMP, leading to muscle relaxation via NO formation; vasodilator	Angina; CHF	Headache; orthostatic hypotension; syncope	Long-acting
Isotretinoin [Accutane]	**Vitamin A analog**	**Severe acne; psoriasis**	**Keratinization; teratogenic**	
Itraconazole [Sporanox]	**Antifungal—inhibits ergosterol synthesis, preventing cell membrane formation**	**Oral for fungal infections (esp. dermatophytoses and onychomycosis)**	**GI disturbances; hepatotoxicity**	
Kanamycin [Kantrex]	**Antibiotic—aminoglycoside; binds** 30S ribosome subunits; **bacteriostatic at low concentration; bactericidal at high concentration**	**Reduction of gut flora**	**Ototoxicity; neurotoxicity**	
Ketamine [Ketalar]	**Anesthetic agent, blocks NMDA-type glutamate receptors**	**General anesthetic**	**Dissociative anesthesia; catatonia; hallucinations**	
Ketoconazole [Nizoral]	**Antifungal—inhibits ergosterol synthesis, preventing cell membrane formation; inhibits adrenal and gonadal steroid synthesis**	**Chronic mucocutaneous candidiasis; blastomycosis; histoplasmosis; coccidiodomycosis; hypercortisolism; prostate carcinoma**	**GI irritation; gynecomastia; thrombocytopenia; hepatotoxic; rash; fever; chills**	**Inhibits cytochrome P450**
Ketorolac [Toradol]	**NSAID—reversibly inhibits cyclooxygenase** (both COX-1 and COX-2) → decreases prostaglandin synthesis; relieves pain and reduces swelling	**Postoperative pain;** severe pain	GI distress, **GI ulcers;** coagulation disorders; aplastic anemia metabolic abnormalities; hypersensitivity; renal damage	
Labetalol [Normodyne, Trandate]	**Antihypertensive—nonselective β and α_1 blocker**	**Hypertension and atrial fibrillation**		
Lactulose [Chronulac]	**Osmotic laxative**	Decreases ammonia in hepatic encephalopathy; constipation	Abdominal bloating, flatulence	
Lamivudine (3TC) [Epivir]	**Antiviral, nucleoside reverse transcriptase inhibitor—cytidine analog** → inhibits viral reverse transcriptase → prevents integration of DNA copy of viral genome into host DNA	**AIDS (Used in HAART)**	**Neutropenia, anemia, peripheral neuropathy, pancreatitis, and lactic acidosis**	

Lamotrigine [Lamictal]	Antiepileptic—blocks Na^+ channels	Add-on drug for epilepsy		
Lansoprazole	**Proton pump inhibitor—irreversibly inhibits H^+/K^+-ATPase in gastric parietal cells →decreases proton secretion by parietal cells**	Peptic ulcer disease, gastritis, esophageal reflux, **Zollinger–Ellison syndrome**		**Inhibits cytochrome P450;** given with **clarithromycin** and **amoxicillin** for ***Helicobacter pylori***
Latanoprost [Xalatan]	Prostaglandin $F_{2\alpha}$; increases aqueous humor outflow	Glaucoma	Blurred vision; burning; hyperemia; itching; hyperpigmentation of iris; keratitis	
Lente [Humulin L, Novolin L]	**Intermediate acting insulin**—*see mechanism for insulin*	**Diabetes mellitus** (typically **Type 1**)	**Hypoglycemia** (diaphoresis, vertigo, and tachycardia); insulin allergy; insulin antibodies; lipodystrophy	
Leucovorin	Allows stem cells to bypass the inhibition of dihydrofolate reductase caused by methotrexate	Treats acute toxicity of methotrexate		
Leuprolide [Lupron]	**GnRH analog**—agonist (when given pulsatile), antagonist (when given continuously)	**Infertility** (given pulsatile), **prostate cancer** (given continuous), **uterine fibroids,** PCOS, endometriosis, precocious puberty	Nausea, vomiting, and antiandrogen effects (testicular atrophy)	
Levamisole [Ergamisol]	Antihelminthic—immunostimulatory to host; helps rid the host of parasite	*Ascaris* (roundworm); *Ancylostoma* (hookworm); therapy for immunodeficiency	GI disturbances; rashes; neutropenia	
Levodopa [Larodopa]	**Antiparkinsonian agent—precursor of dopamine; administered with carbidopa (most often) or benserazide to inhibit carboxylase deactivation of levodopa in periphery**	**0**		**Inhibited by vitamin B_6; do not give with MAOI or pyridoxine**
Levofloxacin [Levaquin]	**Antibiotic—Quinolone; inhibits DNA gyrase** (topoisomerase II) and **topoisomerase IV→** blocks DNA synthesis; bactericidal	**Gram-negative infections (esp. UTI and bone): *Pseudomonas*, Enterobacteriaceae, and *Neisseria*; Gram-positive infections** (*Staphylococcus*, *Streptococcus*); **intracellular: *Legionella***	**GI disturbances; headache; dizziness; phototoxicity; cartilage damage (children, fetus); tendonitis and tendon rupture (adults); myalgias (children)**	**May elevate theophylline to toxic levels, causing seizure; contraindicated in pregnant women**
Levomethadyl [Orlaam]	Opioid agonist	Long-lasting maintenance therapy for heroin addiction		
Levonorgestrel [Plan B]	**Progesterone**—binds progesterone receptors	**Endometrial cancer,** amenorrhea, abnormal uterine bleeding, and **prevention of pregnancy**		Also used to prevent endometrial hyperplasia in postmenopausal women taking estrogen
Levothyroxine (T_4) [Levothroid]	Synthetic analog of thyroxine T_4	**Hypothyroidism**	Tachycardia, heat intolerance, tremors, and arrhythmia	

Therapeutic Agent (common name, if relevant) [trade name, where appropriate]	Class–Pharmacology and Pharmacokinetics	Indications	Side or Adverse Effects	Contraindications or Precautions to Consider; Notes
Lidocaine [Xylocaine]	**Antiarrhythmic (class IB), anesthetic agent—blocks Na^+ channels intracellularly**	**Local anesthetic; ventricular tachycardia**	**Sleepiness; light-headedness; visual/audio disturbances; restlessness; nystagmus; shivering; tonic–clonic convulsion; death**	**Given with epinephrine to maintain locality and increase duration of anesthetic properties via epinephrine-mediated vasoconstriction**
Lisinopril [Prinivil, Zestril]	**Antihypertensive—vasodilator; ACE inhibitor**	**CHF**	**Postural hypotension; renal insufficiency; hyperkalemia; persistent dry cough**	**Pregnancy**
Lispro [Humalog]	**Rapid acting insulin**—*see mechanism for insulin*	**Diabetes mellitus** (typically **Type 1**), **hyperkalemia, and stress induced hyperglycemia**	**Hypoglycemia** (diaphoresis, vertigo, and tachycardia); insulin allergy; insulin antibodies; lipodystrophy	
Lithium **[Eskalith, Lithobid, Lithotabs, Lithonate]**	Antimanic—unclear mechanism; inhibits regeneration of IP_3 and DAG; important for many second-messenger systems	Bipolar disorder, acute manic events	Tremor, hypothyroidism, polyuria, and teratogenesis	Close monitoring of serum levels required due to narrow therapeutic window
Loperamide [Imodium]	**Antidiarrheal—similar to opioid agonist**	**Oral antidiarrheal**		
Loratadine [Claritin]	**Antihistamine**—H_1 blocker (second generation)	**Seasonal allergies**	**Sedating;** rare: headache, dizziness, fatigue, CNS, weak antiandrogenic effect, leukopenia, and reduced sperm count	**Inhibits metabolism or absorption of some drugs;** less sedating than first generation H1 blocker due to decreased CNS entry
Lorazepam [Ativan]	Antianxiety—benzodiazepine; enhances GABA; increases IPSP amplitude	Sedative; hypnotic; antianxiety; antiepileptic; panic attack		
Losartan [Cozaar]	**Antihypertensive—angiotensin II receptor antagonist**	**Hypertension**	**Dizziness; upper respiratory infection; headache**	
Losartan [Cozaar]	**Antihypertensive**—angiotensin II receptor blockers → prevents vasoconstriction from angiotensin II	**Hypertension**	Fetal renal toxicity, **hyperkalemia**	
Lovastatin [Mevacor]	**Lipid lowering agent—HMG-CoA reductase inhibitors**—inhibits synthesis of cholesterol precursor mevalonate; **decreases LDL, increases HDL, and decreases TG**	**High LDL, preventative after thrombotic event (e.g., MI, stroke)**	Reversible increase in LFTs, myositis	**Contraindicated in pregnant or lactating women and children**
α_2-Macroglobulin	Inhibits fibrinolysis			

Magnesium hydroxide [Milk of Magnesia]	**Anatacid, osmotic laxative**—buffers gastric acid by raising pH	Peptic ulcer, gastritis, esophageal reflux, and constipation	**Diarrhea, hyporeflexia, hypotension, cardiac arrest, and hypokalemia**	**Can affect the absorption, bioavailability, or urinary excretion of drugs by changing the gastric pH, urinary pH, or gastric emptying**
Magnesium sulfate, Magnesium citrate	**Osmotic laxative**		Magnesium toxicity (in renal insufficiency)	
Malathion	Organophosphate—inhibits cholinesterase	Least toxic organophosphate		
Mannitol [Osmitrol]	Osmotic diuretic—prevents isosmotic reabsorption of filtrate in **PCT, loop of Henle,** and **collecting tubule**; loss of Na^+ and all other filtered solutes in urine	Shock, drug overdose, decreased intracranial or intraocular pressure; maintenance of urine flow in rhabdomyolysis	Pulmonary edema, dehydration; contraindicated in anuria and congestive heart failure	Results in increased urine volume; readily filtered and not reabsorbed
Maprotiline	Blocks NE uptake	Major depression	Sedation, orthostatic hypotension	
Mebendazole [Vermox]	Antihelminthic—irreversible; inhibits glucose uptake	Hookworm; roundworm; threadworm; some cestodes		
Mecamylamine [Inversine]	Antihypertensive—nicotinic ganglionic blocker	Hypertension emergency; smoking cessation	Decreases GI motility; cycloplegia; hypotension; xerostomia	
Mechlorethamine (nitrogen mustard) [Mustargen]	Antineoplastic—DNA alkylation and cross-linking	Cancer	Nausea; vomiting; bone marrow suppression; alopecia; teratogenicity; carcinogenicity	
Meclizine [Antivert, Bonine]	Antiemetic agent—H_1-blocker	Emesis; vertigo	Teratogenic	
Mefloquine [Lariam]	Antimalarial—uncertain mechanism	Treatment of acute attack of chloroquine-resistant organisms	CNS: dizziness, disorientation, hallucinations, seizure, and depression; GI disturbances; nausea; vomiting; abdominal pain	
Melatonin	Promotes sleep	Clock shifting		Pineal hormone
Melphalan [Alkeran]	Antineoplastic—DNA alkylation and cross-linking	Cancer	Nausea; vomiting; bone marrow suppression (serious); alopecia; teratogenicity; carcinogenicity; pulmonary fibrosis; hypersensitivity	
Menotropin [Pergonal]	Mixture of FSH and LH	Secondary hypogonadism with infertility		
Meperidine [Demerol]	**Opioid agonist**	**Pain;** acute migraine attacks	**CNS excitation at high doses;** histamine release; antimuscarinic effects	**Contraindicated in patients with MAOI** (results in hyperpyrexia)
Mephenesin	Centrally acting muscle relaxant	Muscle spasms; tetanus contractions; orthopedic manipulation	Sedation	

Therapeutic Agent (common name, if relevant) [trade name, where appropriate]	Class–Pharmacology and Pharmacokinetics	Indications	Side or Adverse Effects	Contraindications or Precautions to Consider; Notes
Mepivacaine [Isocaine]	Anesthetic agent—blocks Na^+ channels intracellularly	Local anesthetic	Sleepiness; light-headedness; visual/audio disturbances; restlessness; nystagmus; shivering; tonic–clonic convulsion; death	
Mercaptopurine [Purinethol]	Antineoplastic—inhibits purine synthesis; disrupts DNA and RNA synthesis	Childhood leukemias	Bone marrow suppression	
Meropenem	**Carbapenem**—cell wall inhibitor; same mechanism as penicillin; bactericidal	**Broad spectrum—Gram-positive cocci** (MSSA and *Streptococcus*), **Gram-negative rods** (*Pseudomonas* and *Enterobacter* sp.), **anaerobes,** dormant bacteria	Reduced risk of seizure compared to imipenem	Stable to dihydropeptidase I, unlike imipenem
Metformin [Glucophage]	**Hypoglycemic agent, biguanide**—unknown mechanism, postulated to decrease gluconeogenesis, increase glycolysis → decreases serum glucose levels	Oral treatment for **NIDDM (type II diabetes)**	**Lactic acidosis,** GI upset (diarrhea, nausea, and abdominal pain), metallic taste	Stop use in patients undergoing studies or procedures involving **contrast**; can be used in patients without islet function
Methadone [Dolophine]	**Opioid agonist—synthetic**	**Maintenance therapy for heroin addiction, pain**	Respiratory depression; histamine release; constipation; nausea; miosis	
Methicillin	**Antibiotic—β-lactam, penicillin derivative,** cell wall inhibitor; same mechanism as penicillin; distinguished by activity against **penicillinase producing Staphylococcus**; bactericidal	***Staphylococcus* infections** (except MRSA)	**Hypersensitivity reactions;** interstitial nephritis (methicillin)	Penicillinase resistant; MRSA is resistant to methicillin because of altered penicillin binding protein target site
Methimazole [Tapazole]	**Antithyroid agent—inhibits peroxidase enzyme in thyroid → decreases synthesis of thyroid hormone**	**Hyperthyroidism**	**Agranulocytosis**	**Crosses the placenta; can cause fetal goiter, hypothyroidism, and aplasia cutis (fetal scalp defect)**
Methohexital [Brevital]	Anesthetic agent—barbiturate; prolongs IPSP duration	Antiepileptic; cerebral edema; anesthetic (stage 3 anesthetic)		Ultrashort acting
Methotrexate [Rheumatrex]	Antineoplastic—**dihydrofolate reductase inhibitor; immunosuppressant**	**Rheumatic arthritis;** bone marrow transplant; acute lymphocytic and myelogenous leukemia; choriocarcinoma; lung cancer	Oral and GI ulceration; **bone marrow suppression; thrombocytopenia; leukopenia;** hepatotoxic	**Leucovorin is given as an adjuvant after treatment**
Methoxyflurane [Penthrane]	Anesthetic agent	General anesthetic	Nephrotoxic	No longer used
Methylcellulose [Citrucel]	**Bulk-forming laxative**—dietary fiber	Constipation	Impaction above strictures, fluid overload, gas, and bloating	

Methyldopa [Aldomet]	**Antihypertensive—c**entrally acting sympathetic agent (α agonist) → decreases sympathetic outflow from CNS	**Hypertension**	Sedation, hemolytic anemia	**Positive Coombs test**
Methylphenidate [Ritalin]	CNS stimulant—amphetamine; releases neurotransmitter from synapse	Stimulant; treatment of choice for **attention-deficit hyperactivity disorder**		
Methysergide [Sansert]	**Antimigraine—**5-HT antagonist and weak vasoconstrictor	Prophylaxis of migraine	GI distress; inflammatory fibrosis of kidney, lung, and cardiac valves	**Contraindicated in patients with peripheral vascular disease, coronary artery disease, and pregnancy; patient placed on a drug holiday to prevent tachyphylaxis**
Methyltestosterone [Android, Virilon]	**Androgen**—androgen receptor agonist	**In males: hypogonadism, delayed puberty** (promotes secondary sex characteristics), and impotence; **In females: estrogen receptor positive breast cancer**	**Masculinization (hirsutism), testicular atrophy,** prostate hyperplasia, prostate cancer, impotence, **stunt growth** (premature epiphyseal plate closure), and hyperlipidemia	Decreases testicular testosterone, leading to Leydig cell inhibition and gonadal atrophy
Metoclopramide [Reglan]	**GI stimulant—prokinetic agent; D_2 receptor antagonist; central and peripheral D_2 antagonism at low doses,** weak 5-HT_3 antagonism at high doses; enhances acetylcholine release, increases resting tone, contractility, lower esophageal sphincter tone, and motility (does not affect colon transit time)	**Diabetic** and **postoperative gastroparesis; nausea;** counteracts nausea of **migraine**; increases stomach motility	Sleepiness; fatigue; headache; insomnia; dizziness; nausea; akathisia, **dystonia,** and tardive dyskinesia	Interacts with **digoxin** and **diabetic agents; contraindicated in small bowel obstruction**
Metocurine [Metubine Iodide]	**Nondepolarizing neuromuscular blocker**			
Metolazone [Mykrox, Zaroxolyn]	Diuretic—decreases Na^+ reabsorption in the distal tubule by inhibiting the Na^+/Cl^- cotransporter; reduced peripheral resistance	Hypertension, CHF	Hypokalemia; hyperuricemia; hypovolemia; hyperglycemia (especially in diabetics); hypercalcemia; hypersensitivity reaction; Na^+ excretion in advanced renal failure	
Metoprolol [Toprol XL]	**Antihypertensive,** antiarrhythmic (class II)—β_1-selective blocker	**Hypertension, angina, MI, and antiarrhythmic**	**Impotence, asthma, bradycardia,** AV block, heart failure, sedation, and sleep alterations	

Therapeutic Agent (common name, if relevant) [trade name, where appropriate]	Class–Pharmacology and Pharmacokinetics	Indications	Side or Adverse Effects	Contraindications or Precautions to Consider; Notes
Metronidazole [Flagyl]	**Antibiotic, Antiprotozoal**—penetrates cell membrane and gives off nitro moiety → forms toxic metabolites → reacts and damages DNA; bactericidal	***Bacteroides fragilis*** (esp. for endocarditis and CNS); **Pseudomembrane colitis** (*C. difficile*); **amebiasis; giardiasis; trichomoniasis, bacterial vaginosis** (*Gardnerella vaginalis*), **peptic ulcer disease** (part of *H. pylori* triple therapy)	Nausea; vomiting; **disulfiramlike reaction to alcohol;** metallic taste; paresthesia; stomatitis; carcinogenic and mutagenic	**Contraindicated in pregnancy**
Metyrapone [Metopirone]	Inhibits cortisol synthesis	Diagnosis of pituitary dysfunction		
Mevastatin	Lipid-lowering agent—inhibits **HMG-CoA reductase; lowers LDL**	Hyperlipidemia (esp. type II)	**Liver toxicity; myopathy;** mild GI disturbances	**Contraindicated in pregnant** or lactating women, or in children
Mexiletine [Mexitil]	Antiarrhythmic (class IB)—Na^+-channel blocker			
Mezlocillin [Mezlin]	Antibiotic—β-lactam	Pseudomonas; Proteus		IV
Midazolam [Versed]	**Benzodiazepine; short-acting**	**Preanesthetic medication; produces antegrade amnesia (loss of memory of events after administration), calming down the patient**	Circulatory and respiratory depression	**Flumazenil antagonizes CNS depression caused by benzodiazepines**
Mifepristone (RU-486)	**Antiprogesterone**—synthetic steroid, progesterone receptor blocker → blocks the effects of progesterone → myometrium contraction	**Termination of intrauterine pregnancy** (emergency postcoital contraceptive)	**Heavy bleeding, uterine cramping,** GI effects (nausea, vomiting, and anorexia)	Controversial "Morning after" drug
Miglitol	**Hypoglycemic agent, α-glucosidase inhibitor**—inhibits intestinal brush border enzyme α-glucosidase→ delays sugar hydrolysis and glucose absorption → decreases **postprandial hyperglycemia**	Oral treatment for **NIDDM (type II diabetes)** postprandially	**Flatulence,** cramps, and diarrhea; may reduce absorption of iron	Does not cause reactive hypoglycemia; decreases HbA1c
Milrinone [Primacor]	Inotropic agent—phosphodiesterase inhibitor; increases contractility via increase in intracellular Ca^{2+}	CHF		
Mineral oil [Fleet Mineral Oil Enema]	**Laxative—hyperosmolar agent;** draws water into gut lumen → gut distension → promotes peristalsis and evacuation of bowel	**Preoperative patients;** short-term treatment of constipation		May interfere with the absorption of fat-soluble vitamins

Minoxidil [Loniten, Rogaine]	Antihypertensive—**K^+ channel opener** → hyperpolarizes and relaxes vascular smooth muscle	**Severe hypertension**	**Hypertrichosis**, pericardial effusion	
Mirtazapine	α-2 antagonist → increases release of NE and 5-HT	Major depression (especially with insomnia)	**Weight gain,** dry mouth, increased appetite, and sedation	
Misoprostol [Cytotec]	**Cytoprotectant—PGE_1 analog → increased production and secretion of gastric mucosa barrier, decreased acid production;** cervical dilation, uterine contractions	**Prevents NSAID induced peptic ulcers;** maintains patent ductus arteriosus; **induction of labor**, termination of pregnancy	**Diarrhea**	**Abortion inducing drug,** contraindicated in women of childbearing age
Molindone [Moban]	Antipsychotic—blocks D_2 receptors	Psychosis	Parkinsonism; tardive dyskinesia	
Montelukast [Singulair]	**Leukotriene inhibitor;** reduces inflammation	**Asthma**		Not for acute attacks
Moricizine [Ethmozine]	Antiarrhythmic (class IC)—Na^+ -channel blockers	Ventricular arrhythmia	Dizziness; nausea	
Morphine [Astramorph, Duramorph, Infumorph, Kadian, MS Contin, Oramorph, MSIR, Roxanol]	Opioid agonist—chronic oral dose converted to more potent morphine-6-glucuronide	Severe pain; general anesthetic; antitussive; antidiarrheal	Respiratory depression; histamine release; constipation; nausea; nausea; miosis	
Moxifloxacin	**Antibiotic—Quinolone; inhibits DNA gyrase** (topoisomerase II) and **topoisomerase IV** → blocks DNA synthesis; bactericidal	**Gram-negative infections (esp. UTI and bone): *Pseudomonas*, Enterobacteriaceae, and *Neisseria*; Gram-positive infections** (*Staphylococcus*, *Streptococcus*); **intracellular: *Legionella*; anaerobes**	**GI disturbances; headache; dizziness; phototoxicity; cartilage damage (children, fetus); tendonitis** and **tendon rupture (adults); myalgias (children)**	**May elevate theophylline to toxic levels, causing seizure; contraindicated in pregnant women**
Muromonab (OKT3)	**Immunosuppressant—monoclonal antibody against CD3 on T lymphocytes**	Acute rejection of **renal transplants**		
Muscarine	**Muscarinic agonist**		Abdominal pain; diarrhea; bronchoconstriction	**Contraindicated in patients with peptic ulcer, asthma, hyperthyroidism, and Parkinson disease**
Nabilone [Cesamet]	Antiemetic—unknown mechanism; binds cannabinoid receptors and inhibits vomiting center in medulla	Emesis	Dry mouth; dizziness; inability to concentrate; disorientation; anxiety; tachycardia; depression; paranoia; psychosis	THC derivative
***N*-Acetylcysteine [Mucomyst]**	Breaks disulfide bonds; **mucolytic** (loosens mucus plugs)—**replenishes glutathione**	**Overdose of acetaminophen; liquefies sputum to assist expulsion**	Unpleasant odor during administration	

Therapeutic Agent (common name, if relevant) [trade name, where appropriate]	Class–Pharmacology and Pharmacokinetics	Indications	Side or Adverse Effects	Contraindications or Precautions to Consider; Notes
Norethindrone	**Progesterone**—binds progesterone receptors	**Endometrial cancer,** amenorrhea, abnormal uterine bleeding, and **prevention of pregnancy**		Also used to prevent endometrial hyperplasia in postmenopausal women taking estrogen
Norfloxacin	**Antibiotic—Quinolone; inhibits DNA gyrase** (topoisomerase II) and **topoisomerase IV** → blocks DNA synthesis; bactericidal	**Gram-negative infections** (esp. UTI and bone): *Pseudomonas*, Enterobacteriaceae, and *Neisseria*; **Gram-positive infections** (staphylococci)**; intracellular: *Legionella***	**GI disturbances; headache; dizziness; phototoxicity; cartilage damage (children, fetus); tendonitis** and **tendon rupture (adults); myalgias (children)**	May elevate theophylline to toxic levels, causing seizure
Norgestimate	**Progesterone**—binds progesterone receptors	**Endometrial cancer,** amenorrhea, abnormal uterine bleeding, and **prevention of pregnancy**		Also used to prevent endometrial hyperplasia in postmenopausal women taking estrogen
Nortriptyline [Pamelor]	Tricyclic antidepressants—inhibit **reuptake** of NE and 5-HT at neuronal synapses	Major depression, panic disorder, and anxiety	Sedation, **alpha blocking effects** (orthostatic hypotension), **anticholinergic** (tachycardia, dry mouth, and urinary retention), hallucinations (in elderly), and confusion (elderly); overdose toxicity results in **convulsions, coma, cardiotoxicity** (arrhythmias), respiratory depression, and hyperpyrexia	
NPH [Humulin N, Novolin N]	**Intermediate acting insulin**—*see mechanism for insulin*	**Diabetes mellitus** (typically **Type 1**)	**Hypoglycemia** (diaphoresis, vertigo, and tachycardia); insulin allergy; insulin antibodies; lipodystrophy	
Nystatin [Mycostatin]	Antifungal—binds to cell membrane sterols (esp. ergosterol) → disrupting fungal membranes; fungicidal	**Mucosal candida** infections (skin, vaginal, and GI)	Few	Used topically or as mouth rinse; too toxic for systemic use
Octreotide [Sandostatin]	**Synthetic analog of somatostatin**—decreases release of GH, gastrin, secretin, VIP, CCK, glucagon, and insulin	**Acromegaly; glucagonoma; insulinoma; carcinoid syndrome**	Nausea; cramps; and gallstones	
Ofloxacin [Floxin]	**Antibiotic—Quinolone, DNA synthesis inhibitor; inhibits DNA gyrase** (topoisomerase II) and **topoisomerase IV** → blocks DNA synthesis; bactericidal	**Gram-negative infections** (esp. UTI and bone): *Pseudomonas*, Enterobacteriaceae, and *Neisseria*; **Gram-positive infections** (staphylococci); **intracellular: *Legionella***	**GI disturbances; headache; dizziness; phototoxicity; cartilage damage (children, fetus); tendonitis and tendon rupture (adults); myalgias (children)**	May elevate theophylline to toxic levels, causing seizure

Olanzapine [Zyprexa]	Atypical antipsychotic—blocks D_4, α_1, 5-HT, and muscarinic receptors	Schizophrenia, OCD, anxiety disorder, depression, mania, and Tourette syndrome	Agranulocytosis, **weight gain, diabetes; extrapyramidal** (occurs at a lower rate than typicals), **anticholinergic** (dry mouth, constipation), **alpha blockade** (hypotension), **histamine** (sedation); toxicity results in neuroleptic malignant syndrome (occurs at a lower rate than typicals)	
Omeprazole [Prilosec]	**Proton pump inhibitors—irreversibly inhibits H^+/K^+-ATPase in gastric parietal cells →decreases proton secretion by parietal cells**	Peptic ulcer disease, gastritis, esophageal reflux, and **Zollinger–Ellison syndrome**		**Inhibits cytochrome P450;** given with **clarithromycin** and **amoxicillin** for ***Helicobacter pylori***
Ondansetron [Zofran]	**Antiemetic—serotonin antagonist, 5-HT_3 blocker**	**Nausea** (caused by **cancer therapy** or **postoperative state**)	Headache; constipation; dizziness	
Oprelvekin [Neumega]	**Interleukin-11** stimulates multiple stages of **thrombopoiesis** increasing platelet production	**Thrombocytopenia**		
Orlistat [Xenical]	**Inhibits pancreatic lipases →** alters fat metabolism	**Obesity** (long term)	**Steatorrhea,** GI irritation, reduced absorption of fat soluble vitamins, and headache	**Used in conjunction with modified diet**
Oxacillin [Bactocill]	Antibiotic—β-lactam; penicillinase-resistant	*Staphylococcus* infections		
Oxaprozin [Daypro]	NSAID—mildly uricosuric	Acute gout		Contraindicated in patients with kidney stones
Oxazepam [Serax]	Antianxiety—benzodiazepine; enhances GABA; increases IPSP amplitude	Sedative; hypnotic; antiepileptic, anxiolytic		Recommended for use in elderly
Oxybutynin [Ditropan]	Antimuscarinic	Bladder/GI spasm; decreases acid in ulcer		
Oxycodone [Roxicodone]	**Partial opioid agonist** at mu receptor	Severe pain; general anesthetic	Respiratory depression; constipation; nausea	
Oxytocin [Pitocin, Syntocinon]	**Synthetic analog of oxytocin—stimulates uterine contraction and contraction of breast myoepithelial cells; milk letdown reflex**	**Induces labor; controls uterine hemorrhage**		
Paclitaxel [Taxol]	Antineoplastic—polymerizes tubules	Ovarian and breast cancer		
Pamidronate [Aredia]	Bone stabilizer—pyrophosphate analog; reduces hydroxyapatite crystal formation, growth, and dissolution, which reduces bone turnover	Hypercalcemia of malignancy; Paget disease; osteoporosis; hyperparathyroidism		

Therapeutic Agent (common name, if relevant) [trade name, where appropriate]	Class–Pharmacology and Pharmacokinetics	Indications	Side or Adverse Effects	Contraindications or Precautions to Consider; Notes
Pancuronium [Pavulon]	Nondepolarizing neuromuscular blocker			Minimal histamine release
Paroxetine [Paxil]	Selective serotonin reuptake inhibitors—inhibit **reuptake** of 5-HT at neuronal synapses	Major depression, OCD, anorexia, and bulimia	Inhibits liver enzymes, nausea, agitation, **sexual dysfunction** (anorgasmia), **and** dystonic reactions	Contraindicated with **MAOIs** secondary to **serotonin syndrome** (hyperthermia, muscle rigidity, and cardiovascular collapse); allows time for antidepressant effect, usually takes 2–3 weeks
Penicillamine [Cuprimine, Depen]	Antiarthritis—antigold medicine; not specific; unknown mechanism; arthritis relief	**Rheumatic arthritis; copper poisoning; metal chelator**	Decreases vitamin B6; bone marrow suppression; proteinuria; autoimmune syndrome	
Penicillin	**Antibiotic—β-lactam, cell wall inhibitor; binds PBP → inhibits transpeptidase** cross-linking of cell wall **→ inhibits bacterial cell wall synthesis → activates autolytic enzymes;** bactericidal	**Gram-positive cocci, Gram-positive rods, Gram-negative cocci, some anaerobes, enterococci,** and **spirochetes**	**Hypersensitivity reactions; platelet aggregation problems; hemolytic anemia; CNS effects; superinfection** (pseudomembrane colitis)	Not penicillinase resistant
Pentazocine [Talwin]	Mixed agonist/antagonist of opioids	Analgesia		Only mixed agonist/antagonist available orally
Pentobarbital [Nembutal sodium]	Barbiturate—prolongs IPSP duration	Cerebral edema; anesthetic		
Pergolide [Permax]	Antiparkinsonian—dopamine agonist; inhibits prolactin release	Treats breast engorgement; inhibits lactation		
Phenazocine	Opioid agonist			
Phenelzine	**Antidepressant, monoamine oxidase inhibitors**—inhibit **degradation** of NE and 5-HT at neuronal synapses	**Atypical depression** (with hypersomnia, anxiety, sensitivity to rejection, and hypochondriasis)	**Hypertensive episodes** with ingestion of tyramine-containing foods or beta agonists, hyperthermia, and convulsions	Contraindicated with **SSRIs** and **meperidine** secondary to **serotonin syndrome** (hyperthermia, muscle rigidity, and cardiovascular collapse)
Phenobarbital	**Barbiturate**—prolongs IPSP duration	**Antiepileptic (partial and tonic–clonic); cerebral edema; anesthetic**	Sedation	Many drug interactions
Phenolphthalein [Ex-Lax]	**Stimulant laxative**—reduces absorption of electrolytes and water from gut	Constipation	Tumorigenic	
Phenoxybenzamine [Dibenzyline]	Antihypertensive—α-blocker; long-acting; irreversible	Pheochromocytoma	Nasal congestion; miosis; orthostatic hypotension	

Phentolamine [Regitine]	**Antihypertensive—α-blocker**	**Diagnosis of pheochromocytoma;** hypertension (especially tyrosine-induced)		
Phenylbutazone [Butazolidin]	**NSAID**	**Rheumatic arthritis; acute gout**	**Agranulocytosis; aplastic anemia**	
Phenylephrine [Neo-Synephrine, Nostril]	Nasal decongestant—α_1-agonist	Nasal decongestant	Hypertension	
Phenylzin	Antidepressant—MAOI; nonselective but isoenzyme A most important; irreversible	Depression		
Phenytoin [Dilantin]	**Antiepileptic—decreases Na^+ flux**	**Epilepsy (partial and tonic–clonic); digitalis-induced arrhythmia**	**Decreases folic acid; gingival hyperplasia; hirsutism; nystagmus**	**Induces cytochrome P450; saturable elimination**
Physostigmine [Eserine]	**Inhibits cholinesterase**	**Intestinal or bladder atony; glaucoma**		
Pilocarpine [Ocusert]	**Antiglaucoma—muscarinic agonist**	**Xerostomia; narrow- and open-angle glaucoma**	**Focusing problems; nausea; abdominal pain; sweating; high dose: bradycardia, hypotension**	**Contraindicated in patients with peptic ulcer, asthma, hyperthyroid, and Parkinson disease**
Pioglitazone [Actos]	Hypoglycemic agent, thazolidinedione— improves target cell response to insulin	Oral treatment for **NIDDM (type II diabetes)**	**Weight gain,** edema, hepatotoxicity, increases LDL, and triglycerides	
Pindolol [Visken]	Antihypertensive antiarrhythmic (class II)—β-blocker	Hypertension		
Piperacillin [Pipracil]	**Antibiotic—β-lactam, penicillin derivative,** cell wall inhibitor; same mechanism as penicillin; distinguished by activity against ***Pseudomonas***; bactericidal	**Extended spectrum**—*Pseudomonas*; *Proteus*, and *Enterobacter* species	**Hypersensitivity reactions,** decreased platelet function	Not effective against penicillinase resistant staphylococcus, **combined with clauvulanic acid** (pencillinase inhibitor) to enhance spectrum; **resistant to β-lactamase;** administered IV
Piperazine [Entacyl]	Antihelminthic—causes flaccid paralysis in worm	Ascariasis (roundworm); Oxyuriasis (pinworm)	GI disturbances; urticaria; minor CNS	
Pirenzipine	**Muscarinic antagonist—blocks M1 receptors on ECL cells → decreases histamine secretion; blocks M_3 receptors on parietal cells → decreases acid secretion**	Peptic ulcer	**Tachycardia, dry mouth, and blurry vision** (difficulty accommodating)	
Piroxicam [Feldene]	NSAID			Long-acting; contraindicated in the elderly

Therapeutic Agent (common name, if relevant) [trade name, where appropriate]	Class–Pharmacology and Pharmacokinetics	Indications	Side or Adverse Effects	Contraindications or Precautions to Consider; Notes
Platelet-activating factor (PAF)	Activation of platelets and PMN aggregation; increases vascular permeability			
Plicamycin [Mithracin]	Antineoplastic—inhibits DNA-directed RNA synthesis; decreases protein synthesis needed for bone reabsorption	Paget disease; hypercalcemia		
Polymyxins [Aerosporin]	**Antibiotic—binds to cell membranes** → disrupt osmotic properties; bactericidal	**Gram-negative bacteria: *Pseudomonas* and coliforms; topical only; intrathecal for Pseudomonas meningitis**	**Neurotoxic; nephrotoxic** (acute renal tubular necrosis)	
Potassium	**Depresses ectopic pacemaker in hypokalemia**	**Digoxin toxity**		
Potassium iodide [Thyro-Block]	Expectorant—increases bronchial secretions; high doses decrease release of thyroid hormone	Promotes cough; hyperthyroidism		
Pralidoxime (2-PAM) [Protopam]	**Acetylcholinesterase reactivator**	**Overdose of malathion/parathion organophosphates; must be used before aging occurs**		
Pravastatin [Pravachol]	**Lipid lowering agent—HMG-CoA reductase inhibitor**—inhibits synthesis of cholesterol precursor mevalonate; **decreases LDL, increases HDL, and decreases TG**	**High LDL, preventative after thrombotic event (e.g., MI, stroke)**	Reversible increase in LFTs, myositis	Contraindicated in pregnant or lactating women and children
Praziquantel [Biltricide]	Antihelminthic—increases membrane permeability causing loss of Ca^{2+}	Schistosomes; flukes	GI disturbances; headache; fever; urticaria	
Prazosin [Minipress]	**Antihypertensive—α_1-blocker** → vasodilation → decreases total peripheral resistance	**Pheochromocytoma; hypertension**	**Orthostatic hypotension;** dizziness, headache	First dose orthostatic hypotension
Prednisone [Deltasone]	**Glucocorticoid—inhibits protein synthesis; reduces lymph node and spleen size; inhibits cell cycle activity of lymphoid cells; lyses T cells; suppresses antibody, prostaglandin, and leukotriene synthesis; blocks monocyte production of IL-1**	**Rheumatic arthritis; autoimmune disorders; allergic reaction; asthma; COPD; organ transplantation (esp. during rejection crisis)**	**Osteoporosis; Cushingoid reaction; psychosis; glucose intolerance; infection; hypertension; cataracts**	

Prilocaine [Citanest]	Anesthetic agent—blocks Na^+ channels intracellularly	Local anesthetic	Sleepiness; light-headedness; visual/audio disturbances; restlessness; nystagmus; shivering; tonic–clonic convulsion; death	
Primaquine phosphate [Primaquine Phosphate]	**Antimalarial**—unknown mechanism	**Cures vivax malaria; prophylaxis for falciparum malaria**	GI disturbances; mild anemia; **marked hemolysis in G-6-PD-deficient individuals; prolongs QT interval**	
Probenecid [Benemid]	Antigout—increased secretion of uric acid (uricosuric)—competes with uric acid for **reabsorption in the kidney**	Chronic gout therapy	**Caution: should not be used in patients with sulfa allergies;** rash; GI disturbances; drowsy	Should not be used to treat acute gout or patients with uric acid stones
Probucol [Bifenabid, Lesterol]	Lipid-lowering agent—lowers HDL and LDL; mechanism unknown	Hyperlipidemia	Prolongs QT interval; GI disturbances	Contraindicated in patients with heart disease
Procainamide [Pronestyl, Procanbid]	**Antiarrhythmic (class IA)—Na-channel blocker**	**Ventricular arrhythmia**	**Lupuslike syndrome**	
Procaine [Novocain]	Anesthetic agent—blocks Na^+ intracellularly	Local anesthetic	Sleepiness; light-headedness; visual/audio disturbances; restlessness; nystagmus; shivering; tonic–clonic convulsion; death	
Procarbazine [Matulane]	Antineoplastic—DNA alkylation and strand breakage; inhibits nucleic acid and protein synthesis	Cancer		
Prochlorperazine [Compazine]	**Antiemetic—dopamine (D_2 receptor) antagonist**	**Nausea;** counteracts nausea of **migraine**	Teratogenic	
	Hormone—secretory changes in endometrium and breast; necessary to maintain pregnancy		**Long-lasting suppression of menses; endometriosis; hirsutism; bleeding disorders; nausea; breast tenderness; hyperpigmentation; gallbladder disease; migraines; hypertension**	
Progesterone [Progestasert]	**Progesterone**—binds progesterone receptors	**Endometrial cancer**, amenorrhea, abnormal uterine bleeding, and **prevention of pregnancy**		Also used to prevent endometrial hyperplasia in postmenopausal women taking estrogen
Prolactin	**Hormone—stimulates lactation**			
Promethazine [Phenergan]	**Antihistamine, antiemetic**—D_2-receptor antagonist; H_1-blocker	Counteracts nausea of **migraine**; allergies; **motion sickness**	Sedation; CNS depression; atropine-like effects; allergic dermatitis; blood dyscrasias; **teratogenicity;** acute antihistamine poisoning	
Propafenone [Rythmol]	Antiarrhythmic (class IC)—Na^+-channel blocker			

Therapeutic Agent (common name, if relevant) [trade name, where appropriate]	Class–Pharmacology and Pharmacokinetics	Indications	Side or Adverse Effects	Contraindications or Precautions to Consider; Notes
Raloxifen [Evista]	**Selective estrogen receptor modulator—breast (estrogen antagonist); Endometrium (estrogen antagonist):** prevents proliferation of endometrium; **Bone (estrogen agonist):** decreases bone turnover, increases bone density; **Cardiovascular (estrogen agonist):** decreases LDL	**Osteoporosis; breast cancer**	**Hot flashes;** sinusitis; weight gain; muscle pain; leg cramps; **increased risk of blood clots**	Unlike estrogen, raloxifene **does not decrease HDL**
Ranitidine [Zantac]	**H_2 blocker—blocks histamine H_2 receptors reversibly → decreases proton secretion by parietal cells**	**Peptic ulcer disease, gastritis, and esophageal reflux**	**Gynecomastia, impotence,** decreased libido in males, **confusion, dizziness, and headaches**	**Crosses placenta; decreases renal excretion of creatinine; cytochrome P450 inhibitor**
Repaglinide [Prandin]	Hypoglycemic agent—**meglitinide; acts at pancreatic islet cell** to reduce K^+ efflux, increases Ca^{2+} influx, **increases secretion of insulin**	Oral treatment for **NIDDM** (type II diabetes)	**Hypoglycemia**	
Reserpine [Rauserfia]	Antihypertensive—prevents storage of monoamines in synaptic vesicle	Hypertension	**Mental depression,** sedation, nasal stuffiness, and diarrhea	
RhoGAM	**Rh immunoglobulin**	**Prevents hemolytic disease of the newborn**		
Ribavirin	**Antiviral—guanosine analog;** inhibits IMP dehydrogenase → decreases synthesis of guanine nucleotides	**RSV in children; hepatitis C when given with interferon**	**Hemolytic anemia, teratogen**	
Rifampin [Rifadin]	**Antibiotic—inhibits DNA-dependent RNA polymerase**	**Mycobacterium; reduces resistance to dapsone when used in treatment of leprosy; meningococcal prophylaxis in contacts of children with *H. influenza* type b**	**Turns body fluid orange in color; liver damage**	**Interferes with birth control pills by increasing estrogen metabolism; induces cytochrome P450**
Risedronate [Actonel]	**Bone stabilizer—bisphosphonate; pyrophosphate analog;** reduces hydroxyapatite crystal formation, growth, and dissolution, which reduces bone turnover	**Hypercalcemia of malignancy; Paget disease; osteoporosis; hyperparathyroidism**	**Pill-induced esophagitis**	

Risperidone	Atypical antipsychotic—blocks D_2, 5-HT, α_1, and H_1 receptors	Schizophrenia, useful for positive and negative symptoms	Agranulocytosis, **extrapyramidal** (occurs at a lower rate than typicals), **anticholinergic** (occurs at lower rate than other agents), **alpha blockade** (hypotension), and **histamine** (sedation); toxicity results in neuroleptic malignant syndrome (occurs at a lower rate than typicals)	Second-line agent used for refractory schizophrenia
Ritodrine [Yutopar]	B_2 agonist → uterine relaxation	Inhibits preterm labor		
Ritonavir [Norvir]	**Antiviral, protease inhibitor—** protease responsible for final step of viral proliferation; inhibits protease in progeny virons → assembly of nonfunctional viruses	**AIDS (Used in HAART)**	**GI irritation (nausea, diarrhea), hyperglycemia, and lipodystrophy**	**All protease inhibitors end in -navir; metabolism occurs by CYP450**
Rituximab	Monoclonal antibodies; binds to CD20 receptor on tumor cells, resulting in lysis	Non-Hodgkin lymphoma	Fever, rigor, chills; nausea, hypersensitivity; tumor lysis syndrome; irregular heart rhythms; infection; pancytopenia	
Ropivacaine	Anesthetic agent—blocks Na^+ intracellularly	Local anesthetic	Sleepiness; light-headedness; visual/audio disturbances; restlessness; nystagmus; shivering; tonic–clonic convulsion; death	
Rosiglitazone [Avandia]	Hypoglycemic agent, thazolidinedione—improves target cell response to insulin	Oral treatment for **NIDDM (type II diabetes)**	**Weight gain,** edema, hepatotoxicity, increases LDL, and triglycerides	
Salmeterol [Serevent]	**Antiasthmatic—long-acting β_2 agonist, leads to relaxation of smooth muscle**	Asthma prophylaxis	**Hand tremor;** headache; nervousness; dizziness; cough; stuffed nose; runny nose; ear pain; muscle pain/cramps; sore throat	Not in acute asthmatic attack
Saquinavir [Invirase]	**Antiviral, protease inhibitor—** protease responsible for final step of viral proliferation; inhibits protease in progeny virons → assembly of nonfunctional viruses	**AIDS (Used in HAART)**	**GI irritation (nausea, diarrhea), hyperglycemia, and lipodystrophy**	**All protease inhibitors end in -navir; metabolism occurs by CYP450**
Sargramostim [Leukine]	**Granulocyte-macrophage colony-stimulating factor**	**Recovery of bone marrow (e.g., bone marrow transplant failure)**	Hypertension	
Sarin/Soman	Irreversibly inhibits cholinesterase	Rapidly fatal		"Nerve gas"
Scopolamine	**Anticholinergic—**M_1-muscarinic receptor antagonist	**Motion sickness** prophylaxis	**Dry mouth,** drowsiness, and **vision disturbances**	**Delivered transdermally**

Therapeutic Agent (common name, if relevant) [trade name, where appropriate]	Class–Pharmacology and Pharmacokinetics	Indications	Side or Adverse Effects	Contraindications or Precautions to Consider; Notes
Scorpion toxin	Presynaptic neuromuscular junction blocker; overstimulates ACh release			
Secobarbital [Seconal]	Antiepileptic—anesthetic agent; barbiturate; prolongs IPSP duration	Epilepsy; cerebral edema		
Selegiline [Eldepryl]	Antiparkinsonian—increases dopamine by inhibiting MAO_b irreversibly	Parkinson disease		
Senna [Senokot]	**Stimulant laxative;** increases peristalsis	Constipation	Electrolyte imbalances (chronic use); melanosis coli	
Sertraline **[Zoloft]**	Selective serotonin reuptake inhibitors—inhibit **reuptake** of 5-HT at neuronal synapses	Major depression, OCD, anorexia, bulimia, and anxiety	Inhibits liver enzymes, nausea, agitation, **sexual dysfunction** (anorgasmia), and dystonic reactions	Contraindicated with **MAOIs** secondary to **serotonin syndrome** (hyperthermia, muscle rigidity, and cardiovascular collapse); allows time for antidepressant effect, usually takes 2–3 weeks
Sevoflurane [Sevorane, Ultane]	Anesthetic agent	General anesthetic		
Sibutramine [Meridia]	**Sympathomimetic serotonin and norepinephrine reuptake inhibitor**	**Obesity** (short term and long term)	Hypertension, tachycardia	
Sildenafil [Viagra]	**Phosphodiesterase type 5 inhibitor (cGMP-specific)**—increased cGMP → smooth muscle relaxation → increased blood flow in the corpus cavernosum → penile erection	**Erectile dysfunction**	**Abnormal vision** (impaired blue-green color vision); **UTIs; cardiovascular events; priapism; dyspepsia,** headache, and flushing	Risk of hypotension (fatal) in patient taking nitrates
Simvastatin [Zocor]	Lipid-lowering agent—**HMG-CoA reductase inhibitors**—inhibit synthesis of cholesterol precursor mevalonate; **decreases LDL, increases HDL, and decreases TG**	**High LDL, preventative after thrombotic event (e.g., MI, stroke)**	Reversible increase in LFTs, myositis	Contraindicated in pregnant and lactating women and children
Sodium nitroprusside	Antianginal—direct release of NO → increases cGMP → vasodilator (arterial dilation)	**Hypertensive emergency, CHF, and angina**	Cyanide toxicity; hypotension	Short acting, given IV
Somatostatin [Zecnil]	**Hormone—decreases release of GH, gastrin, secretin, VIP, CCK, glucagon, and insulin**	**Acromegaly; glucagonoma; insulinoma**	**Nausea; cramps; gallstones**	

Sotalol [Betapace]	Antiarrhythmic (class III)—K^+-channel blocker	Torsade de pointes		
Spectinomycin [Trobicin]	**Aminoglycoside antibiotic**—protein synthesis inhibitor; **irreversibly binds 30S ribosome** subunits; **bacteriostatic** at low concentration; **bactericidal** at high concentration	**Broad-spectrum:** Gram-negative rods; good for **bone** and **eye** infections; *Proteus, Pseudomonas, Enterobacter, Klebsiella*, and *E. coli*	**Ototoxicity; renal toxicity; neuromuscular blockade;** nausea; vomiting; vertigo; allergic skin rash; superinfections	Used to treat gonorrhea in those allergic to penicillin
Spironolactone [Aldactone]	Potassium sparing diuretic—binds to intracellular aldosterone steroid receptors in **collecting tubules**; blocks induction of Na^+ channels and $Na^+/$ATPase synthesis or blocks Na channels directly (amiloride, tramterene); loss of Na^+, Cl^- in urine	Hyperaldosteronism, potassium depletion, and congestive heart failure	**Hyperkalemic metabolic acidosis, gynecomastia** (spironolactone), and antiandrogen effects	Results in decreased secretion of K^+ and H^+, which can lead to **hyperkalemic metabolic acidosis;** often given in combination with a thiazide
Stavudine (d4T)	**Antiviral, nucleoside reverse transcriptase inhibitor—thymidine analog→** incorporated into viral DNA by reverse transcriptase →terminates viral DNA synthesis → prevents integration of DNA copy of viral genome into the host DNA	**AIDS (Used in HAART)**	**Neutropenia, anemia, peripheral neuropathy, pancreatitis, and lactic acidosis**	**Good CNS penetration**
Streptokinase [Streptase]	**Thrombolytic—plasminogen activator**	**Lysis of clots**	**Hemorrhage**	
Streptomycin	**Aminoglycoside antibiotic**—protein synthesis inhibitor; **irreversibly binds 30S ribosome** subunits; **bacteriostatic** at low concentration; **bactericidal** at high concentration	**Broad-spectrum:** Gram-negative rods; good for **bone** and **eye** infections; *Proteus, Pseudomonas, Enterobacter, Klebsiella*, and *E. coli;* **tuberculosis and other mycobacteria**	**Ototoxicity; renal toxicity; neuromuscular blockade; nausea;** vomiting; vertigo; allergic skin rash; superinfections	
Strychnine	Acts on the postsynaptic Renshaw cell; binds to glycine receptor (mimics effect of tetanus)	Depression	Fatal seizures	Rat poison
Succinylcholine [Anectine]	**Depolarizing neuromuscular blocker**	**Rapid-sequence intubation**	**Increases intraocular pressure; succinylcholine apnea in genetically defective pseudo-cholinesterase; malignant hyperthermia if given with halothane**	**Contraindicated in patients with glaucoma and patients taking antibiotics**
Sucralfate [Carafate]	Antiulcer—protective coating of GI lining	Reduces the effect of gastric acid on mucosa	Constipation	

Therapeutic Agent (common name, if relevant) [trade name, where appropriate]	Class–Pharmacology and Pharmacokinetics	Indications	Side or Adverse Effects	Contraindications or Precautions to Consider; Notes
Sulfamethoxazole, sulfisoxazole, sulfadiazine	**Antibiotic—sulfonamide, DNA synthesis inhibitor; competitive inhibitor of dihydropteroate synthetase (blocks folic acid synthesis);** bacteriostatic	**Broad-spectrum; Gram-positive UTI; Chlamydia infection of genital tract and eye; treatment of nocardiosis**	**Forms crystals in kidney and bladder, causing damage; hypersensitivity reaction; photosensitivity; kernicterus (in infants); hemolysis (in G-6-PD deficiency)**	Displaces other drugs such as warfarin from albumin
Sulfasalazine	**Anti-inflammatory—sulfapyridine (antibacterial)** and **mesalamine (anti-inflammatory)**	Ulcerative colitis, Crohn disease	Malaise, nausea, **sulfonamide toxicity,** and reversible **oligospermia**	**Activated by colonic bacteria**
Sulfinpyrazone [Anturane]	Antigout—increased secretion of uric acid (uricosuric)—competes with uric acid for **reabsorption in the kidney**	Chronic gout therapy	**Caution: should not be used in patients with sulfa allergies;** GI irritation; hypersensitivity reaction; agranulocytosis	Should not be used to treat acute gout or patients with uric acid stones
Sulindac [Clinoril]	Anti-inflammatory—prodrug sulfide	Chronic inflammation (arthritis)		
Sumatriptan [Imitrex]	**Antimigraine—agonist at 5-HT$_{1d}$ receptors**	**Acute attack of migraine**		
Ipecac (syrup) [Quelidrine]	Expectorant—increases bronchial secretions	Promotes cough		
Tacrine [Cognex]	**Alzheimer agent—noncompetitive cholinesterase inhibitor; muscarinic agonist**	**Alzheimer disease**	**Hepatotoxicity**	
Tacrolimus (FK506) [Prograf]	**Immunosuppressant—blocks activation of T-cell transcription factors; involved in interleukin synthesis**	**Transplant rejection**	**Nephrotoxic; neurotoxic; hyperglycemia; GI disturbances**	
Tamoxifen [Nolvadex]	**Selective estrogen receptor modular—competitively binds estrogen receptors; breast (estrogen antagonist):** prevents proliferation of estrogen receptor positive tumor cells; **endometrium (partial agonist); bone (agonist):** decreases bone turnover, increases bone density	**Treats estrogen-dependent breast cancer in postmenopausal women;** reduces contralateral breast cancer; osteoporosis prevention	**May increase risk of endometrial cancer; hot flashes;** flushing	
Temazepam [Restoril]	Benzodiazepine—enhances GABA; increases IPSP amplitude	Sedative; hypnotic; antianxiety; antiepileptic		

Terazosin [Hytrin]	Antihypertensive—α_1-blocker	Pheochromocytoma; hypertension; benign prostatic hyperplasia	Postural hypotension	
Terbinafine [Lamisil]	Antifungal—inhibits squalene-2,3-epoxidase	Orally for onychomycosis; topically for dermatophytes		
Terbinafine [Lamisil]	Antifungal—inhibits squalene-2,3-epoxidase	Orally for onychomycosis; topically for dermatophytes	Hepatotoxicity	
Terbutaline [Brethine, Bricanyl, Brethaire]	**β_2-agonist**—bronchodilator	**Bronchodilates to treat asthma; inhibits preterm labor; relaxes uterus**		
Tetanus toxin	**Acts at the presynaptic Renshaw cell; prevents glycine release**		Seizures	
Tetracaine [Pontocaine]	Anesthetic agent—blocks Na^+ channels intracellularly	Local anesthetic	Sleepiness; light-headedness; visual/audio disturbances; restlessness; nystagmus; shivering; tonic–clonic convulsion; death	
Tetracycline [Achromycin, Sumycin, Topicycline]	**Tetracycline antibiotic—protein synthesis inhibitor; binds 30S ribosome subunits** → prevents attachment of tRNA; bacteriostatic	**Broad-spectrum including atypical pathogens: *Chlamydia, Rickettsia, Mycoplasma pneumoniae, Vibrio cholerae, Ureaplasma urealyticum, Tularemia, H. pylori,* and *Borrelia burgdorferi*** (Lyme disease)	**Liver toxicity; GI distress; depression of bone/teeth development** (less with doxycycline); **photosensitivity** (less with doxycycline); **superinfections owing to broad-spectrum; Fanconi syndrome**	**Contraindicated in pregnancy and children; divalent cations inhibit gut absorption, therefore cannot take with milk, antacids, or iron-containing preparations; tetracycline is renally eliminated; doxycycline is fecally eliminated and must not be taken in patients with renal insufficiency**
THC (active ingredient in marijuana)	Unknown mechanism; binds cannabinoid receptors and inhibits vomiting center in medulla	Antiemetic	Dry mouth; dizziness; inability to concentrate; disorientation; anxiety; tachycardia; depression; paranoia; psychosis	
Theobromine	Unknown mechanism; stimulates CNS, cardiac muscle; relaxes smooth muscle; produces diuresis; increases cerebral vascular resistance			
Theophylline [Aerolate, Elixophyllin, Respbid, Slo-bid, Slo-Phyllin, Theo-24, Theo-Dur, Theolair, Uniphyl]	Methylxanthines—unknown mechanism; postulated to inhibit phosphodiesterase → decreases cAMP hydrolysis → promotes bronchodilation; stimulates CNS, cardiac muscle; relaxes smooth muscle; produces diuresis; increases cerebral vascular resistance	Asthma	Cardiotoxicity, neurotoxicity	Metabolized by cytochrome P450; narrow therapeutic window; Tolerance develops

Therapeutic Agent (common name, if relevant) [trade name, where appropriate]	Class–Pharmacology and Pharmacokinetics	Indications	Side or Adverse Effects	Contraindications or Precautions to Consider; Notes
Tranexamic acid (AMCHA) [Cyklokapron]	Thrombotic agent—competitive inhibitor of plasminogen activation	Inhibits fibrinolysis; promotes thrombosis		
Tranylcypromine [Parnate]	Antidepressant—MAOI; nonselective, but isoenzyme A most important; reversible	Depression		Only reversible MAOI
Trazodone [Desyrel]	Atypical antidepressant—inhibits reuptake of serotonin	Major depression (especially with insomnia), insomnia	Sedation, nausea, **priapism,** and postural hypotension	
TRH (protirelin) [Relefact TRH]	Stimulates TSH and prolactin release	Diagnosis of thyroid disease		
Triamcinolone	**Glucocorticoid**—inhibits protein synthesis; reduces lymph node and spleen size; inhibits cell cycle activity of lymphoid cells; lyses T cells; suppresses antibody, prostaglandin, and leukotriene synthesis; blocks monocyte production of IL-1	Addison disease; rheumatic arthritis; autoimmune disorders; allergic reaction; asthma; organ transplantation (esp. during rejection crisis)	**Osteoporosis; Cushingoid reaction; psychosis; glucose intolerance; infection; hypertension; cataracts; peptic ulcers**	
Triamterene [Dyrenium]	Potassium sparing diuretic—binds to intracellular aldosterone steroid receptors in **collecting tubules**; blocks induction of Na^+ channels and Na^+/ATPase synthesis and blocks Na channels directly; loss of Na^+, Cl^- in urine	Hyperaldosteronism, potassium depletion, and congestive heart failure	**Hyperkalemic metabolic acidosis, gynecomastia** (spironolactone), and antiandrogen effects	Results in decreased secretion of K^+ and H^+, which can lead to **hyperkalemic metabolic acidosis;** often given in combination with a thiazide
Triazolam [Halcion]	Benzodiazepine—enhances GABA; increases IPSP amplitude	Sedative; hypnotic; antianxiety	Paranoia; violent behavior; antiepileptic	
Trientine	Metal chelator	Copper poisoning; Wilson disease		
Trifluridine [Viroptic]	Antiviral—thymidine derivative; inhibits DNA polymerase; inhibits DNA synthesis	DNA viruses		
Trihexyphenidyl [Artane]	Antiparkinsonian—muscarinic blocker	Parkinson disease		
Triiodothyronine (T_3) [Triostat]	Synthetic analog of thyroid hormone T_3	**Hypothyroidism**	Tachycardia, heat intolerance, tremors, and arrhythmia	
Trimethaphan [Arfonad]	Antihypertensive—nondepolarizing nicotinic blocker	Hypertension (short-term)		

Trimethoprim [Proloprim, Trimpex]	**Antibiotic—DNA synthesis inhibitor; competitive inhibition of dihydrofolate reductase** (blocks folic acid synthesis); bacteriostatic	**Gram-negative UTI; combined with sulfonamides to treat UTI, otitis media, chronic bronchitis, shigellosis, *Salmonella*, and PCP**	Megaloblastic anemia, leukopenia, and granulocytopenia	Supplementation with folic acid may help pancytopenia
Triretinoin [Retin-A]	Retinoids—inhibits microcomedo formation and existing lesions; makes keratinocytes in sebaceous follicles less adherent and easier to remove	Acne; skin cancer	Photosensitivity	
Trovafloxacin [Trovan]	Antibiotic—Quinolone, blocks DNA synthesis by inhibiting DNA gyrase	Gram-negative infections (esp. UTI and bone): *Pseudomonas*, Enterobacteriaceae, and *Neisseria*; Gram-positive infections; intracellular: *Legionella*	GI disturbances; headache; dizziness; phototoxicity; cartilage damage in children	May elevate theophylline to toxic levels, causing seizure
TSH (thyrotropin) [Thyrogen]	**Increases output of thyroid hormone**	**Assesses thyroid function; increases uptake of I-131 in thyroid carcinoma**		
d-Tubocurarine [Tubarine]	**Nondepolarizing neuromuscular blocker**		Paralysis	
Ultralente [Humulin U, Novolin U]	**Long acting insulin**—*see mechanism for insulin*	**Diabetes mellitus** (typically **Type 1**)	**Hypoglycemia** (diaphoresis, vertigo, and tachycardia); insulin allergy; insulin antibodies; lipodystrophy	
Undecylenic acid [Desenex]	Antifungal—unknown mechanism; fungistatic	Topical for dermatophytes (esp. tinea pedis)		
Urofollitropin [Metrodin]	FSH analog	Infertility		
Urokinase [Abbokinase]	**Thrombolytic agent—plasminogen activator**	**Lysis of clots**	**Hemorrhage**	
Valacyclovir [Valtrex]	**Antiviral—guanosine analog;** inhibits DNA polymerase	**HSV, VZV, EBV, and CMV at high doses**	**GI disturbances; CNS and renal problems; headache; tremor; rash**	**Longer lasting than acyclovir**
Valproic acid [Depakene]	**Antiepileptic—blocks Na^+ channels and increases GABA**	**Epilepsy: partial, absence, and tonic–clonic**	**Liver toxicity; pancreatitis; potentially fatal**	
Vancomycin [Vancocin]	**Antibiotic—cell wall inhibitor;** binds to D-alanyl-D-alanine portion of cell wall → inhibits cell wall glycopeptide polymerization → stops bacterial cell wall synthesis; bactericidal	**Serious infections by Gram-positive bacteria: *Streptococcus, Staphylococcus, Pneumococcus*, and some anaerobes (esp. *Clostridium difficile*)**	**Ototoxicity, nephrotoxicity, thrombophlebitis, and diffuse flushing—"red man syndrome"; caused by histamine release**	Can prevent red man syndrome by pretreatment with antihistamines and slow infusion; resistance occurs when bacteria change amino acid in cell wall to D-ala D-lac

Therapeutic Agent (common name, if relevant) [trade name, where appropriate]	Class–Pharmacology and Pharmacokinetics	Indications	Side or Adverse Effects	Contraindications or Precautions to Consider; Notes
Zanamivir, oseltamivir [Tamiflu]	**Antiviral—inhibits neuraminidase** → decreases release of progeny viruses	**Influenza A and B treatment and prophylaxis**		Begin within 2 days of onset of flu symptoms to decrease the duration and intensity of symptoms
Zidovudine (ZDV, formerly AZT) [Retrovir]	**Antiviral, nucleoside reverse transcriptase inhibitor**—inhibits viral reverse transcriptase → prevents integration of DNA copy of viral genome into the host DNA	**AIDS (Used in HAART); HIV pregnant female** to reduce fetal transmission	**Neutropenia, anemia** (megaloblastic anemia), **peripheral neuropathy, pancreatitis, and lactic acidosis**	**Effects of bone marrow suppression, such as neutropenia and anemia, can be reduced by the addition of GM-CSF**
Zileuton	**Antiasthma agent—5-lipoxygenase inhibitor** → inhibits conversion of arachidonic acid to leukotriene → prevents bronchoconstriction and inflammatory cell infiltrate	**Improves asthma**		
Zolpidem [Ambien]	Binds to benzodiazepine receptor, but is not a benzodiazepine	Insomnia		

5-HT, 5-hydroxytryptamine (serotonin); ACE, angiotensin-converting enzyme; ACh, acetylcholine; ACTH, adrenocorticotropic hormone; ADP, adenosine diphosphate; AML, acute myelocytic leukemia; ATPase, adenosine triphosphatase; AV, atrioventricular; BAL, blood alcohol level; BP, blood pressure; BPH, benign prostatic hypertrophy; cAMP, cyclic adenosine monophosphate; CBC, complete blood count; CCK, cholecystokinin; cGMP, cyclic guanosine monophosphate; CHF, congestive heart failure; CMI, cell-mediated immunity; CMV, cytomegalovirus; CNS, central nervous system; CoA, coenzyme A; COPD, chronic obstructive pulmonary disease; COX, cyclooxygenase; DCT, distal convoluted tubule; dCTP, deoxycytidine triphosphate; DHEA, dehydroepiandrosterone; EBV, Epstein–Barr virus; ECG, electrocardiogram, electrocardiography; FAD, flavin adenine dinucleotide; FMN, flavin mononucleotide; FSH, follicle-stimulating hormone; GABA, γ-aminobutyric acid; GH, growth hormone; GI, gastrointestinal; GnRH, gonadotropin-releasing hormone; HDL, high-density lipoprotein; HMG-CoA, 3-hydroxy-3-methylglutaryl coenzyme A; IFN, interferon; IPSP, inhibitory postsynaptic potential; LDL, low-density lipoprotein; L-DOPA, levodopa (levo-3, 4-dihydroxyphenylalanine); LH, luteinizing hormone; LPL, lipoprotein lipase; LTB_4, leukotriene B_4; MAO, monoamine oxidase; MAO_b, monoamine oxidase B; MAOI, monoamine oxidase inhibitor; MHC, major histocompatibility complex; MI, myocardial infarction; NAD, nicotinamide adenine dinucleotide; NADH, reduced nicotinamide adenine dinucleotide; NE, norepinephrine; NIDDM, noninsulin-dependent diabetes mellitus; NO, nitric oxide; NSAID, nonsteroidal anti-inflammatory drug; PCP, phencyclidine; PCT, proximal convoluted tubule; PDA, patent ductus arteriosus; PGE_1, prostaglandin E_1; PGE_2, prostaglandin E_2; PGF_{2a}, prostaglandin F_{2a}; PMN, polymorphonuclear; PTH, parathyroid hormone; PTT, partial thromboplastin time; Rh, rhesus [factor]; RSV, respiratory syncytial virus; SLE, systemic lupus erythematosus; SSRI, selective serotonin reuptake inhibitor; TCA, tricyclic antidepressant; TG, triglycerides; THC, tetrahydrocannabinol; TSH, thyroid-stimulating hormone; UTI, urinary tract infection; VIP, vasoactive intestinal peptide; VLDL, very low density lipoprotein.

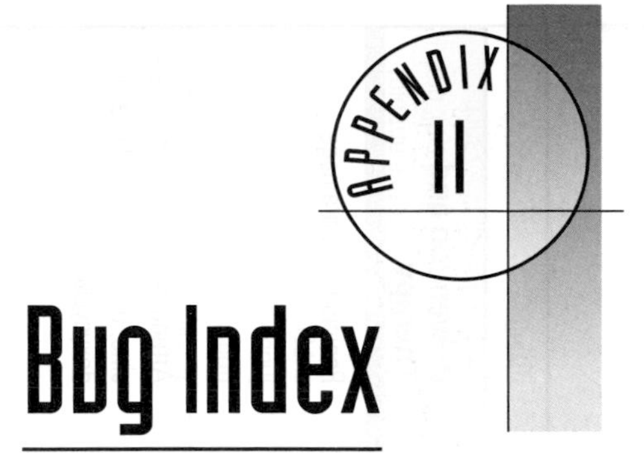

Bug Index

Name	Morphology	Pathogenesis	Description of Disease	Laboratory Findings, Notes	Transmission	Prevention and Therapy
Clostridium perfringens	Gram +; rod; spore former; anaerobic	α-Toxin (damages cell membranes); γ-toxin (tissue necrosis and hemolysis); choleralike heat-labile enterotoxin (food poisoning—watery diarrhea); spores establish in GI and produce entertoxins	Gas gangrene; food poisoning; anaerobic cellulites	Large rods found in food; double-zone of hemolysis	Grows in traumatized tissue (muscle); spores in food and soil germinate in reheated foods (stews, soups)	Clean and debride wounds; cook food well
Clostridium tetani	Gram +; rod; spore former (tennis racquet shaped); anaerobic	Tetanus toxin (exotoxin)—blocks release of inhibitory neurotransmitters	Tetanus: Lockjaw (trismus), spastic paralysis (opisthotonos), and sardonic grin (risus sardonicus)	Usually not recovered by culture	Spore entry via wound (e.g., a rusty nail)	Toxoid vaccine (2, 4, 6, and 18 months) booster every 10 years; tetanus immunoglobulin (passive immunity); penicillin
Corynebacterium diphtheriae	Gram +; rod; club shaped; arranged in V or L; not spore former	Exotoxin-A subunit ADP ribosylates EF-2, and B subunit binds toxin to the cell; phage conversion	Diphtheria—pseudomembrane forms in the throat; bull neck; systemic toxemia	Tellurite plate (Löffler's medium) grows black colonies	Airborne droplets	Inactivated toxoid vaccine; antitoxin (neutralizes unbound toxin); penicillin; erythromycin
Coxiella burnetii	Obligate intracellular	Unknown	Q fever	Only rickettsia not transmitted to humans by an arthropod vector; occupational hazard for tanners, sheep shearers, dairy farmers	Inhalation of aerosols of urine, feces; transplacental	Tetracycline
Enterococcus faecalis	Gram +; cocci	Lipoteichoic acid	Urinary, biliary, and cardiovascular infections; endocarditis	Catalase-negative; bacitracin resistant; variable hemolysis; grows in 6.5% NaCl/Lancefield group D	Normal flora of gut gaining access to blood	Penicillin and an aminoglycoside
Escherichia coli	Gram –; bacilli	Endotoxin—septic shock; heat-labile (LT) enterotoxin: Increased cAMP leads to diarrhea; heat-stable (ST) stimulates guanylate cyclase to cause diarrhea; pili: Adhere to epithelium especially in UTIs; Verotoxin (O157:H7): Shigellalike toxin in EHEC that inhibits 28S rRNA to cause bloody diarrhea	UTIs; sepsis; neonatal meningitis; enteropathogenic *E. coli* (EPEC): Traveler's diarrhea; enterotoxigenic *E. coli* (ETEC): Watery diarrhea; enteroinvasive *E. coli* (EIEC): Dysentery; enterohemorrhagic *E. coli* (EHEC): Bloody diarrhea, hemolytic uremic syndrome	Oxidase—cysteine agar	Transplacental; fecal–oral route; foodborne	UTIs: Trimethoprim-sulfamethoxazole; sepsis: Cephalosporins; traveler's diarrhea: Rehydration

Francisella tularensis	Gram –; rod; intracellular	Capsule; intracellular within macrophages; granuloma formation	Painful lymph nodes; glandular and ocular ulcers	Serology	Zoonotic via rabbits and ticks	Live attenuated vaccine; streptomycin; thorough cooking of meat
Gardnerella vaginalis	Gram variable; bacillus; anaerobic	Unknown	Vaginosis—watery discharge, fishy odor	Clue cells (epithelial cells coated with bacteria); whiff test	Sexually transmitted	Metronidazole
Haemophilus ducreyi	Gram –; bacilli	Virulence via pili	Chancroid with pain and purulent exudate	Lesions similar to those of syphilis; lymphadenopathy	Sexually transmitted	Nafcillin; erythromycin
Haemophilus influenzae	Gram –; coccobacilli; polysaccharide capsule (polyribitol phosphate)	IgA protease degrades antibody and attaches to respiratory tract; capsule (type B) prevents phagocytosis	Infantile meningitis; epiglottitis; No. 2 cause of otitis media and sinusitis	Needs heme (factor X) and NAD (factor V) to grow; chocolate agar; check CSF	Respiratory droplets	Hib vaccine (b-type capsule conjugated to diphtheria toxoid as a carrier protein); ceftriaxone
Helicobacter pylori	Gram –; bacilli; motile; flagella	Urease results in ammonia production and subsequent gastric damage	Peptic ulcers (type B gastritis)	Microaerophilic; Campy plate; urea breath test; urease +; serology ELISA; biopsy	Ingestion	Triple therapy: Amoxicillin, omeprazole, and clarithromycin; Quadruple therapy; bismuth, tetracycline, metronidazole, and omeprazole
Klebsiella pneumoniae	Gram –; bacilli; capsule; + quellung reaction	Large capsule hinders phagocytosis	Pneumonia, particularly in malnourished alcoholics; UTI; bacteremia	Currant-jelly sputum (thick bloody sputum)	Aspiration of respiratory droplets	Cephalosporins
Legionella pneumophila	Gram –; bacilli	Endotoxin affects smokers, alcoholics, and those older than 55 years of age	Legionnaire disease (atypical pneumonia)	Dieterle silver stain; cysteine required for culture; urine test for Legionella antigen	Aerosol from environmental water sources, contaminated air conditioning system	Erythromycin
Listeria monocytogenes	Gram +; rod; arranged in V or L; tumbling motility; not spore former	Grows intracellularly in macrophages; listeriolysin-O cytotoxic	Meningitis and sepsis in newborns and immunocompromised	Small, gray colonies; β-hemolysis; motility; serology	Transferred to humans by animals or their feces; unpasteurized milk; contaminated vegetables, cheese, and cabbage	Ampicillin and gentamicin
Moraxella catarrhalis	Gram –; diplococcus		Upper respiratory tract infection; No. 3 cause of otitis media and sinusitis		Transmitted by respiratory secretions	Azithromycin; penicillin resistant (100% strains make β-lactamase)
Mycobacterium *avium-intracellulare (MAC)*	Acid-fast bacilli	Unknown	Tuberculosis-like disease in the immunocompromised		From the soil and water to the immunocompromised individuals	Amikacin plus doxycycline

Name	Morphology	Pathogenesis	Description of Disease	Laboratory Findings, Notes	Transmission	Prevention and Therapy
Staphylococcus aureus	Gram +; cocci; capsule; protein A in the cell wall; yellow, creamy, grapelike clusters on culture	Rapid growth; protein A (antiphagocytic); enterotoxin (watery diarrhea); toxic shock syndrome toxin; exfoliation; α-toxin; coagulase	Abscesses; pyogenic infections (endocarditis, osteomyelitis); food poisoning; toxic shock syndrome; scalded skin syndrome	Coagulase +; catalase +; β-hemolytic; novobiocin-sensitive; ferment mannitol	Via the hands from the skin, nasal mucosa; entertoxin: Ham, chicken salad, cottage cheese, processed food	Hand washing; 80% penicillin-resistant (make β-lactamase); vancomycin; cephalosporin
Staphylococcus epidermidis	Gram +; cocci; white, creamy, grapelike clusters on culture	Surface glycocalyx	Endocarditis; infection on catheters and implant sites; sepsis in neonates	Coagulase –; catalase +; no hemolysis; novobiocin-sensitive	On skin; IV drug users	Vancomycin
Staphylococcus saprophyticus	Gram +; cocci; creamy, grapelike clusters	Selectively adheres to transitional epithelium	UTIs in young women	Coagulase –; catalase +; no hemolysis; novobiocin-resistant	Many sexual partners	Quinolones
Streptococcus agalactiae	Gram +; cocci; diploid; Group B Streptococcus	Capsular antigen (contains sialic acid blocks opsionization)	No. 1 cause of neonatal sepsis and meningitis	Catalase –; bacitracin-resistant; β-hemolysis; Lancefield group B; hippurate hydrolysis +	Genital tract of some women	Ampicillin before delivery; penicillin G
Streptococcus pneumoniae	Gram +; cocci; lancet shaped; in pairs; polysaccharide capsule (85 different types)	Capsule prevents phagocytosis; IgA protease; adheres to mucosa	Pneumonia; meningitis; bacteremia; upper respiratory infection; otitis media	Catalase –; α-hemolysis bile soluble; inhibited by Optochin; quellung reaction (capsular swelling)	Noncommunicable	Polysaccharide capsular vaccine available for high-risk groups; penicillin and erythromycin
Streptococcus pyogenes	Gram +; cocci; chains or pairs; rough or smooth hyaluronic acid capsule	M protein (pili); streptokinase (dissolves fibrin); DNase; hyaluronidase; hemolysins: Erythrogenic toxin (scarlet fever rash); streptolysin-O and -S; exotoxin A (superantigen causing TSS-like syndrome)	Pharyngitis; cellulitis; rheumatic fever; acute glomerulonephritis; TSS-like syndrome	Catalase –; bacitracin (A disk)-sensitive; (β-hemolytic; antistreptolysin-O for serotyping; Lancefield group A; rapid antigen detection test	Normal flora of skin, throat causing disease when in blood	Penicillin G

Treponema pallidum	Spirochete	Multiplication followed by blood vessel involvement	Syphilis—primary with painless sores, purulent exudate, and induration; secondary with a rash; tertiary (rare) includes CNS involvement and aortitis	Darkfield microscopy; screen with RPR or VDRL test for cardiolipin (non-treponemal tests); confirm with FTA-abs or MHA-tp (treponemal specific test); systemic illness can occur with treatment (Jarisch–Herxheimer reaction)	Sexually transmitted; transplacental	Penicillin
Tropheryma whippelii	Gram +; rod actinomycete	Foamy macrophages found in the lamina propria of the jejunum	Whipple disease—steat-orrhea, lymphadenopathy, fever, and cough	Visualization of the organ-ism in a biopsy of the small bowel	Unknown	Trimethoprim–sulfamethoxazole
Vibrio cholerae	Gram –; comma-shaped rod; polar flagella ADP ribosylates G protein	Pili adhere to gut mucosa; phage-coded cholera toxin: 2 A active subunits and 5 B binding units (A subunit in-creasing cAMP and causing movement of ions and water out of the cell)	Rice-water stools	Fecal specimens culture; agglutination assays	Fecal–oral route via water and food	Vaccine ineffective; rehydration; tetracycline, chloroamphenicol
Vibrio parahaemolyticus	Gram –; comma-shaped rod	Toxin	Explosive diarrhea; cramps; nausea	High-infective dose required	Shellfish; raw or under-cooked seafood	Self-limiting
Yersinia pestis	Gram –; bacillus; intracellular	V and W antigens (active within macrophages); fibrinolysin; F1 protein inhibits phagocytosis	Bubonic plague (with lymph node swelling and bubo); fever; conjunctivitis	Cultures are hazardous and precautions must be taken	Zoonotic via rat fleas	Vaccine; streptomycin

ADP, adenosine diphosphate; bCG, bacille Calmette–Guérin; cAMP, cyclic adenosine monophosphate; CNS, central nervous system; CSF, cerebrospinal fluid; DNase, deoxyribonuclease; EHEC, enterohemorrhagic *Escherichia coli;* EIEC, enteroinvasive *Escherichia coli;* ELISA, enzyme-linked immunosorbent assay; EPEC, enteropathogenic *Escherichia coli;* ETEC, enterotoxigenic *Escherichia coli;* FTA-abs, Flurescent treponemal Antibody absorption test; GI, gastrointesti-nal; Hib, *Haemophilus influenza* type b; IV, intravenous; LPS, lipopolysaccharide; MHA-tp, Microhemoglutination test; MP, metalloproteinase; Mp, macrophage; NAD, nicotinamide–adenine dinucleotide; PID, pelvic inflammatory disease; PMN, polymorphonuclear neutrophils; PPD, purified protein derivative; RPR, rapid plasma reagin; TSS, toxic shock syndrome; UTI, urinary tract infection; U.S., United States; VDRL, Venereal Disease Research Laboratory.

Name	Morphology	Description of Disease	Pathogenesis	Laboratory Findings, Notes	Transmission	Prevention and Therapy
Human immunodeficiency virus	Enveloped RNA virus; diploid; single stranded; + polarity; reverse transcriptase, retrovirus	AIDS	Infects and kills helper T cells via the CD4 receptors and gp120 protein	Screen with ELISA; Western blot test confirms	Sexual, body fluids, transplacental; blood products	AZT to HIV-infected mothers and newborns; AZT, ddI, ddC; treat opportunistic infections like pneumonia or Kaposi sarcoma
Influenza virus	Enveloped RNA virus; segmented; single stranded; – polarity; polymerase in virion	Influenza	Infects the epithelium of the respiratory tract via hemagglutinin and neuraminidase on surface spikes; antigenic shift and drift of surface spikes lead to epidemics	Cell culture; hemagglutination inhibition; complement fixation; H and N protein spikes	Respiratory droplets; vaccine composed of inactivated strains of current virus which causes disease	Amantadine or Rimantadine for both prevention and treatment; vaccine composed of inactivated strains of current virus which causes disease
Measles virus	Enveloped RNA virus; single stranded; – polarity; polymerase in virion	Measles; subacute sclerosing panencephalitis (SSPE)	Infection spreads via the bloodstream from the upper respiratory tract to the organs; maculopapular rash caused by an immune response (Koplik spots)	Usually not done	Respiratory droplets	Attenuated vaccine; no treatment
Mumps virus	Enveloped RNA virus; single stranded; – polarity; polymerase in virion	Mumps; sterility owing to bilateral orchitis **MNEMONIC:** I got bumps from my mumps	Spreads from the upper respiratory tract to the organs (parotid glands, testes, ovaries, and CNS) via the bloodstream	Cell culture and hemadsorption; rise in antiviral antibody	Respiratory droplets	Attenuated vaccine; no treatment
Norwalk virus	Nonenveloped; RNA virus; single stranded; linear; + polarity	Gastroenteritis	Binds to cells of intestinal brush border; prevents absorption of water and nutrients; blunted villi in jejunum; infiltration with mononuclear cells	Not performed; serology; ELISA for Ag; stool EM	Fecal-oral	Symptomatic treatment
Papillomavirus	Nonenveloped DNA virus; circular; double stranded	Papillomas (warts); condylomata acuminata; cervical and penile carcinoma	dsDNA incorporates into host DNA; E1 and E2 promote DNA replication; E6 and E7 early viral genes inhibit activity of p53 and Rb tumor suppressor genes, respectively	Koilocytes (squamous cell with perinuclear clearing) in lesions; to define type use in situ DNA hybridization	Sexual via direct contact with genital lesions	Interferon-α; liquid nitrogen for warts; vaccine; annual Pap smear for cervical cancer screening

Parainfluenza	Enveloped; single stranded –RNA virus	Upper respiratory tract infection; croup (laryngotracheobronchitis); bronchiolitis; pneumonia	Two major surface glycoproteins fusion and HN; replication limited to respiratory epithelial cells		Direct person-to-person contact and large droplet aerosols	Ribavirin
Parvovirus B19	Nonenveloped; DNA virus; single stranded; linear	Erythema infectiosum (fifth disease)—characterized by "slapped cheek" appearance; may cause aplastic crisis in sickle cell disease	Erythema infectiosum—virus causes immune-complex deposition; aplastic anemia: Virus infects immature RBCs and kills them	Parvovirus-specific IgG/IgM antibody levels; laboratory analysis for viral DNA	Unknown—may be respiratory or direct contact	Self-limited
Poliovirus	Nonenveloped RNA virus; single stranded; + polarity	Abortive poliomyelitis; aseptic meningitis (more common); paralytic poliomyelitis; progressive potpoliomyelitis muscle atrophy (very rare)	Replicates in the pharynx and GI tract and spreads to the CNS; death of the anterior horn cells in the spinal cord; neurotropic for motor cortex	Isolation from CSF	Fecal-oral	Salk vaccine: Inactivated; Sabin vaccine: Attenuated, given in childhood immunizations; no treatment; **MNEMONIC:** Saber tooth tiger is alive and eats (Sabin vaccine is live oral vaccine)
Rabies virus	Enveloped RNA virus; bullet shape; single stranded; – polarity RNA; polymerase in virion	Rabies	ACh receptor of neuron binds virus; the virus follows the retrograde direction to invade the CNS and brain, resulting in encephalitis	Negri bodies (eosinophilic inclusion in nerve cell)	Animal (skunks, bats) bites; domestic dogs in developing countries	Before exposure: Vaccine; after exposure: Antirabies immunoglobulin plus inactivated vaccine from human cell culture; no treatment
Reovirus (Rotavirus)	Nonenveloped RNA virus; 11 segments; double stranded; RNA polymerase in virion	Gastroenteritis in children	Resistant to stomach acid, thus infects the small intestine	ELISA detects the virus in stool	Respiratory droplets; fecal–oral route	Rehydration with fluids and electrolytes
Respiratory syncytial virus	Enveloped RNA virus; single stranded; – polarity; polymerase in virion	Pneumonia or bronchiolitis in children	Immune response to lower respiratory tract infection	Multinucleated giant cells	Direct person-to-person contact	Ribavirin
Rhinovirus	Nonenveloped RNA virus; single stranded; + polarity; numerous serotypes	Common cold	Upper respiratory tract mucosa and conjunctiva infected; replicates at temperatures <37 °C; killed by stomach acid	None	Aerosol droplets with hand-to-nose transmission	None

Parasites and Protozoa

Name	Morphology	Pathogenesis	Description of Disease	Laboratory Findings, Notes	Transmission	Prevention; Therapy
Ascaris lumbricoides	Intestinal parasite	Larvae in the lung and a heavy worm burden in gastrointestinal tract	Ascariasis—intestinal obstruction, abdominal pain, coughing, nausea	Eosinophilia; eggs in feces	Contaminated food or soil	Maintain sanitary conditions; mebendazole
Entamoeba histolytica	Intestinal protozoan; cigar-shaped cysts; four nuclei	Trophozoite form invades the colon	Amebic dysentery; liver abscess; flask-shaped ulcers	Trophozoites seen in stool	Fecal-oral	Maintain sanitary conditions; metronidazole with diloxanide; steroids exacerbate
Enterobius vermicularis	Intestinal parasite	Worms and eggs (passed in feces) result in perianal pruritus	Pinworm infection—anal pruritus, vaginal irritation, and cystitis	Eggs on "Scotch tape" test (tape applied to the anus and then viewed under a microscope)	Reinfection by self; fecal-oral contact; egg ingestion	Mebendazole
Giardia lamblia	Intestinal protozoan; pear shaped; flagella; tumbling motility; two nuclei; four flagella	Interfere with fat and protein absorption	Giardiasis—acute diarrhea	Visible in stool	Fecal-oral	Maintain sanitary conditions; metronidazole
Leishmania donovani	Protozoan	Organs of the reticuloendothelial system are destroyed by macrophages infected with the protozoan	Visceral leishmaniasis (kala azar)—hyperpigmentation of the skin, massive splenomegaly, fever, anemia, and malaise	Biopsy of reticuloendothelial tissue shows the infected macrophages	Female Phlebotomus sandfly transmits the disease from the infected host to a human	Protection from sandfly bites; sodium stibogluconate (antimony compound)
Plasmodium sp.	Blood and tissue protozoan; signet ring trophozoites in RBCs; Schüffner dots (red-yellow dots in RBCs); banana-shaped gametocytes	Sporozoites from bite enter the bloodstream and invade hepatocytes (exoerythrocytic phase); merozoites invade the RBCs (erythrocytic phase)	Malaria—fever, chills, hepatomegaly, splenomegaly; symptoms in cyclical pattern (3 days for *P. malariae;* 2 days for *P. ovale, P. falciparum, P. vivax*); tissue anoxia	Blood smear shows organisms; *P. falciparum* is acute and needs immediate treatment	Female *Anopheles* mosquito	Protection from bites; chloroquine; quinine; mefloquine; insecticides
Schistosoma sp.	Blood fluke; eggs have spine (*S. mansoni* has large lateral spine, *S. haematobium* has a terminal spine, *S. japonicum* has a small lateral spine); two sexes	Eggs lead to inflammation, fibrosis, and granuloma formation	Schistosomiasis—pipestem fibrosis of liver; *S. haematobium* affects the bladder; *S. mansoni* affects the colon	Eggs in the stool or urine	Penetration of the skin by cercariae	Maintain sanitary conditions; praziquantel

Taenia sp.	Cestode: *T. solium*—pork tapeworm; *T. saginata*—beef; *Diphyllobothrium latum*—fish; four suckers and circle of hooks; 5–10 uterine branches	Encyst in tissue (eyes, brain, muscle) resulting in mass lesions	Taeniasis and cysticercosis	Gravid proglottids in stool	Eating raw or undercooked meat	Cook meat and maintain sanitary conditions; niclosamide
Toxoplasma gondii	Tissue protozoan	Infects macrophages; infects the brain, liver, eyes	Toxoplasmosis	Serologic; high morbidity and mortality	Ingestion of cysts; transplacental; cat feces	Cook meat; sulfonamides
Trichinella spiralis	Intestinal parasite	Muscle inflammation	Trichinosis—periorbital edema, myositis, fever, and diarrhea	Larvae on muscle biopsy; eosinophilia by 14th day; double-barreled egg	Eating raw or undercooked meat	Cook meat; thiabendazole
Trichomonas vaginalis	Urogenital protozoan; pear shaped; flagella; trophozoites	Attaches to the wall of the vagina	Trichomoniasis—itching and burning with yellow discharge from the vagina (strawberry cervix)	Visible in secretions	Sexual transmission	Treat both partners; metronidazole
Trypanosoma brucei (African)	Blood and tissue protozoan	Infects the brain and leads to encephalitis	Sleeping sickness—Winterbottom sign, blank look, fever, edema, and epilepsy	Visible in the blood	Tsetse fly (in Africa);	Protection from bites; insecticide; suramin
Trypanosoma cruzi (American)	Blood and tissue protozoan	Amastigotes attack cells, especially cardiac muscle cells	Chagas disease—CHF; Romaña sign	Visible in the blood	Reduviid bugs (in Latin America)	Protect from bites; insecticide; nifurtimox

CHF, congestive heart failure; RBC, red blood cell.

DKA • Diabetic ketoacidosis

Donovan bodies • Clusters of blue or black-staining chromatin condensations seen in mononuclear cells infected with *Calymmatobacterium granulomatis* (granuloma inguinale)

DVT • Deep vein thrombosis

Dysmenorrhea • Painful menses

Dyspnea • Shortness of breath

ECC • Endocervical curettage

Eclampsia • Preeclampsia (hypertension, proteinuria, and edema) and seizures; occurs during pregnancy

Eczema • Acute or chronic inflammation of the skin described as edematous, papular, vesicular, and crusting; often very itchy

Epitope • Simplest antigenic determinant

Erythema chronicum migrans • A spreading circular red rash with a clear center at the bite site; found in Lyme disease

Erythema marginatum • Distinctive rash, often involving the trunk and extremities; rheumatic fever

Erythema multiforme • Macules, papules, or subdermal vesicles often on the hands and arms; can be an allergic or drug-induced reaction; called Stevens–Johnson syndrome if severe

Ewing sarcoma • Malignant neoplasm of bone usually found in young men; associated with chromosome 11:22 translocation

Exstrophy • A congenital defect resulting in a hollow organ with inside grossly visible, as in exstrophy of the bladder

Ferruginous bodies • Foreign body in the lungs coated with hemosiderin; found in asbestosis or mesothelioma

FEV • Forced expiratory volume

FEV_1 • Volume expired in the first second of forced expiration

FLP • Fasting lipid panel

Foam cell • Histiocytes that have ingested lipid; found characteristically in hypercholesterolemia

Gardner syndrome • Autosomal dominant inherited disease characterized by multiple tumors of the colon, osteomas of the skull, epidermoid cysts, and fibromas that occur before 10 years of age

Genomic imprinting • Differences in the expression of a gene that depend on whether it has been inherited from the mother or the father

Goiter • Enlarged thyroid gland

Gower maneuver • Using the arms to stand from a prone position because of muscle weakness in the legs; found in muscular dystrophy

Gravid • Pregnancy; cumulative number of times a woman has been pregnant

Grey Turner sign • Flank ecchymosis in a butterfly pattern in the retroperitoneum; found in acute hemorrhage of the pancreas

Hapten • Antigen that must be combined with a carrier protein to induce antibody production

Harrison groove • Rib deformity; found in rickets

Heinz bodies • Intracellular inclusions of denatured hemoglobin in red blood cells; found in thalassemia, enzyme defects, and hemoglobinopathies, especially glucose-6-phosphate dehydrogenase deficiency

HELLP • Hemolysis, elevated liver enzymes, low platelets; associated with eclampsia or preeclampsia

Hematochezia • Bloody stool

Hemoptysis • Coughing up blood

Henoch-Schönlein purpura • Purpuric lesions, joint pain and swelling, colic, and bloody stools; usually found in children

Heterophil antibodies • Antibodies found in mononucleosis, caused by Epstein–Barr virus

Hirsutism • Excessive male pattern body and facial hair found in women

Homer-Wright pseudorosettes • Characteristic arrangement of tumor cells often seen in medulloblastomas

Idiotype • Antigenic determinant in their hypervariable regions, unique to a clonal cell line of antibody-producing cells (e.g., IgG antibodies to measles and mumps viruses are idiotypes)

Impetigo • Superficial infection of the skin caused by *Staphylococcus* or *Streptococcus;* begins as a vesicle that ruptures and becomes yellow and crusty; often occurs on the face

Involucrum • Sheath of new bone that forms around necrotic bone (sequestrum)

Isotype • Antigenic differences of immunoglobulins in their constant regions, but they are found in all members of a given species (e.g., IgM and IgG are isotypes)

IVDU • Intravenous drug use

Jarisch-Herxheimer reaction • Inflammatory reaction induced by antibiotic treatment of syphilis

JVD • Jugular venous distention

Kartagener syndrome • Situs inversus, bronchiectasis, chronic sinusitis, impaired cilia; causes reduced fertility in women and sterility in men; autosomal recessive disease of the dynein arms

Kawasaki disease • Fever, conjunctivitis, pharyngitis, cervical lymphadenopathy, acute necrotizing vasculitis; can lead to coronary artery aneurysms; found in children, especially in children who are younger than 2 years of age

Kayser-Fleischer rings • Green pigment encircling the cornea; found in Wilson disease

Keratin pearls • Characteristic microscopic findings in squamous cell carcinoma

Kimmelstiel-Wilson nodules • Characteristic glomerular nodules found in diabetic nephropathy

Koilocytes • Cells with a clear perinuclear halo, characteristic of hepatitis B virus infection

Koplik spots • Red lesions with a blue-white center on the buccal mucosa; characteristic of early measles

Kussmaul breathing • Deep, rapid breathing with an increase in both tidal volume and respiratory rate; often seen in diabetic ketoacidosis or other types of metabolic acidosis

Kussmaul sign • Increase in jugulovenous pressure with inspiration; cardiac tamponade

Lhermitte sign • Flexing of the head causes electric-like shocks to be felt down the spine

Libman-Sacks endocarditis • Aseptic endocarditis with warty lesions of the cardiac valves, found in systemic lupus erythematosus

Lichen planus • Flat, shiny papules on buccal mucosa, male genitalia, and flexor surfaces; unknown cause

Lichen sclerosis • White atrophic patches (leukoplakia) of vulva

LLQ • Left lower quadrant

Lou Gehrig syndrome • Also called amyotrophic lateral sclerosis; disease of the motor tracts of the lateral columns of the spinal cord that causes muscular atrophy

LUQ • Left upper quadrant

Macrosomia • Abnormally large body size

Malar • Cheek or cheek bones

Mallory-Weiss syndrome • Tear of the lower esophagus associated with bloody vomitus, usually found in alcoholics

McBurney point • Located two thirds of the way down on a line connecting the umbilicus with the anterior superior iliac spine; a point of pain in appendicitis

Meigs syndrome • Ovarian fibroma, ascites, and hydrothorax

Menorrhagia • Profuse bleeding during menses

Menorrhalgia • Painful menses

Metrorrhagia • Irregular bleeding from the uterus between menstrual cycles

MMPI • Minnesota Multiphasic Personality Test

Molluscum contagiosum • Disease of the skin caused by a virus characterized by pearl-colored papular lesions

MRSA • Methicillin-resistant *Staphylococcus aureus*

Mycosis fungoides • Progressive lymphoma and inflammatory process of the skin

Myotome • Mesoderm that gives rise to skeletal muscle; innervated by a common nerve

NEC • Necrotizing enterocolitis

Negri bodies • Cytoplasmic inclusion bodies found in nerve cells in rabies; eosinophilic and sharply demarcated

Neurofibrillary tangles • Found in Alzheimer disease

NIFS • Noninvasive flow study

NPO • Latin (nil per os) for "nothing by mouth"

NSS • Normal saline solution

Obturator sign • Right lower quadrant pain on external rotation of the hip; usually associated with appendicitis

OCP • Oral contraceptive pills

OOBTC • Out of bed to a chair

Opsonization • Process by which bacteria are made easier to phagocytize

Orthopnea • Shortness of breath on lying down

Pancoast tumor • Tumor of the apex of the lung resulting in Horner syndrome and brachial plexus compression

Pannus • Grayish membrane that covers the upper portion of the cornea; found in trachoma

Parity • Having given birth to a child

Pemphigus vulgaris • Serious illness marked by flaccid vesicles over the entire body

PFOF • Posterior fontanelle open and flat

PFT • Pulmonary function tests

PICC • Peripherally inserted central catheter

Pleurisy • Inflammation of lung pleura

Plummer-Vinson syndrome • Dysphagia with esophageal webs and hypochromic microcytic anemia

PND • Paroxysmal nocturnal dyspnea; often a symptom of heart failure

PO • Latin (per os) for "by mouth"

Polymenorrhea • Increased frequency of menstrual cycles

Pott disease • Tuberculosis of the spine

Precision • Degree to which a measurement is reproducible, but not necessarily correct (e.g., a thermometer that always shows a temperature that is 5 degrees higher than the actual temperature is precise but not accurate)

Psammoma bodies • Microscopic hyalinized concretions surrounded by cells; found in ovarian serous papillary cystadenocarcinoma, thyroid papillary adenocarcinoma, meningioma, and mesothelioma

Pseudocyesis • False pregnancy; psychiatric phenomenon affecting women with a strong unfilled desire for children in which these women exhibit symptoms of pregnancy

Psoas sign • Right lower quadrant pain on hip flexion; often associated with appendicitis

Psoriasis • Reddish maculopapules with silvery scaling; occurs on the flexor surfaces, scalp, and trunk

PVD • Peripheral vascular disease

Rachitic rosary • Junction of the ribs with cartilage looks like beads on a string; found in children with rickets

Raynaud phenomenon • Spasm of arteries of the hand causing blanching, numbness, and pain in the fingers; found in CREST syndrome

Reed-Sternberg cells • Binucleate cells, "owl eyes"; found in Hodgkin lymphoma

Reinke crystals • Rod-shaped crystals with pointed or rounded ends present in Leydig cell tumors

Wermer syndrome • Multiple endocrine neoplasia (MEN) type I: characterized by tumors of the parathyroid, pancreatic islets, and pituitary or other endocrine organ

Wernicke aphasia • Inability to comprehend the spoken word, even though normal hearing is intact

Whipple disease • A disease characterized by steatorrhea, lymphadenopathy, arthritis, fever, and cough; foamy macrophages are found in the jejunum

Winterbottom sign • Lymphadenopathy of the posterior cervical chain found in African trypanosomiasis (African sleeping sickness)

Wire-loop glomeruli • Thickened basement membrane of glomeruli; characteristic lesion found in patients with systemic lupus erythematosus

WNL • Within normal limits

y/o • Years old

Zollinger-Ellison syndrome • Gastrin hypersecretion and a tumor of the noninsulin-producing cells of the pancreatic islets

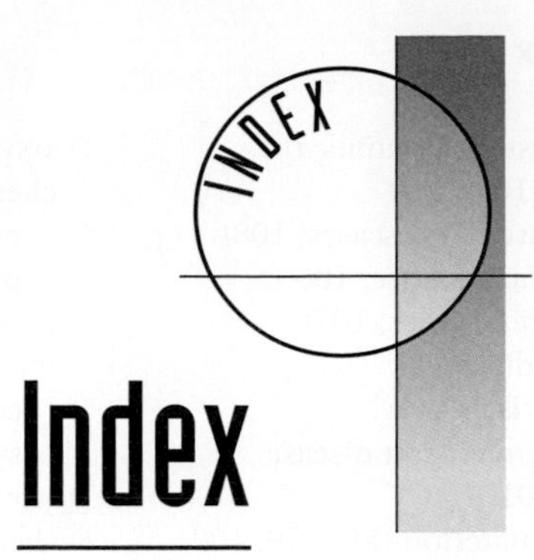

Index

A
Abdominal aorta aneurysm (AAA), 98
Acetaminophen, 262
Achalasia, *139,* 140
Acidosis, 171t
Acquired immunodeficiency syndrome (AIDS), 237
Acute renal failure (ARF), 177–179
Acute tubular necrosis (ATN), 179
Adrenal glands
- congenital adrenal hyperplasia (CAH), 204, *204*
- Cushing syndrome, 205–206, *206*
- development, 187
- hormones, *192*
- pathology, 205–206
- therapeutic agents, 207

Adrenocorticotropic hormone (ACTH), 133
Adult polycystic kidney disease (APKD), *182,* 183
Adult respiratory distress syndrome (ARDS), 114, 121t
Age-related macular degeneration, *59*
Alkalosis, 171t
Amenorrhea, *225*
- causes, *224*
- primary, 223
- secondary, 223–224
- treatment, 226

Androgen insensitivity syndrome (AIS), 225
Anemia, *302*
- classification, 296t
- laboratory blood studies, 300t
- macrocytic anemia, 298–299
- microcytic anemia, 295, 297, 301t
- normocytic anemia, 297–298
- peripheral blood smear findings, 300t

Angiotensin-converting enzyme (ACE), 84, 179
Antiarrhythmics, *89,* 90t–91t
- atrial fibrillation, 87
- digitalis toxicity, 91
- drugs, *89*
- supraventricular tachycardia, 87
- Torsade de pointes, 91
- ventricular fibrillation, 87
- ventricular tachycardia, 87

Antidepressants, 71, 75t–76t, *76*
Antidiuretic hormone (ADH), 84
Antiepileptic agents, 65t
Antihypertensive agents, 95t–96t
- α-blockers, 94
- β-blockers, 94, 97t
- calcium-channel blockers, 97

Anti-infective agents
- antibiotics, 27t–30t
  - aminoglycosides, 31
  - chloramphenicol, 31–32
  - β-lactam agents, 26, 31
  - lincosamides, 32
  - macrolides, 32
  - quinolones, 32–33
  - quinupristin/dalfopristin, 33
  - sulfonamides, 32
  - teicoplanin, 33
  - tetracyclines, 31
  - trimethoprim, 32
  - vancomycin, 33
- antifungal agents, 33, 35t
- antimycobacterial agents, 33, 34t
- antiviral agents, 33–34, 36t

Antiparkinsonian agents, 65, 67t
Antipsychotics, 76, 77t–78t
Arginine vasopressin (AVP), 84
Arthritic joint disease, 252, 254t
Atrial natriuretic peptide (ANP), 84
Autosomal recessive mutation, 132

B
Bacteria
- cell wall components, 15, 19
- genetic transfer, 20t
- genome, 19
- mutation, 19–20

Benign prostatic hyperplasia (BPH), 233
Biostatistics and epidemiology
- biases, 40–41
- disease prevention, 41
- general statistics, 43
- incidence and prevalence, 39t
- research study designs, 40, 41t
- sensitivity and specificity, 39t
- statistical methods, 42–43
- statistical variable relationship, 39–40
- testing, 42–43

Blood urea nitrogen (BUN), 166

C
Caisson disease, 256
Cardiovascular system
- aneurysms, 98t
- arrhythmias
  - antiarrhythmics, 87–91
  - conduction anomalies, 89t
  - ECGs, *88*
- atherosclerosis
  - characterization, 91
  - pathogenesis, 92
  - risk factors, 91–92
- cardiac neoplasms, 109
- congestive heart failure (CHF), 102t
  - ACE inhibitors, 103
  - acute MI, 101
  - angiotensin II receptor blockers (ARBs), 103–104
  - cardiomegaly, *103,* 104
  - digitalis, 104
  - diuretics, 104
  - dobutamine, 104
  - pulmonary edema, *103*
- crunch time review, 308
- development
  - arterial vessels, 81
  - congenital defects, 82t–83t
  - fetal circulation, *82*
  - heart, 80
  - venous vessels, 81
- drugs, adverse effects, 111
- familial dyslipidemias, 92t
- hypertension
  - antihypertensive agents, 94–97
  - essential, 93
  - malignant hypertension, 94
  - secondary hypertension, 93–94
- intrinsic diseases
  - cardiomyopathies, 107t
  - endocarditis, 105–106
  - murmurs, 107t

Cardiovascular system *(continued)*
myocarditis, 105
peripheral vascular diseases, 108t
rheumatic heart disease, 106
valvular heart diseases, 107t
ischemic heart disease
angina pectoris, 99
chronic ischemic heart disease (CIHD), 101
myocardial infarction (MI), 99, *100*
sudden cardiac death, 101
lipid lowering agents, 93t
pericardium diseases
cardiac tamponade, 109
pericarditis, 109–110
physiology and pathology
blood pressure control mechanisms, 84, *85*
cardiac myocytes, 81, *83*
cardiac output, 86, *87*
heart anatomy and signal conduction, 81, *84*
physiologic function, 86, *86*
shock, 110
systemic diseases, 111t
Cholecystokinin (CCK), 140
Chronic obstructive pulmonary disease (COPD)
therapeutic agents, asthma, 122–125
types, 123t
Chronic renal failure (CRF), 180–181
Clonidine, 97
Common sleep disorders, 64
Complement system
activation, 280
complement deficiencies, 281
cytokines, 281t–282t
function, 280
properties, 280–281
Congenital diaphragmatic hernia (CDH), 113
Congestive heart failure (CHF), 102t
ACE inhibitors, 103
acute MI, 101
angiotensin II receptor blockers (ARBs), 103–104
cardiomegaly, *103,* 104
digitalis, 104
diuretics, 104
dobutamine, 104
pulmonary edema, *103*
Corticosteroids, 123, 125
Cretinism, 208–209
Cushing syndrome, *206*
Cyclo-oxygenase (COX) inhibitors, 179
Cystic fibrosis (CF), 132–133
Cystitis, 177

D
Degenerative diseases, 65, 66t
Dementia, 69t
Demyelinating diseases, 67, 68t
Deoxyribonucleic acid (DNA)
chemical components
nucleotide structure, *12*
purines and pyrimidines, *11*
packaging, 14
replication
cell cycle, *12,* 13
synthesis, *13,* 14
Depression, 241
Diabetes
diabetes insipidus, 202, 203t
diabetes mellitus, 197
chronic symptoms, 199t
diagnosis, 198t
DKA and NKH states, 199t
treatment, 198, 201–202 199t–201t
type 1 *vs.* type 2, 198t
nodular glomerulosclerosis, *173*
retinopathy, *59*
Diarrhea, 144
bacteria, 145t
inflammatory bowel disease (IBD), 146t
protozoa, 146t
virus, 145t
Diffuse proliferative lupus nephritis, *175*
DiGeorge syndrome, 187
Disseminated intravascular coagulopathy (DIC), 179
Dysfunctional uterine bleeding (DUB), 223

E
Ectopic pregnancy, 228
Endocrine system (*see also* Adrenal glands; Pituitary gland)
adrenal glands, 204–206
blood glucose levels
hyperglycemia, 196
hypoglycemia, 194, 196, *197*
calcium homeostasis, *194*
congenital malformations, 188
crunch time review, 311t
development, 187–188
diabetes insipidus, 202, 203t
diabetes mellitus, 197
chronic symptoms, 199t
diagnosis, 198t
DKA and NKH states, 199t
treatment, 198, 201–202 199t–201t
type 1 *vs.* type 2, 198t
hormones, 189t–190t
adrenal gland, *192*
hypothalamic-pituitary axis, *191*
second-messenger system, 188, 192t, *193*
insulin, 191, 193, *194–195*
multiple endocrine neoplasia syndromes, 213t
obesity, 202, 203t
parathyroid disorders, 212
pituitary disorders, 202, 203
thyroid gland
cretinism, 208–209
formation, 207–208
Graves disease, 209–210
Hashimoto thyroiditis, 209
myxedema, 207–208
neoplasms, 212
subacute (de Quervain) thyroiditis, 209
therapeutic agents, 210
thyrotoxicosis, 210–211, *211*
Enzyme kinetics
chemical reaction, *37*
Lineweaver–Burk plots, 37–39, *38*
Michaelis–Menten equation, 37, *38*
Epidemiology (*see* Biostatistics and epidemiology)
Epidural hematoma, 50, *51*

F
Functional residual capacity (FRC), 113

G
Gardner syndrome, 252
Gastrointestinal (GI) system (*see* Hepatobiliary system)
absorption, *143*
bugs, 159
clinical disorders, 143, 144t
congenital malformations, 136, 137t
crunch time review, 310t
diarrhea, 144
bacteria, 145t
inflammatory bowel disease (IBD), 146t
protozoa, 146t
virus, 145t
food storage, 137–138
food transport, 137
hormones, *136*
innervation and blood supply, *135*
large intestine and rectum, 142
malabsorption syndromes, 148t–149t
motility disorders, 140
muscular layer, *141*
neoplastic disorders, 139t
neoplastic polyps, 149t–150t
nonneoplastic disorders, 138t
small intestine, 140–141, *142*
therapeutic agents
constipation, 162t–163t
Crohn disease, 161t
diarrhea, 161t
heartburn, 160t–161t
nausea, 163t
ulcerative colitis, 161t
Germ cell tumors, 231
Glomerular diseases
glomerular deposits, *176*
nephritic syndrome, 174t, *175*

nephrotic syndrome, 172t, *173*
nonnephritic and nonnephrotic, 176t
Glycogen storage disorders, *270*
Graves disease, 209–210
Guanosine 5'-triphosphate (GTP), 15
Gynecomastia, 232

H
Haemophilus influenzae, type B, 69
Hematopoietic–lymphoreticular system
anemia, *302*
classification, 296t
laboratory blood studies, 299, 300t
macrocytic anemia, *298,* 298–299
microcytic anemia, 295, 297, 301t
normocytic anemia, 297–298
peripheral blood smear findings, 300t
cells, 274, 275t
chemotherapeutics, 303–306
coagulation disorders, 292, 293t
abnormal bleeding, *294*
schistocytes, *295*
complement system
activation, 280
complement deficiencies, 281
cytokines, 281t–282t
function, 280
properties, 280–281
crunch time review, 313
development, 274
hypersensitivity reactions, *283,* 283t
immunodeficiencies
acquired immunodeficiencies, 285t
congenital B-cell deficiencies, 284t
congenital combined T- and B-cell deficiencies, 285t
congenital T-cell deficiencies, 284t
phagocyte deficiencies, 285t
plasma cell abnormalities, 285t
immunoglobulins, 279, *279*
immunosupressants, 286t
leukemia, 295, 296t
lymphocyte differentiation, 278
lymphoma, 295, 296t
myeloproliferative disorders
chronic myelogenous leukemia, 303
essential thrombocythemia, 302–303
myelofibrosis, 302
polycythemia vera, 302
organs
gut-associated lymphatic tissue, 277
liver, 277
lymph, 276
lymph nodes, 274, *276*
spleen, *276,* 277
thymus, 274
platelet destruction, 299, 301
red blood cell physiology, 277, *277,* 278
thrombosis
anticoagulants, 292
antithrombotics, *289,* 290t–291t, 289, 292
clotting cascade, *287*
direct thrombin inhibitors, 292
multiple myeloma, *288–289*
platelet inhibitors, 289, 292
thrombolytics, 292
Hemolytic uremic syndrome (HUS), 179
Hepatobiliary system
bilirubin excretion, *151*
biochemical pathways, *152*
cirrhosis, 155t–156t
clinical disorders, 156t, *157–158*
defective enzyme diseases, 153t
enterohepatic cycling, *151*
glycolysis *vs.* gluconeogenesis *vs.* glycogenolysis, 151, 153t
microscopic organization, *150*
pancreas, 158t
viral hepatitis, 154t, *155*
Horner syndrome, 261
Human immunodeficiency virus (HIV)
etiology, *235,* 235–236
pathology, 236–237, 237t
treatment, 238t–239t, 239
Hyperglycemia, 196–197
Hypoxemia, 117t

I
Immunosupressants, 286t
Interferon therapy, 68
Interstitial lung disease (ILD), 125, 126t
Intravenous (IV) corticosteroids, 68
Isoniazid (INH) therapy, 130–131

K
Karatanger syndrome, 120

L
Large intestine, 142
common clinical disorders, 143, 144t
diarrhea, 145t–146t
Lesch–Nyhan syndrome, 260
Listeria monocytogenes, 70
Liver (*see* Hepatobiliary system)
Lumbar puncture (LP), 67, 70
Lung neoplasms, 133t–134t

M
Meningitis
cerebrospinal fluid evaluation, 70t
common causes, 69t
Microcytic anemia, 295, 297, 301t
Minnesota multiphasic personality inventory (MMPI) test, 240
Multiple endocrine neoplasia (MEN) syndromes, 213
Multiple myeloma, *288–289*
Musculoskeletal system
bone
diseases, 251, 252t
hormonal control, 251
joint diseases, 254t–255t
metabolic and infectious disease, 252, 253t
osteoblasts, 249, *250*
osteoclasts, 251
osteocytes, 249
tumors, 253t–254t
brachial plexus, *258*
lesions, 259t
nerve damage and regeneration, *260*
connective tissue disorder, 256, 257t
crunch time review, 312
development, 247–248
inguinal canal
anatomy, *271,* 271t
hernias, 272t
lumbosacral plexus, *261*
peripheral nerve functions, 259, 262t
segmental nerve functions, 259, 261t
traumatic injuries, 262
muscle
glycogen storage disorders, *270*
muscle fibers, 266, 268t
myocyte contraction, *266–267*
neuromuscular blocking agents, 266–268
neuromuscular disorders, 269t
tumors, 266, 269t
pain management
acetaminophen, 259–260
nonsteroidal anti-inflammatory drugs (NSAIDs), 260, 263, *263*
opioids, 263
therapeutic agents, 264t–265t
skin disorders, 272t
cancers and premalignant conditions, 273t
characteristics, 272
Myelofibrosis, 302–303
Myxedema, 207–208
Myxomas, 109

N
Neisseria meningitidis, 69
Neonatal respiratory distress syndrome (NRDS), 116, 121t
Nephroblastoma, 183
Nervous system
acute meningitis
cerebrospinal fluid evaluation, 70t
common causes, 69t

Nervous system *(continued)*
antiepileptic agents, 65t
antiparkinsonian agents, 65, 67t
brain, blood supply, *49*
brain stem and cerebrum
cerebellar pathway, 55
corticobulbar tract, 55
taste and limbic system, 58
trigeminothalamic pathway, 54
vestibulocochlear pathways, 55, 56t
visual pathways, 56, *57–58*
cavernous sinus, *63*
cerebrum (*see also* brain stem and cerebrum)
cerebrospinal fluid flow, *48*
cerebrovascular disease, 46, 50t
cortex lesions, *52*
congenital malformations, 45t
cranial nerves, 61t–62t
crunch time review, 307
degenerative diseases, 65, 66t
dementia, 69t
demyelinating diseases, 67, 68t
development
central nervous system (CNS), 44
peripheral nervous system (PNS), 44–45
epidural hematoma, 50, *51*
ethics and physician role, 78–79
hypothalamus, *60*
interferon therapy, 68
meninges, *48*
multiple sclerosis (MS), 67
ocular pathology, *59*, 59t
pathologic trauma, *48*
primary headache syndromes, 71t
psychiatry and behavioral science
antidepressants, 71, 75t–76t, *76*
antipsychotics, 76, 77t–78t
defense mechanisms, 72t–73t
drugs abuse and dependence, 72t
nonpharmacologic therapeutic modalities, 79t
personality disorders, 73t
psychoses and neuropsychiatric disorders, 74t–75t
receptors, *47*
neurotoxins and effects, *48*
parasympathetic nervous system, 45, 46t
sympathetic nervous system, 45, 46t
seizures, 64t
sleep
cycles, 63
disorders, 64
spinal cord, *53*
corticospinal tract, 54
dorsal column medial lemniscus pathway, 52
lesions, *60*
posterior white column, 52, 54
spinothalamic tract, 54
subdural hematoma, 50, *51*
thalamus, *61*
tumors, 70t
Neurotoxins, *48*
Nonsteroidal anti-inflammatory drugs (NSAIDs), 262
Normocytic anemias, 297–298
Nucleoside triphosphates (NTP), 12
Null hypothesis (H_0), 42–43
Nystagmus, 55, 56t

O
Obesity, 202, 203
Operons, 15, *18*
Opioids, 265
Osteoarthritis, 259
Osteosarcoma, 252

P
Pancreatitis, 212
Paraneoplastic syndromes, 134
Paraphilias, 242t
Parathyroid hormone (PTH), 133
Pharmacology
absorption, *22*, 23
distribution, 23
elimination, 25
metabolism, 25
older patients, 25
pediatric patients, 25–26
pharmacogenetics, 26
pharmacokinetics
antagonists, *24*
disease, 25
dose-response curve, *23*
effective dose (ED), 23, *24*
lethal dose (LD), 23, *24*
side effects, *316*, 317t
toxicology, 26t
Pituitary gland
development, 187
disorders, 202, 203t
hormones, 189–191
Sheehan syndrome, 202
therapeutic agents, 207t
Plasma cell abnormalities, 285t
Pneumoconiosis, 126, 127t
Pneumonia
bacterial pneumonia, 128t
clinical diagnosis, 129t–130t
clinical manifestations, 127
fungal pneumonia, 129t
mycoplasma, 128t
pathogenesis, 126–127
pathological location, 127
viral pneumonia, 128t
Pneumothorax, 121
Podocyte foot processes, *173*
Polycystic ovary syndrome, 224
Primary headache syndromes, 71t
Protein
post-translational folding, 15
synthesis, 15, *16–17*
Pyelonephritis, 177

R
Rapid eye movement (REM) sleep, 63
Rectum, 142
common clinical disorders, 143, 144t
diarrhea, 145t–146t
Renal cancers, 183
Renal system
acute renal failure (ARF), 177–179
adult polycystic kidney disease (APKD), *182*, 183
cancers, 183t
chronic renal failure (CRF), 180–181
crunch time review, 311t
description, 164–165, *166–167*
development, 164, 165t
glomerular diseases
glomerular deposits, *176*
nephritic syndrome, 174t, *175*
nephrotic syndrome, 172t, *173*
nonnephrotic and nonnephritic, 176t
kidney function
electrolyte balance, 168, *170*, 171t–172t
filtration fraction (FF), 168
glomerular filtration rate (GFR), 165–168
hormones, *169*
innervation and hormones, 168
nephron, *169*
renal blood flow (RBF), 165
renal plasma flow, 165
volume change effects, fluid levels, 168, 169t
kidney stone formation, 182
therapeutic agents
diuretics, *184*, 185t
gout, 185, 186t
uremia, 180–181
urinary tract infections, 177
Reproductive system
breast pathology, 230, 233t
congenital malformations, 215, 218–219t
crunch time review, 321t
development, 214–215, *215–216*
family unit and related concepts, 240–241
fertilization (*see* menstruation and fertilization)
genetic abnormalities
abnormal sex chromosomes, 216, 220t
abnormal somatic chromosomes, 216, 219t
gynecologic diagnostic tests, 229
human immunodeficiency virus

etiology, *235*, 235–236
pathology, 236–237, 237t
treatment, 238–239t, 239
menarche, 216, 220
menopause, 226
menstruation and fertilization
amenorrhea, 223, *224–225*
dysfunctional uterine bleeding (DUB), 223
endometriosis, 224
hormone formation and function, 220, *221*, 222
menstrual cycle, 222–223
polycystic ovary syndrome, 224
oral contraceptives, 226–227
ovarian neoplasms, 230, 230t
pregnancy, 227–229
prostate, *233*
psychosocial development, 240
sex determination, 214
sexuality
gender, 241–242
rape, 243
sexual dysfunction, 242–243
suicide, 243
sexually transmitted diseases, 230t
testicular pathology, 233, 234t
therapeutic agents, 244t–246t
tumors
uterus, 232t
vulva and vagina, 232t
Respiratory carcinomas, 134
Respiratory system
ARDS and NRDS, 120, 121t
breathing control
depth and rate, 118–119
gas exchange, 119–120
medulla, 118
chronic obstructive pulmonary disease (COPD)
therapeutic agents, asthma, 122–125
types, 123t
crunch time review, 309
cystic fibrosis (CF), 132–133
development
bronchial stages, 113
diaphragm muscle, 113
tracheoesophageal (TE) fistula, *112*
drugs, adverse effects, 134
environmental lung diseases, 126, 127t
interstitial lung disease (ILD), 125, 126t
lung defenses, 120
lung neoplasms, 133t–134t
physics and function
airway resistance, 116
compliance, 113–116
lung volumes, 113, *114–116*
ventilation and perfusion, 117, *118*
pneumothorax, 121
pulmonary vascular diseases, 121, 122t
respiratory infections
pneumonia, 126–127, 128t–130t
therapeutic agents, 131, 132t
tuberculosis and its treatment, *130*, 131
upper respiratory infections, 131
Rhabdomyoma, 109
Ribonucleic acid (RNA)
chemical components
nucleotide structure, *12*
purines and pyrimidines, *11*
mRNA synthesis, 14–15
Rifampin, 130–131

S
Sexually transmitted disease (STD), 230t
Sheehan syndrome, 202
Shortness of breath (SOB), 121, 125
Sickle cell disease, 297
Sleep-wake cycles, 63
Small intestine
carbohydrates, 140
common clinical disorders, 143, 144t
diarrhea, 145t–146t
fats, 141, *142*
malabsorption syndromes, 148t–149t
protein, 141
Sodium nitroprusside, 97
Somatostatin, 191
Spirometry, 115
Starling forces, 166, *167*
Streptococcus pneumoniae, 69
Subacute (de Quervain) thyroiditis, 209
Subdural hematoma, 50, *51*
Systemic lupus erythematosus (SLE), 179, 256

T
Testicular neoplasms, 234t
Thalassemia, 297
Thrombosis
anticoagulants, 292
antithrombotics, 290t–291t
clotting cascade, *287*
direct thrombin inhibitors, 292
multiple myeloma, *288–289*
platelet inhibitors, 289, 292
thrombolytics, 292
Thrombotic thrombocytopenic purpura (TTP), 179
Thyroglossal duct cysts, 187
Thyroid gland
cretinism, 208–209
formation, *208*
Graves disease, 209–210
Hashimoto thyroiditis, 209
myxedema, 207–208
neoplasms, 212
subacute (de Quervain) thyroiditis, 209
therapeutic agents, 210
thyrotoxicosis, 210–211, *211*
Thyrotoxicosis, 210–211, *211*Tracheoesophageal (TE) fistula, *112*
Transposons, 19, *20*
Trimethoprim (TMP), 179
Tuberculosis, *130*, 131

U
Uremia, 180–181
Urinary tract infections, 177
USMLE Step 1 exam
National Board of Medical Examiners (NBME), 1
online resources, 9t
personalized study schedule, *10*
preparation
materials, 5–6
schedule, 6–8, 6t–8t
study strategies, 9
registration, 5
test
content, 3
environment, 3
interface, 3, *4*
scoring, 4, *5*
structure, 1–2, 2t, 2

V
Vasodilators, 97
Virus
replication, 21–22
structure, *21*
vs. cells, 20t, 21

W
Wilms tumor, 183